365
SEX MOVES

The Ultimate Book for Couples with 365
Beginners and Advanced Sex Positions

DAY BY DAY

1. Park It Here 8
2. Hug Me, Honey 9
3. Tangled Vines 10
4. Last Licks 11
5. The Hot Seat 12
6. The Strip, Whip, and Drip 13
7. So Happy to Tether 14
8. Tilt Steering 15
9. The Sit and Spin 16
10. On Bended Knee 17
11. The Easy Chair 18
12. The Reverse Piggyback 19
13. How's It Hangin'? 19
14. The Bull Rider 20
15. The Leg Up 21
16. The Hydrant Hump 22
17. Pedal Pleasure 23
18. The Outsider 24
19. Backstage Pass 25
20. The Tight Deadline 26
21. Oral Obedience 27
22. The Standing Ovation 28
23. The Love Shacks 29
24. The Sweet Caress 30
25. Passing Ships 31
26. Feeding the Flames 32
27. The Chair Lift 33
28. Side-by-Side Sensation 34
29. The Tender Trap 35
30. The Burning Bench 36
31. Triple Treat 37
32. Winters Passion 38
33. Extended Bliss 39
34. The Multitasker 40
35. The Lap Wrap 41
36. The Pleasure Plateau 42
37. Sitting Pretty 43
38. The Graceful Grind 44
39. Locked and Loaded 45
40. Safe at Home 46
41. Bottoms Up 47
42. The Shock Absorber 48
43. Up and Away 49
44. The Main Squeeze 50
45. Hearts on Fire 51
46. The Bobsled 52
47. Spanks for the Memories ... 53
48. The Jump Hump 53
49. The Frisky Filly 54
50. X-Rated 55
51. Two for One 56
52. The Deep "C" Dive 57
53. Puppy Love 58
54. Taking Dictation 59
55. The Acrobats 59
56. BJ and the Bare 60
57. Bridge and Tunnel 61
58. The Getaway 62
59. Full Access 63
60. The Alpine Slide 64
61. Over the Edge 65
62. Graceful Union 65
63. In Like a Lion ....
64. The Bent Spoon ....
65. Bridge Diving ....
66. The Hipster ....
67. Hot and Cold ....
68. The Flight Attendant ......
69. Garden of Eden ....
70. The Ironing Board ....
71. The Wishbone ....
72. The Feather Report ....
73. Blind Faith ....
74. The Sensual Scissors .....
75. The Mountie ....
76. Three for All ....
77. Lay Me Down ....
78. Close Encounter ....
79. The Turning Point ....
80. The Kneel Deal ....
81. Take Me Now ....
82. Too Hot to Handle ....
83. Behind the Scenes ....
84. Full Exposure ....
85. Heavy Petal ....
86. The Lick and Lift ....
87. The "Oh My!" Tie ....
88. Riding Blind ....
89. The Hood Ornament ......
90. Pulling Passion ....
91. The Hand Maiden ....
92. Going Down? ....
93. The Grabber ....

#	Title	Page
94.	How Deep Is Your Love?	95
95.	Ride the Tiger	96
96.	Four on the Floor	97
97.	Sexual Boost	97
98.	Coochie, Coochie, Coo	98
99.	Coochie Coo to You, Too	99
100.	The Queen's Throne	100
101.	Roll Play	101
102.	The Laid-Back Lap Dance	102
103.	Give Her a Hand	103
104.	Come as You Are	103
105.	Slip Service	104
106.	Celestial Bodies	105
107.	The Drill Press	106
108.	Hog-Tie Heaven	107
109.	Twin Benches	108
110.	The Helping Hand	109
111.	The Hot Spot	109
112.	The Miner	110
113.	The Fallback	111
114.	Nirvana's Edge	112
115.	The Hot Pretzel	113
116.	Down and Dirty	114
117.	Blow Me Down	115
118.	Strangers in the Night	115
119.	Side and Seek	116
120.	Lost Contact	117
121.	The Headliner	118
122.	Twist and Shout	119
123.	The Sexy Sway	120
124.	Spring Fling	121
125.	"C" Is for Control	121
126.	The Levitating Lady	122
127.	The Wild Mustang	123
128.	Leg Show	124
129.	Cuff Love	125
130.	Outta Sight	126
131.	The Curious Cat	127
132.	Moving Day	128
133.	The Final Frontier	129
134.	The Half and Half	130
135.	The Pony Ride	131
136.	Fab Abs	132
137.	Sit-Up Sex	133
138.	Let's Face It	134
139.	Cushioned Connection	135
140.	Forbidden Fruit	135
141.	The Lucky Catch	136
142.	Open Sesame	137
143.	Sweet Skinsation	138
144.	The Iceman Cometh	139
145.	The Wicked Windmill	140
146.	Stuck in the Middle With You	141
147.	The Hip Swivel Shake	142
148.	The Rumble Seat	143
149.	Rock, Scissors, Pleasure	144
150.	The Love Locker	145
151.	Wang Beneath My Wings	146
152.	The Rocket Locket	147
153.	Clothes Encounter	147
154.	Star-Crossed Lovers	148
155.	Command Central	149
156.	Southern Exposure	150
157.	She's Gotta Have it	151
158.	Carnal Capture	152
159.	The Drop Zone	153
160.	Get Down	154
161.	The Last Grasp	155
162.	The Crossroads	156
163.	Feel the Heat	157
164.	Tuned In and Turned On	158
165.	Rock Around the Clock	159
166.	Cheek to Cheek	160
167.	Missionary Man	161
168.	The Erotic Escalator	162
169.	The Kinky Coil	163
170.	Electric Outlet	164
171.	The Tight Twosome	165
172.	Flesh Dance	166
173.	Leopard's Lair	167
174.	Summer Sensation	167
175.	Let's Get Nuts	168
176.	Linked In	169
177.	Lickety Split	170
178.	The Mechanic	171
179.	The Pelvic Pulse	172
180.	Bent Friends	173
181.	The Strip Search	173
182.	The Chair Essentials	174
183.	The Happy Hostage	175
184.	The Balancing Act	176
185.	Good-Night Spoon	177
186.	Choosing Up Sides	178

187. Bending Beauty........... 179	218. The Silk Scarf........... 206	249. The Stabilizer........... 234
188. The Hang Glider........... 179	219. The Leg Lock........... 207	250. All You Can Eat........... 235
189. The Stimulus Package..... 180	220. The Lookout........... 208	251. Oh What a Knight......... 235
190. The Wimbledon........... 181	221. Bad Kitty........... 209	252. Jack and Jill........... 236
191. Open All Night........... 182	222. The Silent Partner......... 210	253. Body Surfing............. 237
192. Backdoor Man........... 183	223. The Serpent........... 211	254. The Grind............. 238
193. Love Lift Us Up........... 184	224. Bridging the Gap......... 212	255. Lean on Me............. 239
194. Hop in the Sack........... 185	225. That's a Wrap........... 213	256. Table for Three........... 240
195. You Scratch My Back....... 185	226. Peaks and Valleys......... 214	257. Bound for Glory........... 241
196. The Busy Bee........... 186	227. Get Your Kicks........... 215	258. Kneel Appeal........... 241
197. Sideways Satisfaction..... 187	228. Split Decision........... 216	259. Calf Roping............. 242
198. The Next Step........... 188	229. Cruise Control........... 217	260. The Rolling Bone......... 243
199. The Casual Lovers......... 189	230. Arc of Triumph........... 217	261. Floating on Air........... 244
200. Love Letters........... 190	231. The Alley Cat........... 218	262. Sensational Sunrise....... 245
201. The Holding Company..... 191	232. The Captain and the Squeal 219	263. The Hollywood Ending...... 246
202. The Standing Sponge Bath 191	233. The Chinese Rings......... 220	264. Overtime Action........... 247
203. Box Seat........... 192	234. The Backdown........... 221	265. Downward Dong......... 247
204. Taking Charge........... 193	235. The Speakeasy........... 222	266. The Happy Landing....... 248
205. Higher Power........... 194	236. Stand and Deliver......... 223	267. The Championship Belt..... 249
206. The Cheeky Monkey....... 195	237. The Tripod........... 223	268. The Rubberneckers........ 250
207. Tuck Buddies........... 196	238. The Cold Shoulder......... 224	269. The Floor Exercise......... 251
208. Falling for You........... 197	239. The Object of Desire...... 225	270. The Scorching Slide....... 252
209. The Cannoli........... 197	240. Touch You All Over......... 226	271. Scary Good Sex........... 253
210. Elevated Expectations..... 198	241. The Feeling Is Mutual...... 227	272. The Bucket Lust.......... 253
211. Mirror, Mirror........... 199	242. The Screw Top........... 228	273. Dracula's Kiss........... 254
212. Planting Season........... 200	243. Breathless........... 229	274. Sculpted Beauty.......... 255
213. Seated Seduction......... 201	244. The Pow Wow........... 229	275. Play Ball!........... 256
214. Lady and the Clamp....... 202	245. The Welcome Guest....... 230	276. String Duet........... 257
215. The Swan........... 203	246. Down Boy........... 231	277. The Scratching Post....... 258
216. Tie for Two........... 204	247. The Daredevils........... 232	278. Core-pulation........... 259
217. Hidden Desire........... 205	248. No Ifs, Ands, or Butts...... 233	279. Spanks a Lot........... 259

...BY DAY

280. The Shoulder Stand........ 260
281. The Pushing Match........ 261
282. Docking Bay............. 262
283. The Filing Extension....... 263
284. Pushing Pleasure......... 264
285. The Playful Kitten........ 265
286. Come to Papa............ 265
287. Doggy Delivery........... 266
288. The Happy Hooker........ 267
289. Climbing Climax.......... 268
290. Inner Beauty............. 269
291. Slap Happy.............. 270
292. Like a Prayer............ 271
293. Take a Plow............. 271
294. Up, Up, and Away........ 272
295. The Chair-Raising Adventure. 273
296. The Hair Salon........... 274
297. Baby Got Back........... 275
298. Over, Under, Sideways, Down. 276
299. The Jackhammer.......... 277
300. The Seat Saver.......... 277
301. Lost in You.............. 278
302. G-Spot Roulette......... 279
303. Easy Does It............ 280
304. The Neck Brace.......... 281
305. Stepping It Up........... 282
306. On Your Toes............ 283
307. Points of Interest........ 283
308. The Hedge Trimmer....... 284
309. The Triple-Decker Sandwich. 285
310. Inside and Out........... 286
311. The Merger.............. 287
312. The Honey Pot........... 288
313. Kick Your Feet Up........ 289
314. The Bell Ringer.......... 289
315. Is This Seat Taken?....... 290
316. The Curl Friend.......... 291
317. The Rose Garden......... 292
318. Dangerous Curves........ 293
319. "A" for Arousal.......... 294
320. The Love Tug............ 295
321. I Got Your Back.......... 296
322. Come Fly with Me........ 297
323. The Knockout........... 298
324. Frisky Business.......... 299
325. The Slow Burn........... 300
326. Coming Attractions....... 301
327. The Lusty Lounge........ 302
328. Growing Attraction....... 303
329. Blind Man's Muff......... 303
330. The Straddle Royale...... 304
331. The Cocoon............. 305
332. The Whipped-y Nine...... 306
333. Role Reversal........... 307
334. The Buzz Saw........... 308
335. Pump You Up........... 309
336. The Pulley Party......... 309
337. The Feats of Strength.... 310
338. Can't Let You Go......... 311
339. The Passionate Push-Up... 312
340. Captain Crunch......... 313
341. Chin Music.............. 314
342. Winter Warmth.......... 315
343. The Nectar Detector...... 315
344. Tuck, Tuck, Goose........ 316
345. The Butter Churn........ 317
346. Bind Man's Buff.......... 318
347. The Hot Button.......... 319
348. Dirty Dancing........... 320
349. Spellbound............. 321
350. The Bermuda Triangle.... 322
351. Can You Squeeze Me in?.. 323
352. Hoe Motion............. 324
353. The Lusty Lotus......... 325
354. Cross My Heart.......... 326
355. Mr. Clean............... 327
356. The Wash 'n' Blow........ 327
357. Hopping Spree.......... 328
358. Hum's the Word......... 329
359. Parallel Parking......... 330
360. The Homegirl Hang....... 331
361. Go for Stroke........... 332
362. Doggie Treat........... 333
363. The Lowdown........... 334
364. Splendid Sprinter........ 335
365. Endless Embrace........ 336

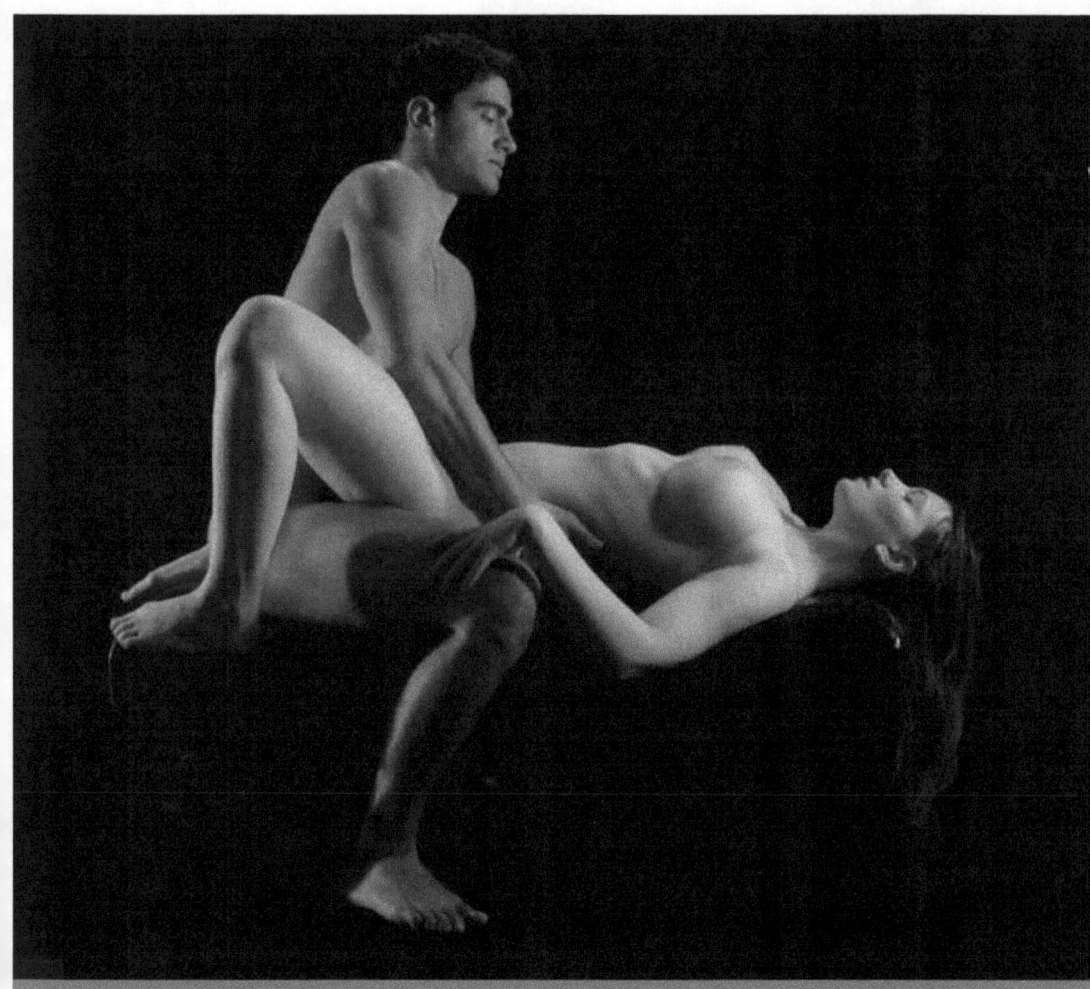

DAY 1

PARK IT HERE

She lies back across a bench while her partner sits facing her with his legs straddling the bench. As he enters her, he's in a perfect position to stimulate her clitoris or he can lean in for deeper penetration and some up-close time with her breasts.

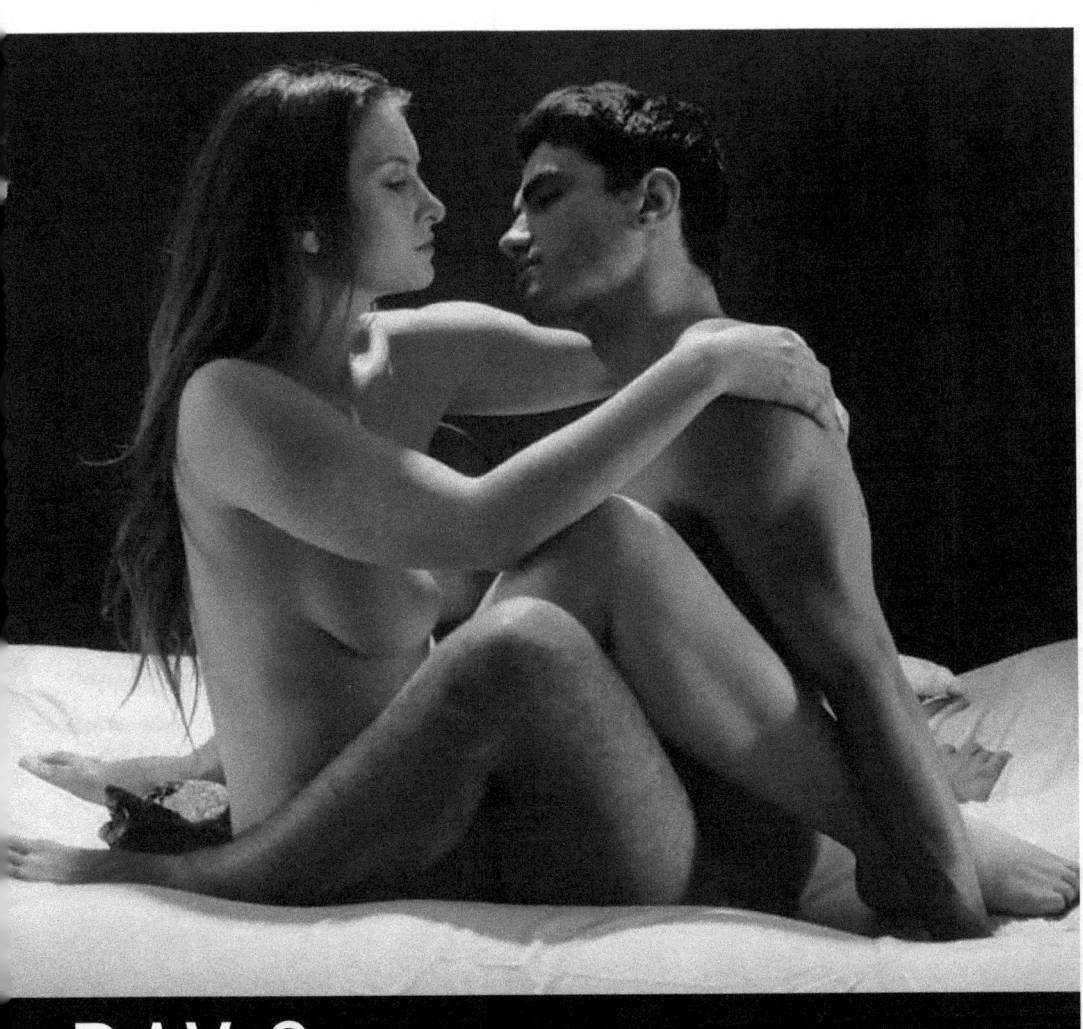

DAY 2

HUG ME, HONEY

The couple sit facing each other on the bed. She brings her legs over his as he slides himself up into her. She hugs her partner as they calmly, languidly move toward climax.

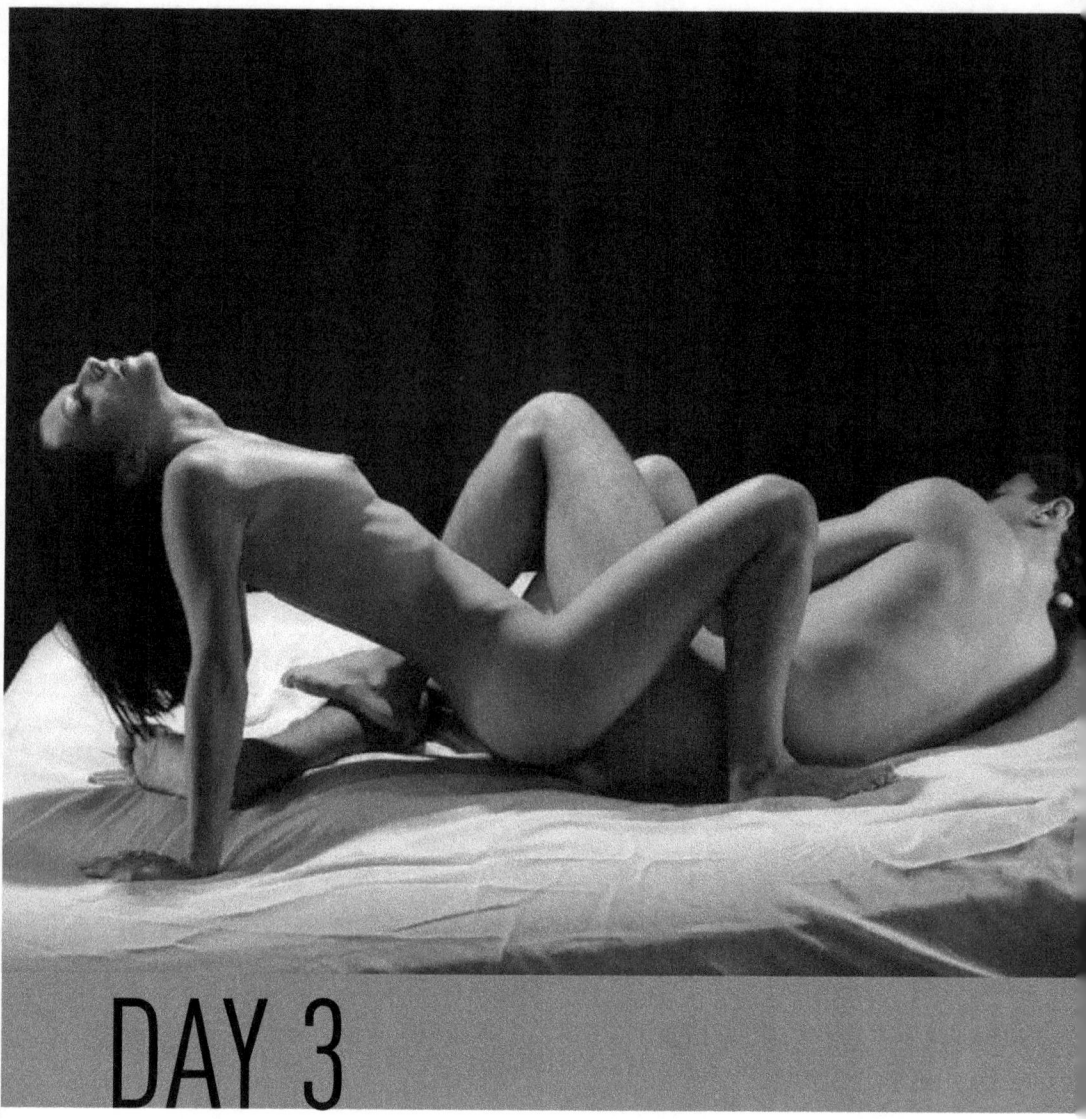

DAY 3

TANGLED VINES

He lies on his side, keeping his bottom leg straight while bending his top leg. His partner shifts her weight back on her hands to giver herself leverage so that she can slide into the open space between his legs, allowing his penis to penetrate her vagina.

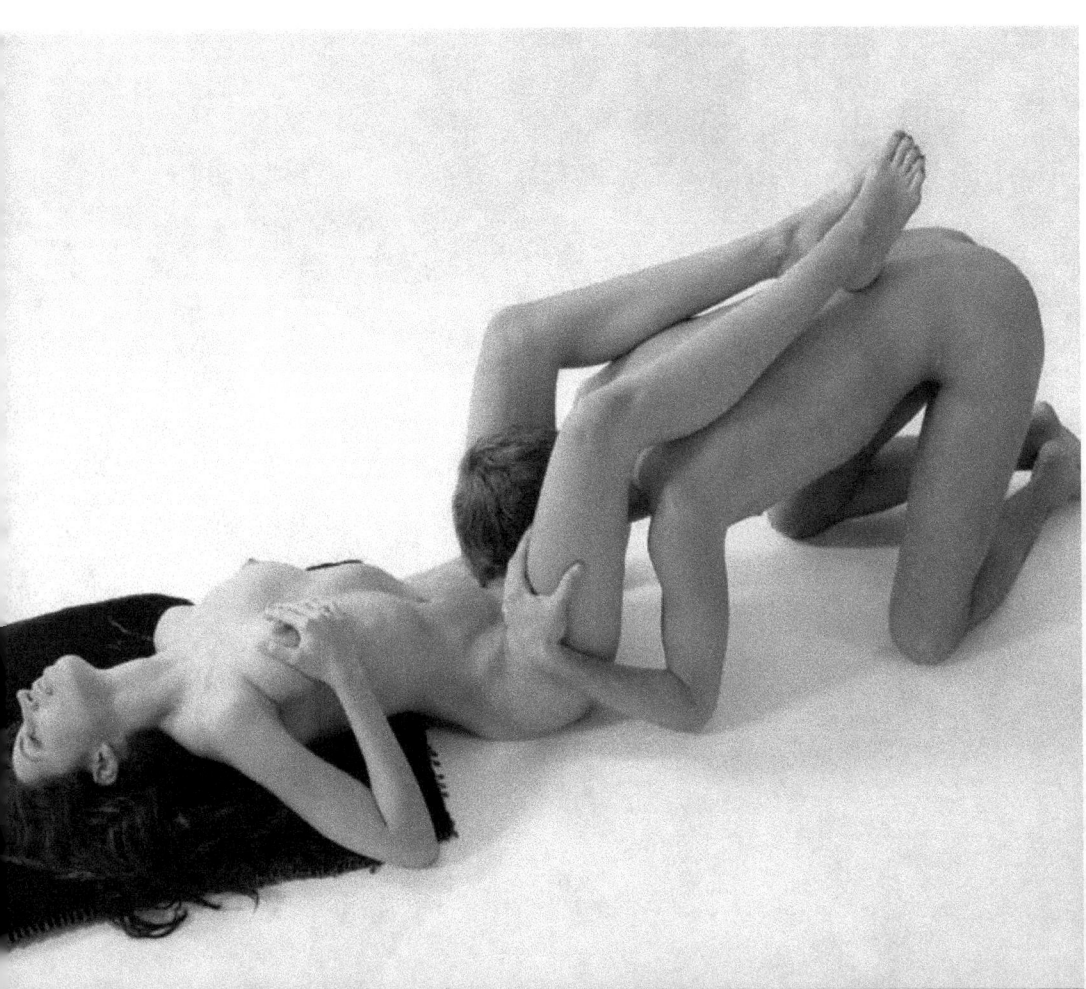

DAY 4

LAST LICKS

She's on the floor resting her head and torso on a pillow. He kneels down in front of her and stimulates her vagina with his mouth and tongue. She kicks up her feet in anticipation of climax.

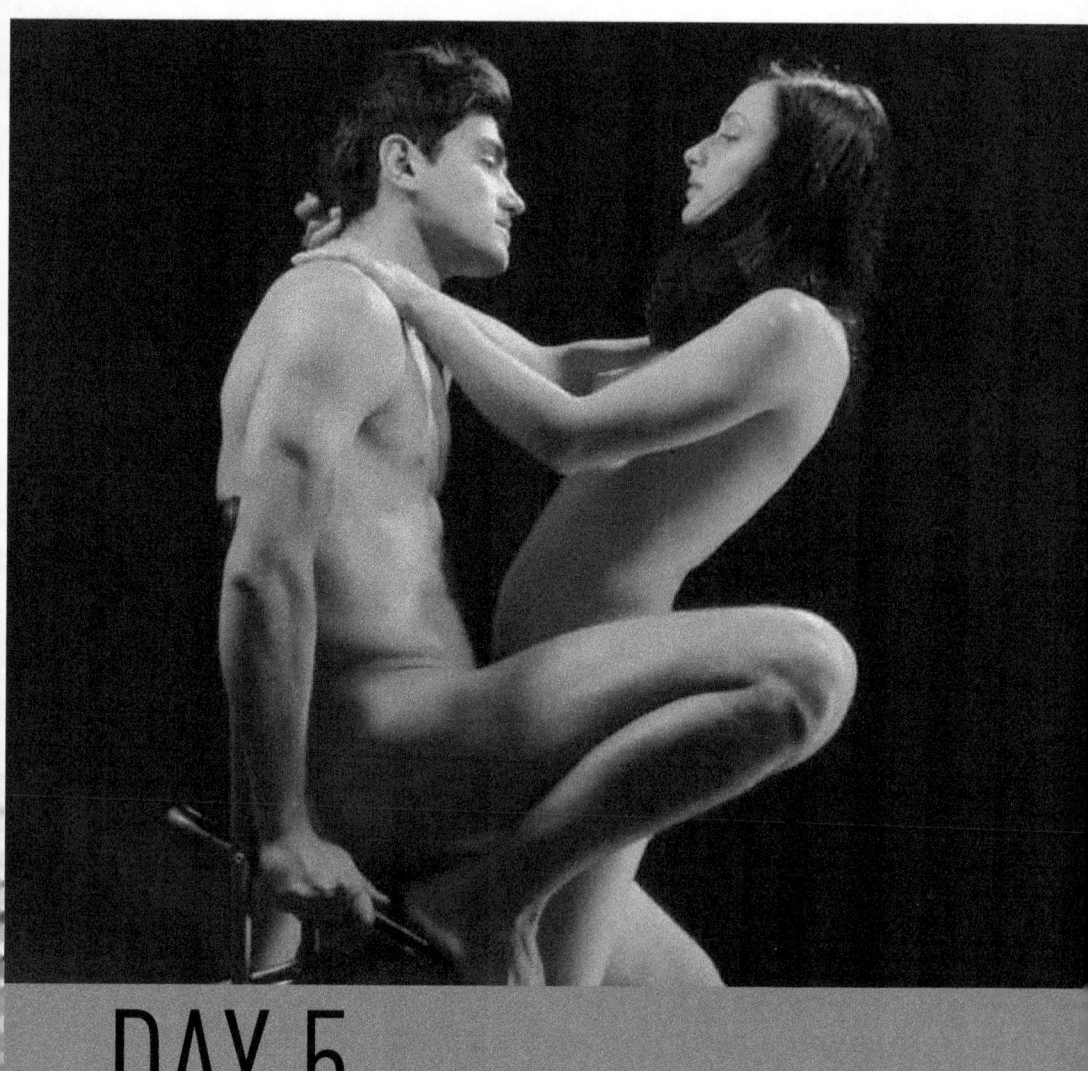

DAY 5

THE HOT SEAT

He climbs into a chair and bends his knees to bring his feet to the edge of the seat. She moves in between his legs to grasp his penis between her thighs from a standing position. Add a bit of self-warming lubricant, and their bumping and grinding will generate some real heat.

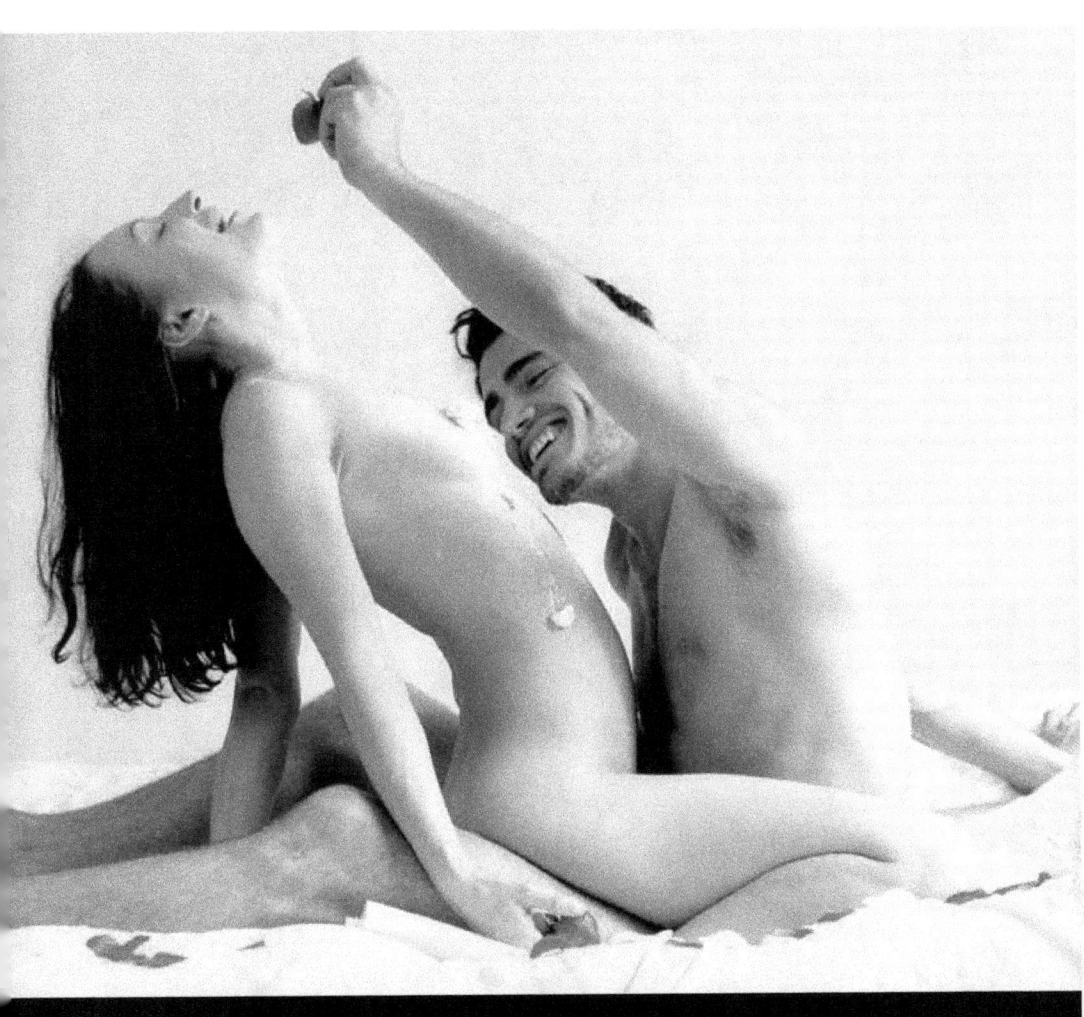

DAY 6

THE STRIP, WHIP, AND DRIP

Having fun while having sex is one of the great joys in life. As the woman straddles her partner, he playfully teases her with a strawberry, even as he attempts to lick whipped cream off of her breasts. Laughter fills the room. They'll worry about cleaning up later.

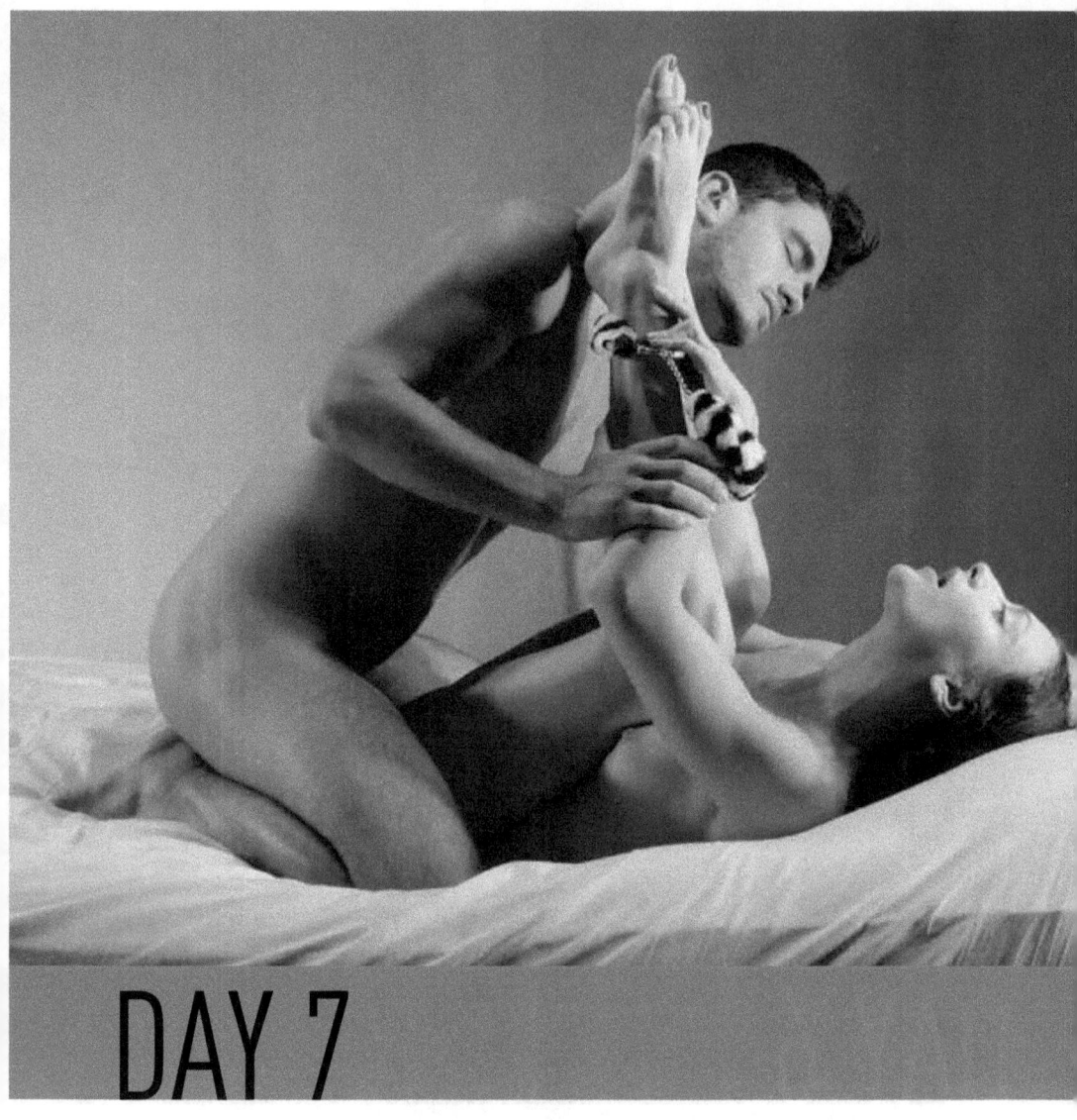

DAY 7

SO HAPPY TO TETHER

She's on her back with her hand cuffed to her ankle. She uses her arm to lift and pull her leg back making it easy for her lover to enter her from a kneeling position. Once there, he may also want to run his hand between the edges of her furry handcuffs and her skin.

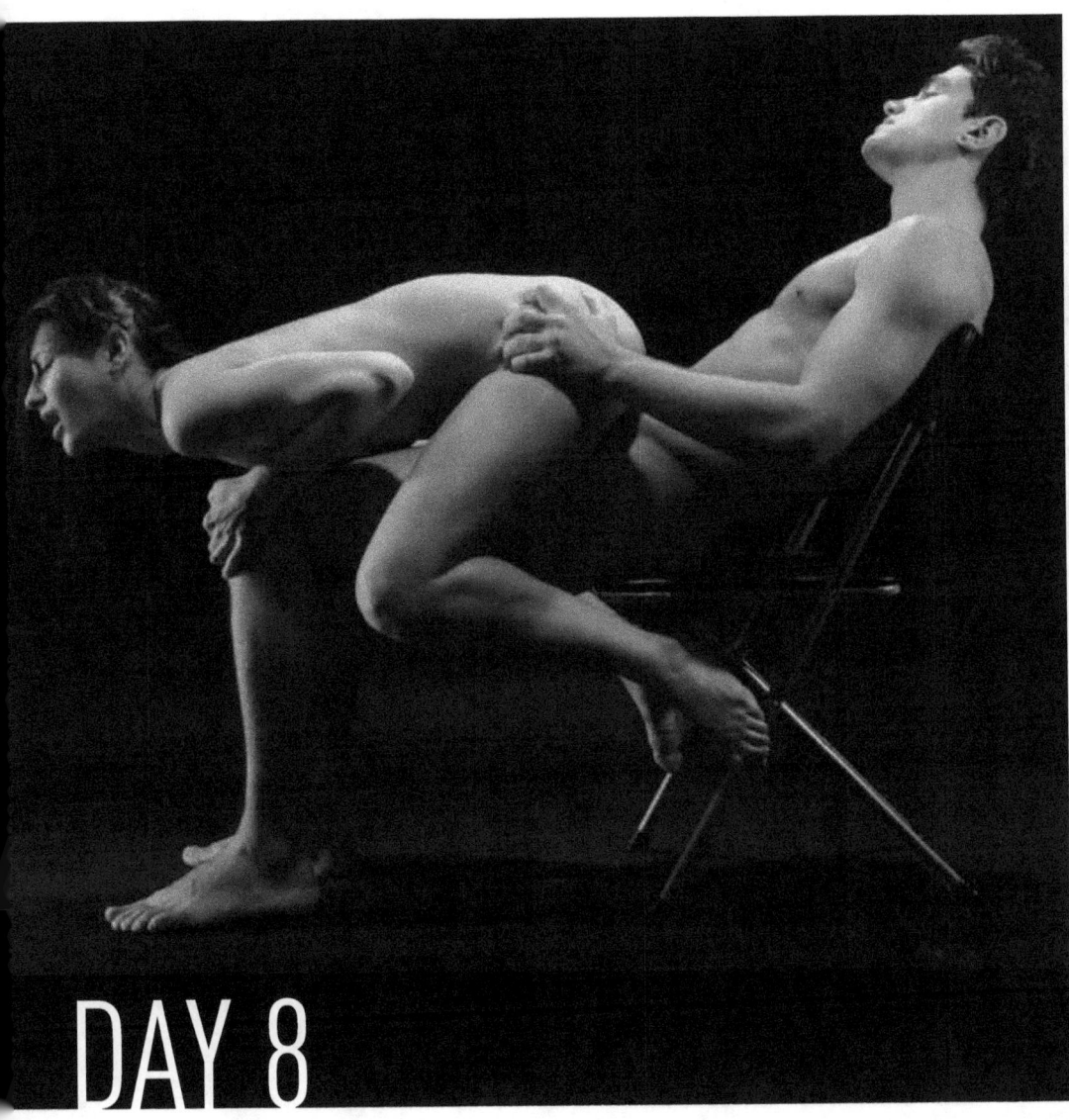

DAY 8

TILT STEERING

He's seated low in a chair with his knees bent and feet flat on the floor. Facing away from her lover, she lowers herself onto his penis. She extends herself forward and rocks back and forth.

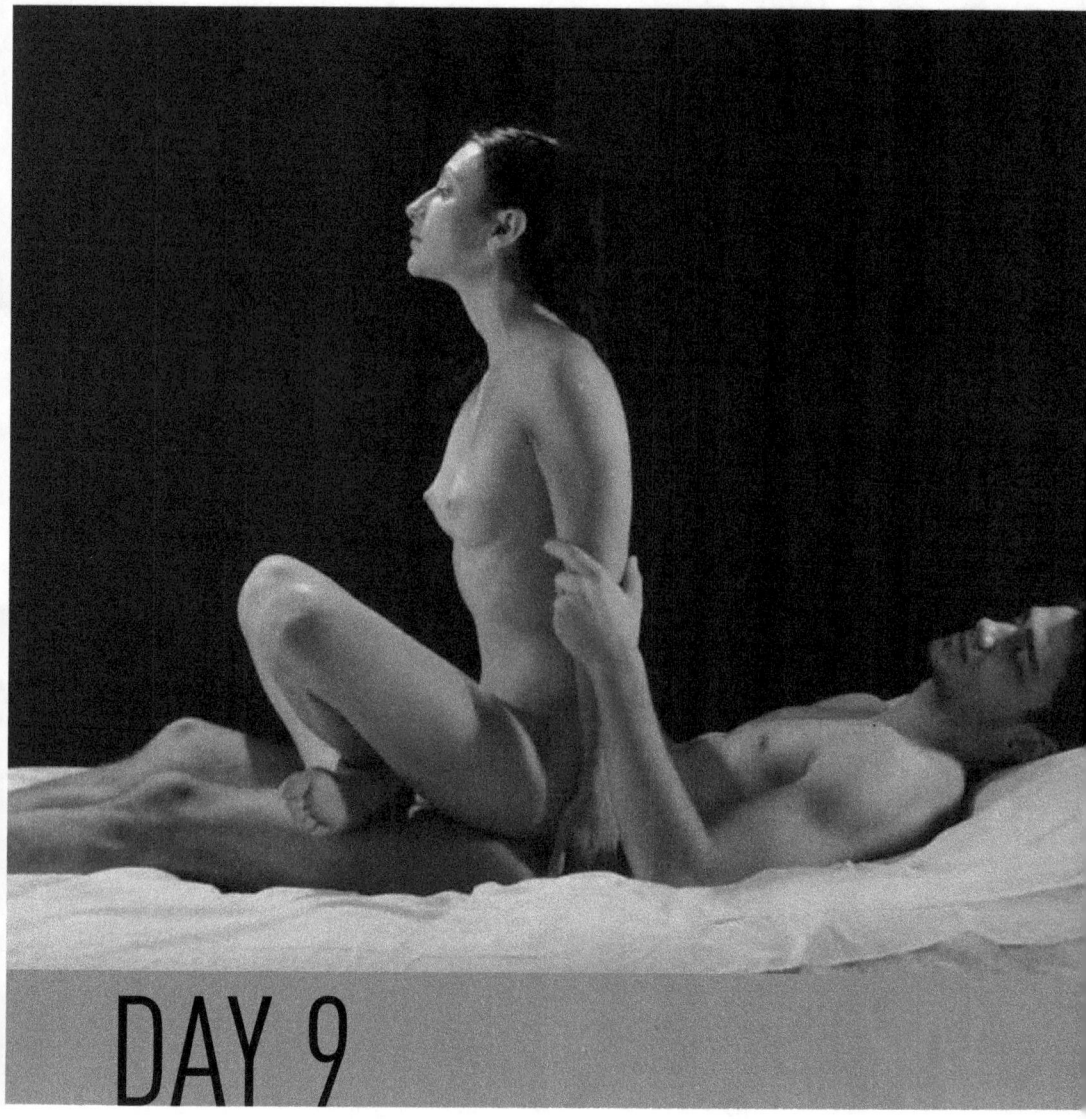

DAY 9

THE SIT AND SPIN

He lies back on the bed with his legs stretched out. Facing away from him, she mounts her lover and crosses her legs. They can both use their hands to rotate her position without breaking the pleasurable penetration.

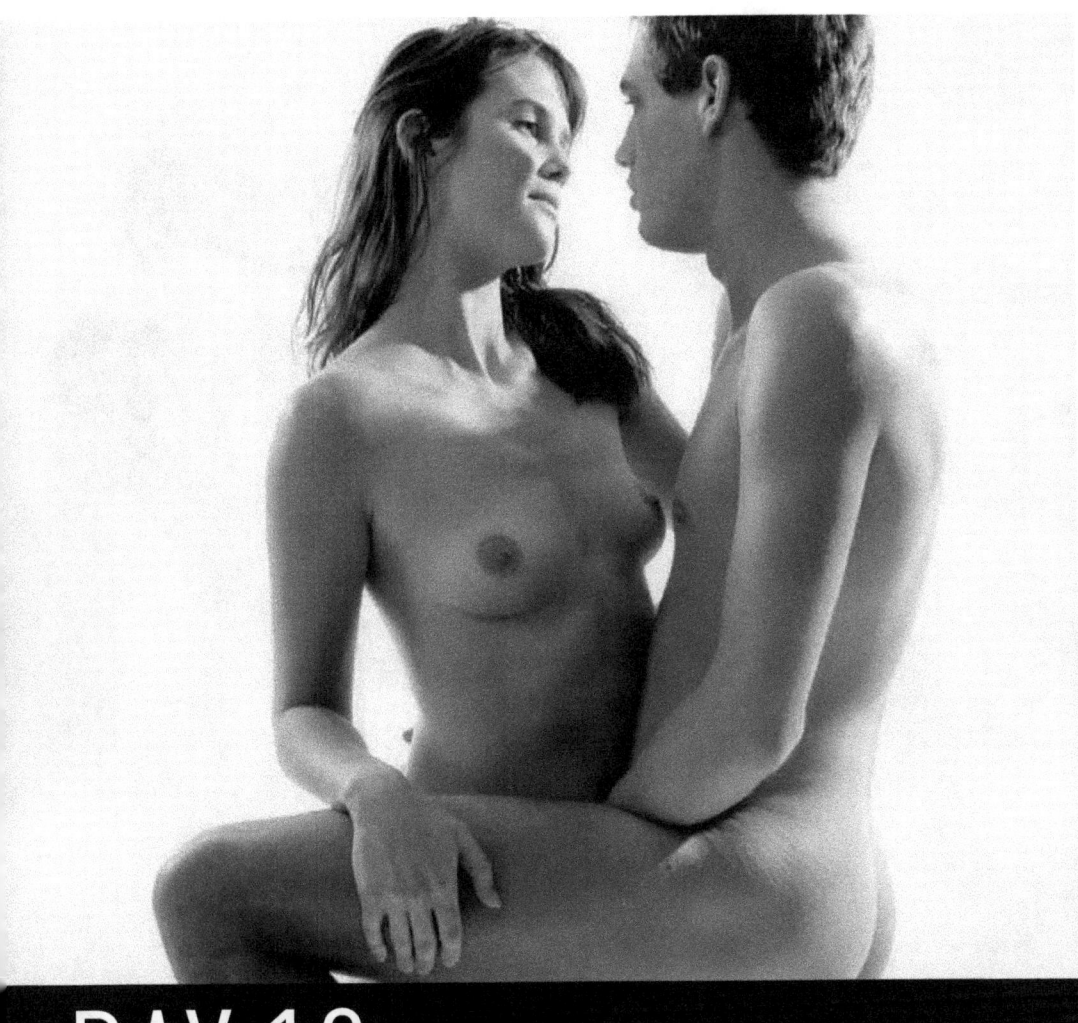

DAY 10

ON BENDED KNEE

The man gets down on one knee and faces his partner as she kneels on both of hers. She opens her kneeling position a bit wider for easier penetration. Be careful, this pose can easily be mistaken as a prelude to a proposal.

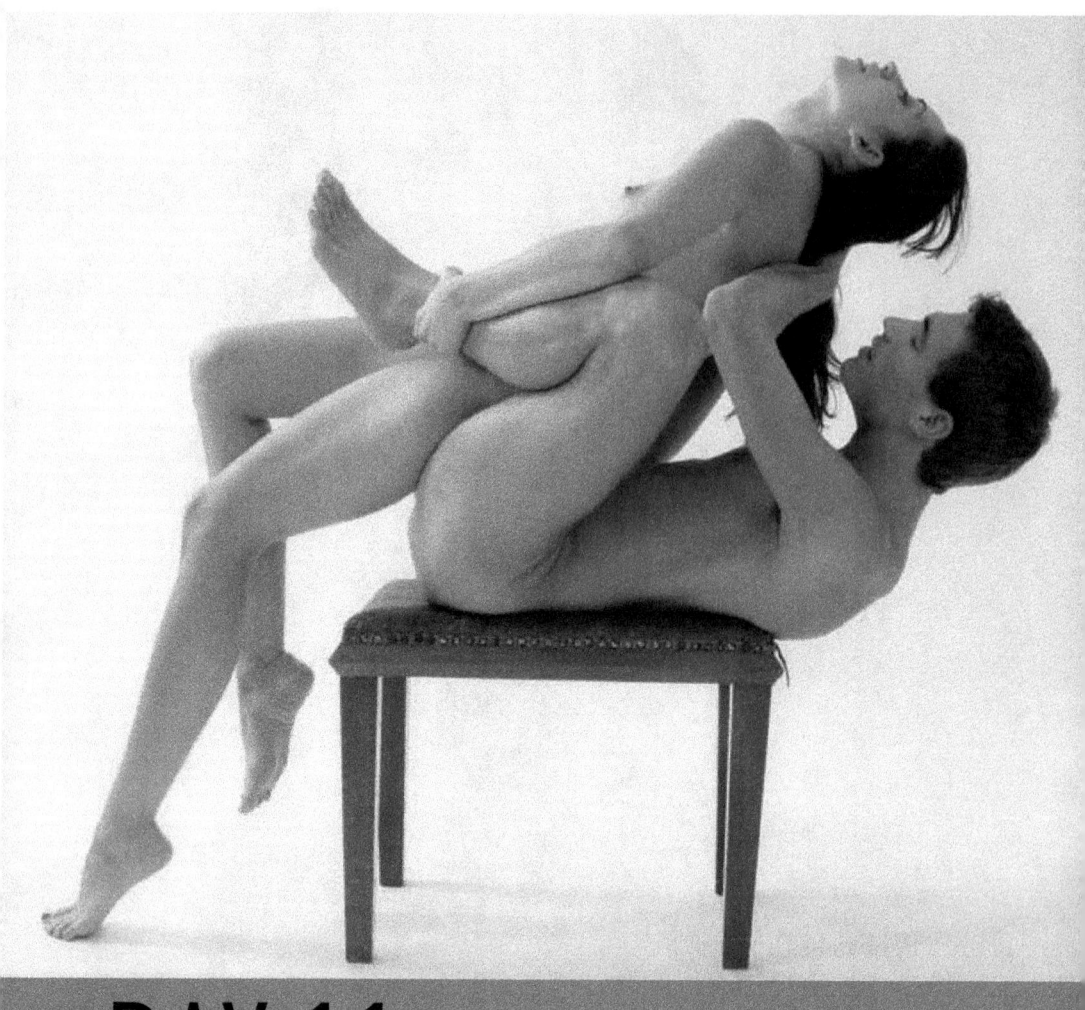

DAY 11

THE EASY CHAIR

He lies back on a low-lying piece of furniture while opening his legs and bringing his knees towards his chest. She mounts her lover, stretching out her legs and reclining her torso back so that he has full access to her breasts.

DAY 12

THE REVERSE PIGGYBACK

He stands straight up with the back of his legs against a table or ottoman. She wraps her arms around her lover's neck and mounts him, placing her feet on the furniture. They can stay where they are or take their passion elsewhere.

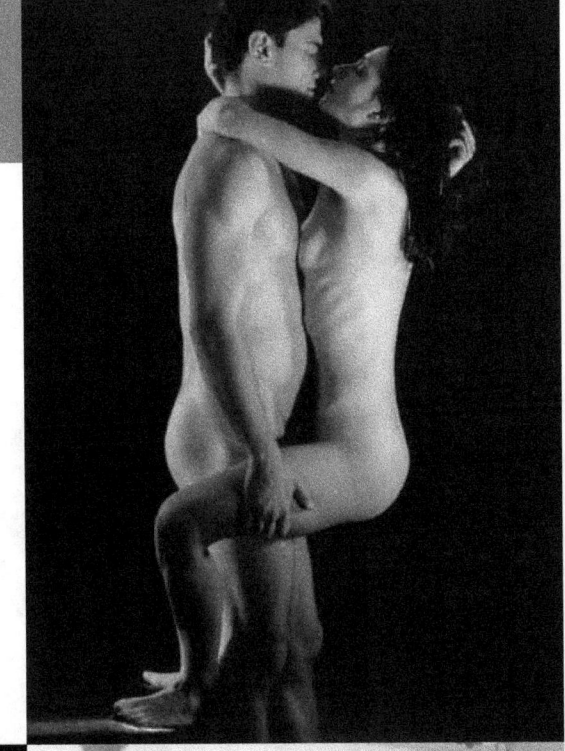

DAY 13

HOW'S IT HANGIN'?

The man hangs from a chin-up bar or support pole as his lover wraps her arms around his neck and allows him to penetrate her. She can keep her feet planted or hang off of him while opening and closing her legs.

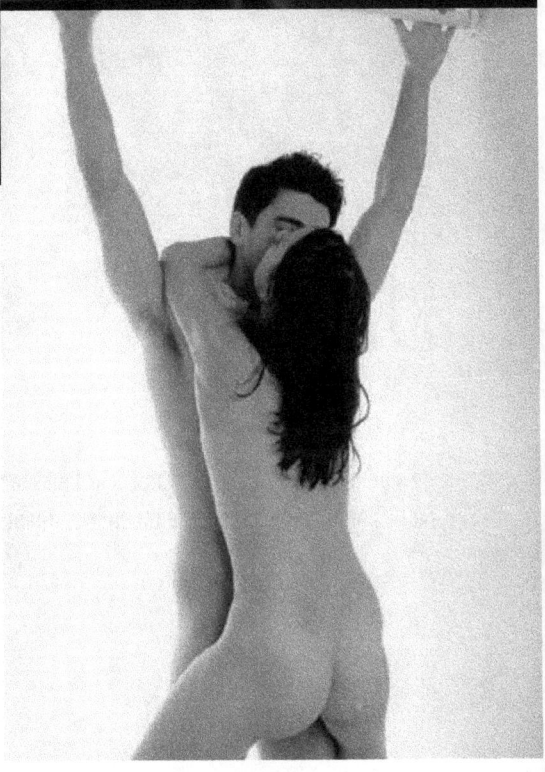

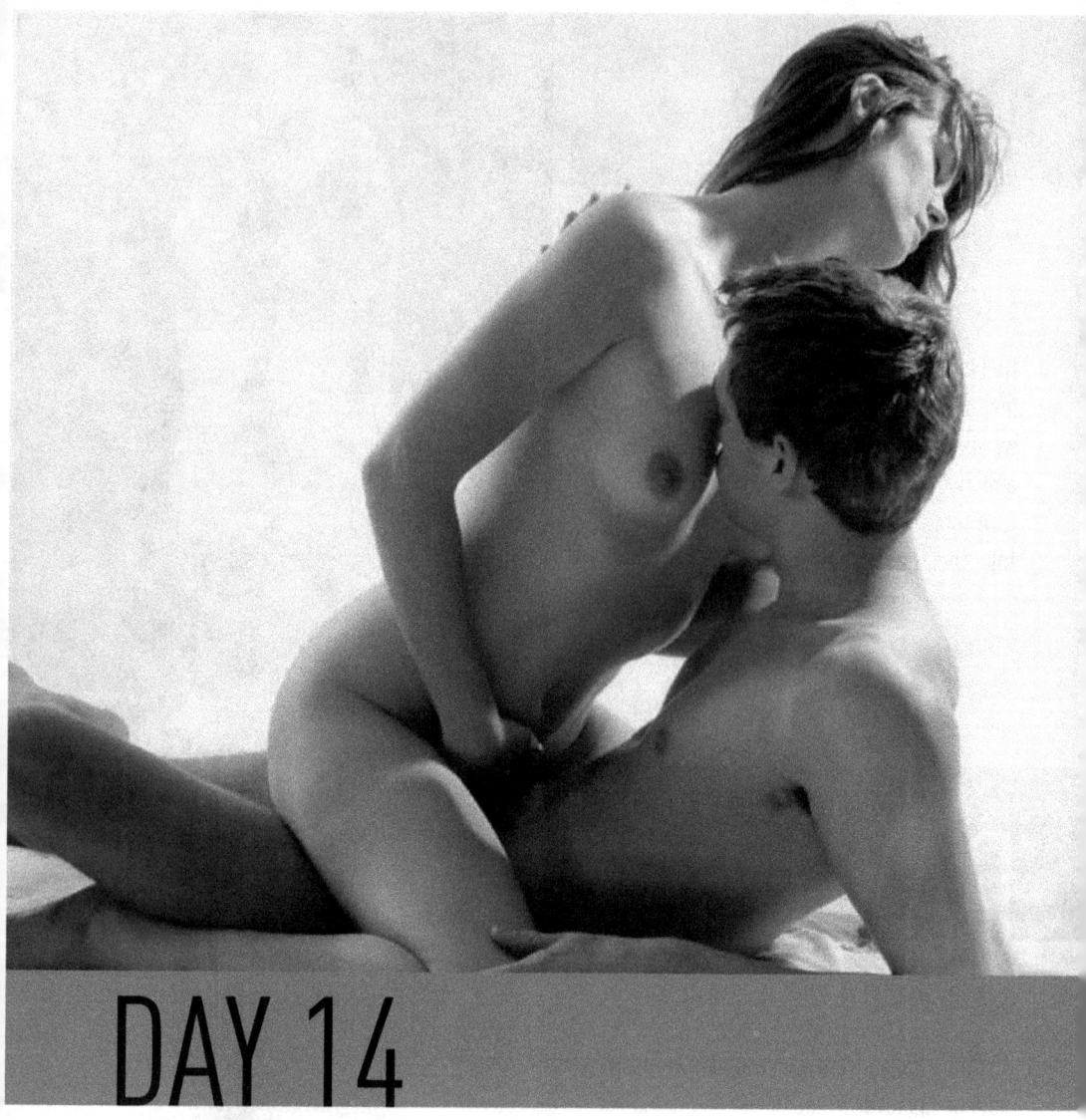

DAY 14

THE BULL RIDER

He's on his back as she climbs aboard and faces him. As she rides him for all he's worth, he has ample opportunity to touch her breasts and stimulate her clitoris.

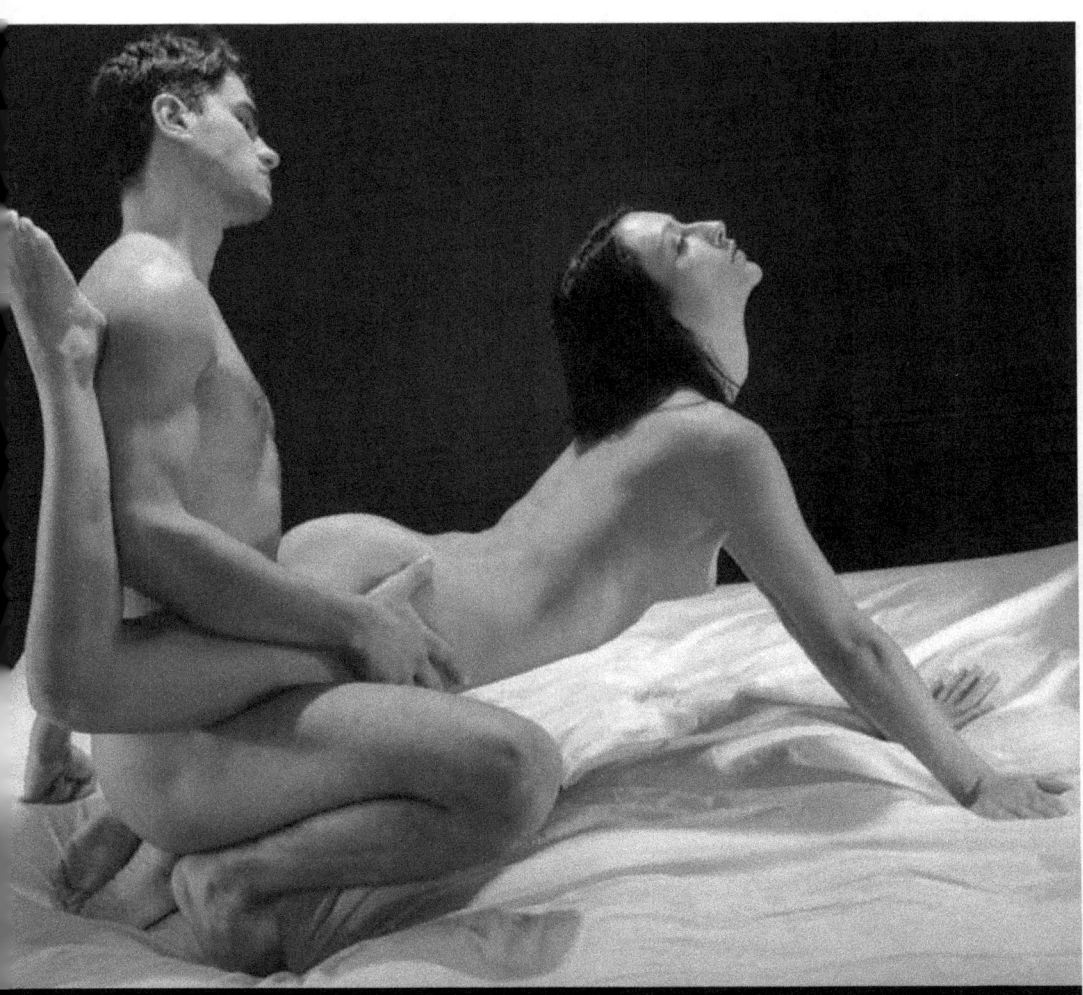

DAY 15

THE LEG UP

The woman gets on all fours as her partner squats down and enters her. As he thrusts she lifts one leg up and brings it against his back, opening herself up for even deeper penetration.

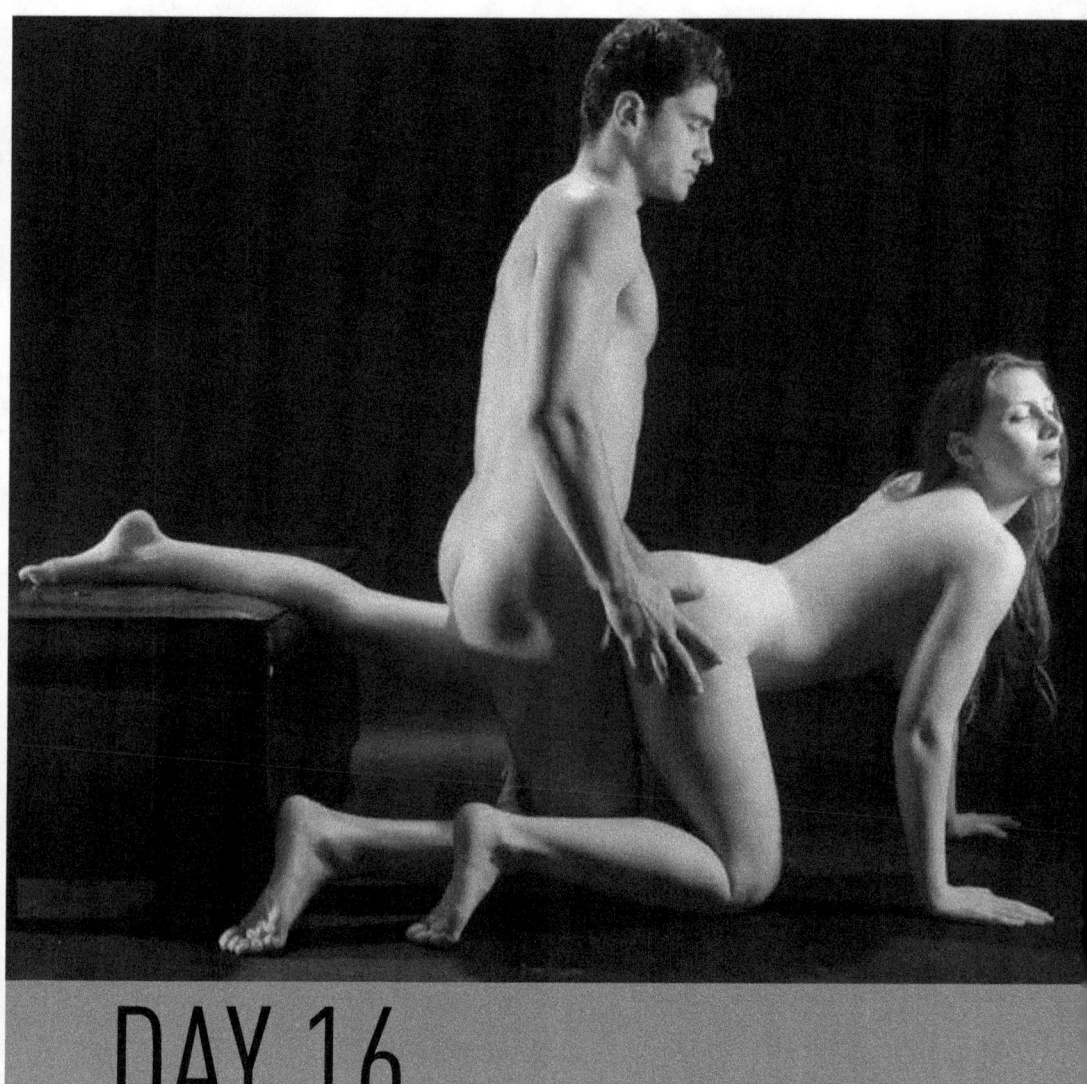

DAY 16

THE HYDRANT HUMP

She kneels on all fours and brings one of her legs straight back to rest across a bench or ottoman. Her lover enters her deeply from a kneeling position. His hands are free to caress her buttocks and breasts.

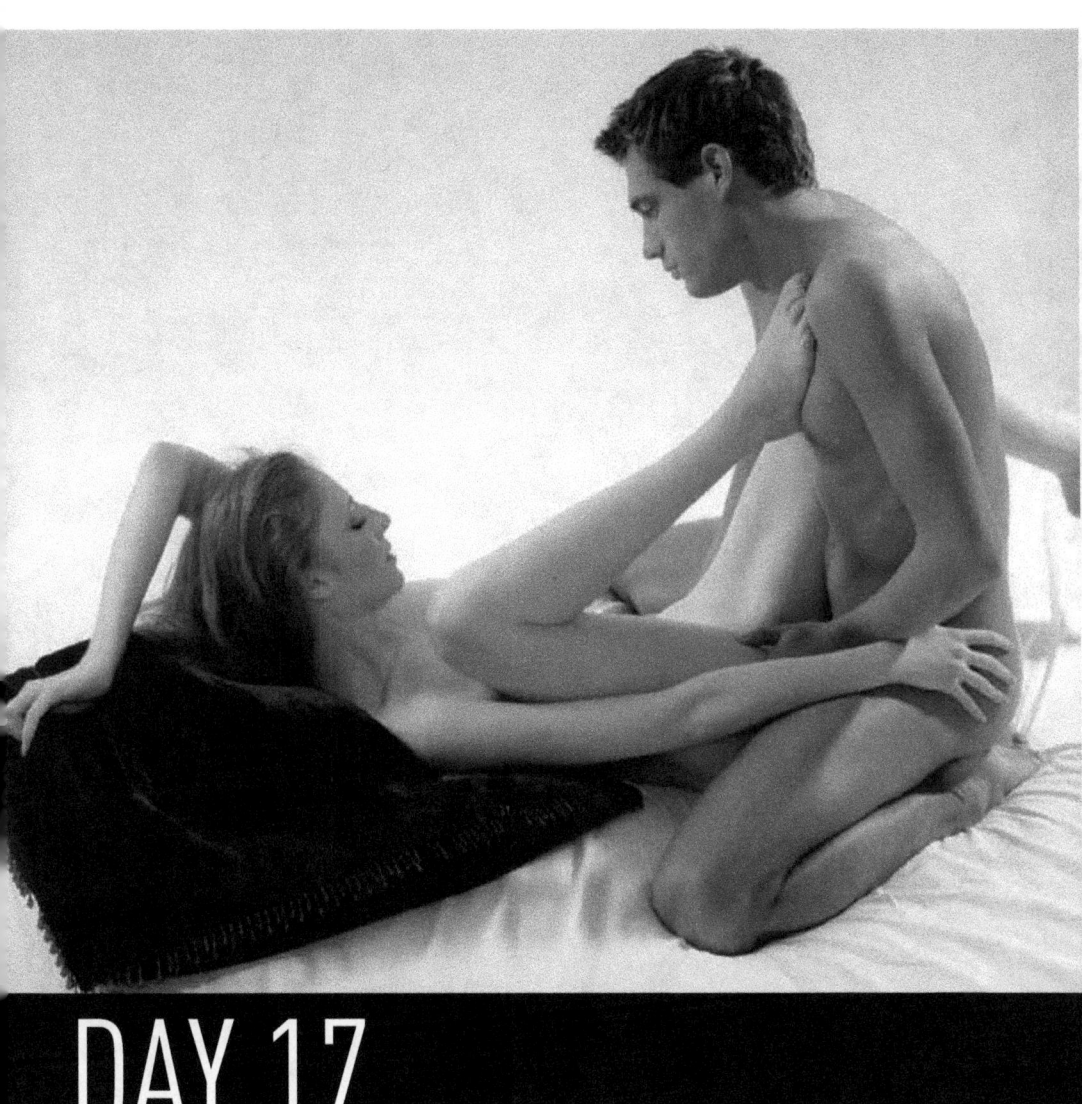

DAY 17

PEDAL PLEASURE

The woman lies on her back with one foot on her partner's chest and the other extended straight out to the side. He bends his knees and mounts her, though she's the one who looks like she's pedaling a bike.

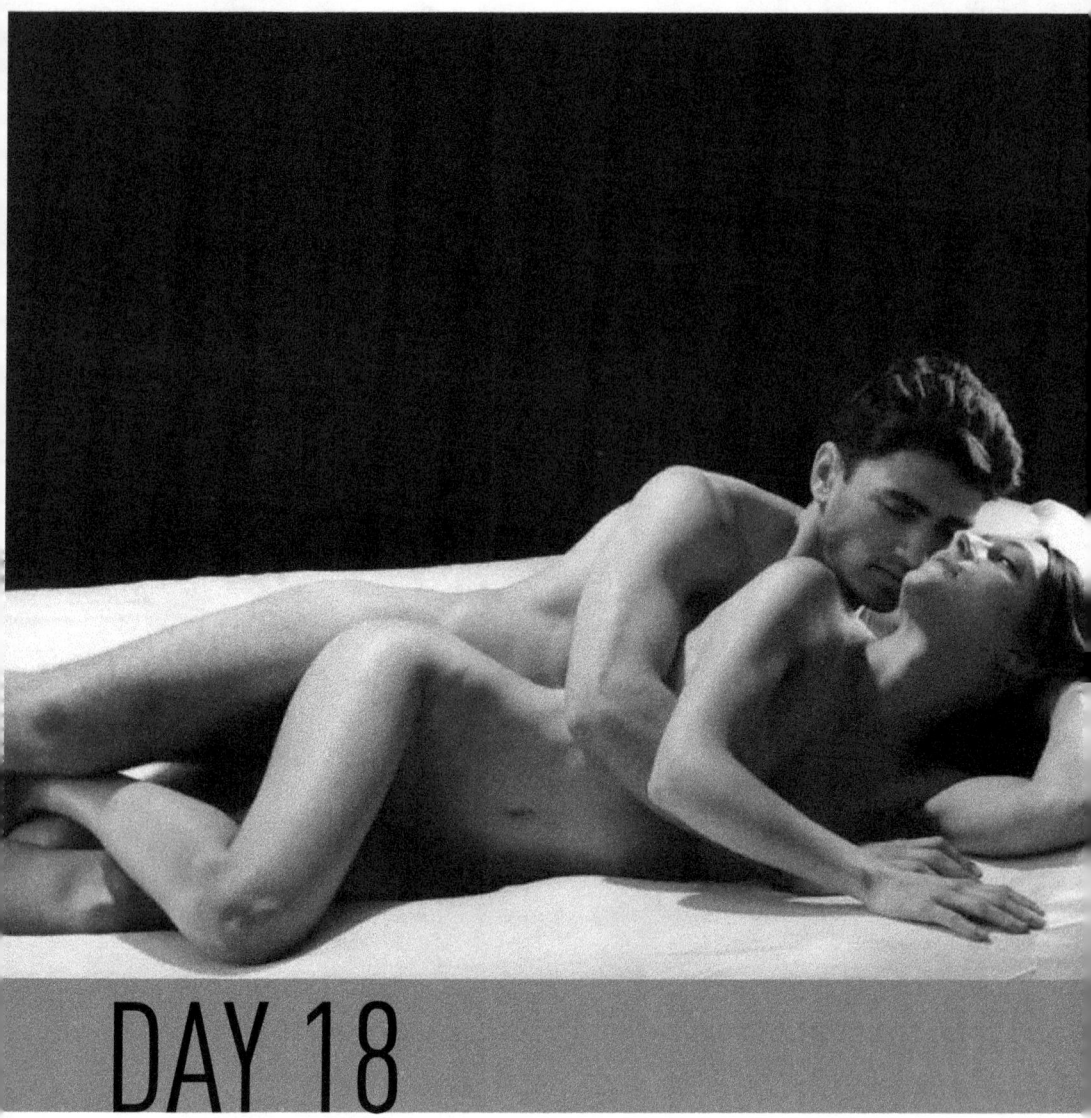

DAY 18

THE OUTSIDER

The lovers get on their sides with the man behind the woman. His legs are outside of hers as he penetrates her vaginally. She complements his thrusts with circular hip movements.

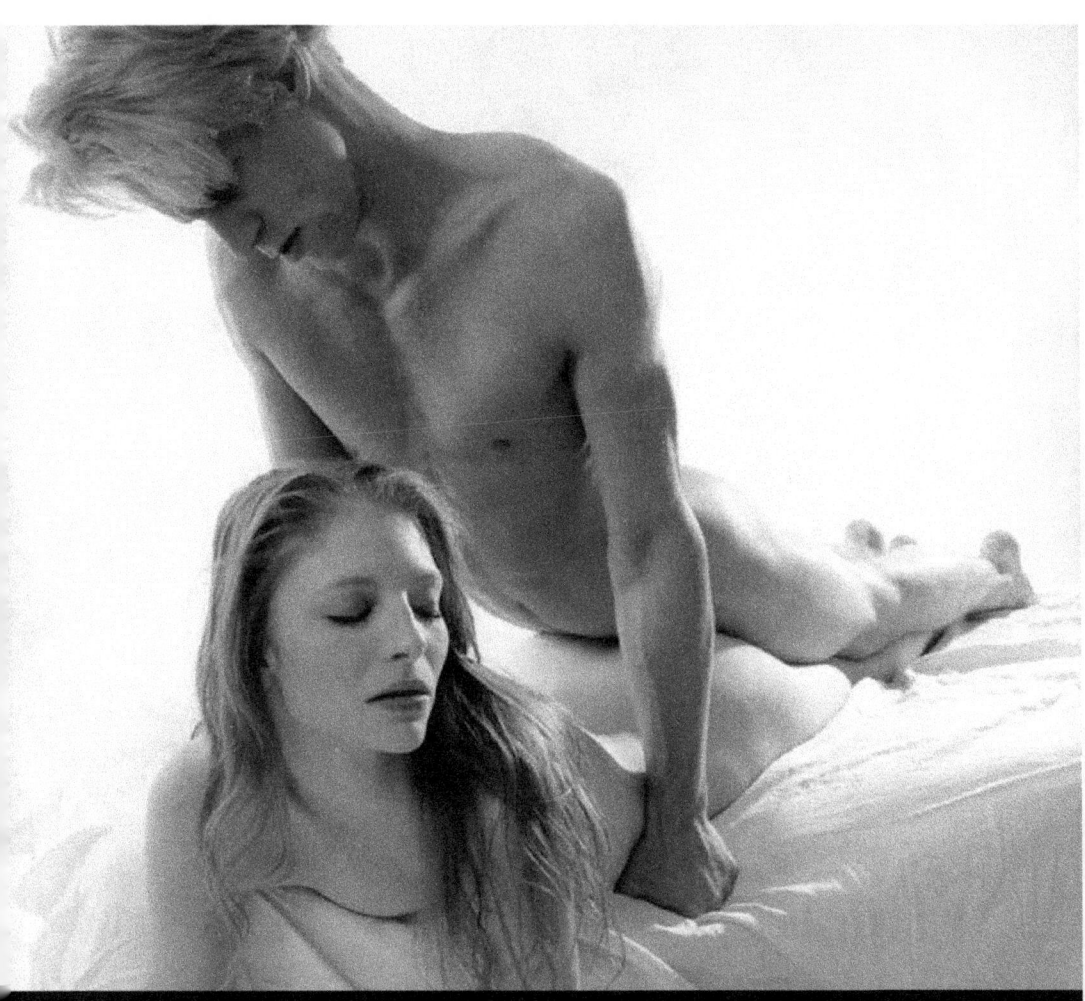

DAY 19

BACKSTAGE PASS

The woman lies on her stomach near the edge of the bed so that her hands hang off and touch the floor. The man stretches out on top of her, lifting his chest up as he enters her from behind.

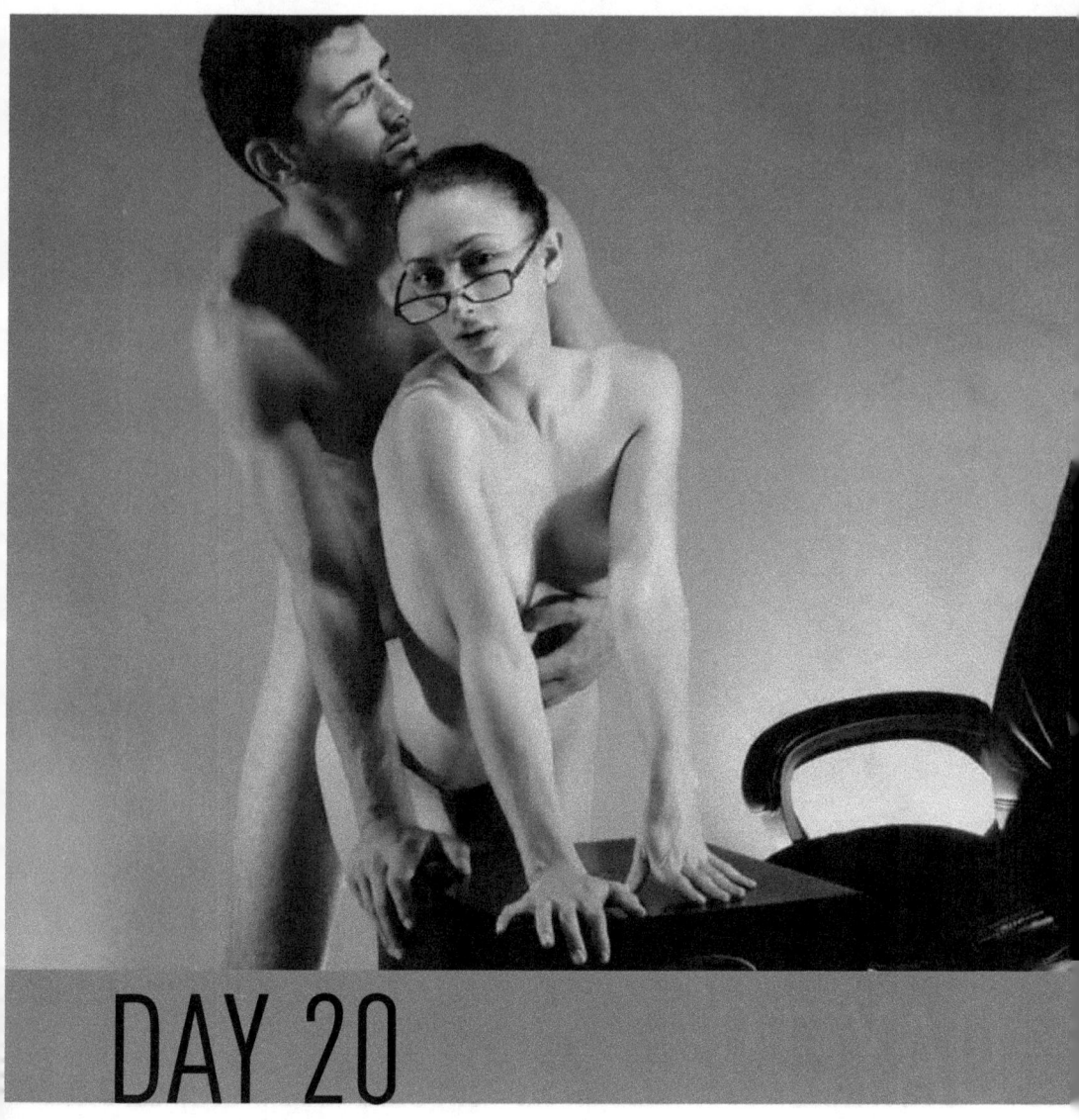

DAY 20

THE TIGHT DEADLINE

Work-related role play is one of the most popular fantasies for couples. The woman places her hands on the file cabinet offering her backside up to her lover. As he penetrates her from behind, she brings her legs closer together, making for a tighter sensation for both.

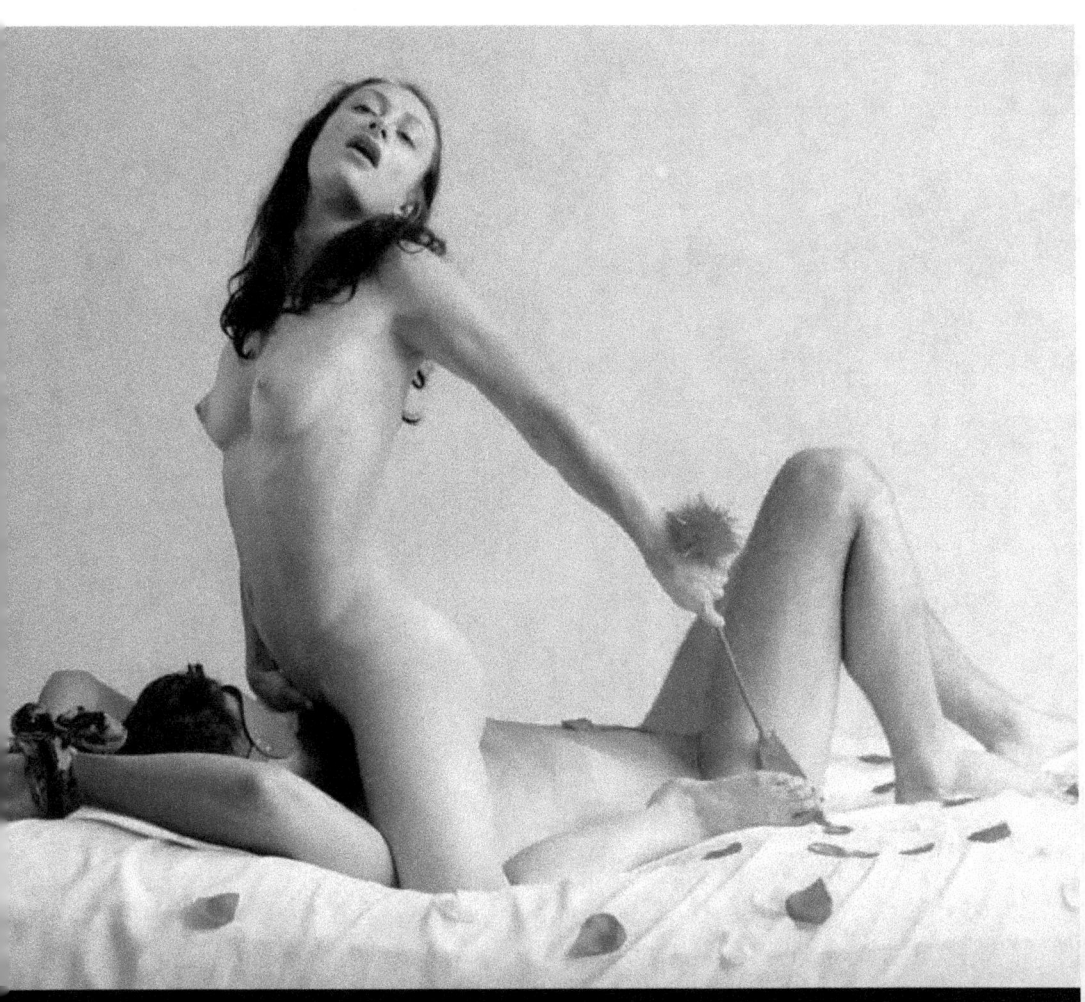

DAY 21

ORAL OBEDIENCE

The man lies back on the bed with his eyes blindfolded and hands bound above his head. His lover wields a riding crop as she straddles his face. She makes no secret as to what she wants him to do with his tongue.

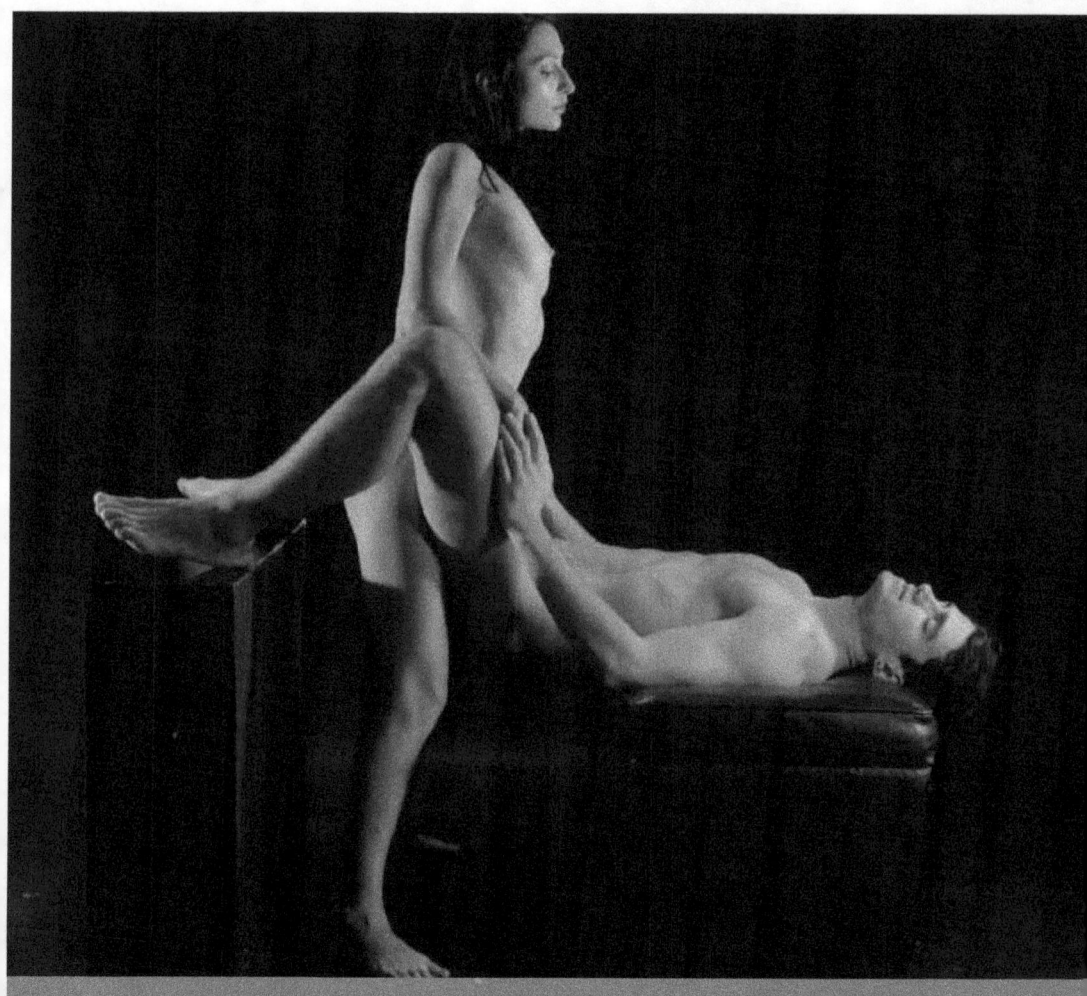

DAY 22

THE STANDING OVATION

The man positions himself between two pieces of low-lying furniture with his head and torso supported on one and his feet on the other. The woman stands in the space between and maneuvers herself so that she can enjoy an exciting new angle of entry from her partner.

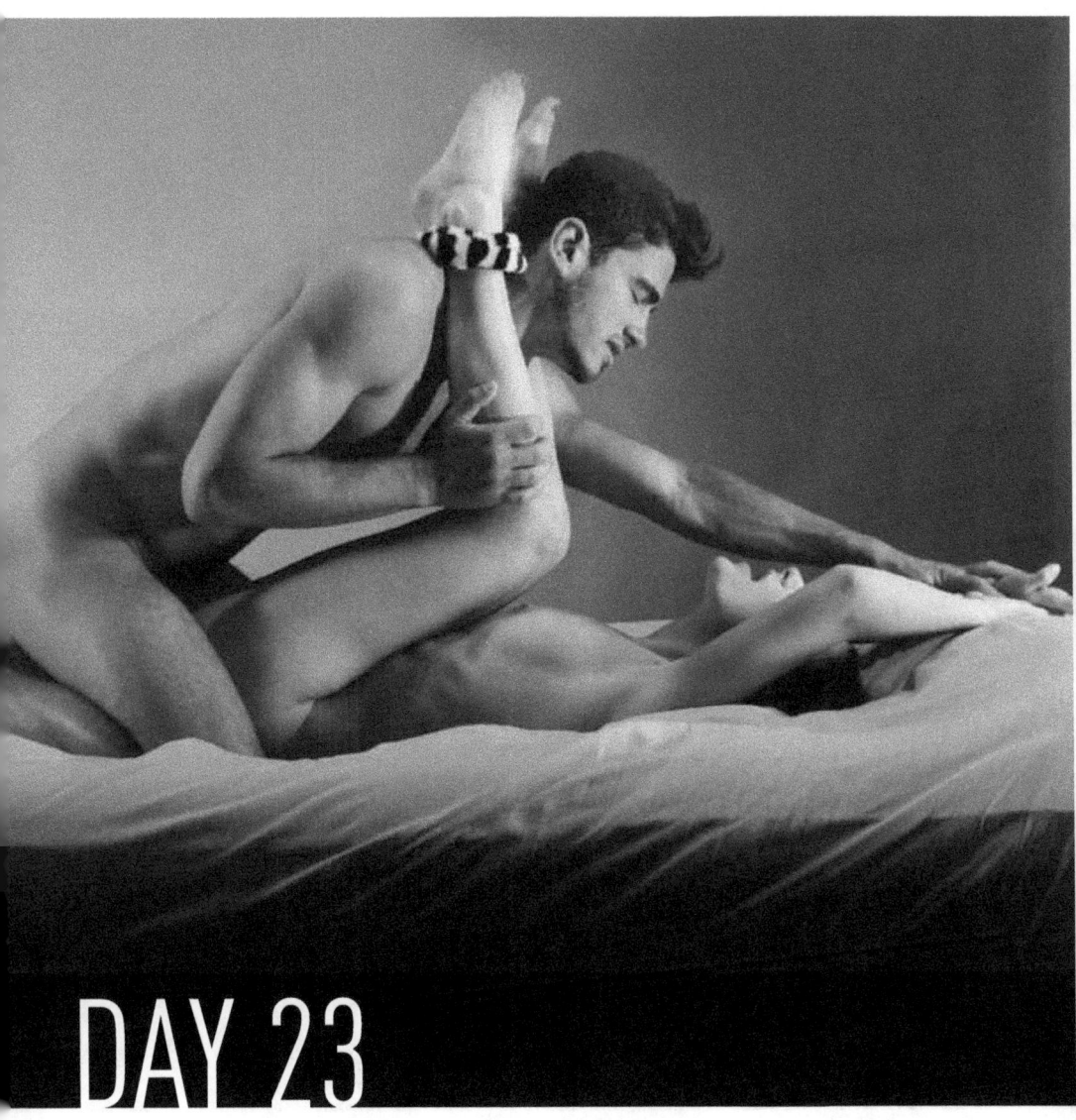

DAY 23

THE LOVE SHACKS

The woman lies back on the bed as her lover helps shackle her feet together. She raises her legs high so that she can slip the cuffs behind his neck. He's her prisoner now as he enters her vagina from a kneeling position.

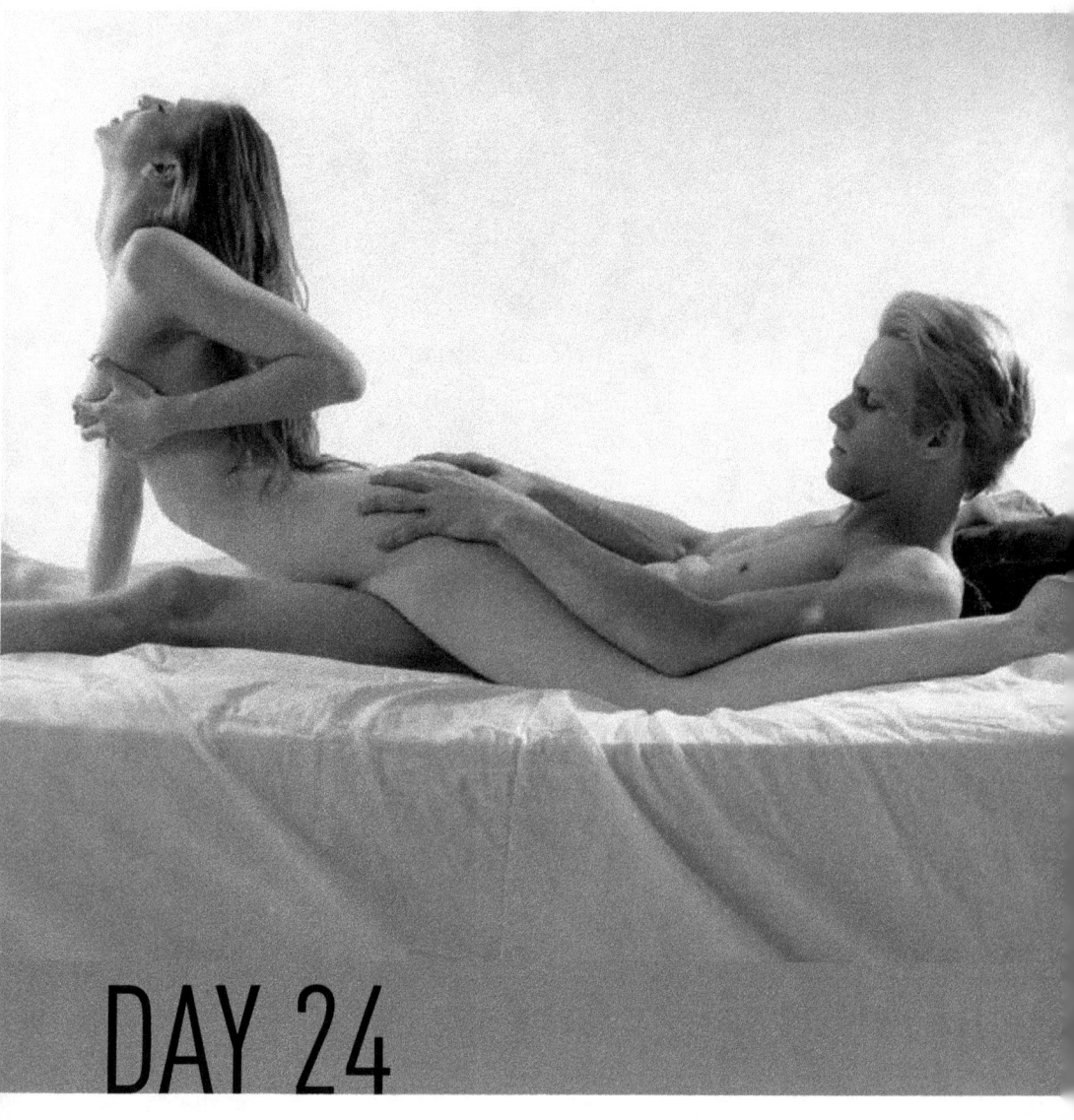

DAY 24

THE SWEET CARESS

The man lies back with his legs fully extended while his partner mounts him and extends in the opposite direction. Her beautiful bottom is right there waiting for his tender touch.

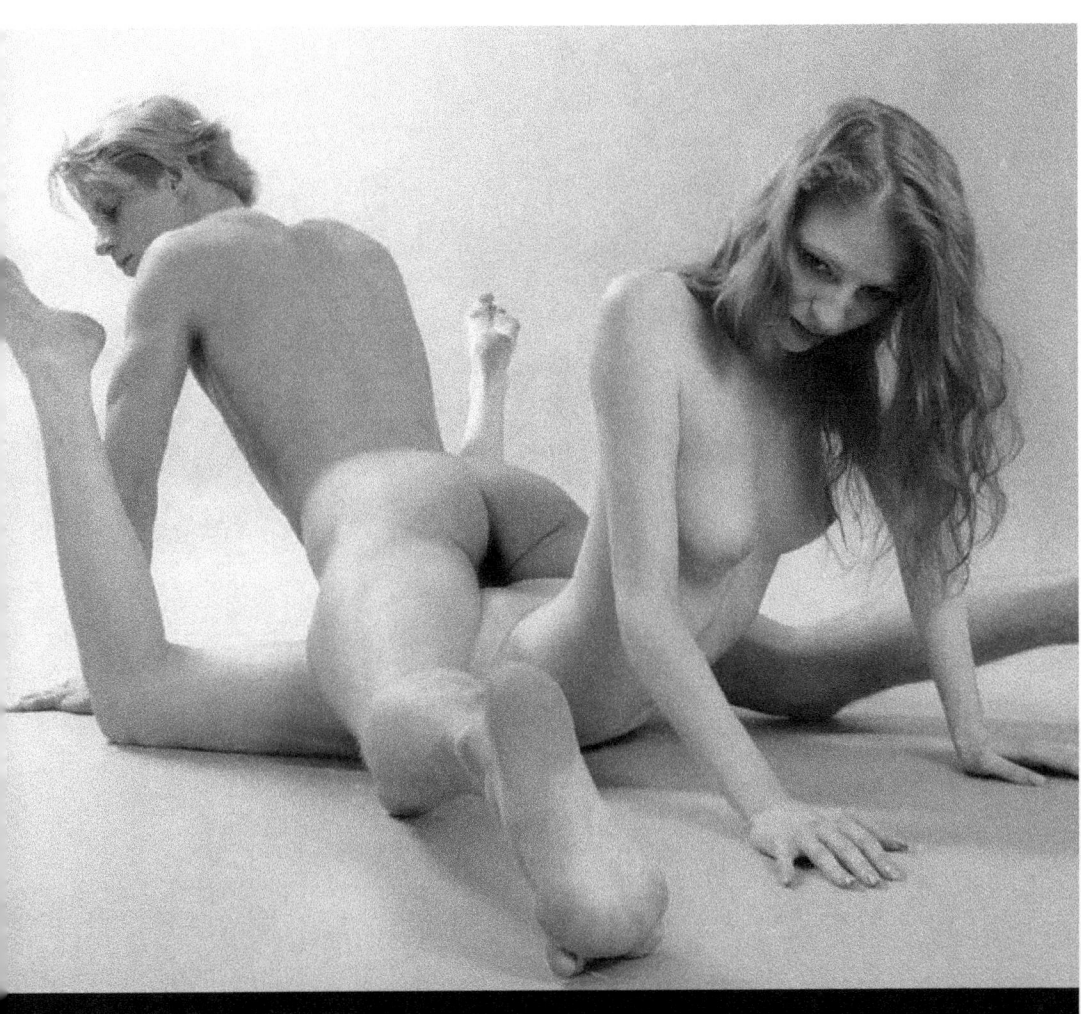

DAY 25

PASSING SHIPS

The woman lies out straight, supporting her weight on her arms. Her partner enters her anally from above while extending his legs back in a V formation. She can then hook her legs back, connecting them further.

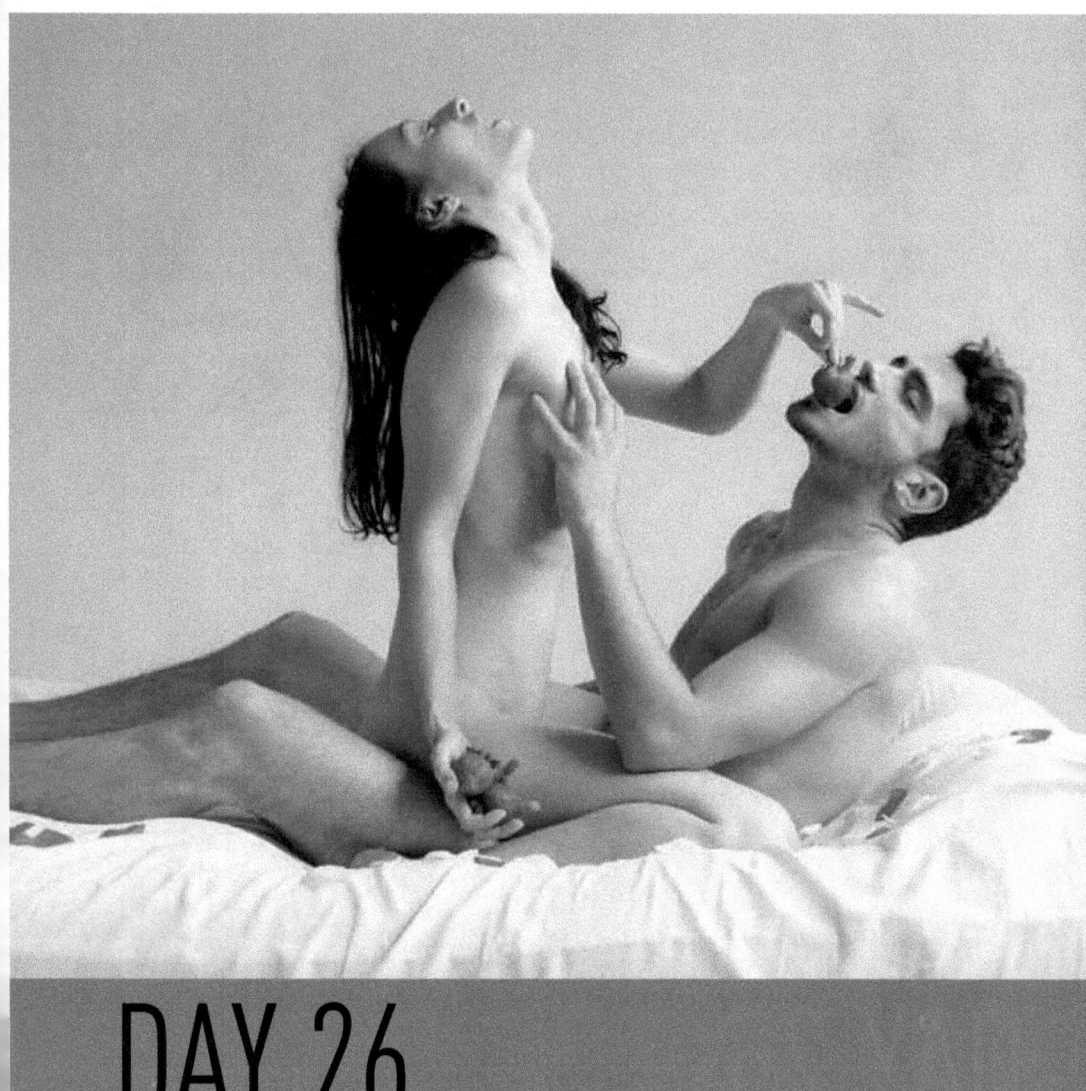

DAY 26

FEEDING THE FLAMES

There has long been an erotic element to food and eating, so it's no surprise when certain culinary elements make their way into the bedroom. Here, the man sits up with his legs extended as his lover straddles him. As he enters her she feeds him strawberries, nourishing him for the long night of lovemaking ahead.

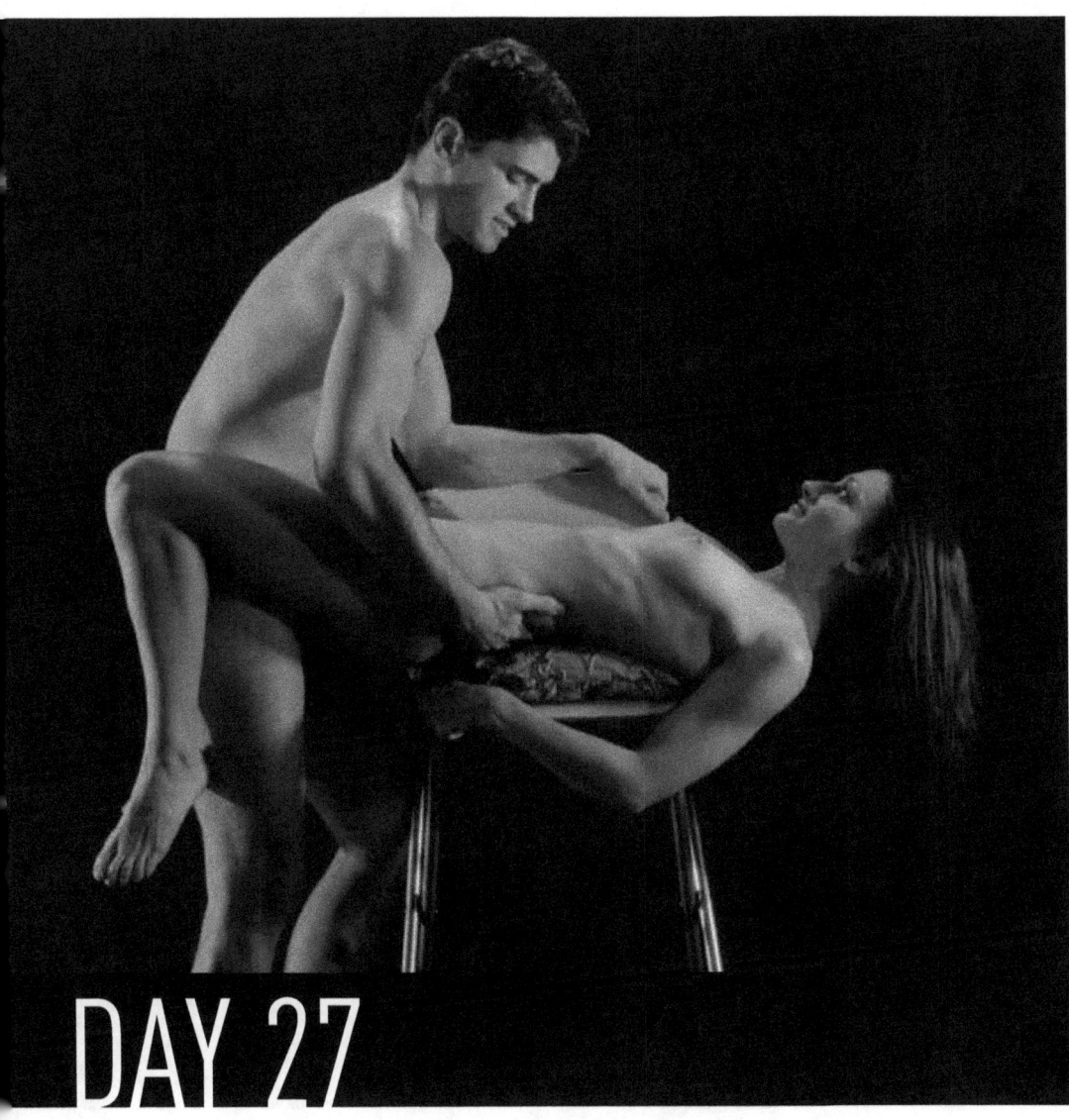

DAY 27

THE CHAIR LIFT

She positions herself back across the seat of a chair or high stool, opening her legs. Her lover enters her from a standing posture while simultaneously using his arm to support, and help arch, her back.

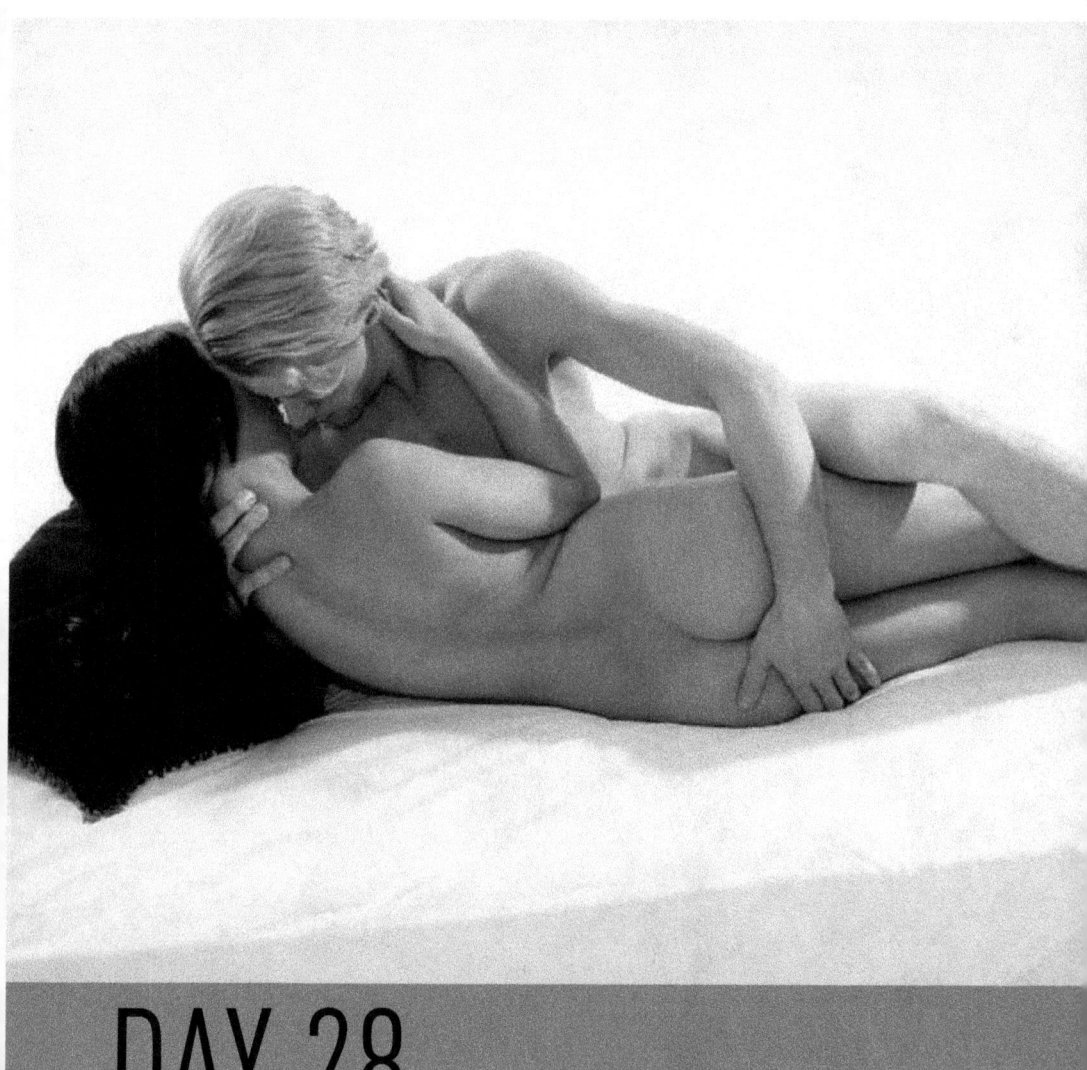

DAY 28

SIDE-BY-SIDE SENSATION

In this classic bedroom favorite, the lovers position themselves on their sides and face each other. Both have a free hand to use at their whim.

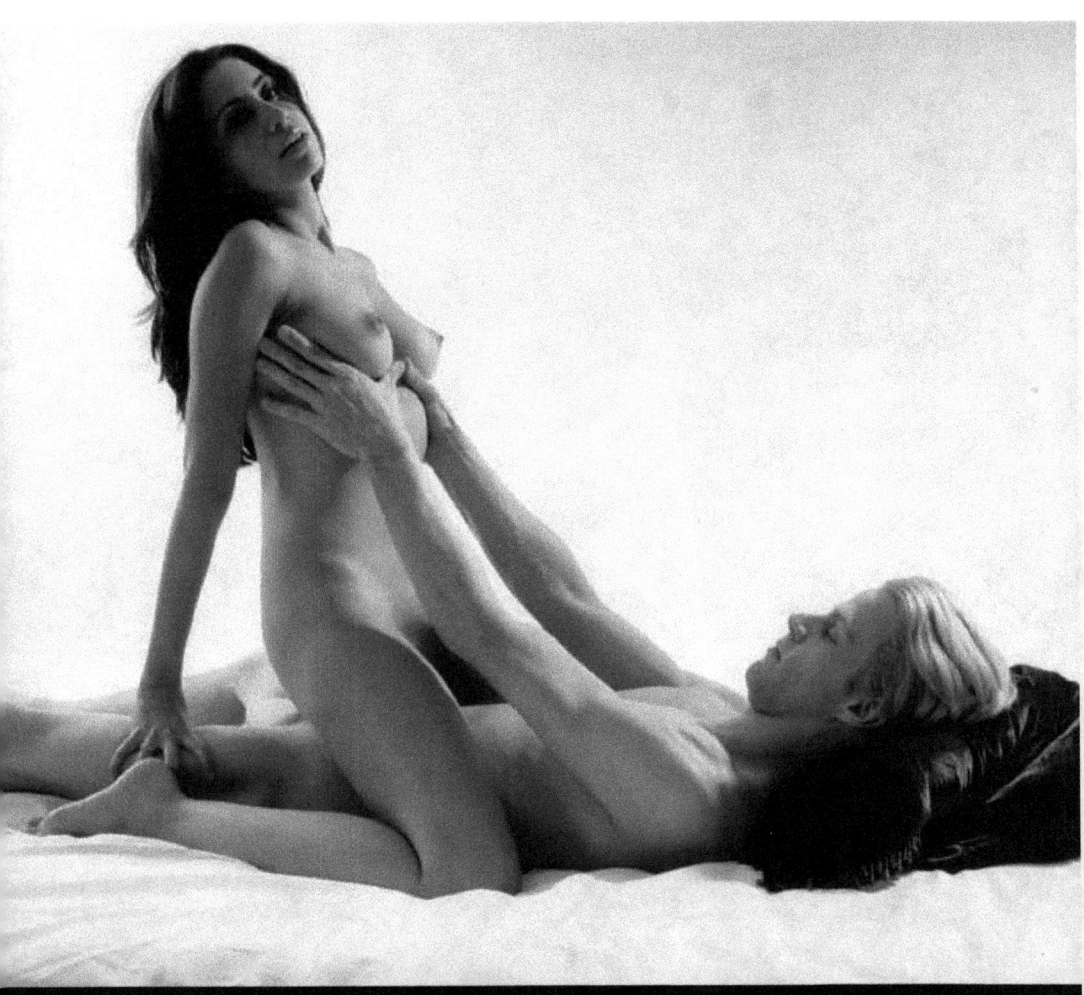

DAY 29

THE TENDER TRAP

She's got him right where she wants him. The man lies flat on his back, with legs outstretched, and the woman mounts him from the top. Once there she can hold him deep in her vagina by squeezing her legs together. A power play that's fun for both.

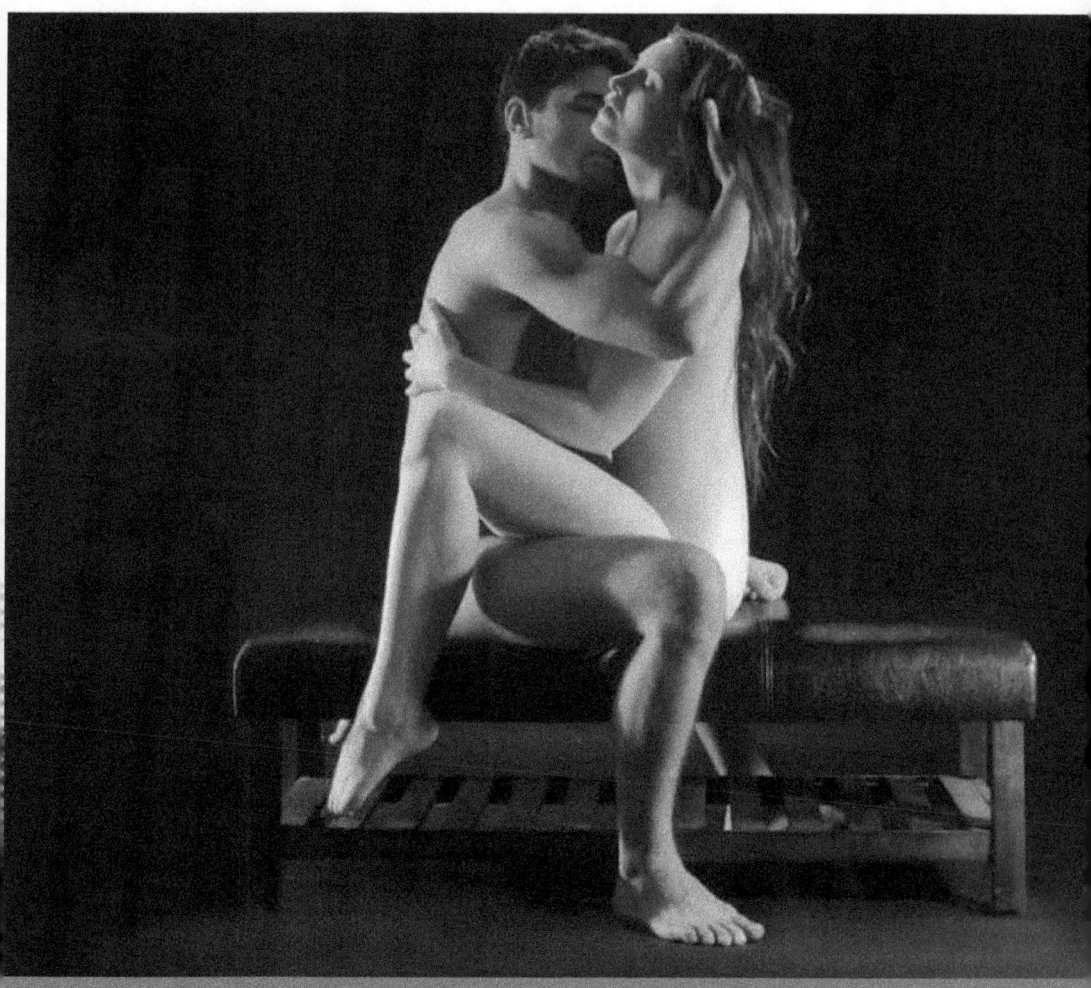

DAY 30

THE BURNING BENCH

The lovers sit on a bench facing each other. He plants both feet firmly on the floor as she straddles his thighs. As he enters her there is plenty of eye contact and gentle touching.

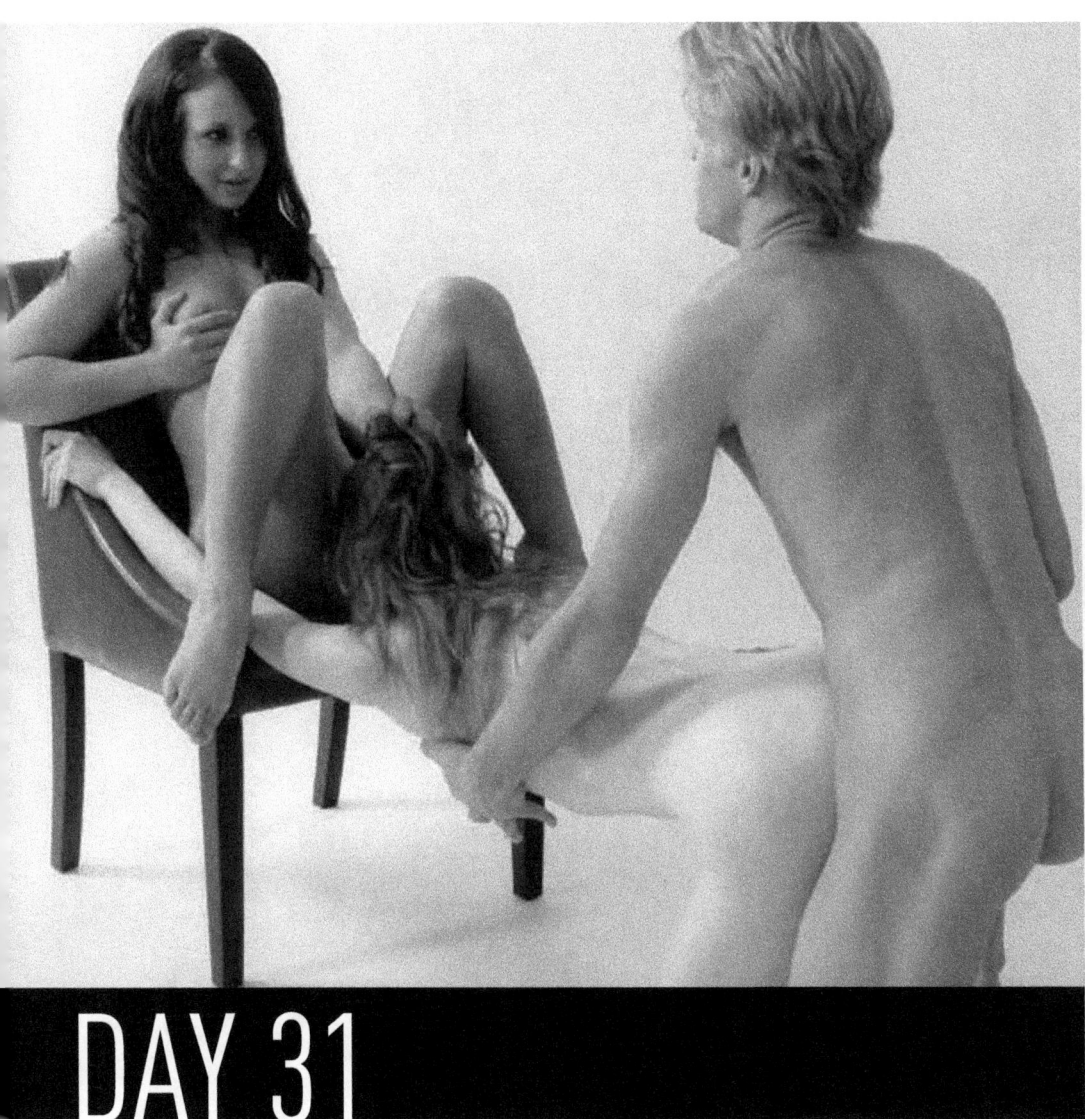

DAY 31

TRIPLE TREAT

For those looking to turn their twosome into a trio. One woman sits in a chair and parts her legs as her female counterpart services her orally. Not to be left out, their male companion enters the lucky maiden in the middle from the rear.

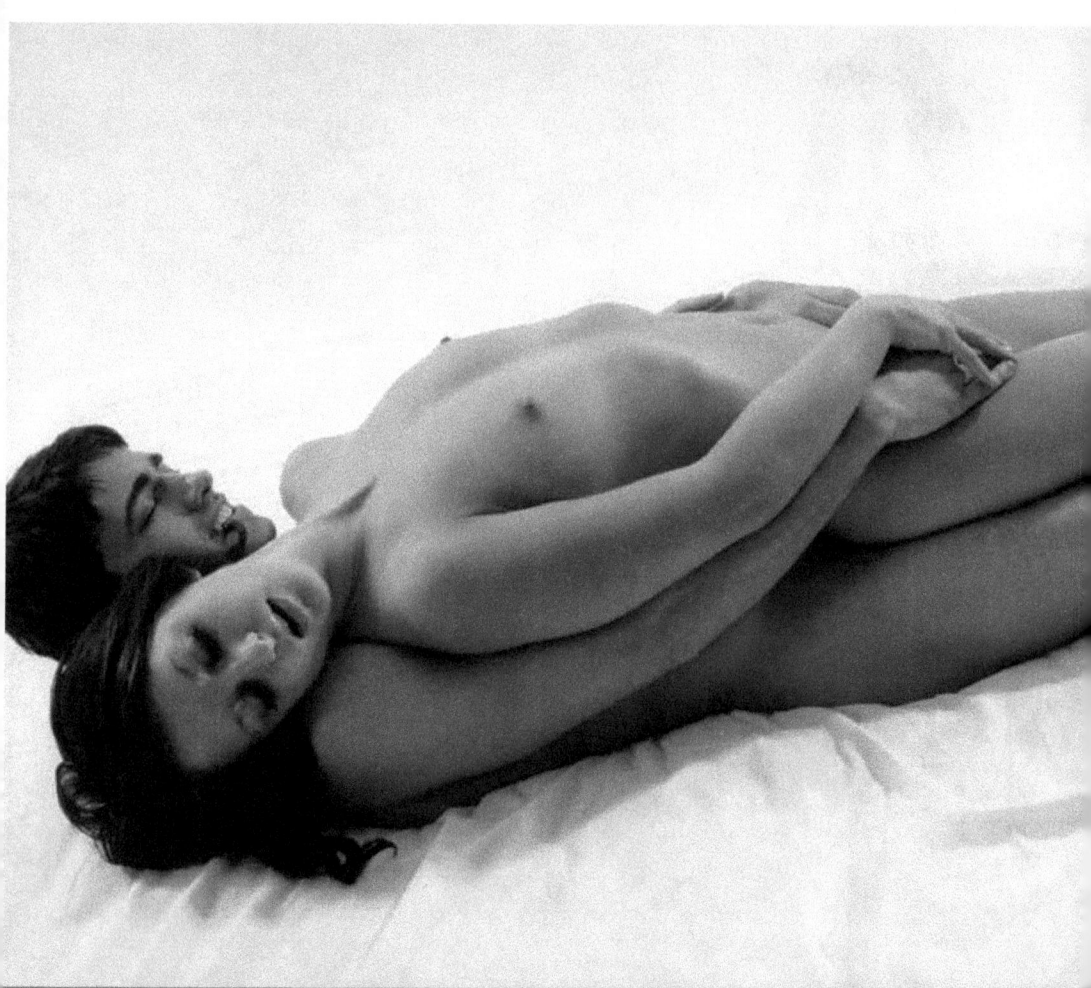

DAY 32

WINTERS PASSION

When outdoor temperatures drop it's the perfect time to heat things up indoors. In this position the woman lies on top of her partner with her back facing him. As both recline his hands are free to stimulate her clitoris.

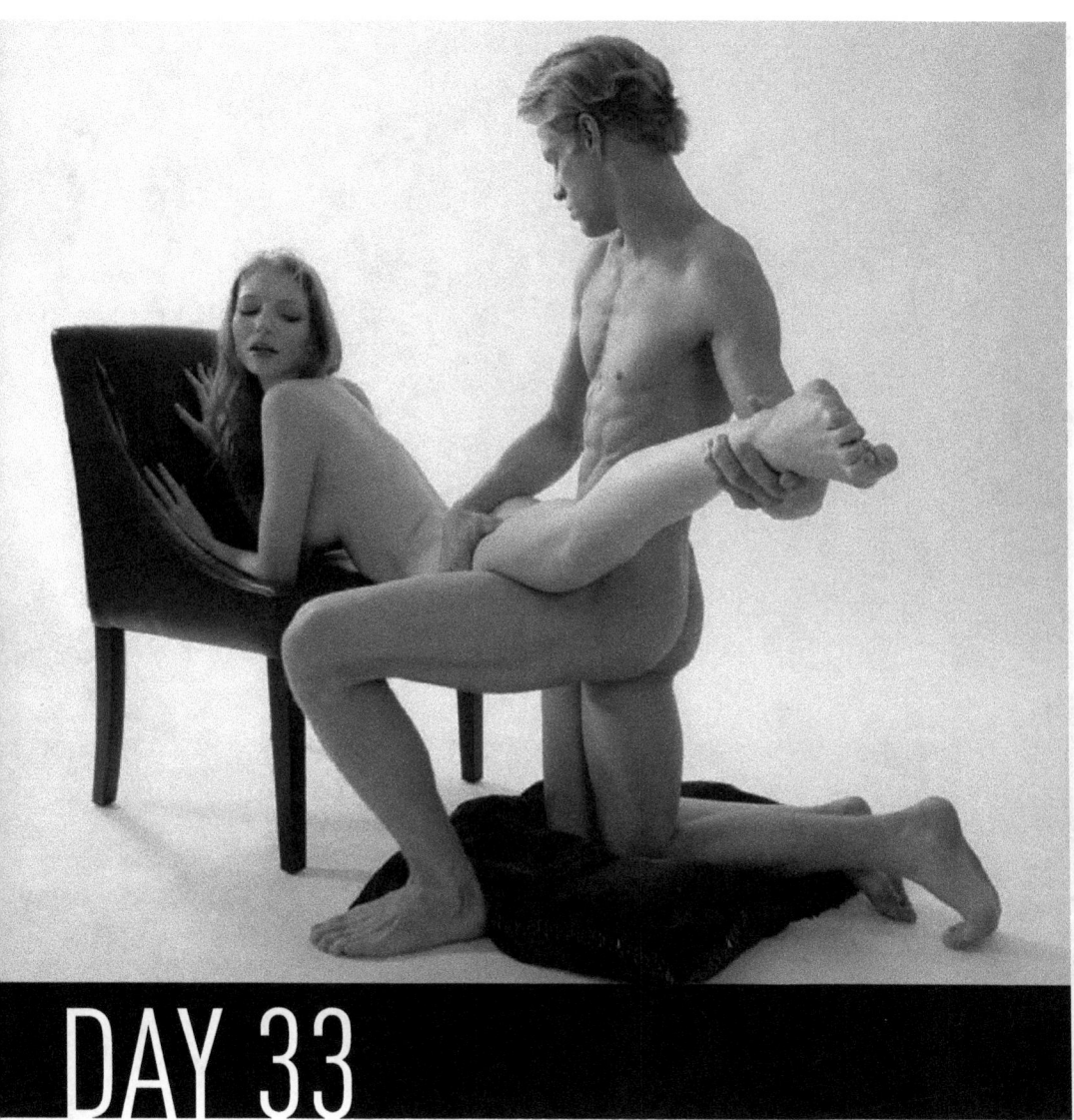

DAY 33

EXTENDED BLISS

She gets on her knees and rests her upper body in a chair. He partner lifts one of her legs and extends it straight back as he mounts her from behind. Using a pillow with this position really is a knee-saver.

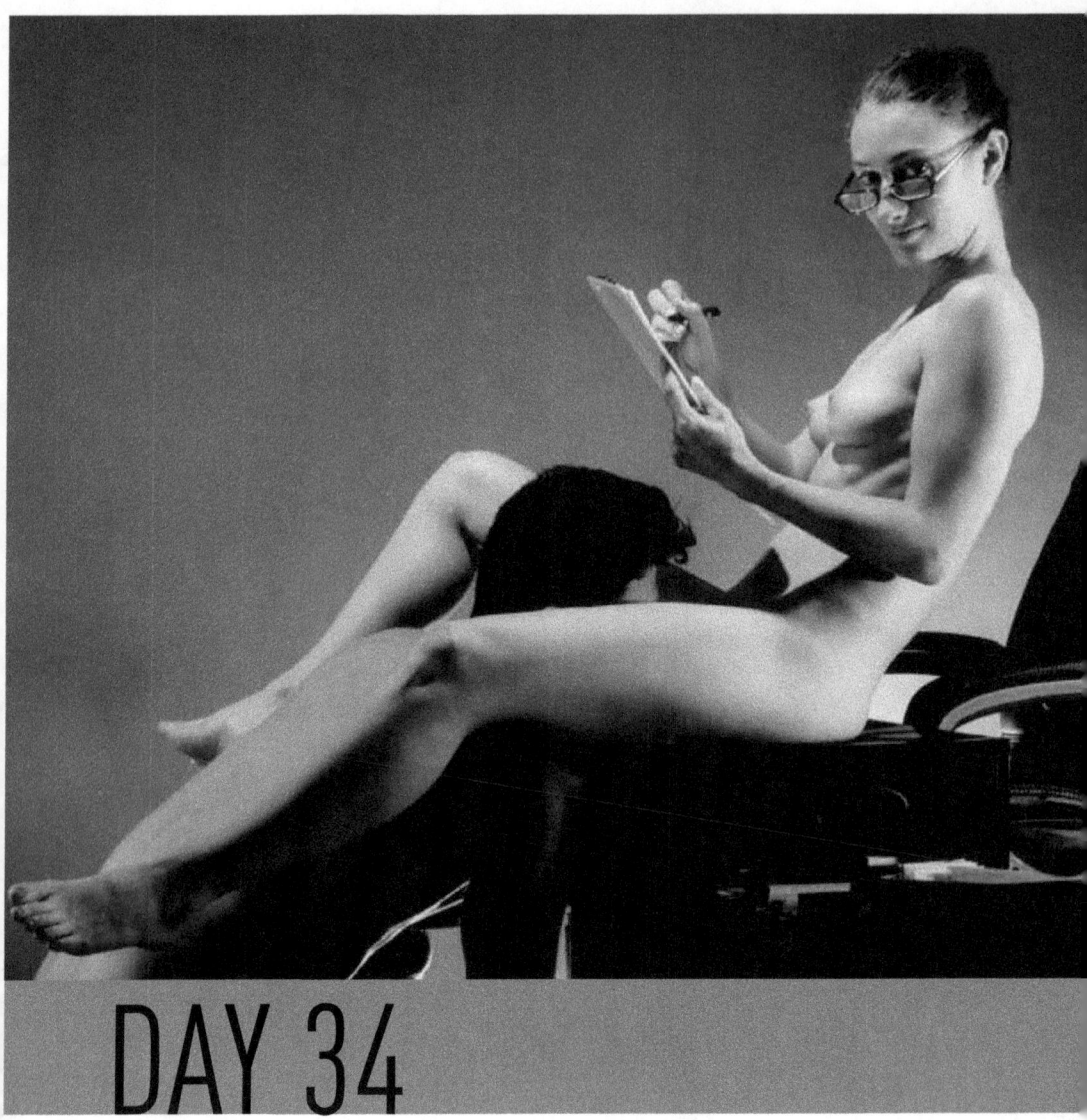

DAY 34

THE MULTITASKER

She perches on top of a file cabinet and spreads her legs. She's working on a report, but her lover knows what she really wants. He pleasures her orally until she says it's quitting time.

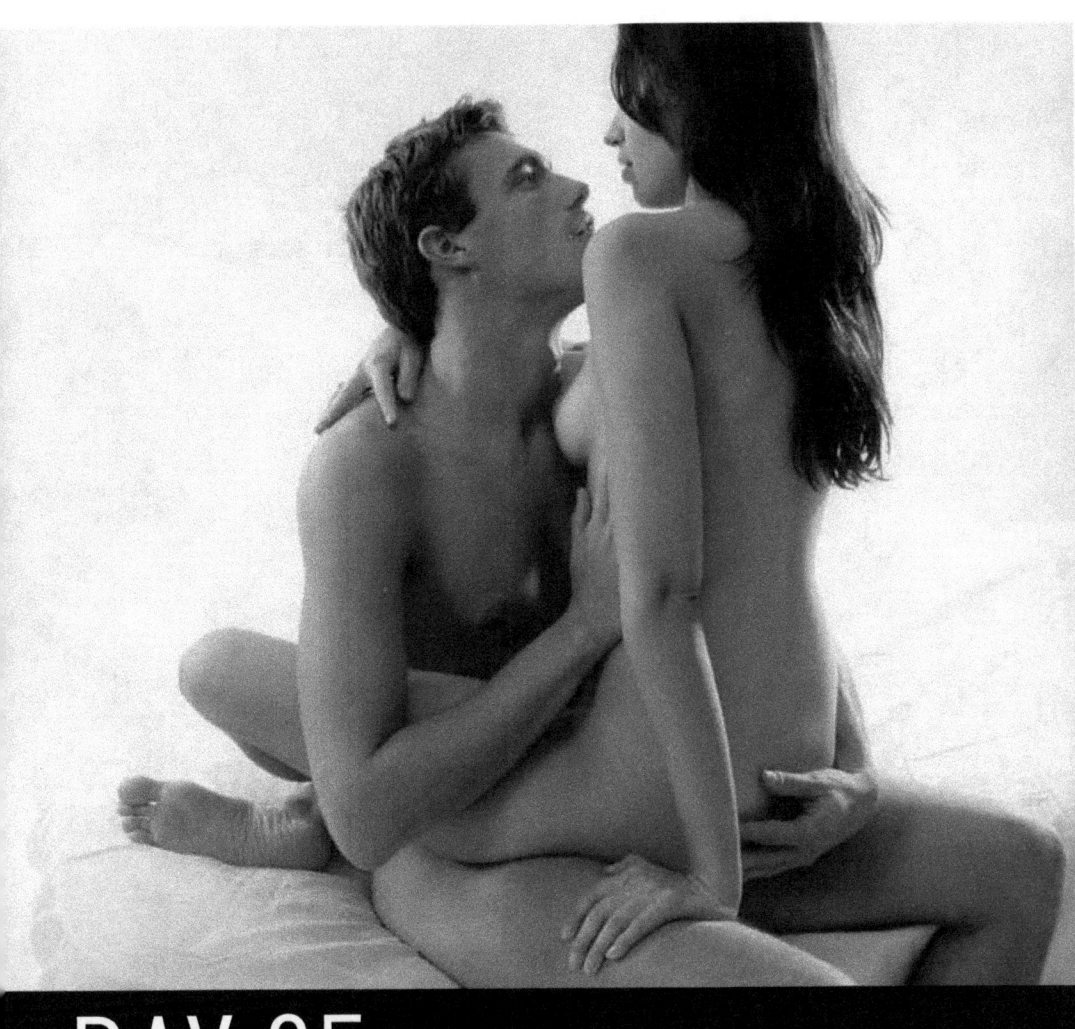

DAY 35

THE LAP WRAP

The man sits on the edge of the bed with his feet on the floor. His partner positions herself in his lap, facing him. There's no shortage of sexy eye contact as she clasps her legs around his waist and, using his thigh for leverage, slowly and tantalizing grinds down on his penis.

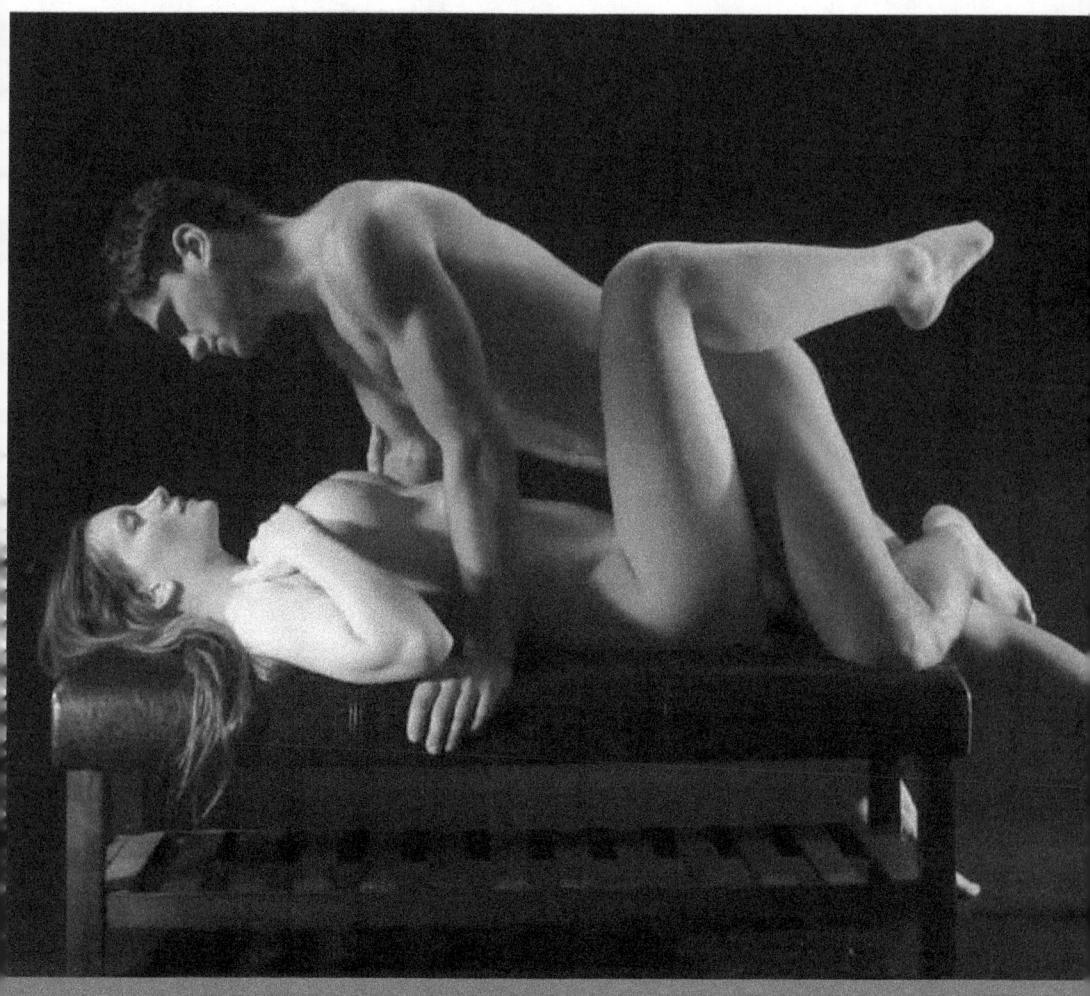

DAY 36

THE PLEASURE PLATEAU

The woman lies back against a padded bench or ottoman. Her lover plants one knee on the bench and enters her. He has ample freedom to thrust to his heart's content.

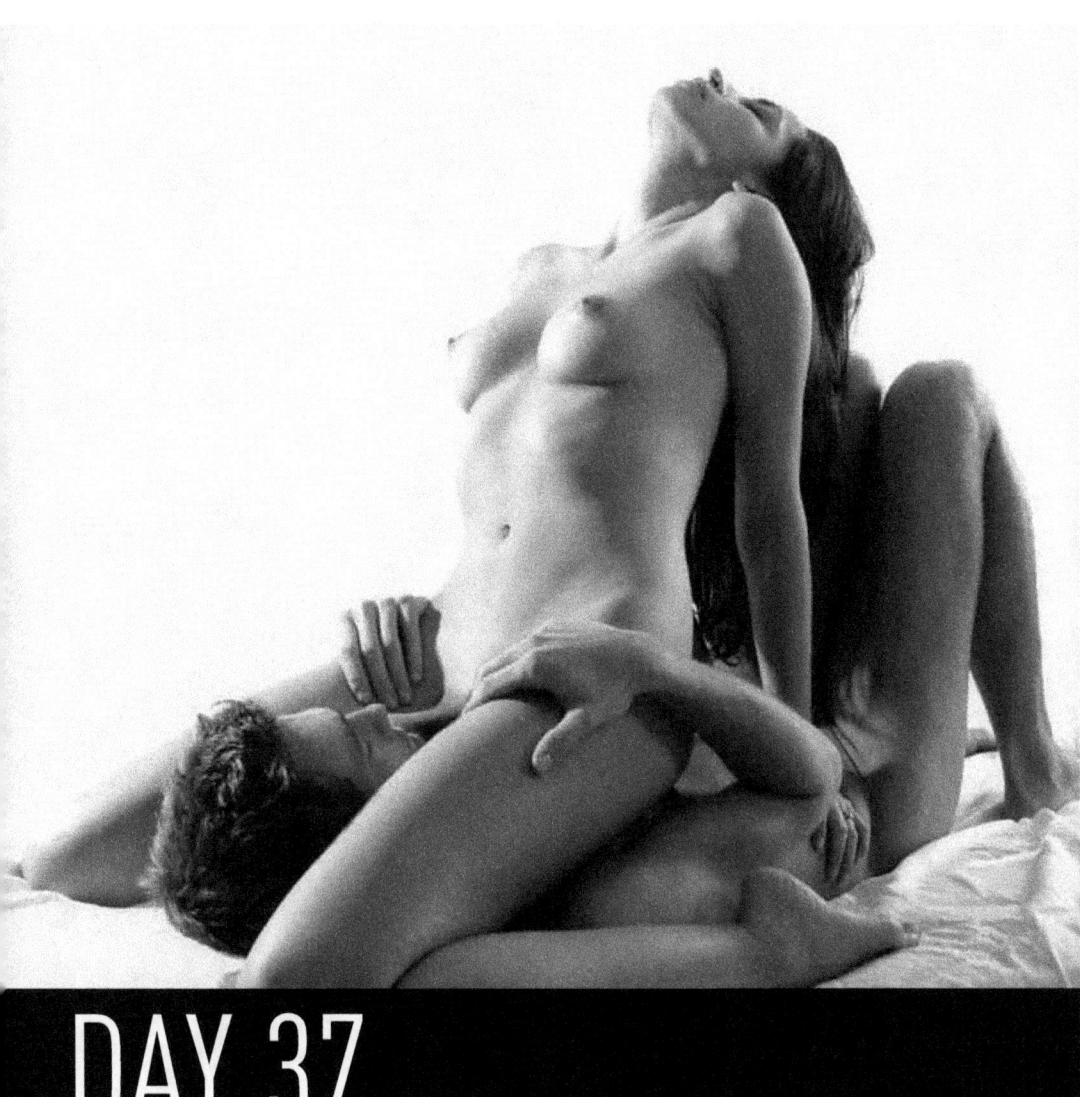

DAY 37

SITTING PRETTY

They don't get much more straightforward than this one. He lies on the bed as she straddles his face, placing her vagina over his mouth. She's looking away from him. He's not going anywhere until she gets what she wants.

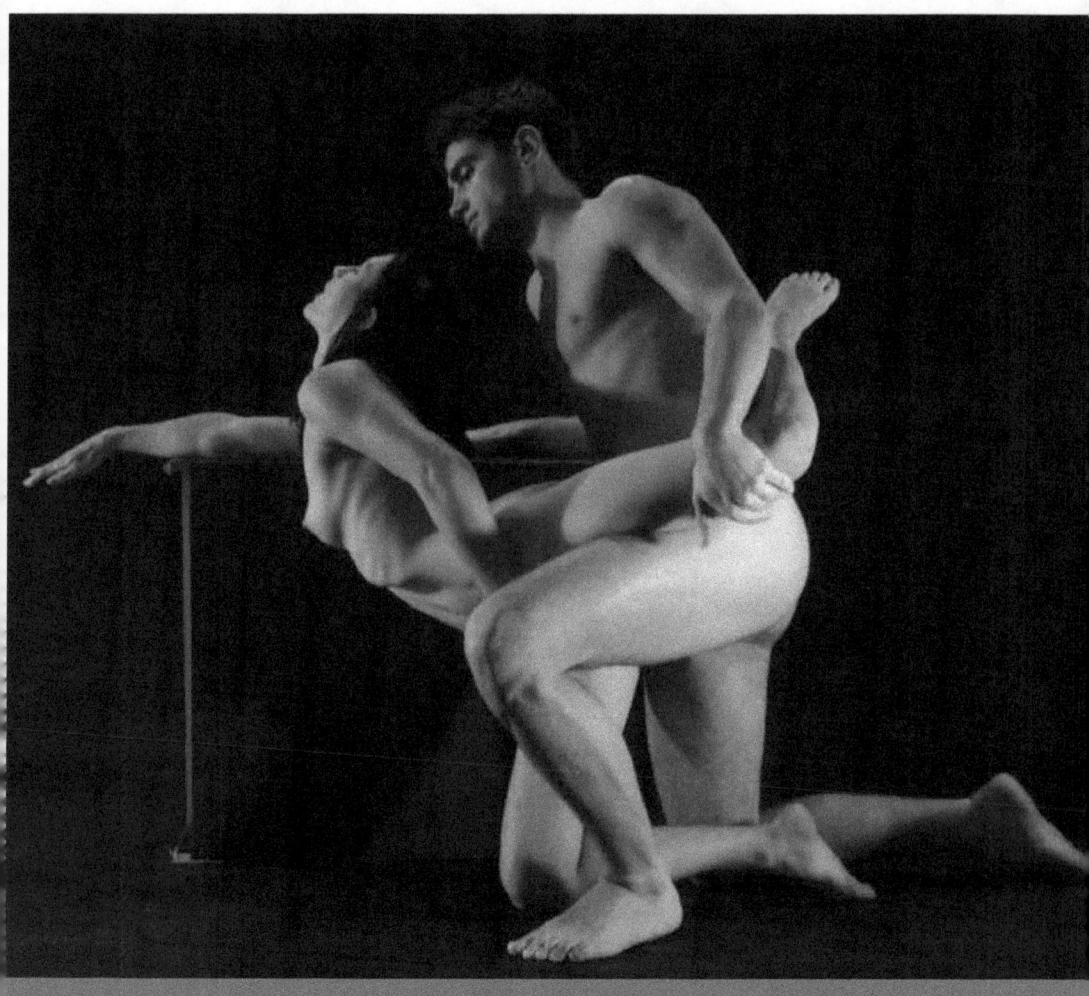

DAY 38

THE GRACEFUL GRIND

Starting on her knees, the woman rests one hand across a table or chair to steady herself for the action to come. Her partner gets down on one knee and penetrates her as he lifts one of her legs up across his thigh. She has a free hand to stroke her clitoris or touch his testicles.

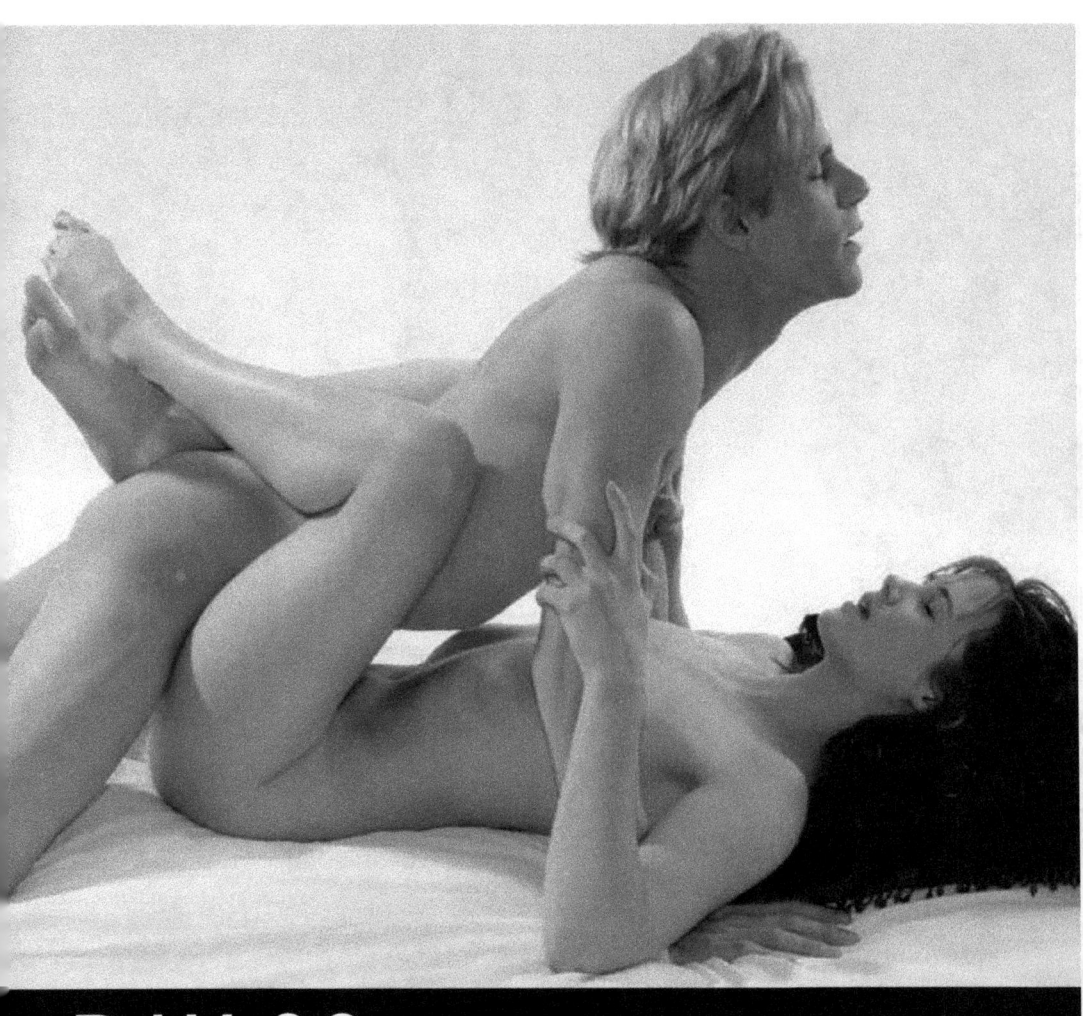

DAY 39

LOCKED AND LOADED

The man kneels and leans forward, supporting his weight with his hands, while the woman locks her legs around his waist and backside. The result is a combustible connection.

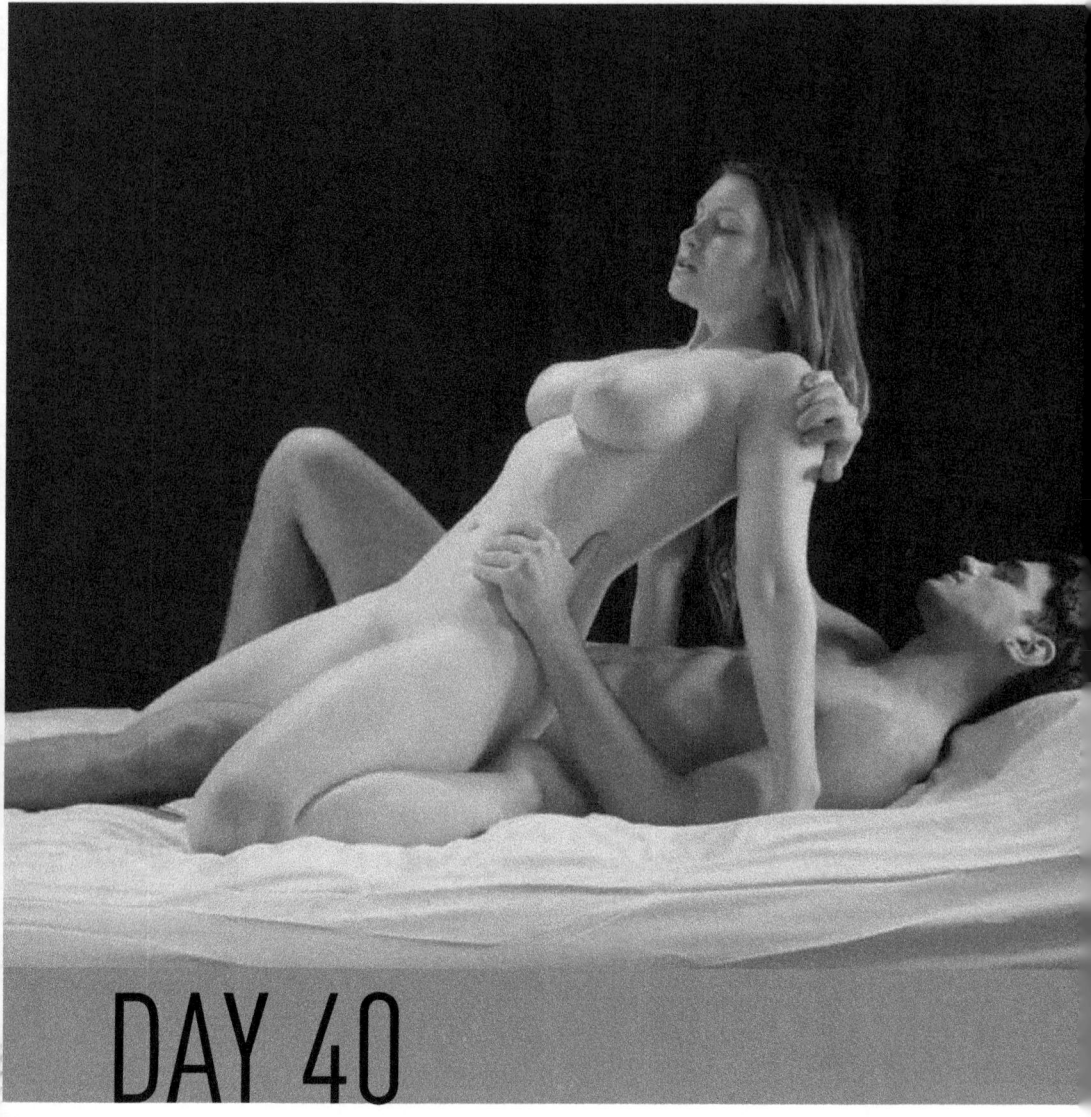

DAY 40

SAFE AT HOME

He's comfortably on his back with one leg bent at the knee and the other fully extended. She straddles his straight leg as he penetrates her. She has little trouble finding a rhythm as she slides up and down.

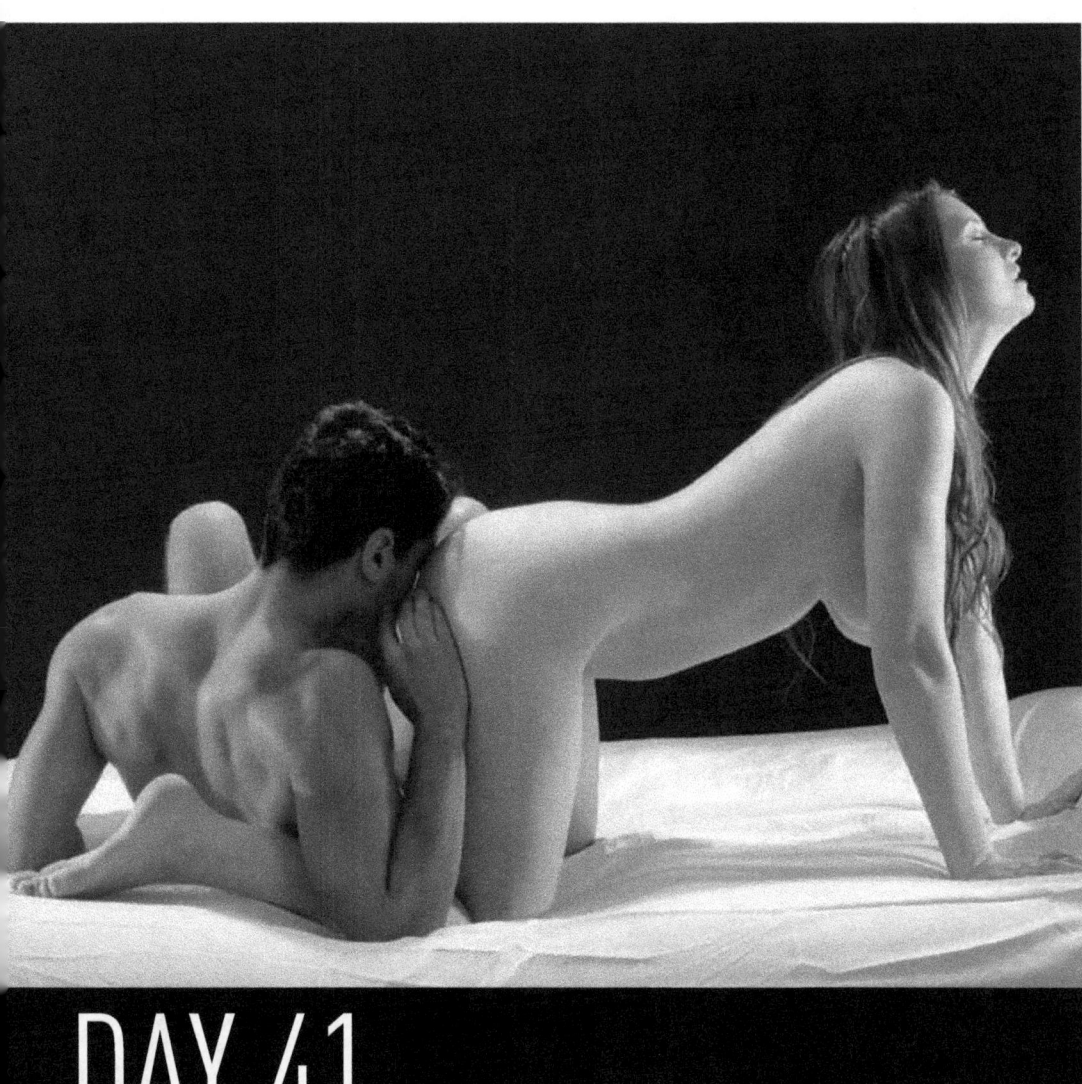

DAY 41

BOTTOMS UP

The man parks himself on his buttocks with his knees bent near the bottom edge of the bed. His partner positions herself perpendicularly at his side with her back turned and buttocks upturned. As he pleasures himself he liberally lashes her vagina from behind.

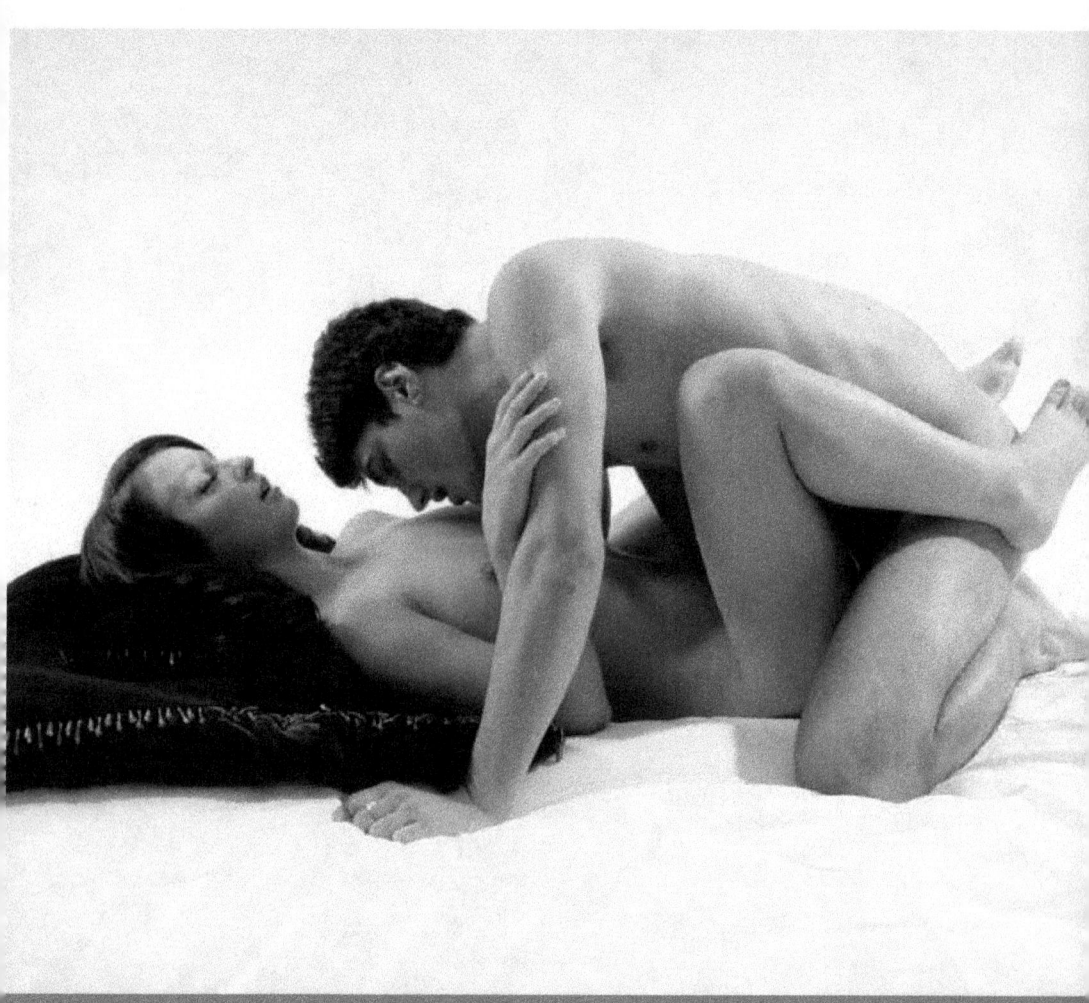

DAY 42

THE SHOCK ABSORBER

Fasten your seat belts! The woman brings her knees in toward her chest as her lover enters her from a kneeling position. Deep penetration and a rocking rhythm are the order of the day (or night).

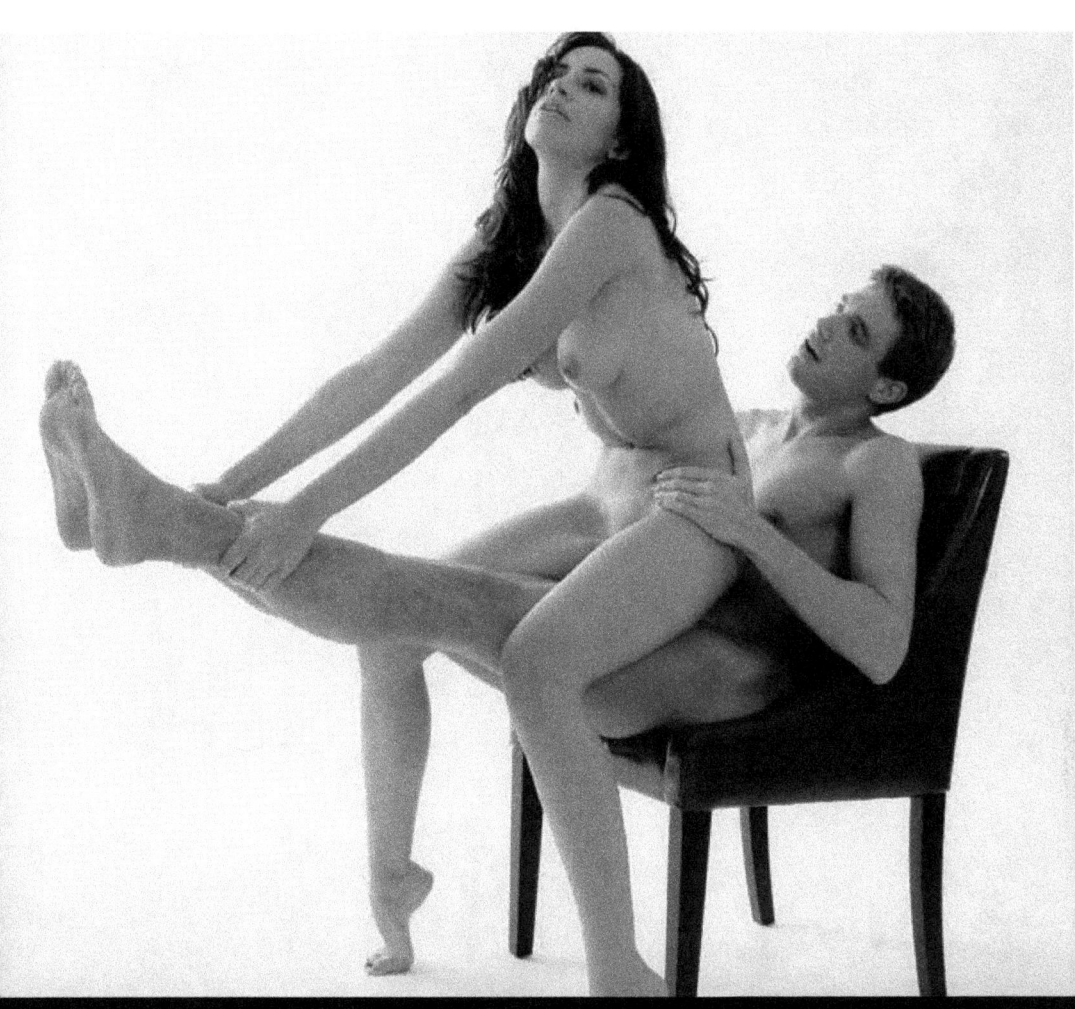

DAY 43

UP AND AWAY

He's seated in a chair with his legs pointing straight out. She mounts her lover, facing away from him, with her hands holding his legs. They blissfully rock up and down.

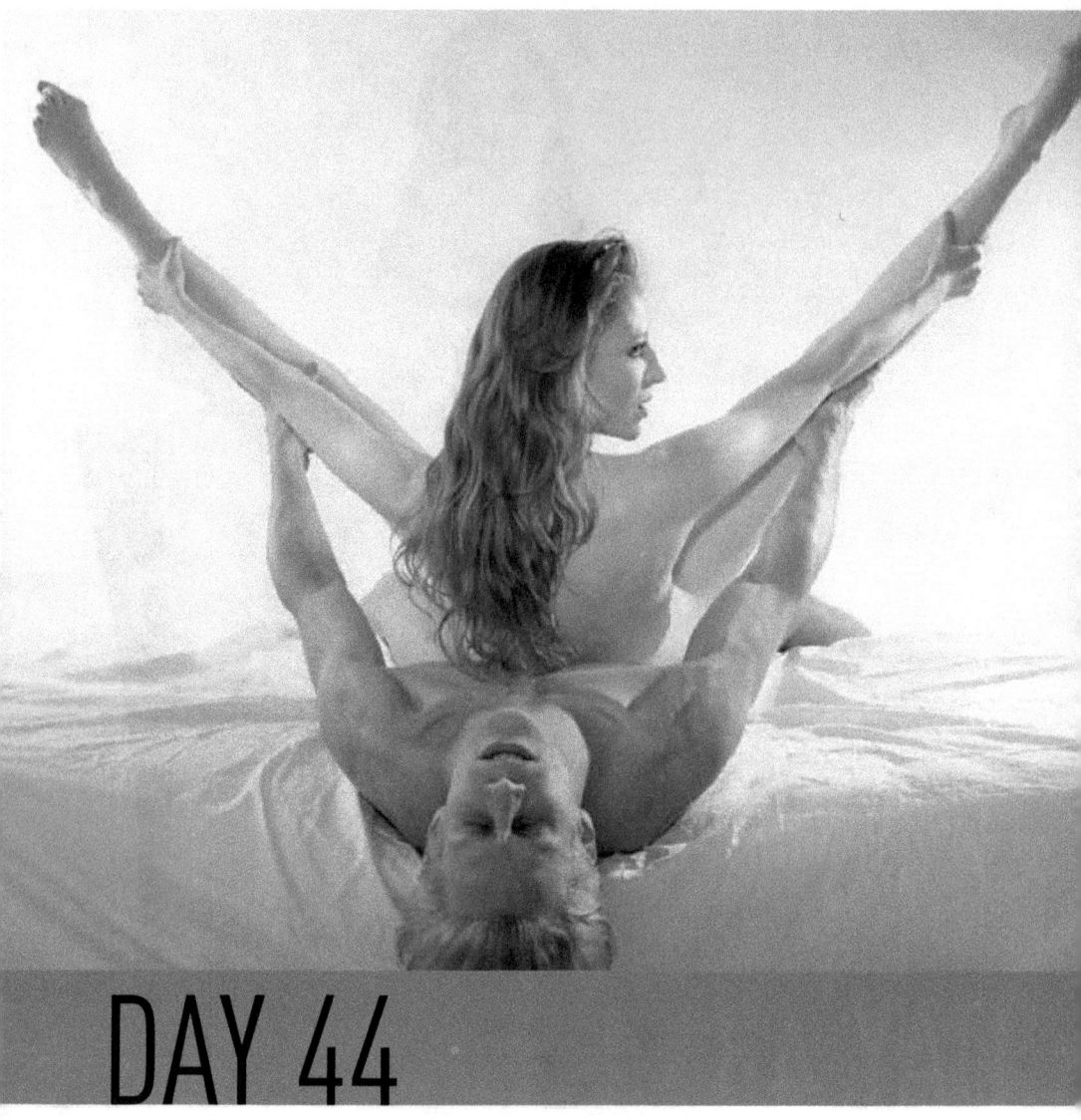

DAY 44

THE MAIN SQUEEZE

The man lies back on the bed with his legs open. The woman gets on top with her back facing her partner and legs spread open. As he penetrates her, he can manipulate her legs open and closed to vary the sensations for both of them.

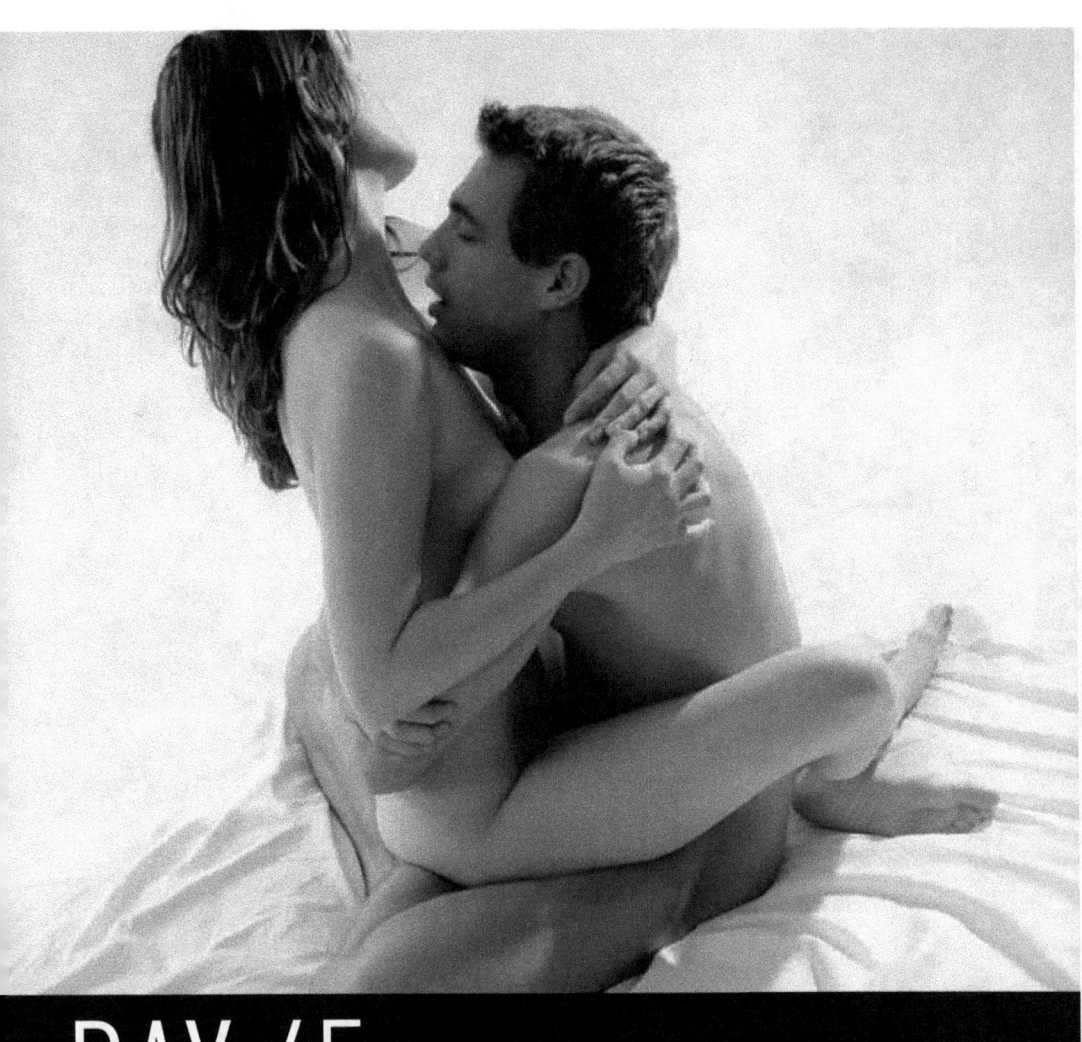

DAY 45

HEARTS ON FIRE

The perfect position for Valentine's Day—or any day to celebrate love. The man sits cross-legged as his lover sits in his lap and coils her legs around his back. When things get this close you can almost hear your partner's heartbeat.

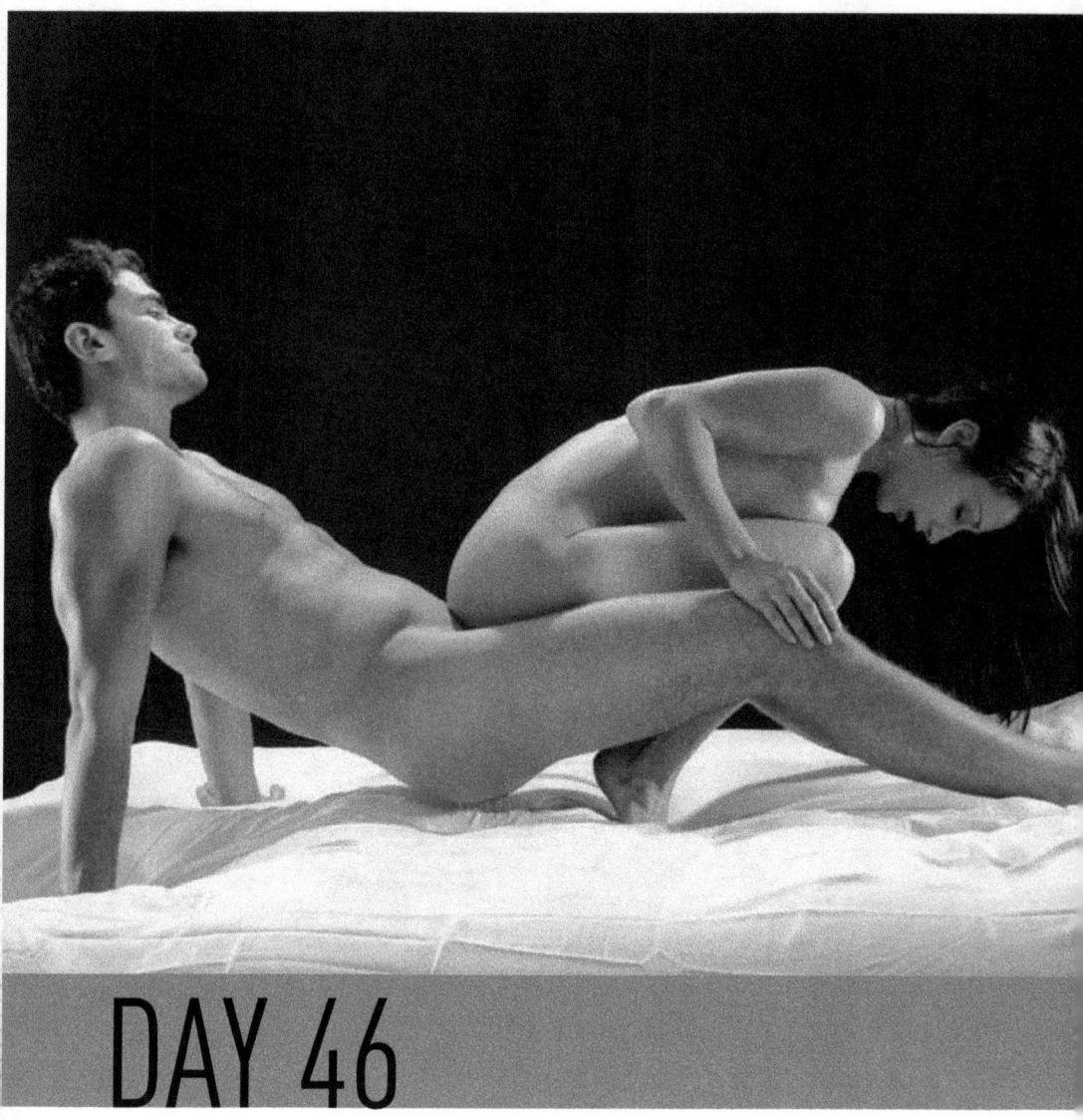

DAY 46

THE BOBSLED

The man places himself on the bed in something of a reverse plank with his arms back and down and legs extended and open. His partner backs in between his legs and takes a seat on his erect penis. Using his knees for support she's doing the driving.

DAY 47

SPANKS FOR THE MEMORIES

The man penetrates the his partner from behind, as she lies on her back across an ottoman and engages in some mutual oral 69ing with her girlfriend. He administers some playful spanks, urging her to keep up her torrid pace.

DAY 48

THE JUMP HUMP

Though some standing positions can be a bit taxing, they can also be a lot of fun. He stands up straight as his lover leaps into his arms and wraps her hands around his neck. She uses his hands as stirrups for her feet as the pair bounce towards climax.

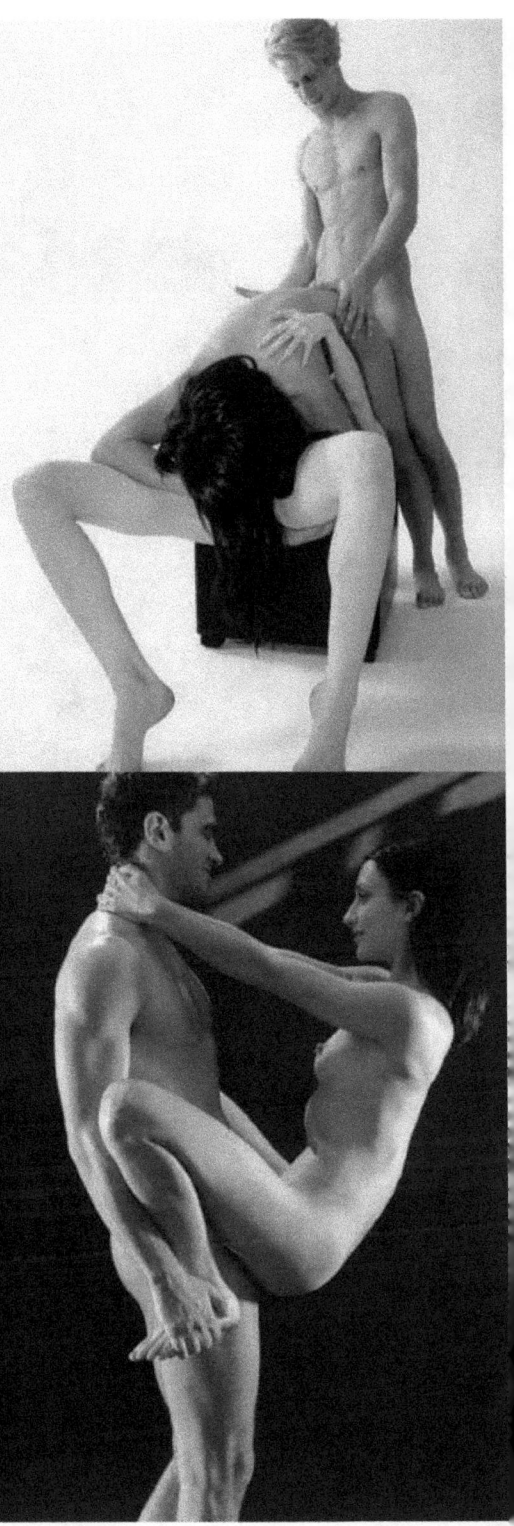

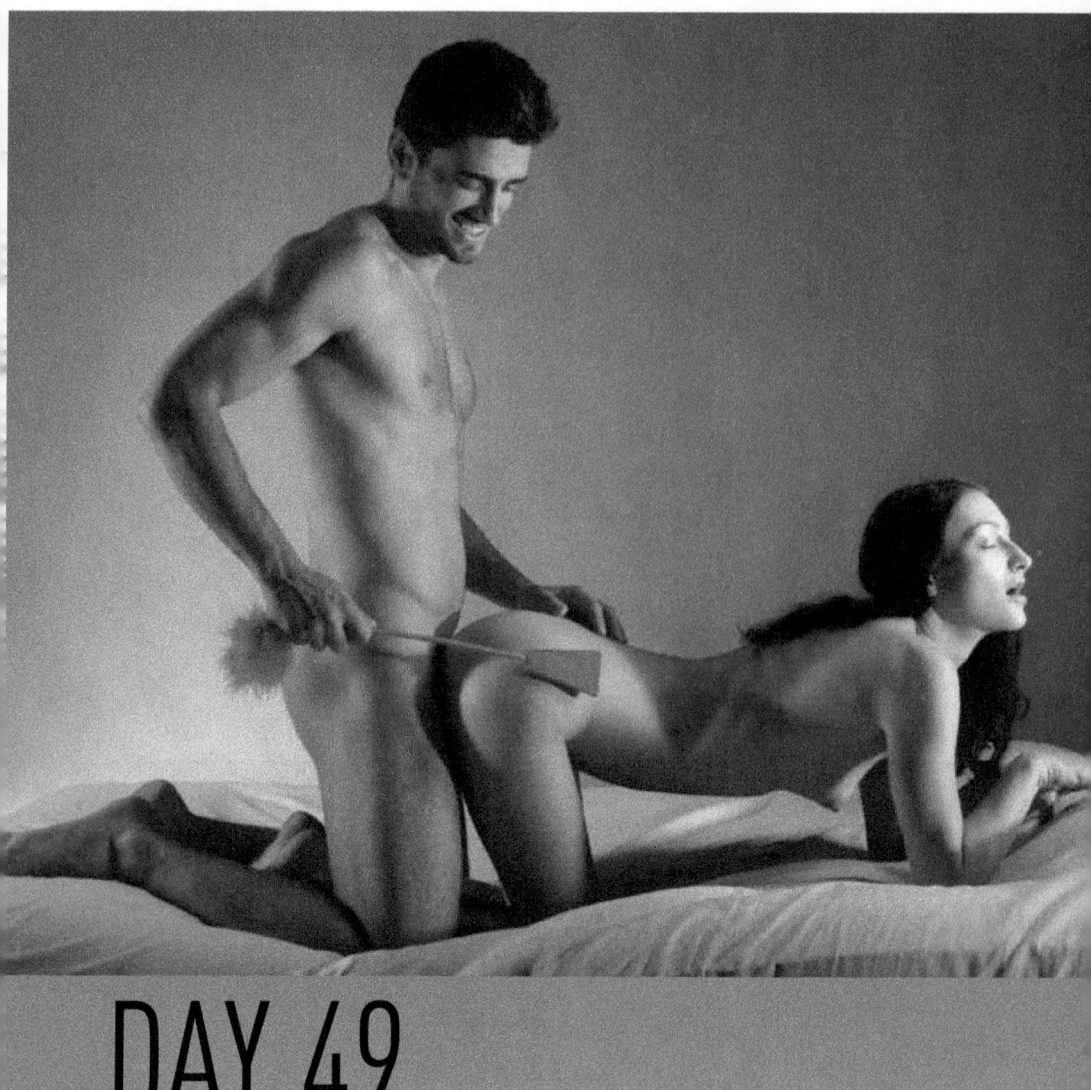

DAY 49

THE FRISKY FILLY

She climbs up on the bed and assumes a doggie position, letting her lover know that he's going to have to tame her. He knows just the thing, and grabs a riding crop as he enters her from behind. As she bucks her hips he playfully taps her buttocks and thighs with the crop to dictate the action.

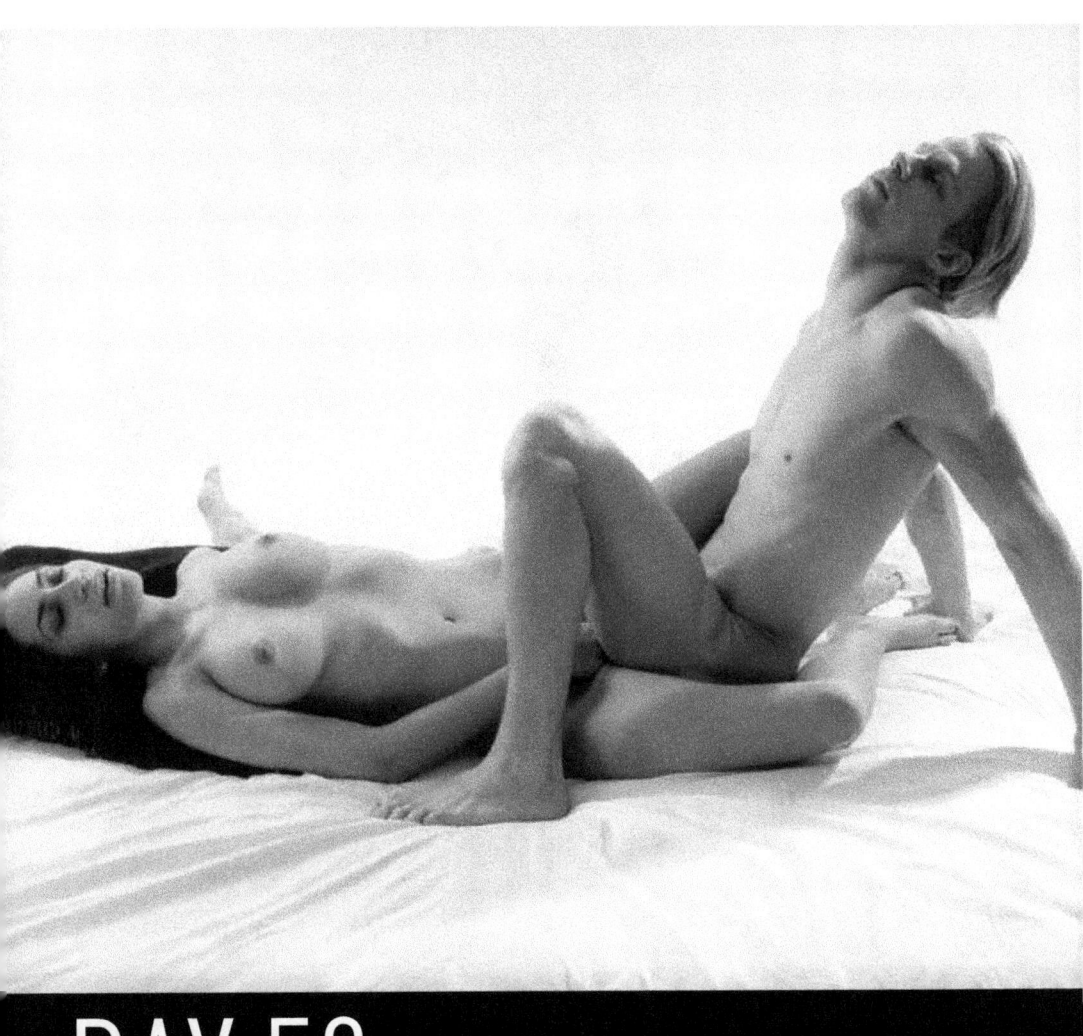

DAY 50

X-RATED

She's on her side with her legs apart. He comes up to meet her in a slightly reclined pose. They lace their legs under and over, making an "X." Penetration angles can be altered with the slightest of movements.

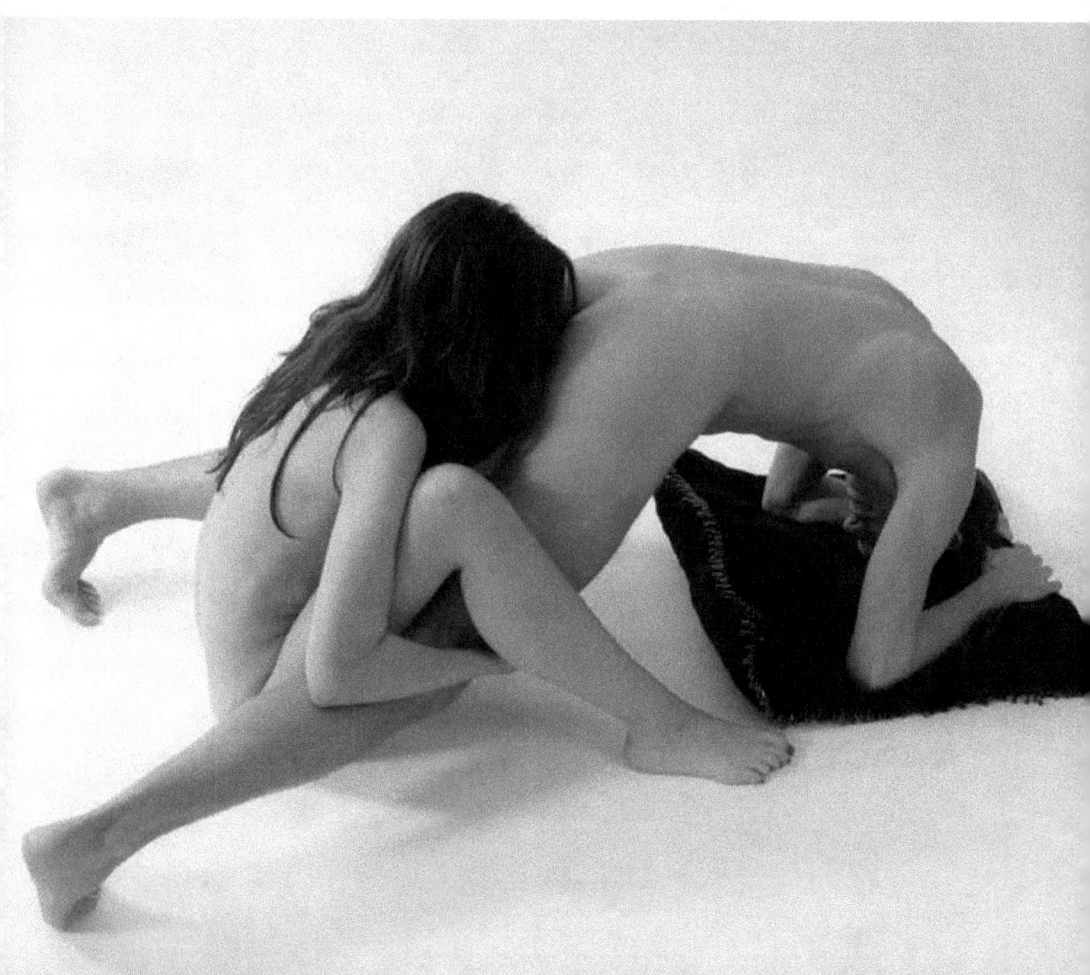

DAY 51

TWO FOR ONE

He bends at the waist resting his forearms on the floor and extending his legs back with knees slightly bent. His lover gets herself in a sitting position between his legs with her legs draped over his. She pleasures his anus with her mouth while using her hands to stimulate his penis and testicles.

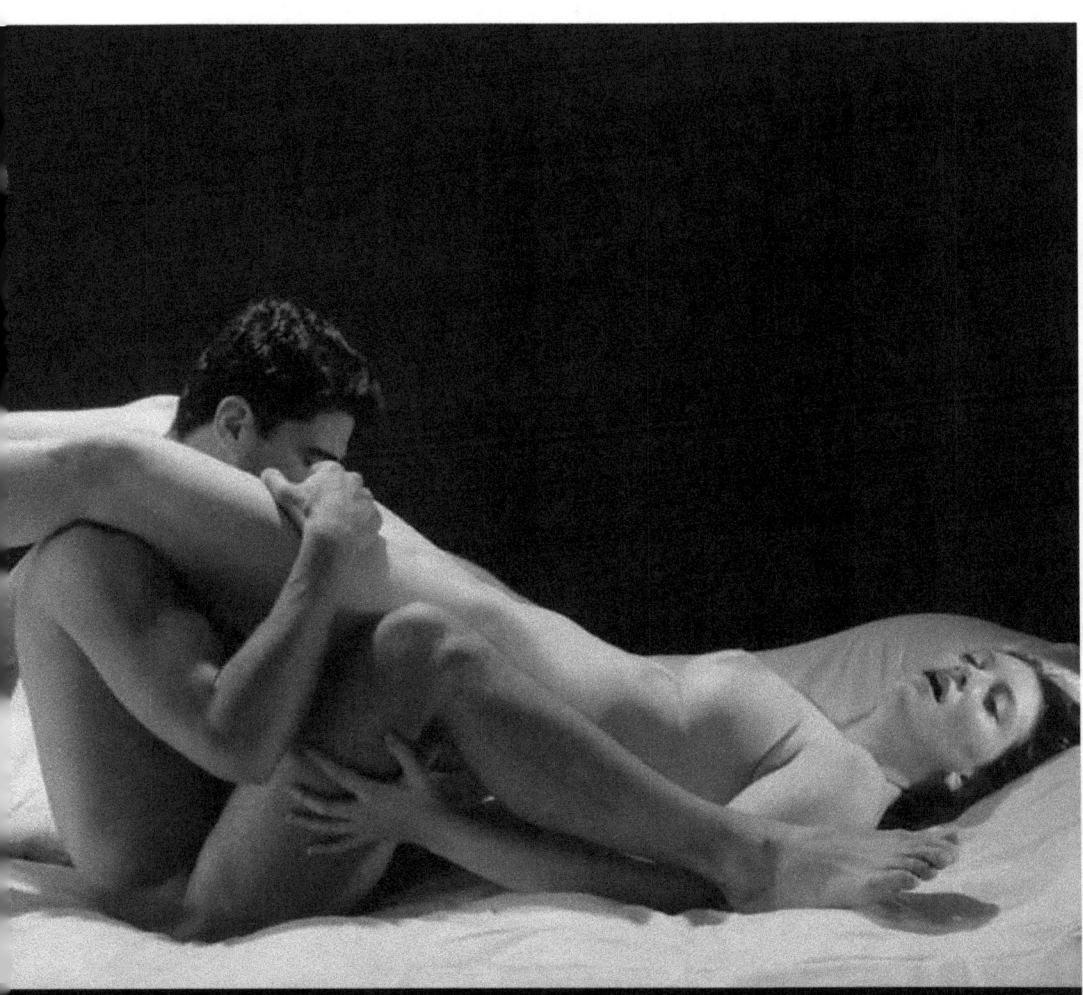

DAY 52

THE DEEP "C" DIVE

She stretches out on the bed as her lover sits on his butt and moves himself in between her legs. She brings her legs up over his shoulders making it all the more easy for him to deliver an earth-shattering round of oral ecstasy.

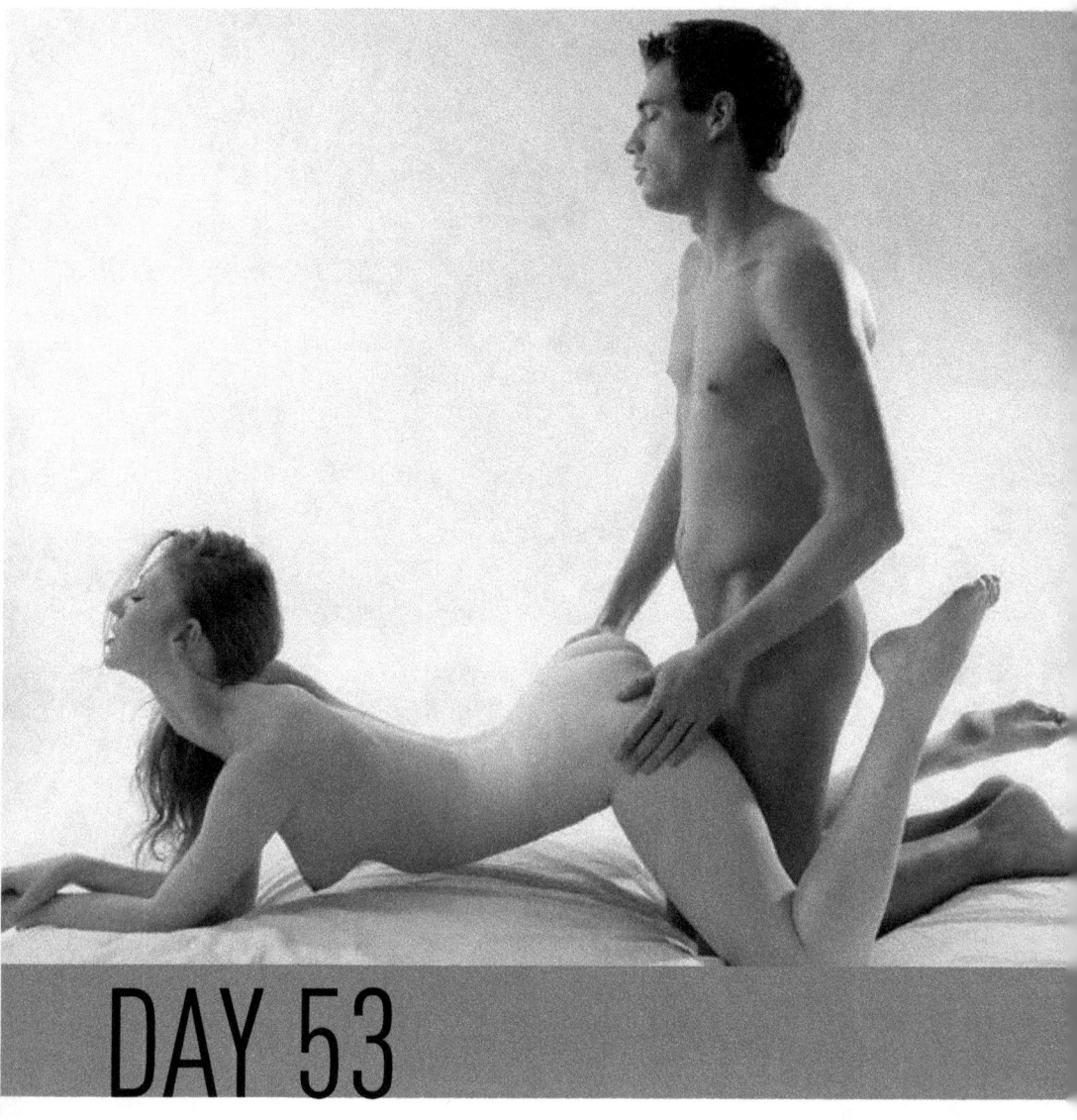

DAY 53

PUPPY LOVE

Here's the classic doggy-style position. She's on all fours as her lover, on his knees, enters her from behind. He can move as fast and as hard as he wants, until she yelps for more.

DAY 54

TAKING DICTATION

He situates himself atop a low-lying file cabinet with one foot resting up against its side. She drops to her knees and gives his penis a thorough tongue-lashing.

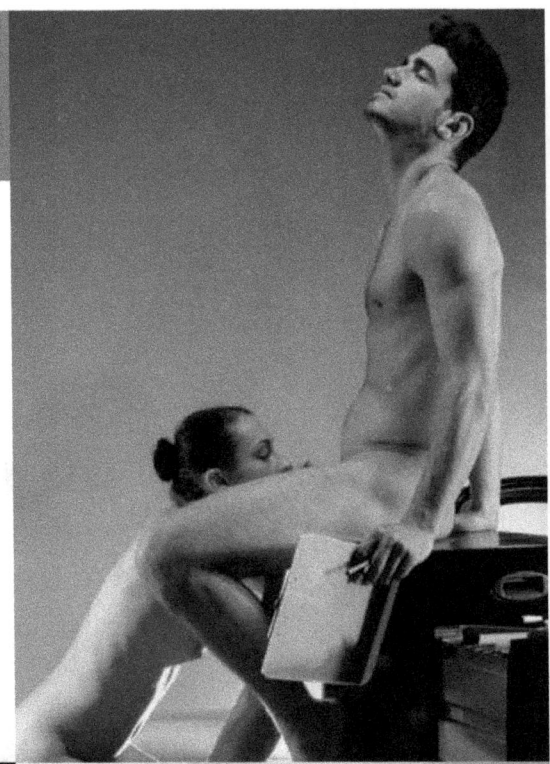

DAY 55

THE ACROBATS

Like a little danger with your lovemaking? In this pose the couple uses a support bar, which they hold onto as the man penetrates his lover from behind. They can both rest their feet on a nearby chair or she can throw caution to the wind and dangle her legs freely. Covering the floor with cushions isn't a bad idea either.

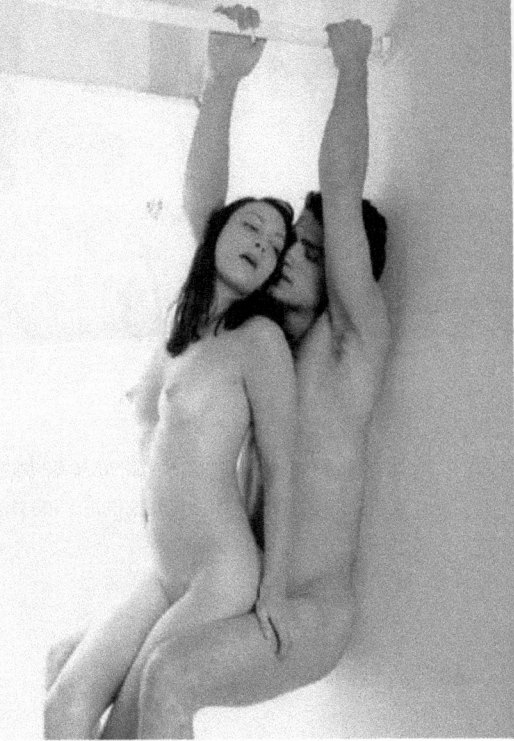

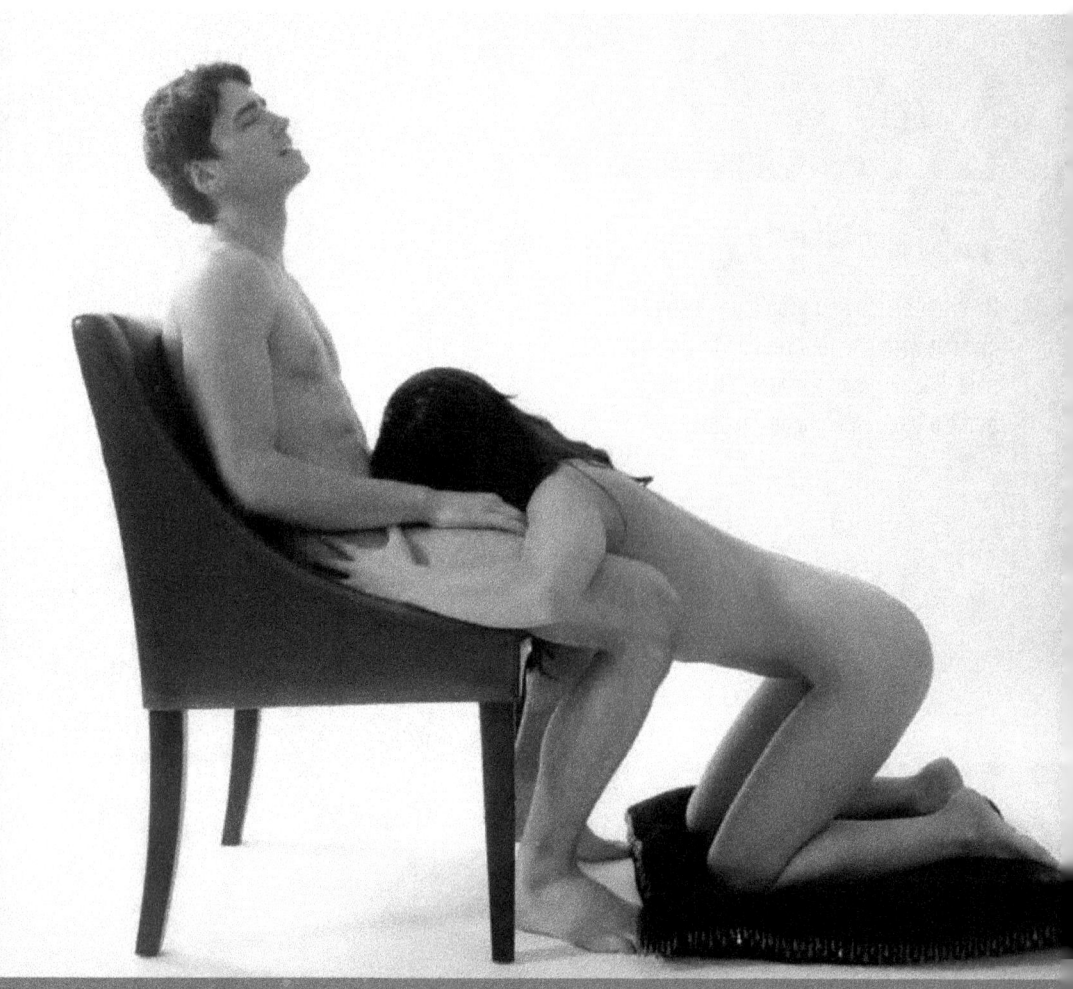

DAY 56

BJ AND THE BARE

The couple get completely naked as he takes a seat. His lover gets on her knees and takes his penis in her mouth. His hands gently massage her back and play with her hair.

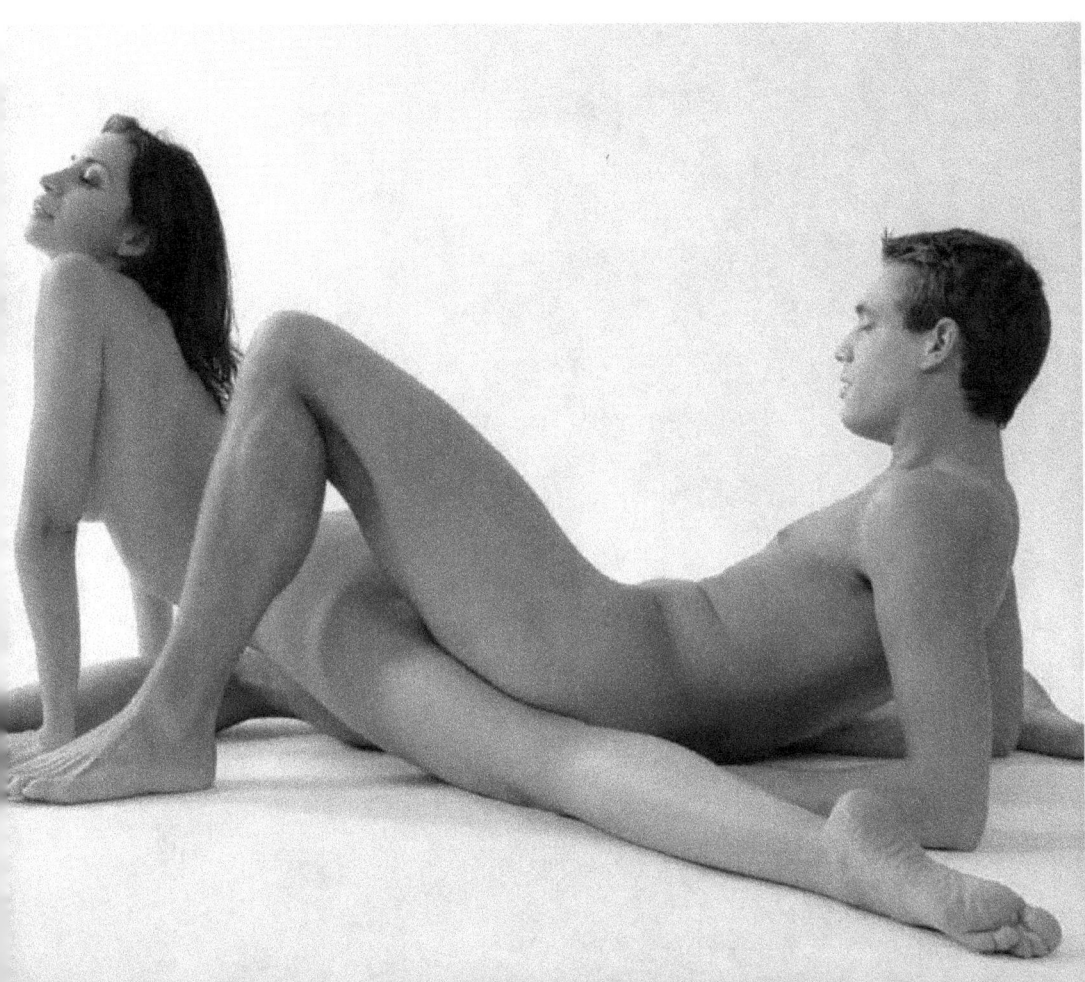

DAY 57

BRIDGE AND TUNNEL

The man rests back on his forearms and arches his back as he enters his partner. She's facing the away from him, her legs extended back, as they drive each other wild with passion.

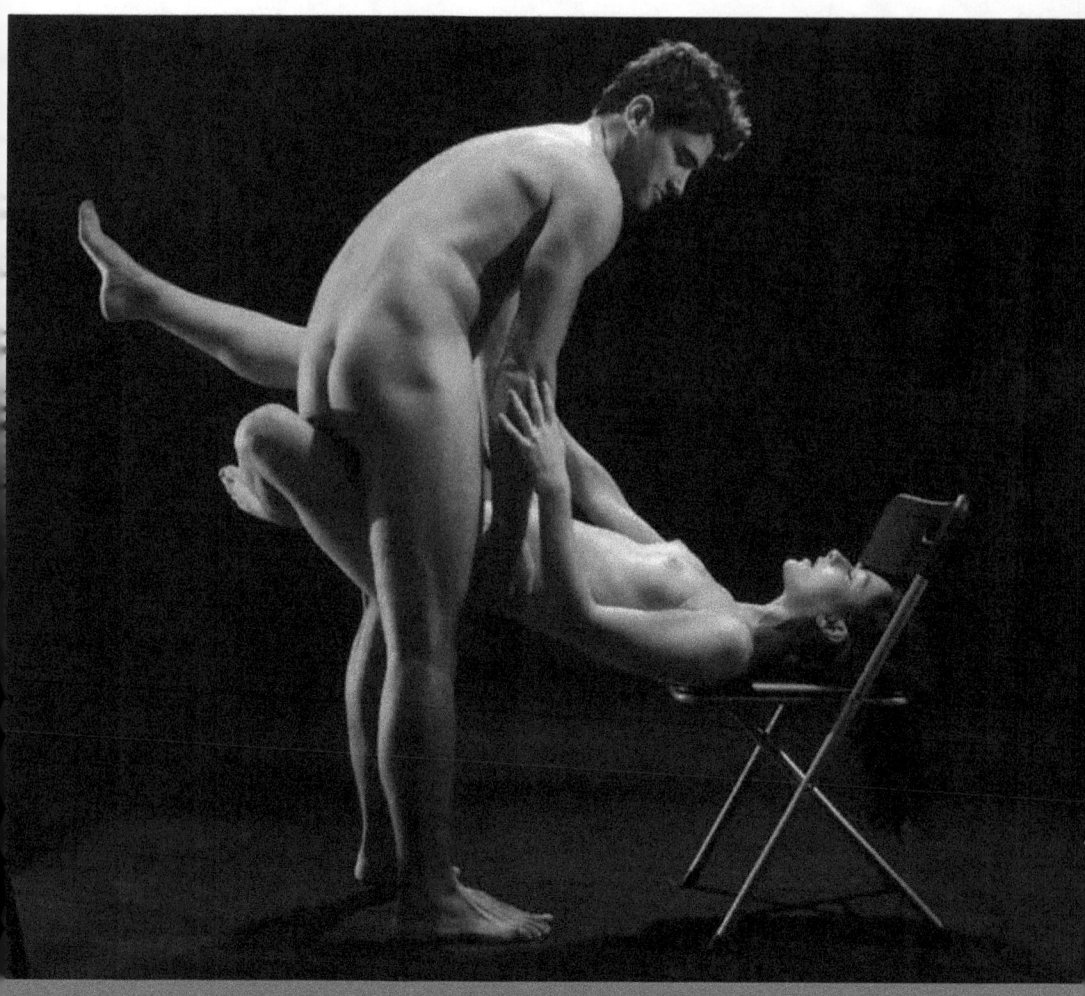

DAY 58

THE GETAWAY

This one is pretty quirky. She supports her head and torso in a chair while swiveling her hips toward her standing lover. As he penetrates her she can pump her legs, as though she's running, to promote other pleasurable sensations.

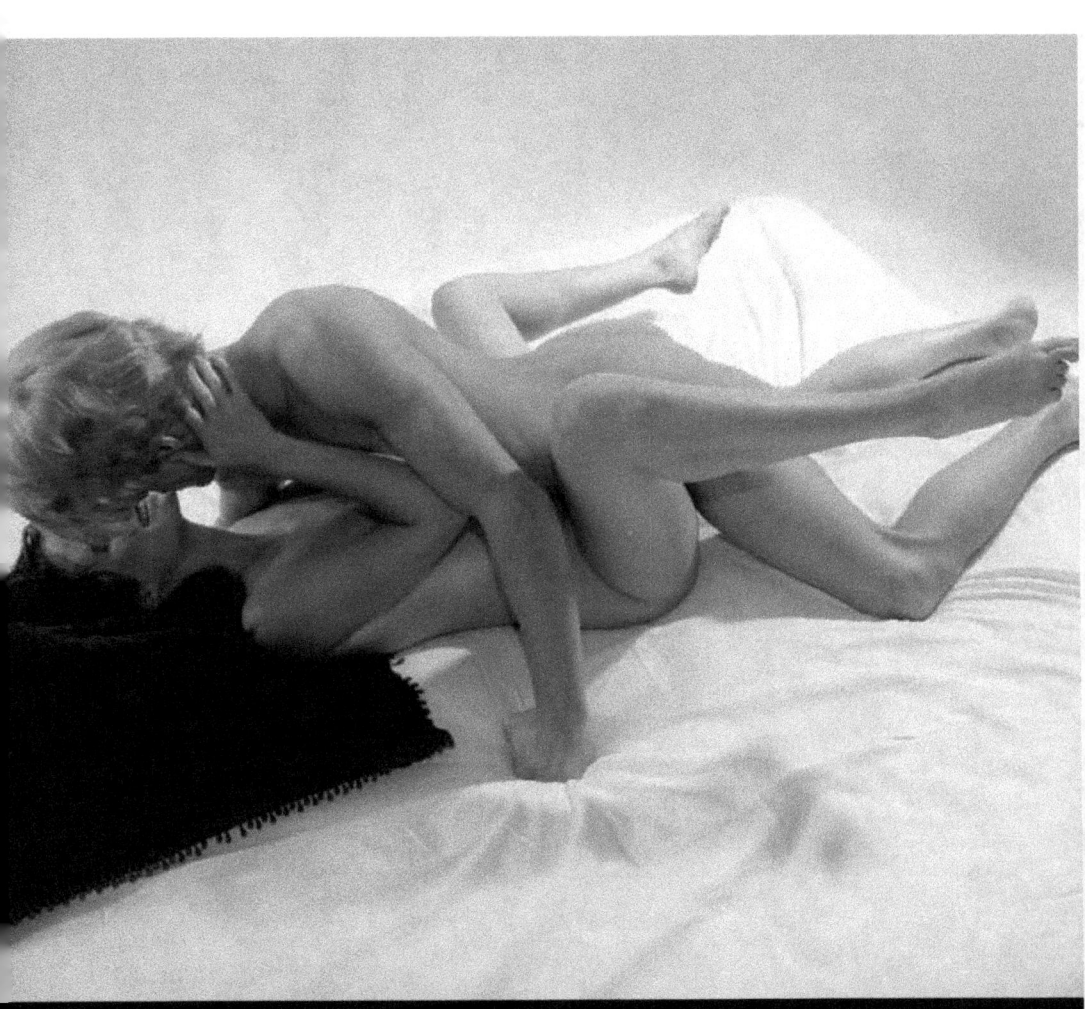

DAY 59

FULL ACCESS

The key component of this missionary variation is the woman moving her thighs outward, away from her lover. This seemingly minor move allows for a not-so-subtle increase in penetration.

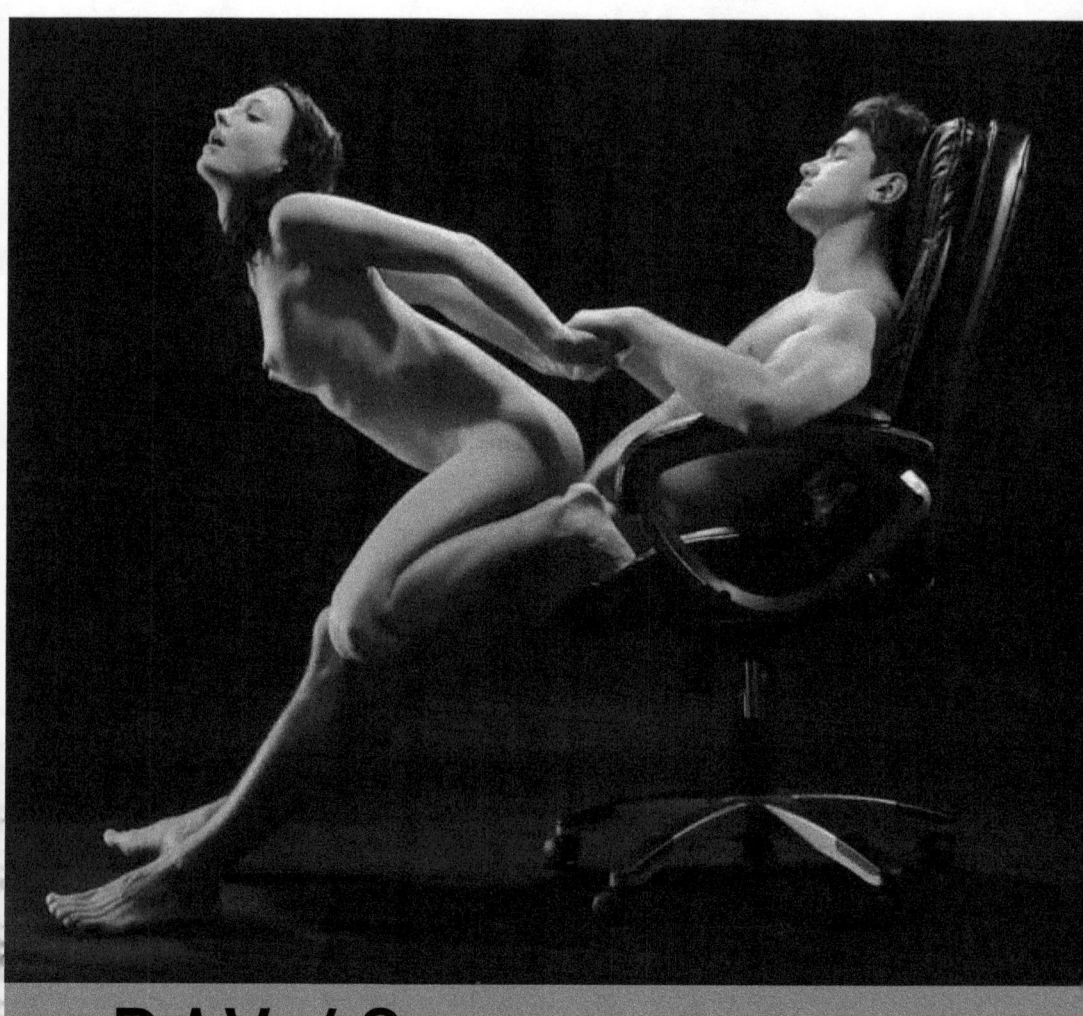

DAY 60

THE ALPINE SLIDE

The man sits low in a chair with his legs extended out diagonally to the floor. His lover mounts his penis and tucks her legs up and back as he holds her arms for support.

DAY 61

OVER THE EDGE

The man sits on the edge of the bed as his partner brings her legs around his back and her hands down to the floor. He can use his hands to caress her buttocks and back.

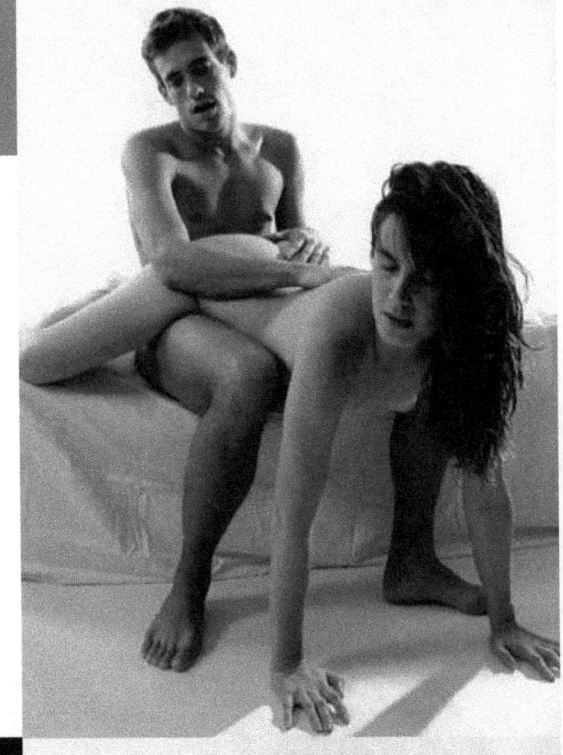

DAY 62

GRACEFUL UNION

Facing away from her lover, the woman places her palms on the floor and brings one leg up to his shoulder while the other rests on the bed. In another variation, the woman can bring both legs up.

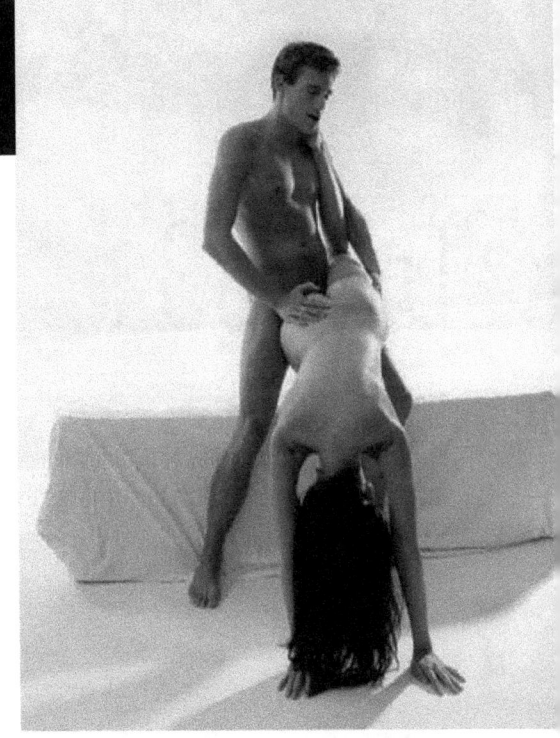

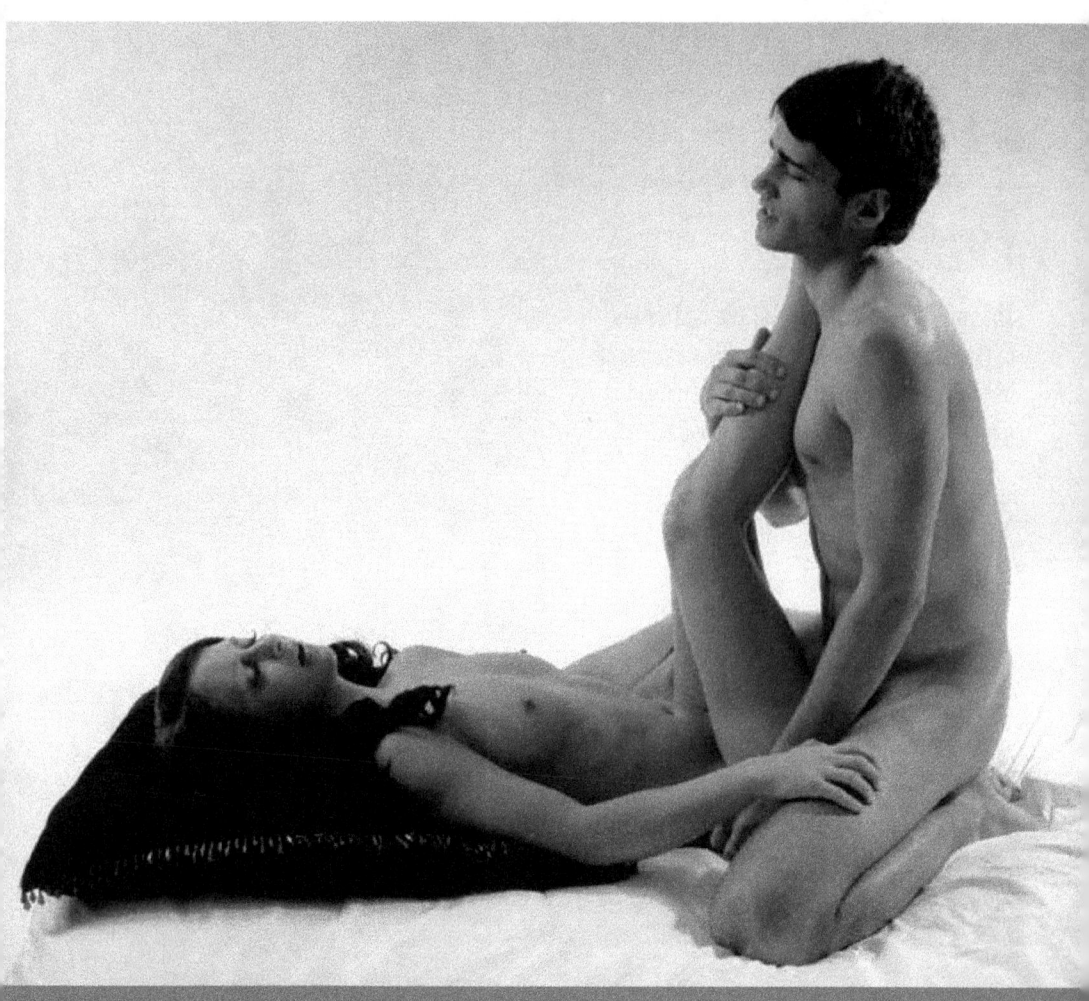

DAY 63

IN LIKE A LION

She lies on her back, brings both of her legs up, and rests them on one of his shoulders. As he enters her, his hands are free to stroke her legs and playfully paw at the rest of her body.

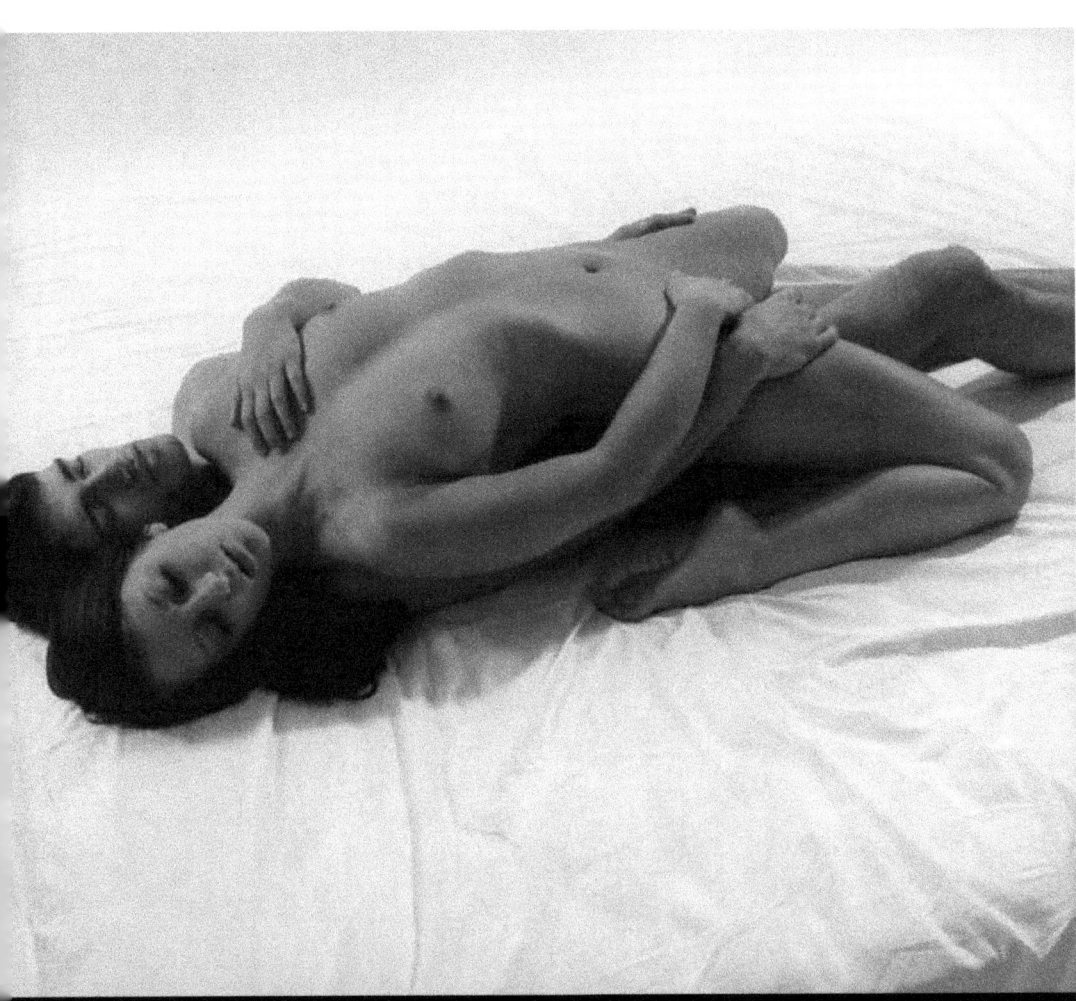

DAY 64

THE BENT SPOON

In this take on a classic spooning pose, the woman is on top with her legs tucked underneath her. It makes for a very different angle of penetration and for plenty of clitoral attention.

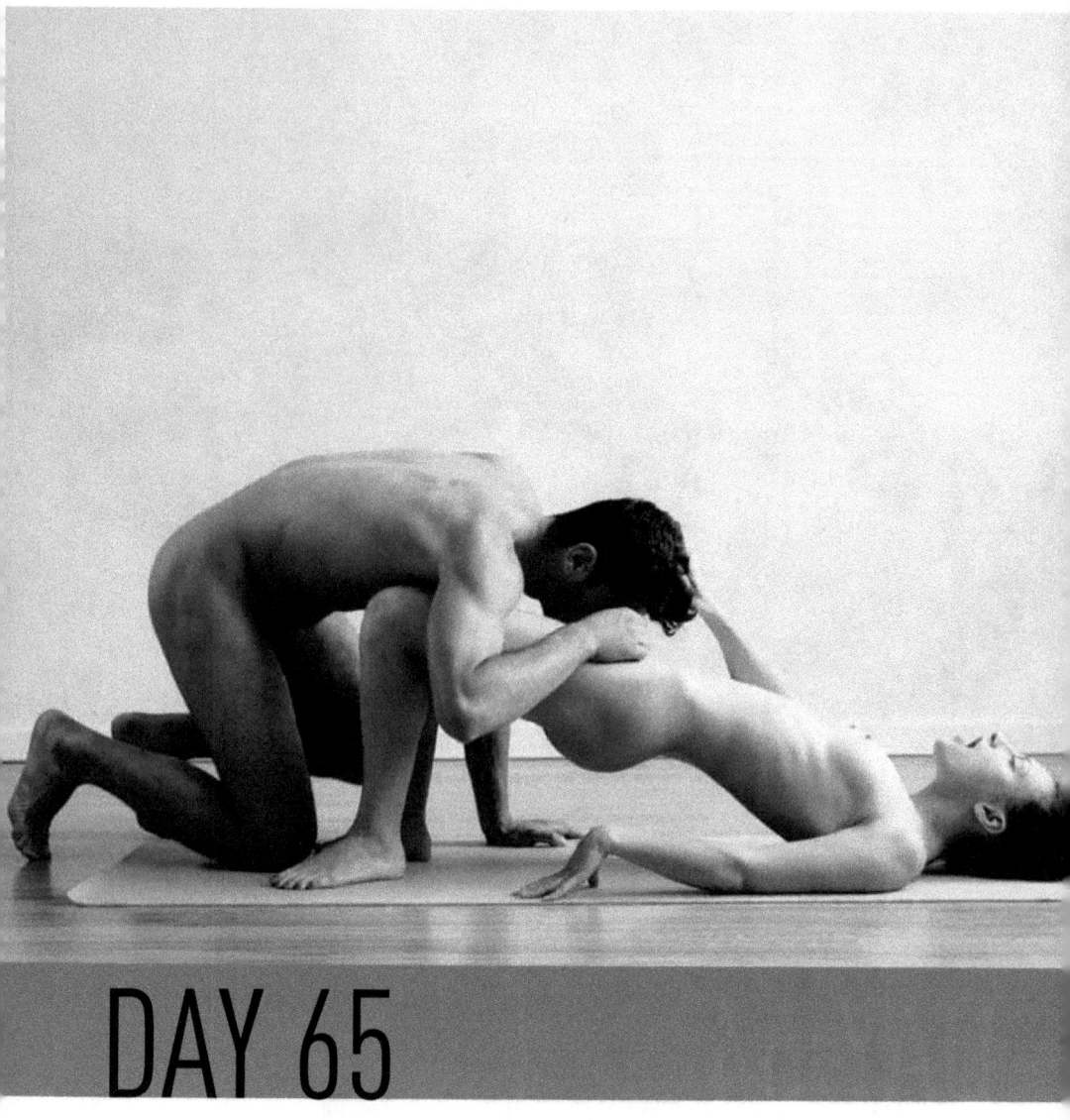

DAY 65

BRIDGE DIVING

The woman lies flat on the floor and brings her body into a bridge position. With she works her abs and glutes, her lover moves in between her legs and samples her sweet nectar.

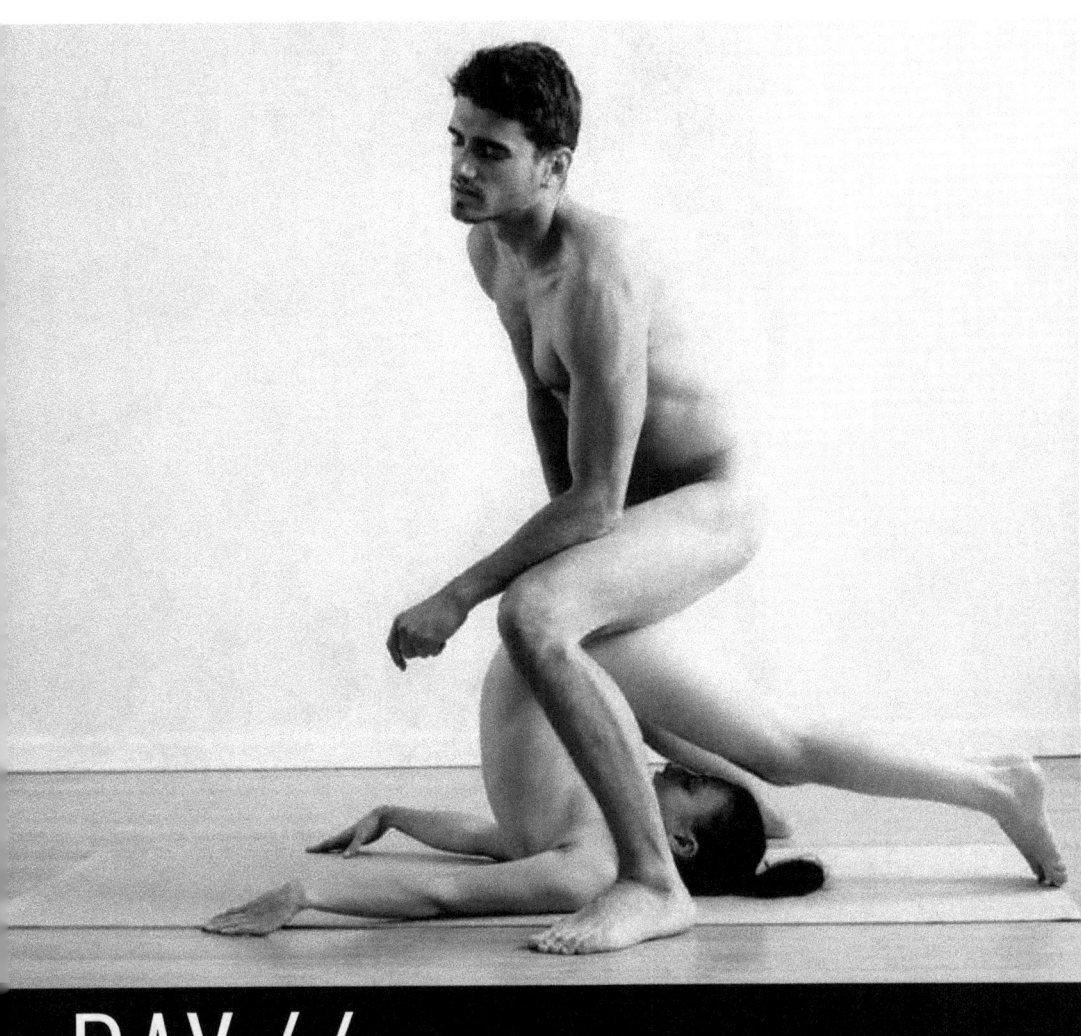

DAY 66

THE HIPSTER

She lies flat on the floor or an exercise mat while raising her hips up and slowly allowing her legs to come back behind her head. As her hands remain in contact with the floor, her lover enters her from above, facing in the other direction. The penetration is deep, but his movement is slow and deliberate in order to avoid putting undue stress on her back.

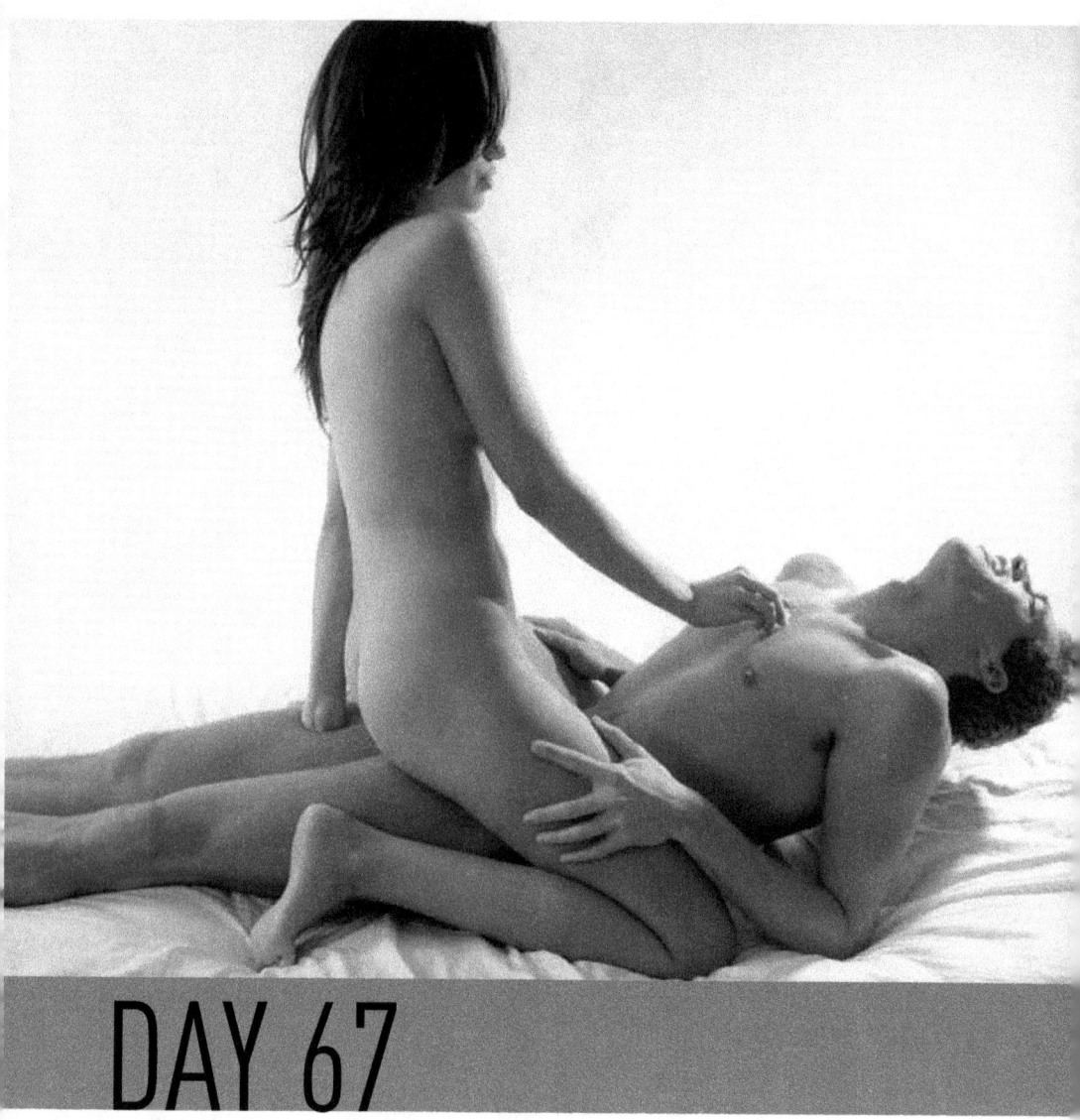

DAY 67

HOT AND COLD

The woman straddles her prone partner, allowing him to enter her deeply. He's utterly at her mercy as she languidly runs an ice cube down his chest, bringing an invigorating chill to all the heat they're creating.

DAY 68

THE FLIGHT ATTENDANT

This one starts with the woman lying on her stomach near the edge of the bed. Her partner penetrates her from behind and lifts her up by the hips as she grabs on to his arms for support. It's the only way to fly.

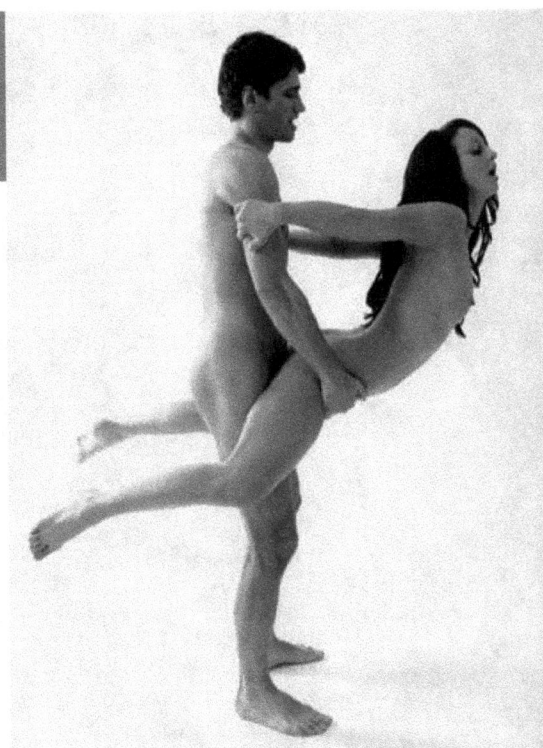

DAY 69

GARDEN OF EDEN

The woman and man stand facing each other completely naked. They slowly explore each other's bodies with light touching and kissing. They wrap their arms around each other as he penetrates her. And it feels like the first time.

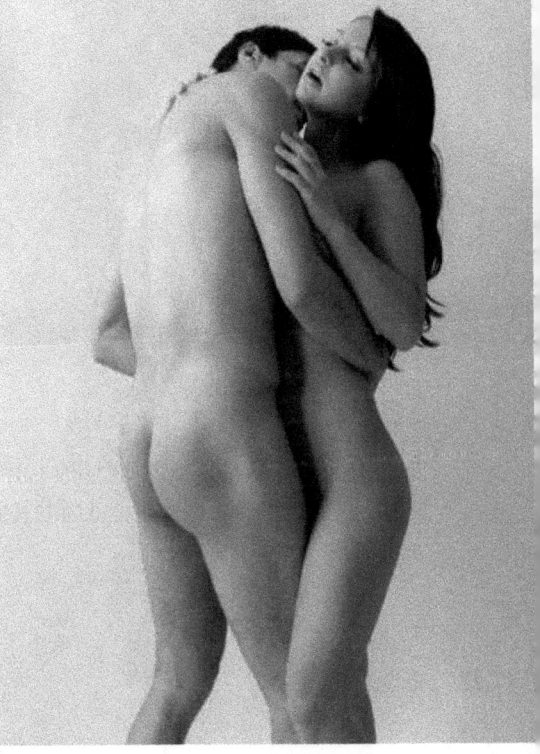

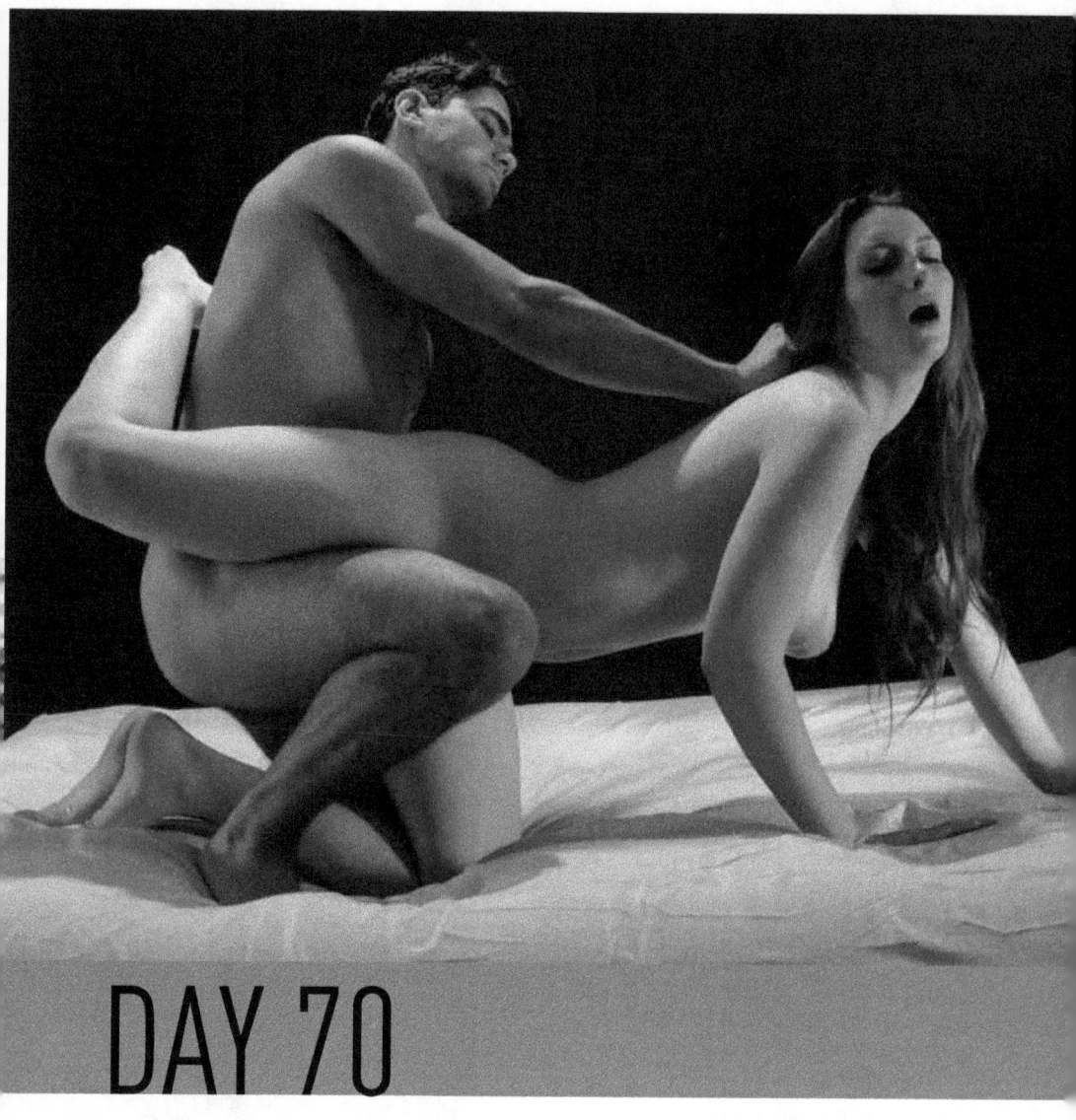

DAY 70

THE IRONING BOARD

She gets up on all fours on the bed. Her partner gets on one knee and penetrates her from behind as she brings one leg up and curls it around his back. As he thrusts he smooths his hand gently down her back.

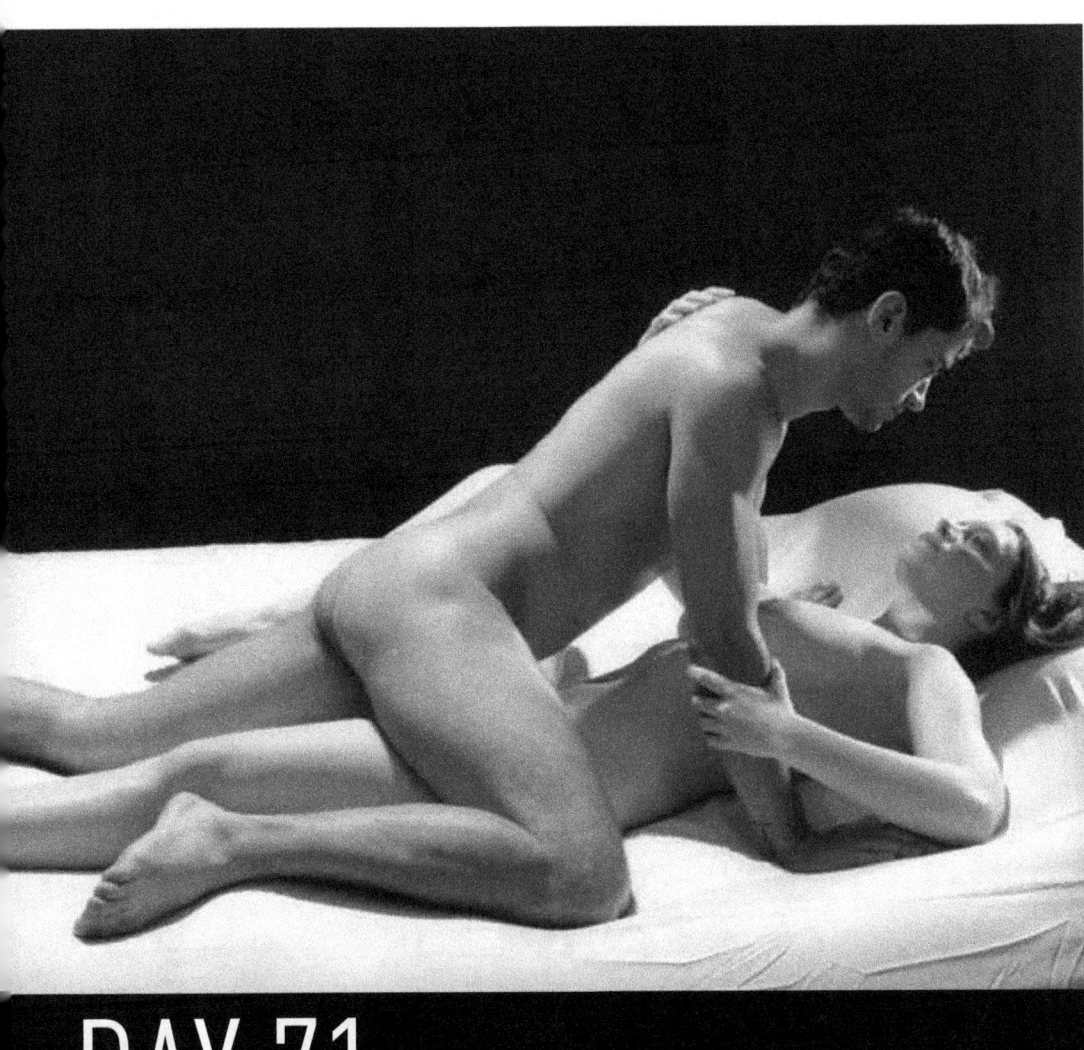

DAY 71

THE WISHBONE

The woman lies back on the bed as her partner straddles one of her legs and penetrates her vagina. He occasionally breaks rhythm to stimulate her clitoris with his penis.

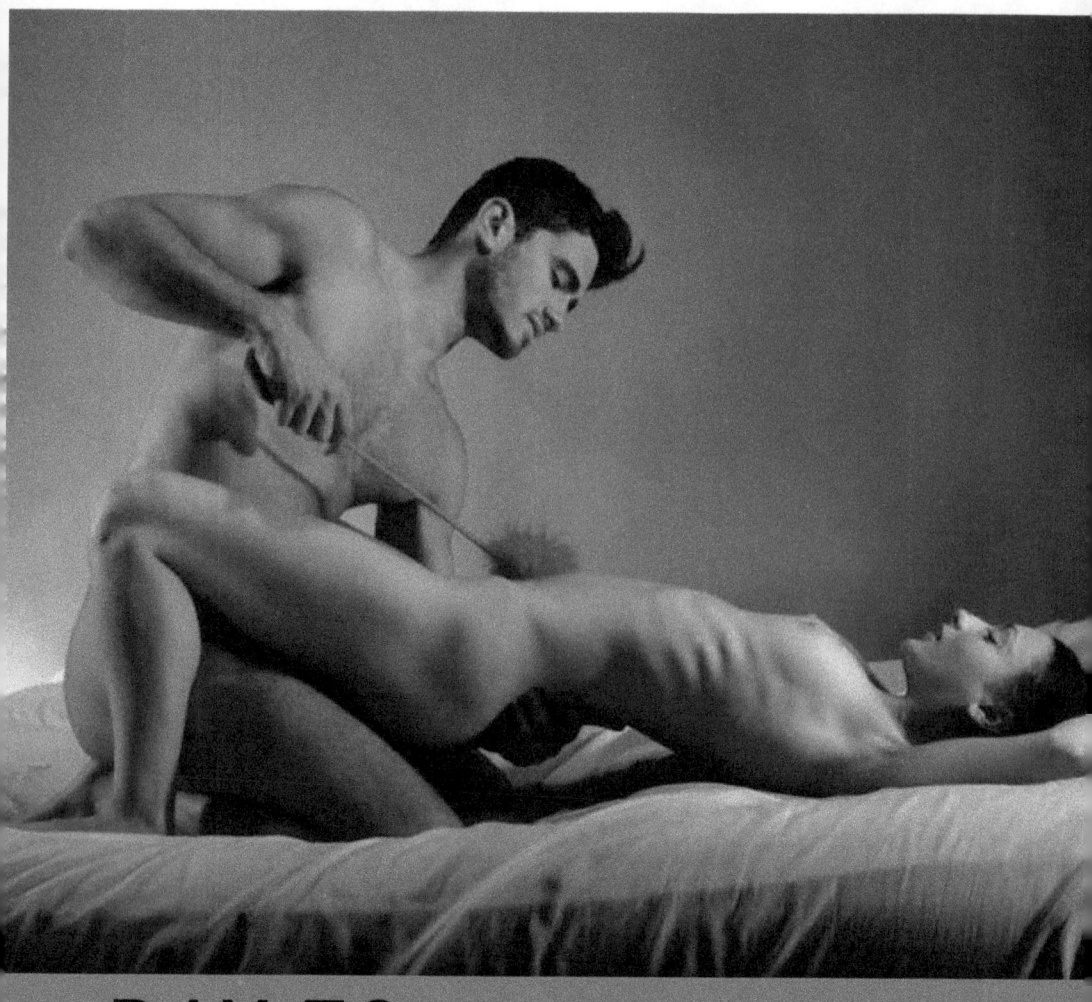

DAY 72

THE FEATHER REPORT

She lies back on the bed, lifting her back and buttocks so that her partner can slide in and enter her from his knees. While he's inside her he traces her breasts with a feather tickler and slowly brings it down the length of her body. He offers additional support by placing his free hand under the small of her back.

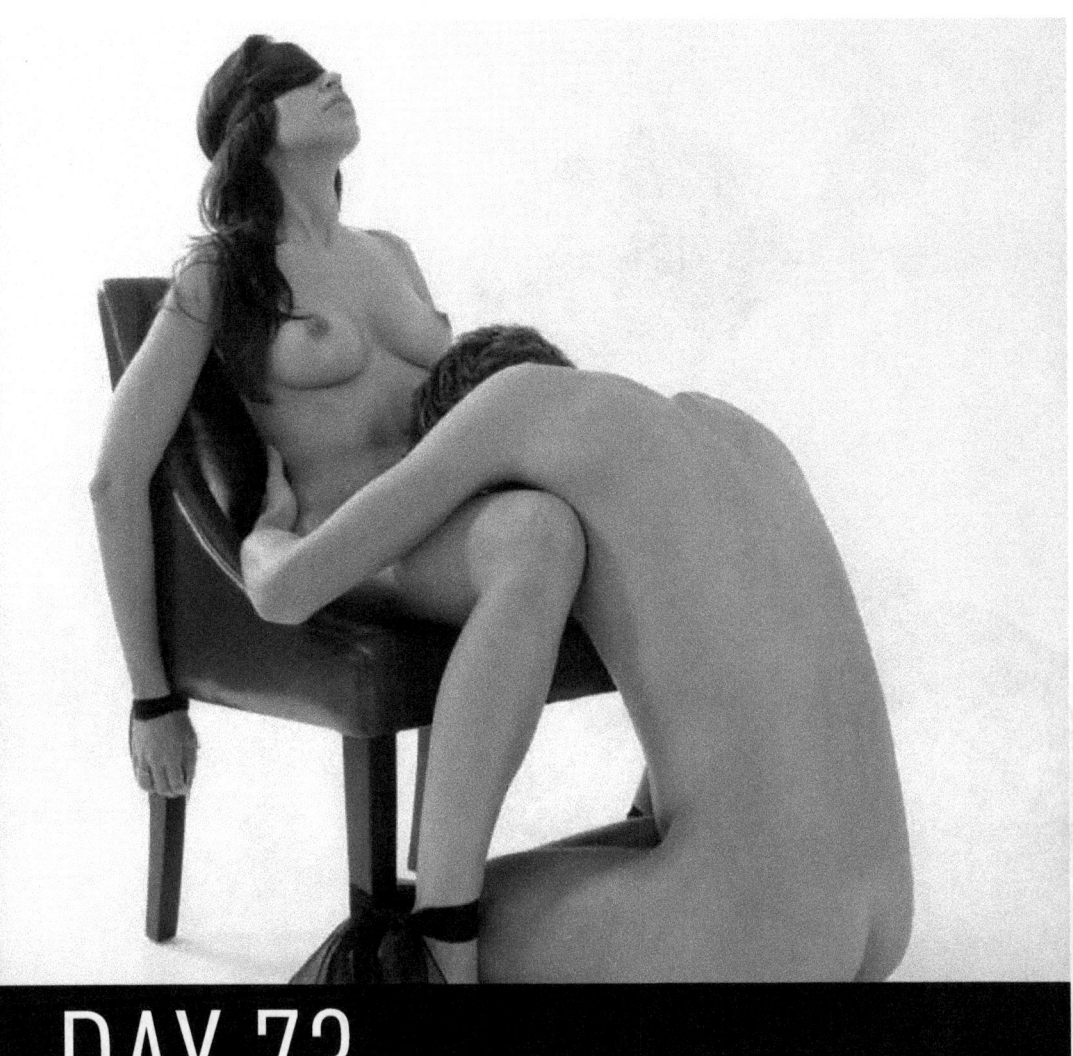

DAY 73

BLIND FAITH

The woman is at her lover's mercy, with her eyes blindfolded and hands bound to a chair.
He rewards his agreeable captive by going down on her until she reaches a trembling climax.

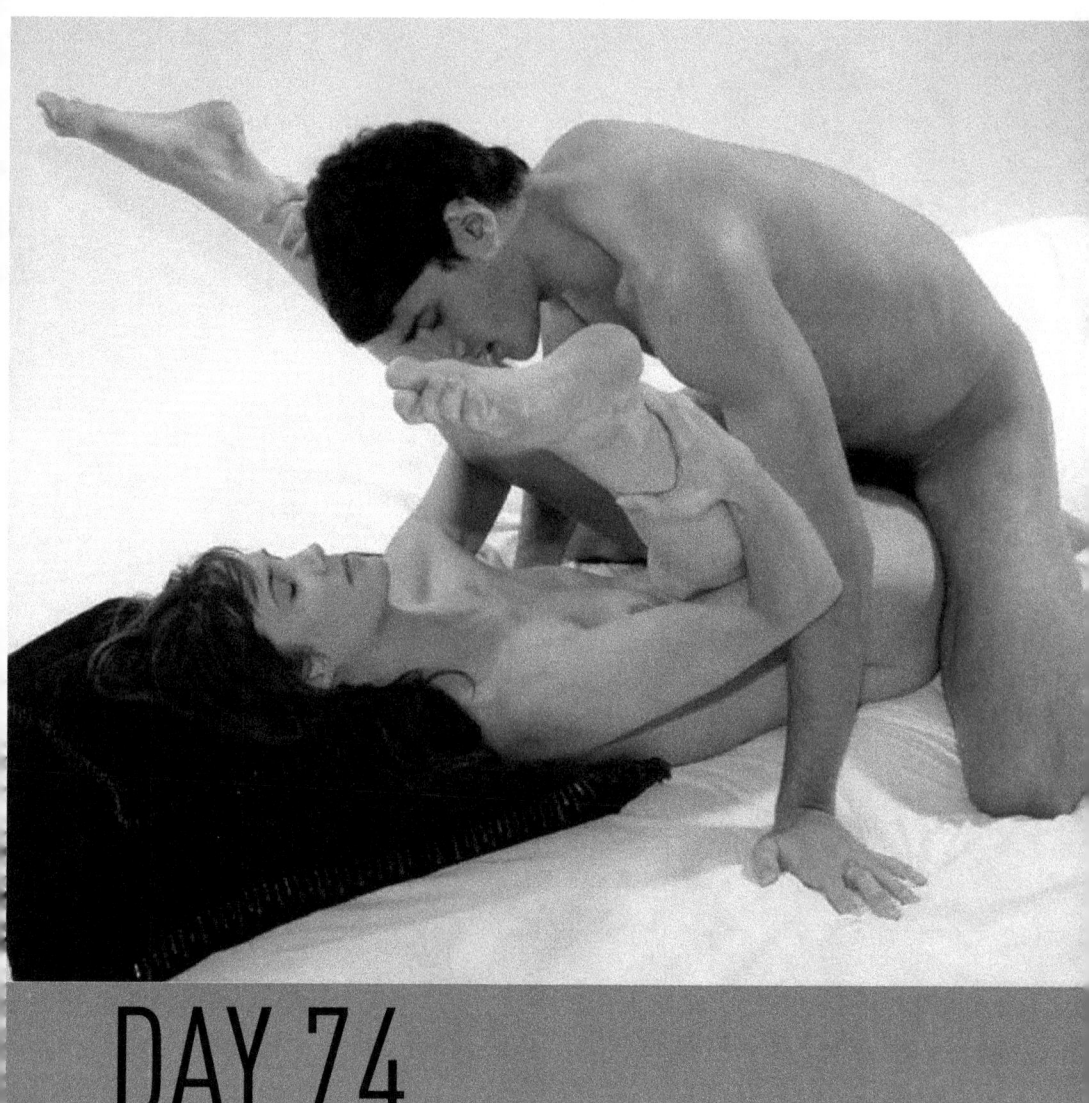

DAY 74

THE SENSUAL SCISSORS

She's got him on his knees, in more way than one. Her legs raised and inside of his arms, she's free to move them back and forth as he enters her. The resulting squeezing sensation is one he won't soon forget.

DAY 75

THE MOUNTIE

The man starts on his back and raises himself up with his feet and hands into a reverse plank position. She climbs atop, keeping her weight on the balls of her feet, ready to ride.

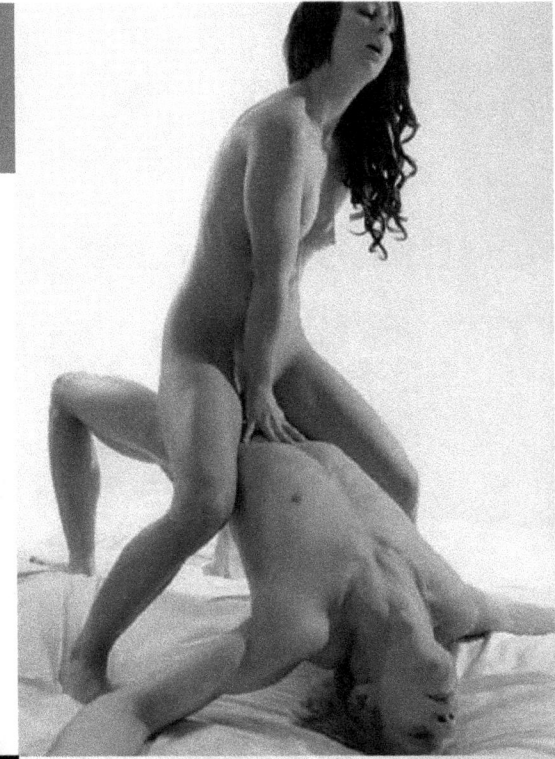

DAY 76

THREE FOR ALL

The man gets up on one knee and enters his partner from behind. As he thrusts away, she's free to explore the vagina and anus of the frisky friend who is up in a chair looking forward to her oral exam.

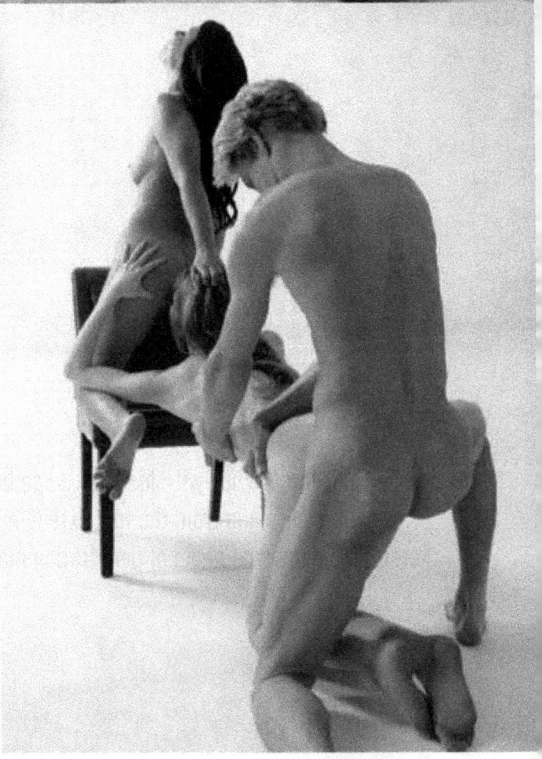

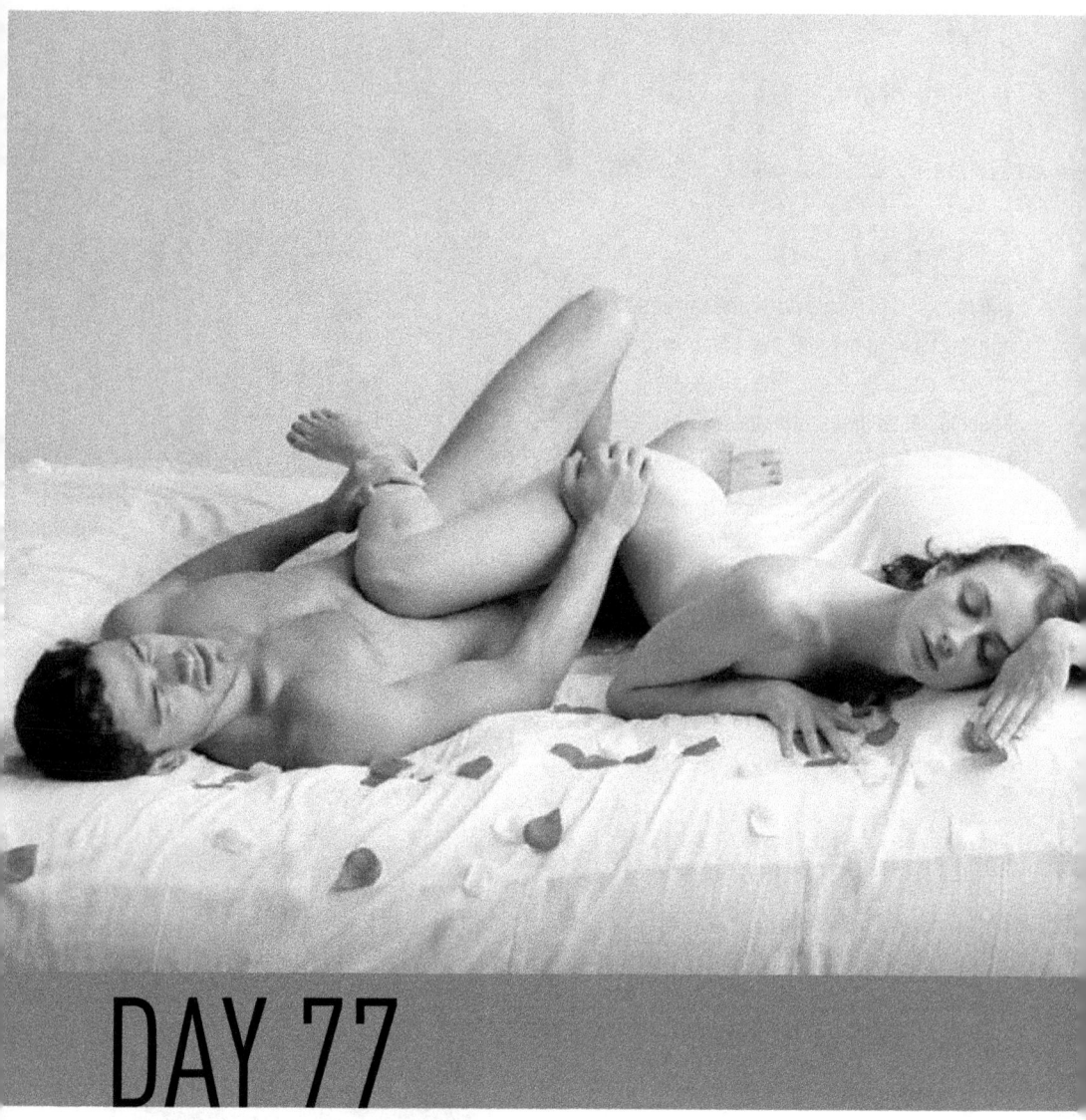

DAY 77

LAY ME DOWN

He lies back on the bed with his outer knee bent. She positions herself perpendicular to her lover and mounts him from the top, extending herself forward so that her head is resting on her arm. The unusual angle of penetration makes for a pleasurable experience for both.

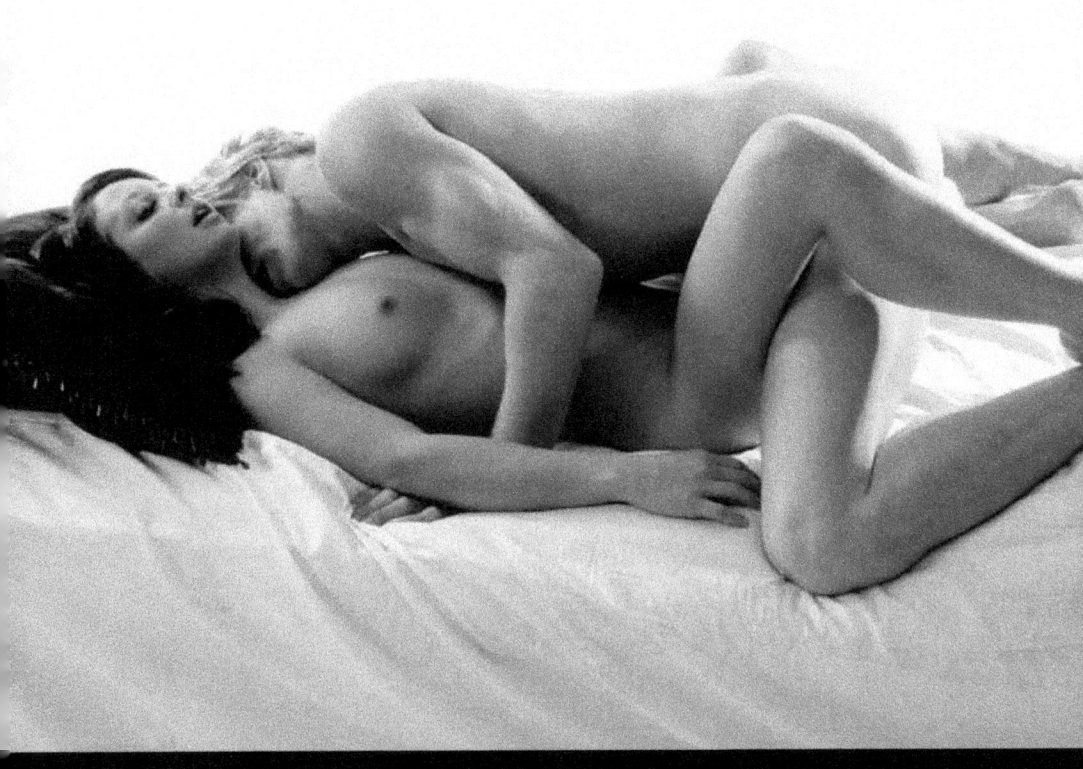

DAY 78

CLOSE ENCOUNTER

Virtually every position allows for some spirited initiative on either partner's part. Here, with the man on top, the woman lifts her legs around him for an even deeper connection as he kisses her neck.

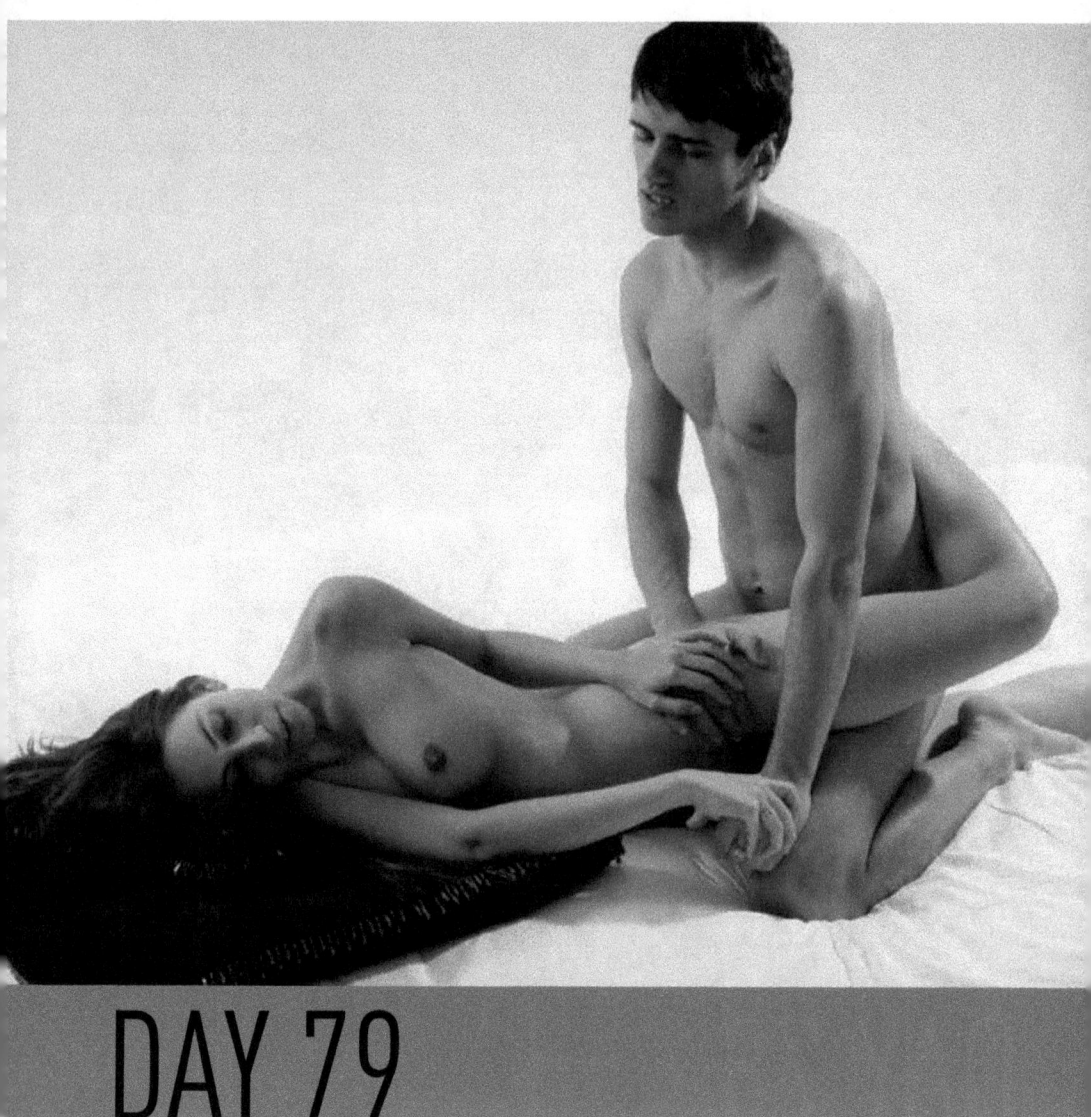

DAY 79

THE TURNING POINT

From her side, the woman brings her top leg over her lover's thigh and around his back while he enters her from a kneeling position. This perpendicular pose still allows for plenty of face time and free-handed fun.

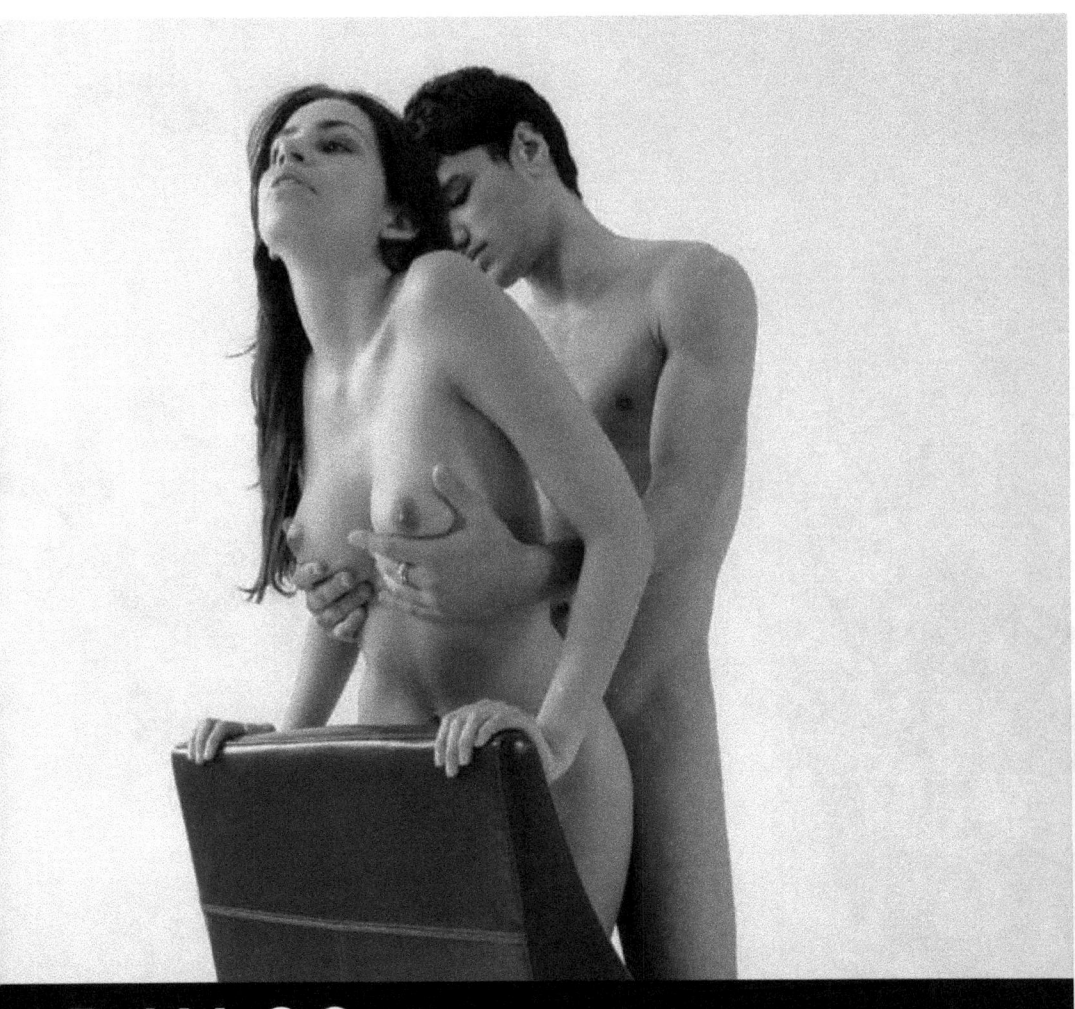

DAY 80

THE KNEEL DEAL

She kneels on a chair with her hands firmly grasping its back. He kneels close behind her and penetrates. His hands can play with her breasts or rub her clitoris.

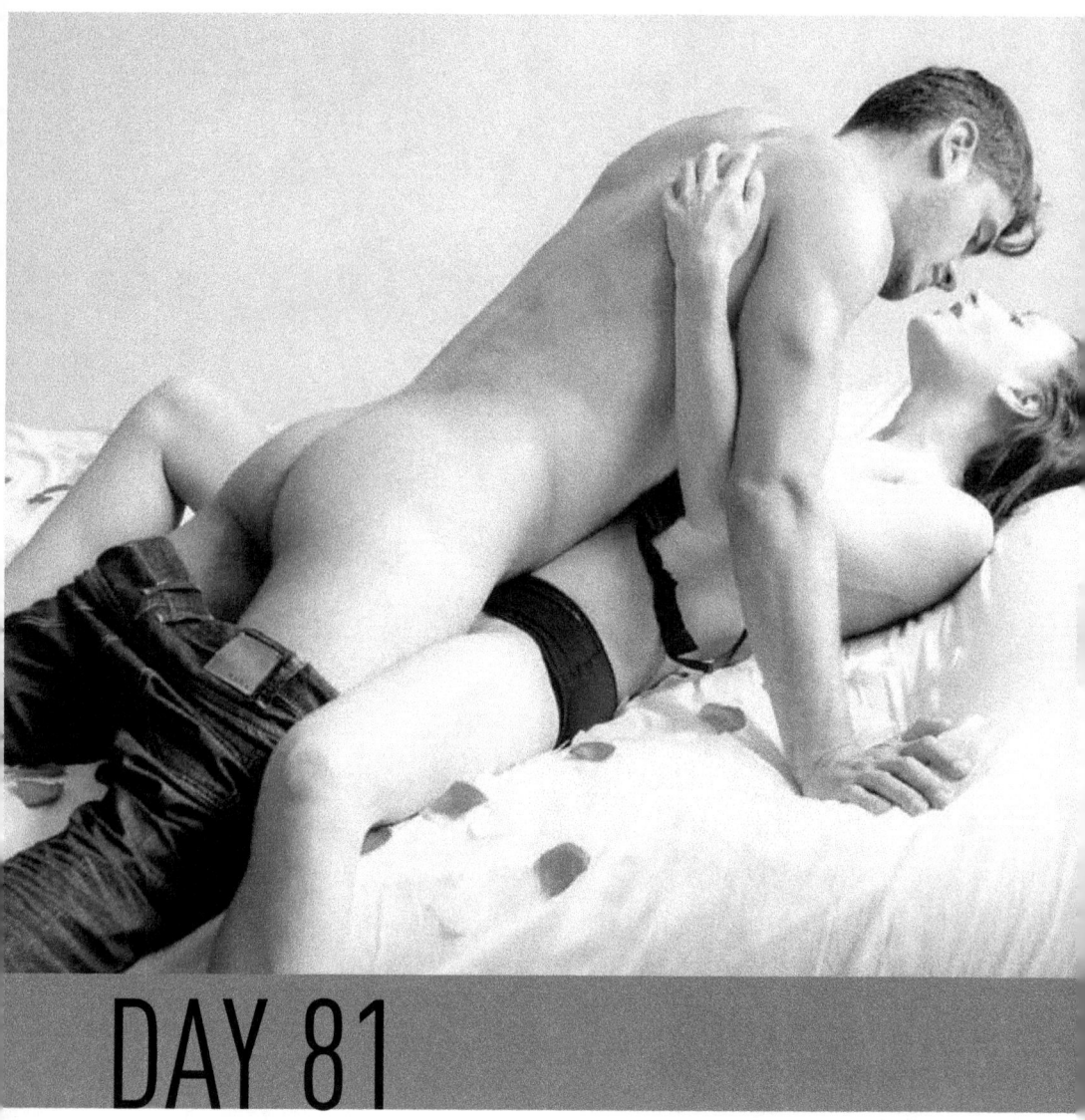

DAY 81

TAKE ME NOW

When it comes to sex, sometimes you just can't wait. The woman lies back and pulls her panties to the side, giving her partner a clear path to penetration. He doesn't need to be asked twice, as he pulls his jeans down and enters her.

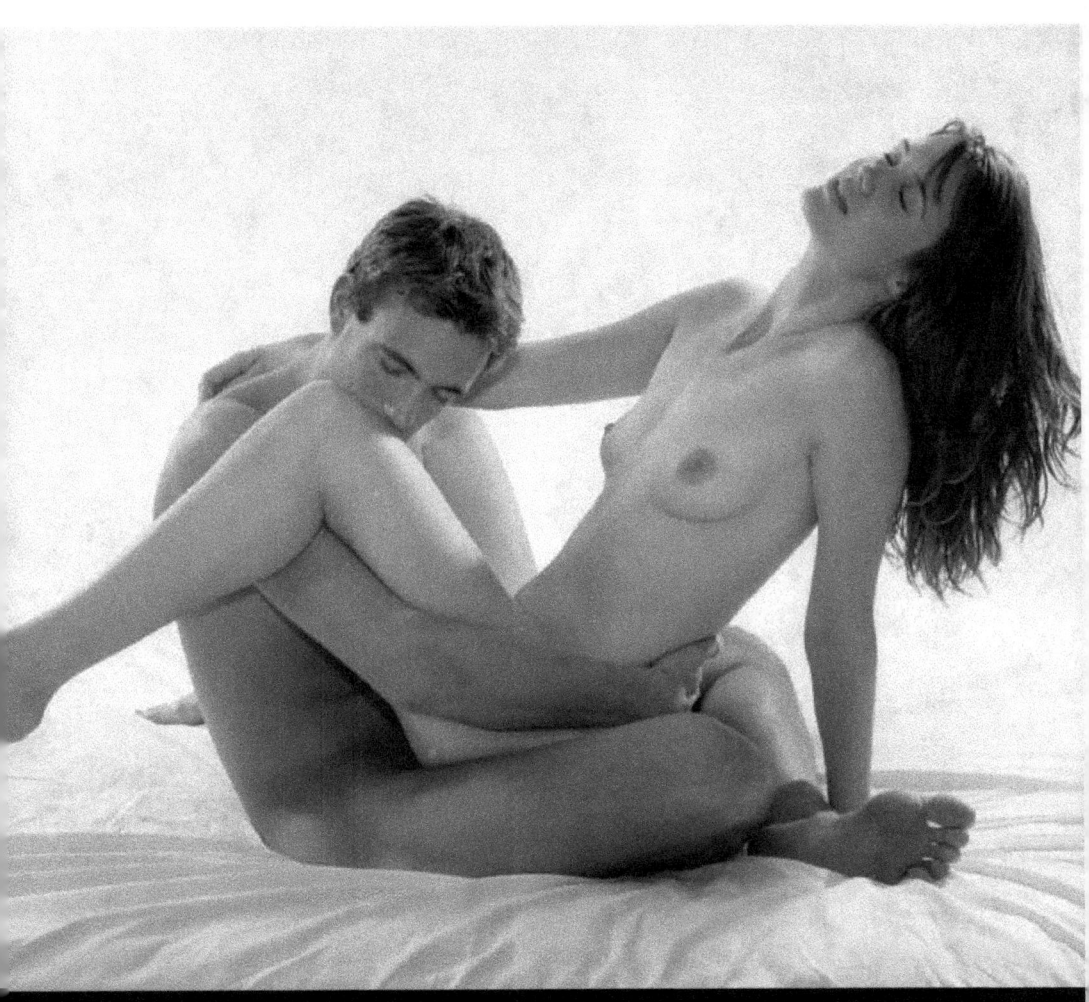

DAY 82

TOO HOT TO HANDLE

He's cross-legged as she sits in his lap and drapes one leg over his arm. This subtle move changes the angle of entry and the sensations that follow.

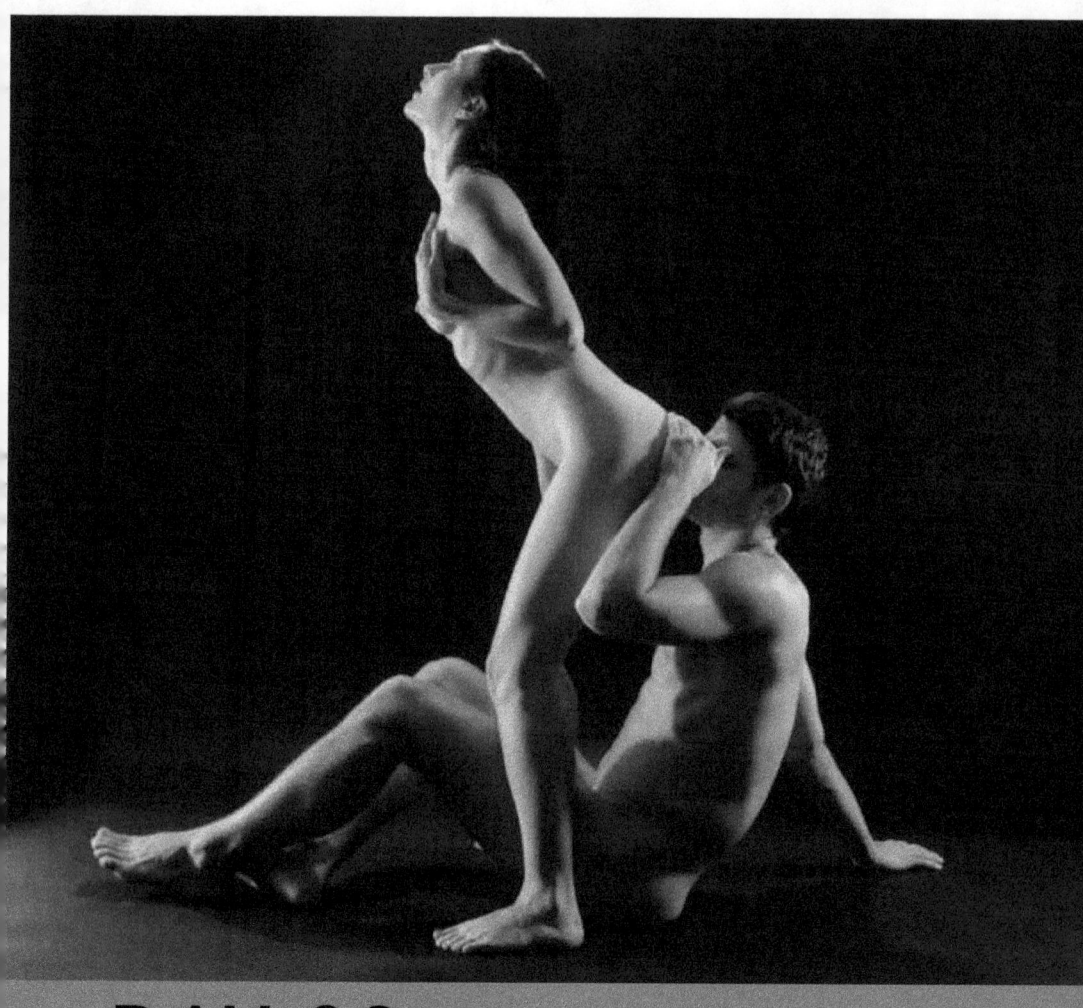

DAY 83

BEHIND THE SCENES

The man sits on the floor with his legs together and knees bent as his lover playfully presents her buttocks for his inspection. His lips and tongue probe every inch of her backyard.

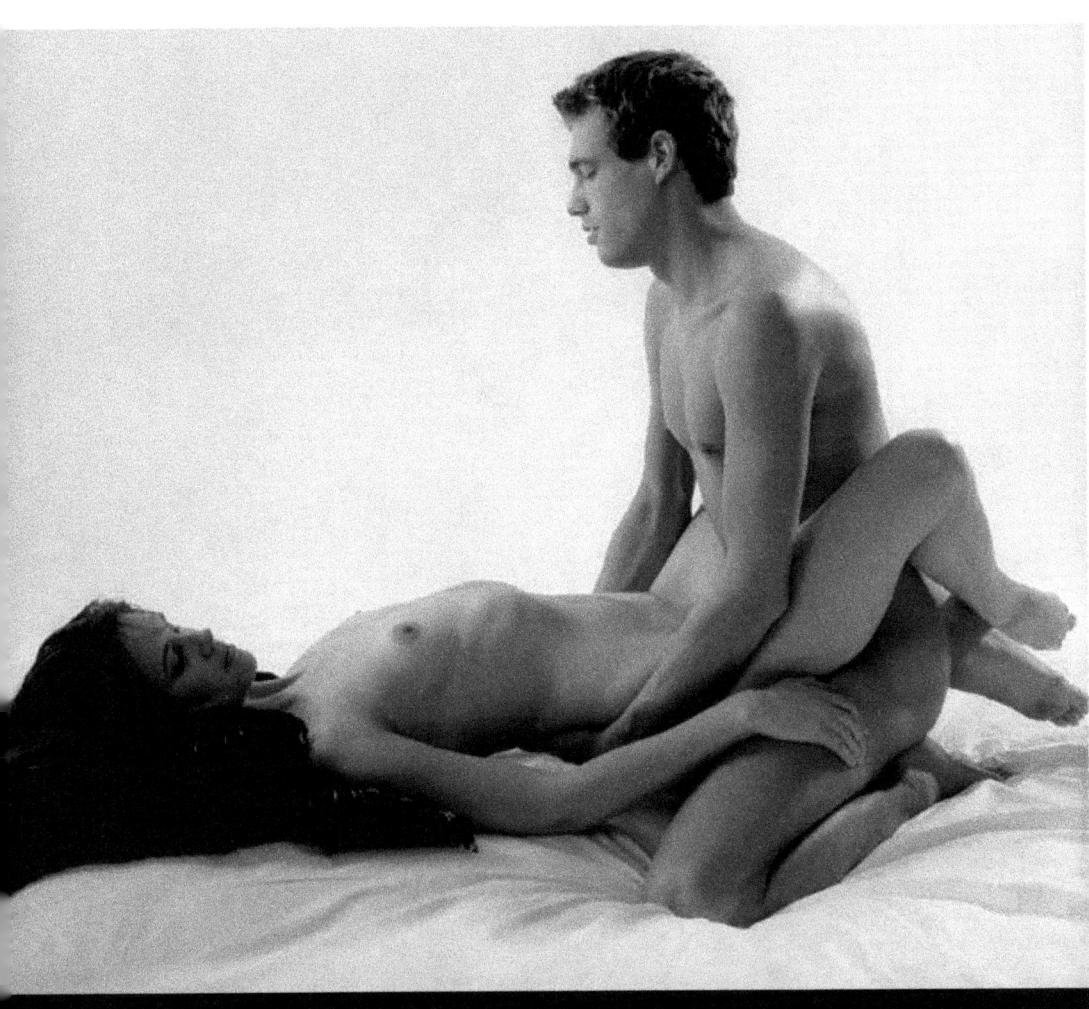

DAY 84

FULL EXPOSURE

She starts in his lap facing her partner. As she leans backward, she locks her legs around his back. He can massage both her breast and clitoris.

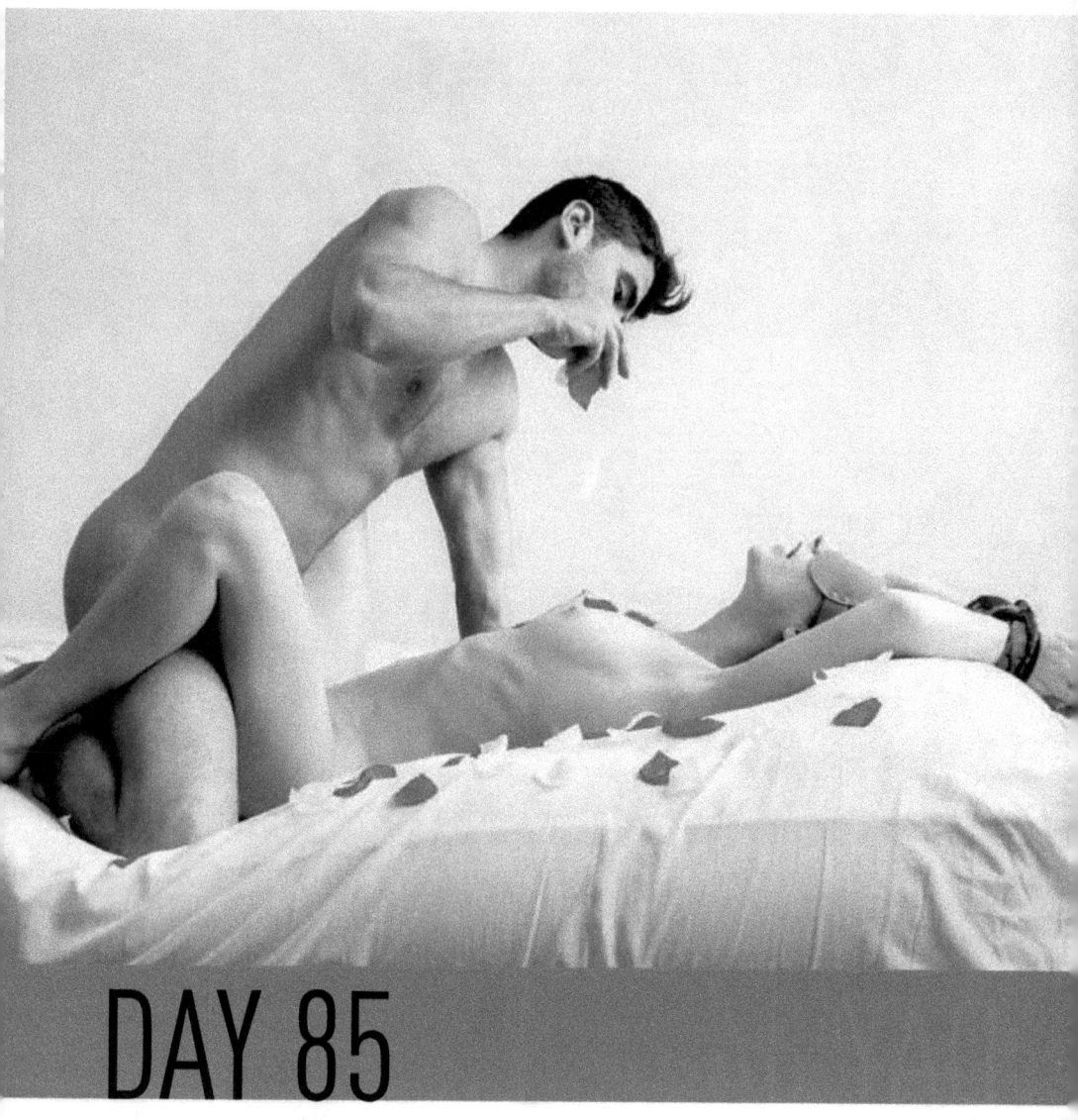

DAY 85

HEAVY PETAL

The woman dons a blindfold and lies back on the bed as her partner ties her hand together over her head. As he enters her from a kneeling position, he gently drops rose petals on to her chest and stomach, heightening her sensory experience.

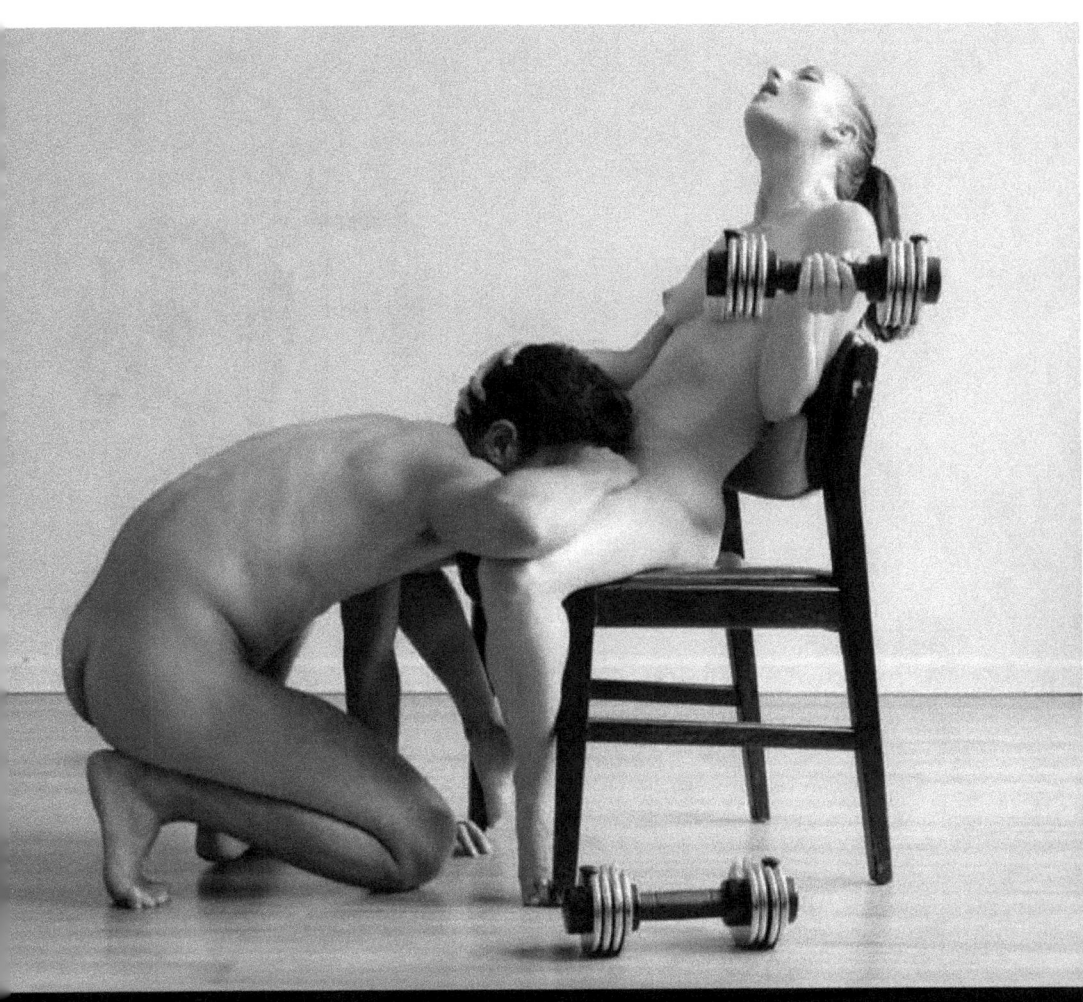

DAY 86

THE LICK AND LIFT

She sits in a chair with her legs spread wide open and a dumbbell in one hand. As her lover services her vagina with his tongue and lips, she can alternate lifting with each hand while stroking his hair with the other.

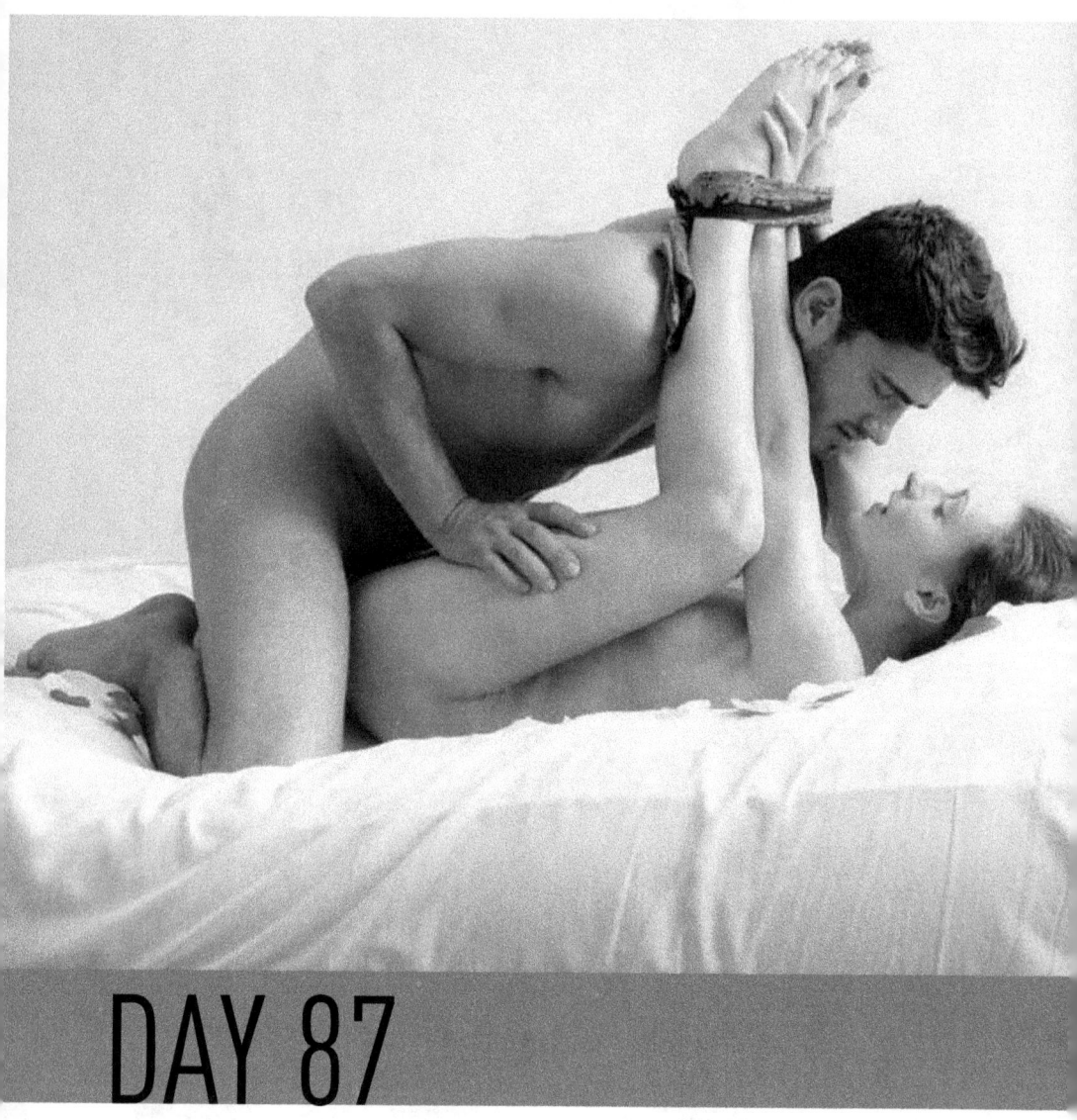

DAY 87

THE "OH MY!" TIE

She's on her back with her hands and feet bound together around her lover's neck. He enters her from a kneeling position as they gaze into each other's eyes.

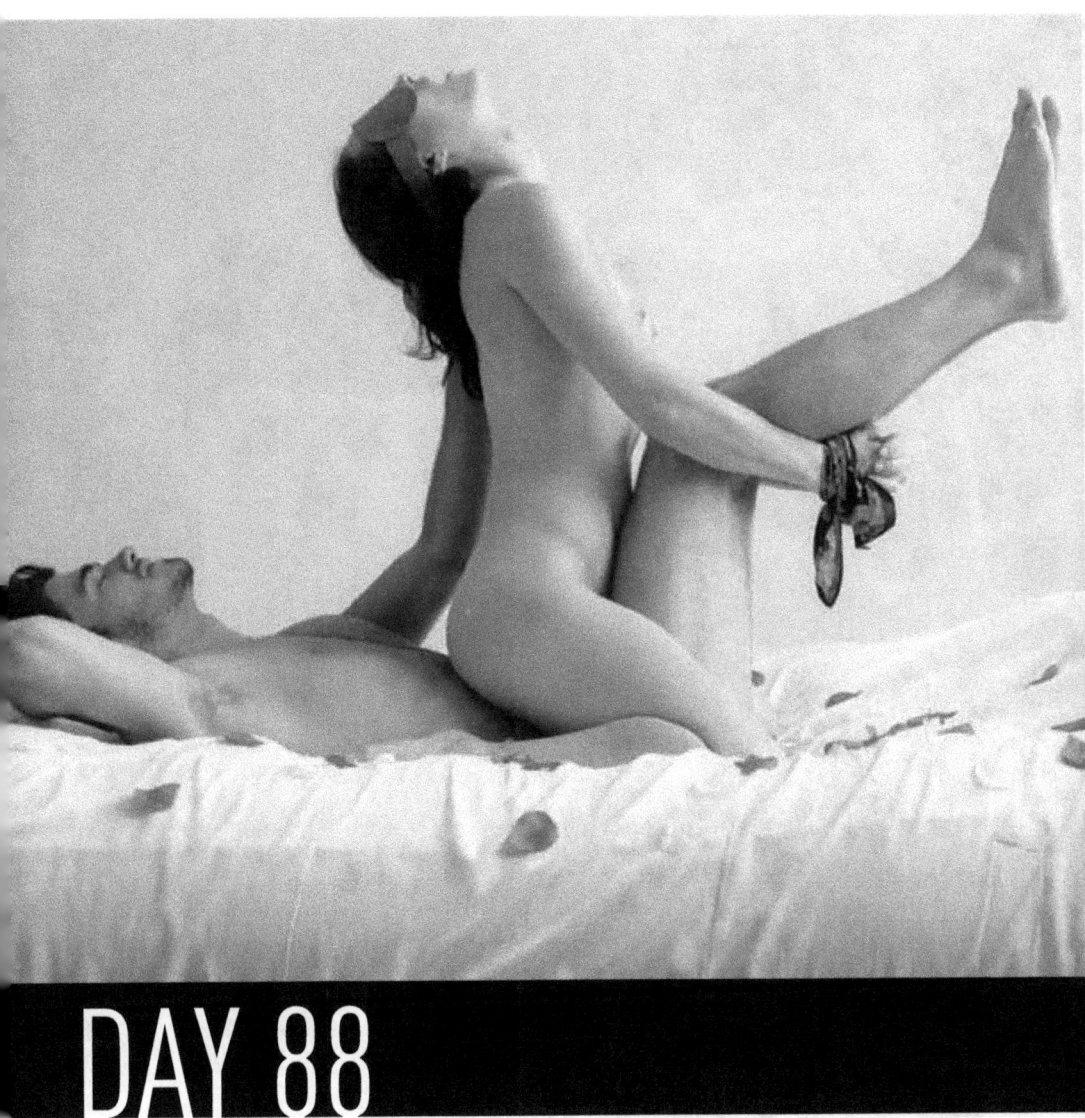

DAY 88

RIDING BLIND

The man starts in a sitting position, helping to tie his blindfolded lover's hands together. As he reclines on the bed, he lifts his legs so that her hands fall around the back of his knees. She straddles him as he penetrates and bucks like a bronco.

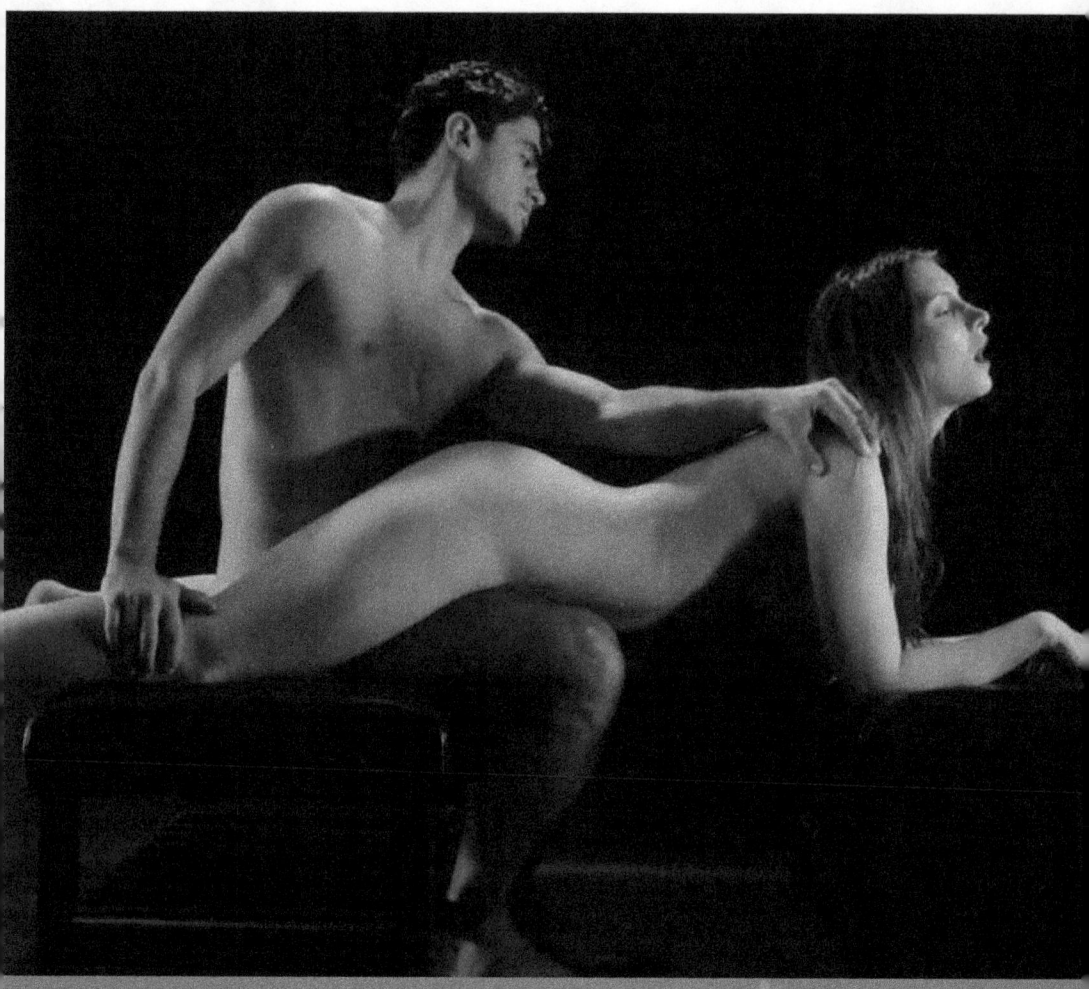

DAY 89

THE HOOD ORNAMENT

The lovers position themselves between two low-lying pieces of furniture. He's in a sitting position as his partner mounts him, facing away, and slowly lowers herself down so that her feet are up on his seat and her forearms are resting on the other object. He's got a great view of her butt as he enters her.

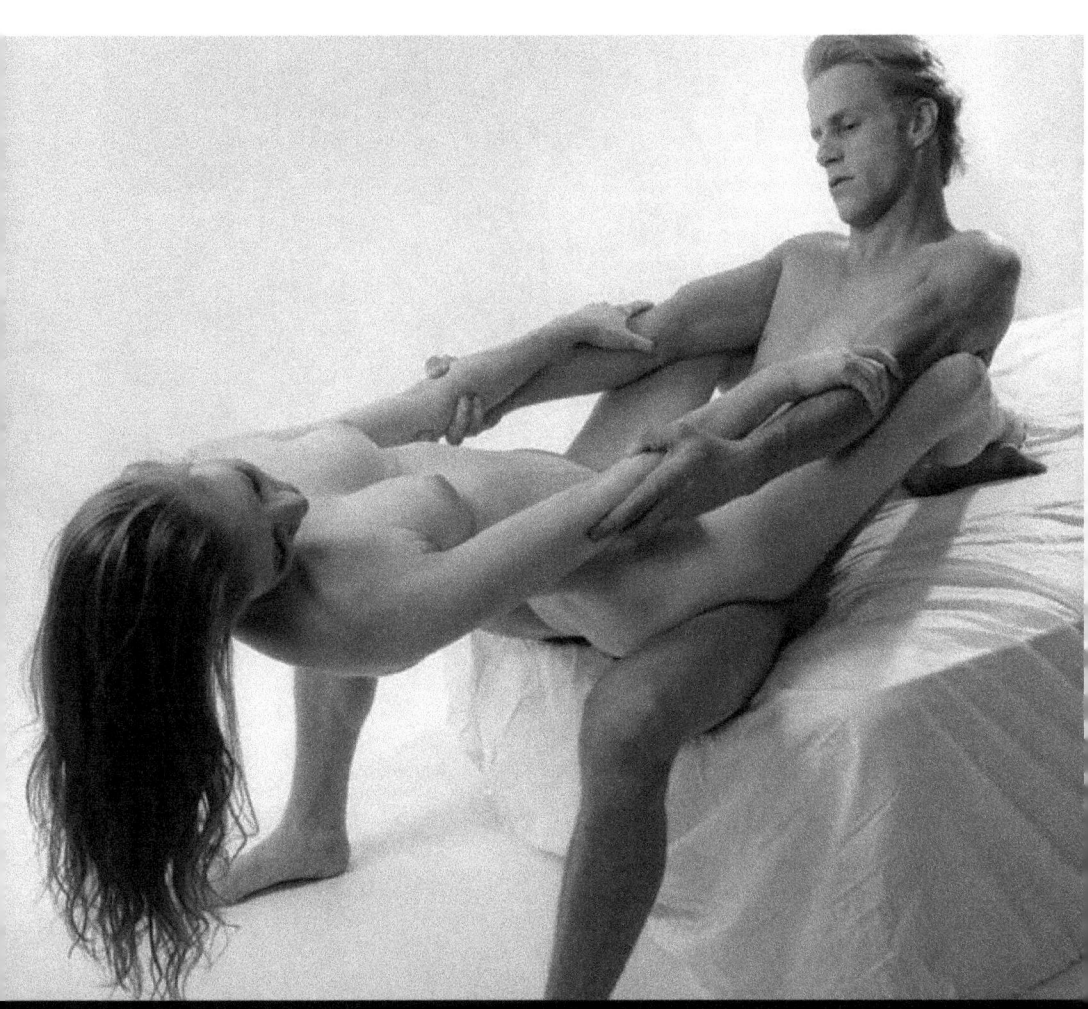

DAY 90

PULLING PASSION

The man sits down at the edge of the bed with his feet on the floor. His lover mounts him, wrapping her legs around his back. They grasp each other's arms and lean back. The tug of war that follows is pure bliss.

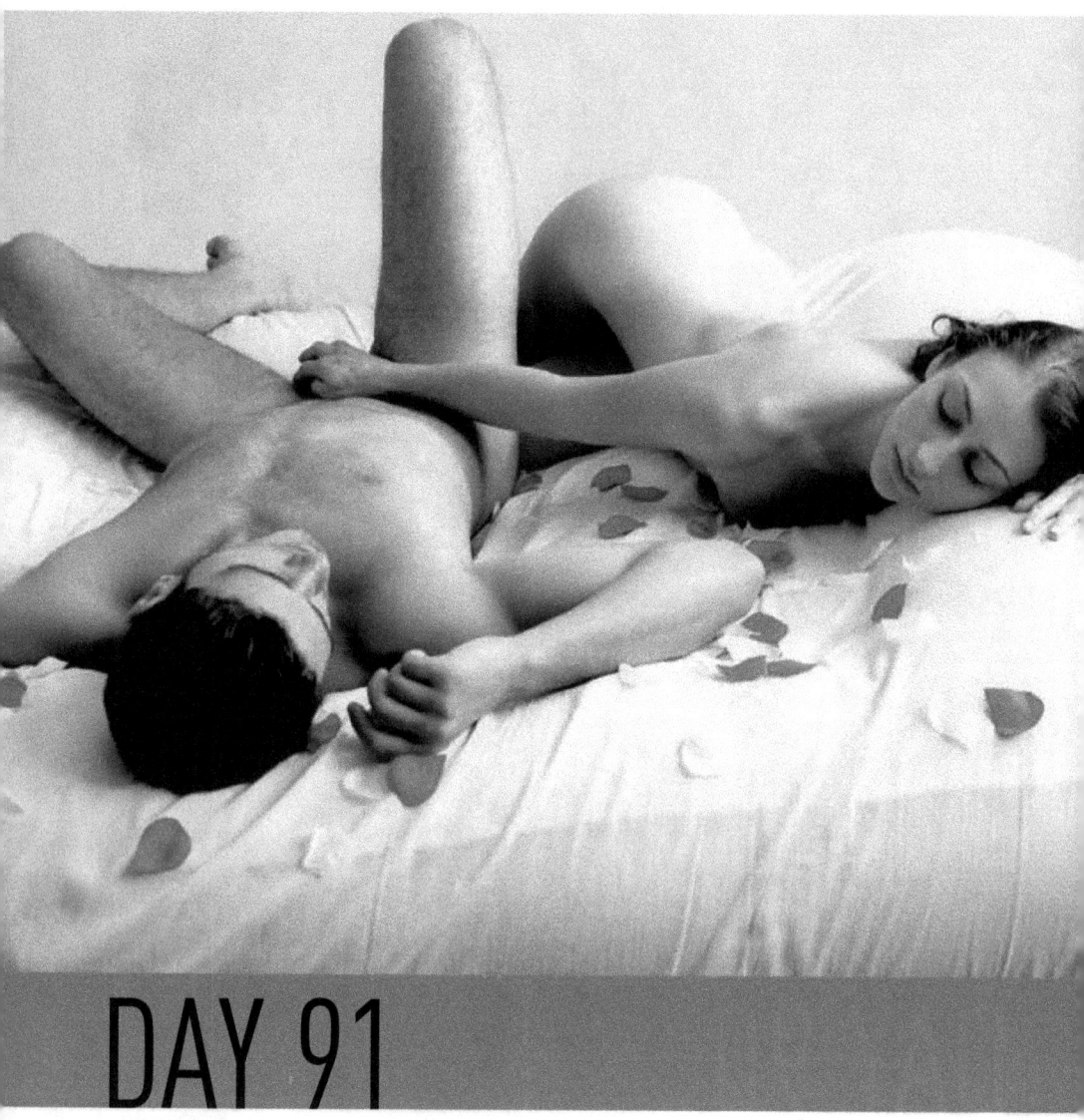

DAY 91

THE HAND MAIDEN

After a bout of more vigorous lovemaking, the couple make themselves comfortable on a rose-covered bed. He lies back, completely relaxed, as his lover positions herself beside him and strokes his penis with her hand until he reaches climax.

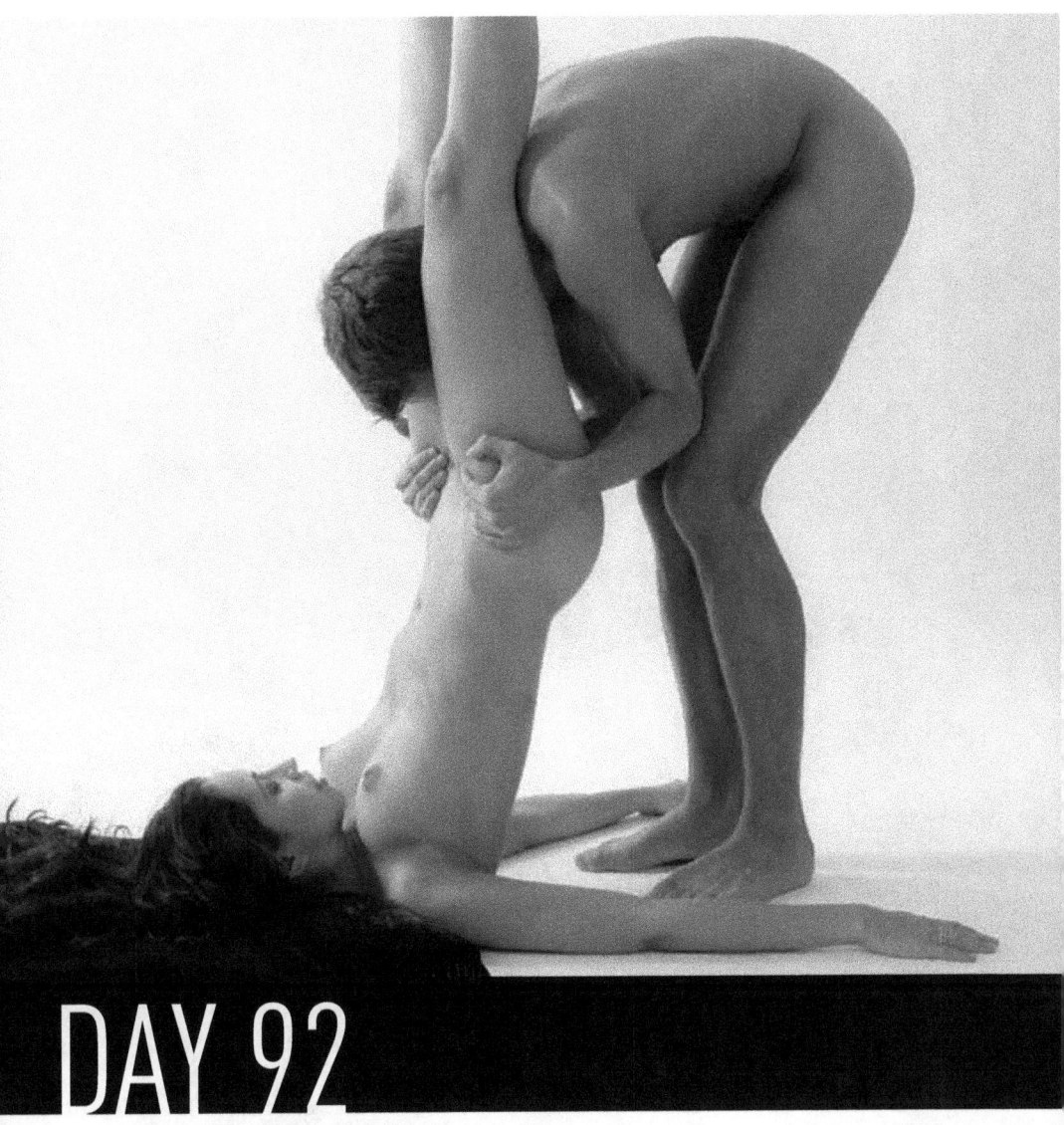

DAY 92

GOING DOWN?

The woman lies flat on the floor with her arms and palms down and moves into a shoulder stand with her legs pointed up. Her partner bends at the waste, grabbing her hips with his hands. His mouth has little problem finding its way down to her vagina.

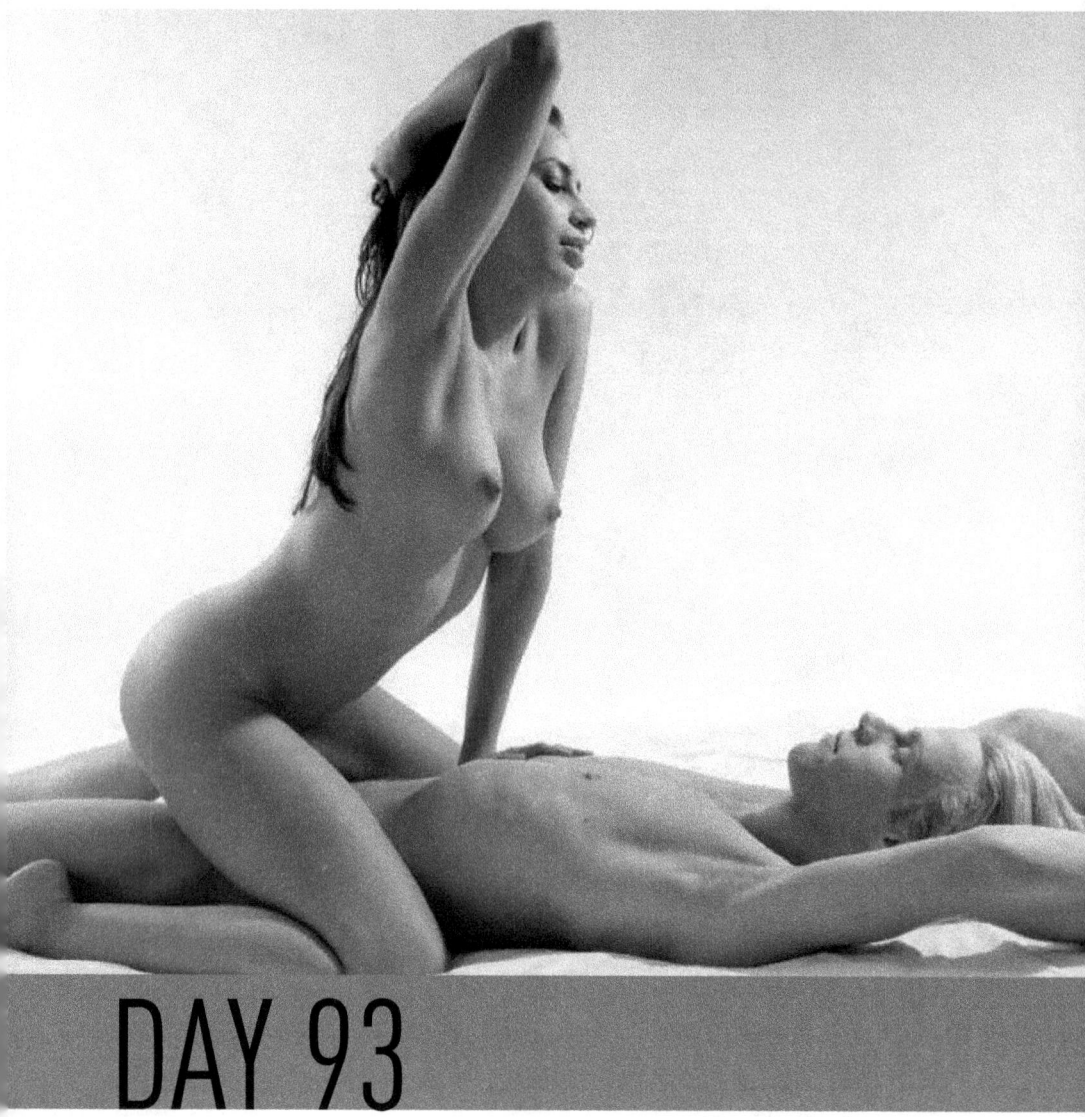

DAY 93

THE GRABBER

The man lies on his back while his lover mounts him. Once she's on top she can grab his penis by manipulating her vaginal muscles as well as her thighs. Her hands are also free to play with all sorts of other things.

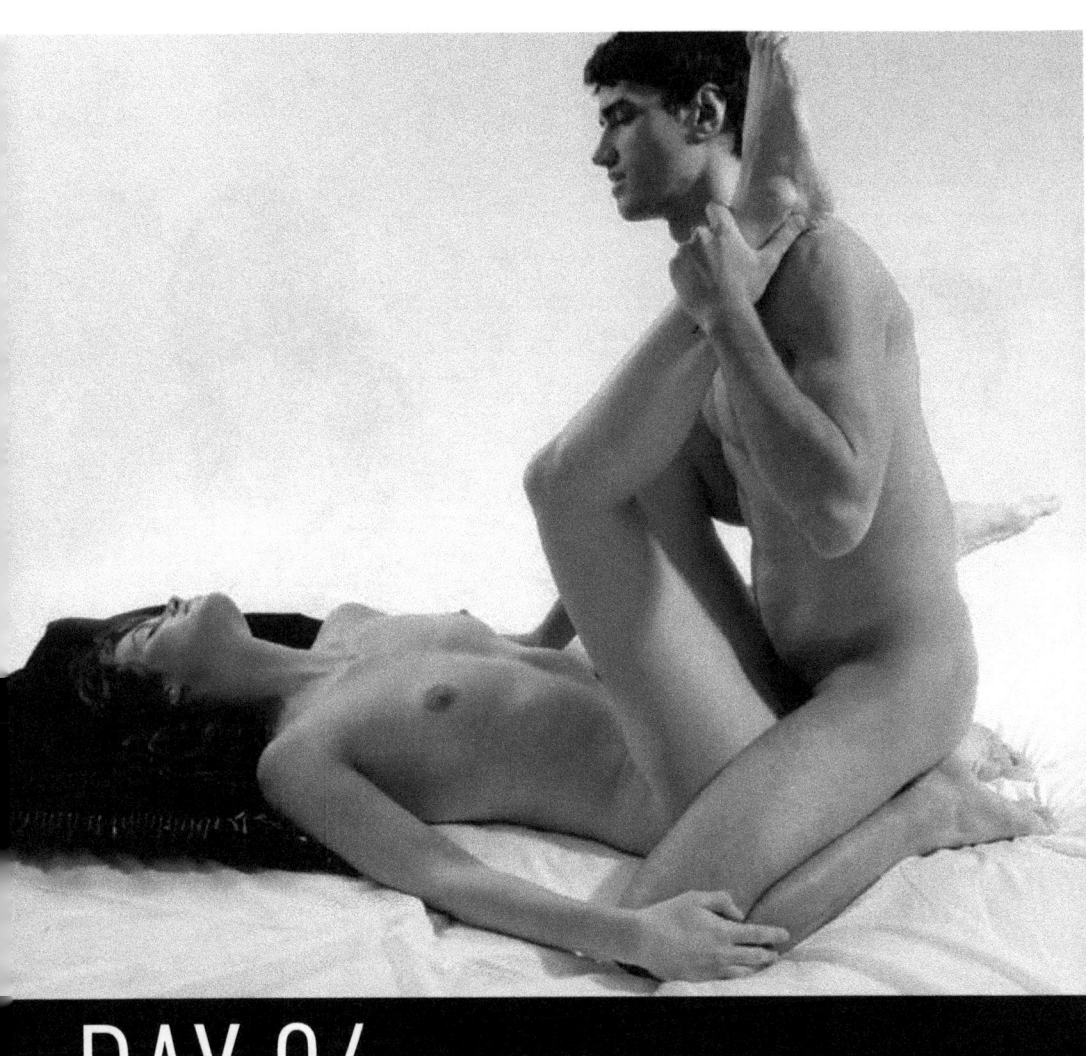

DAY 94

HOW DEEP IS YOUR LOVE ?

Get a leg (or two) up on your lover in this highly satisfying partnership. From her back, the woman can rest one or both of her legs on his shoulders. The result is mutually satisfying penetration and an increased sense of intimacy.

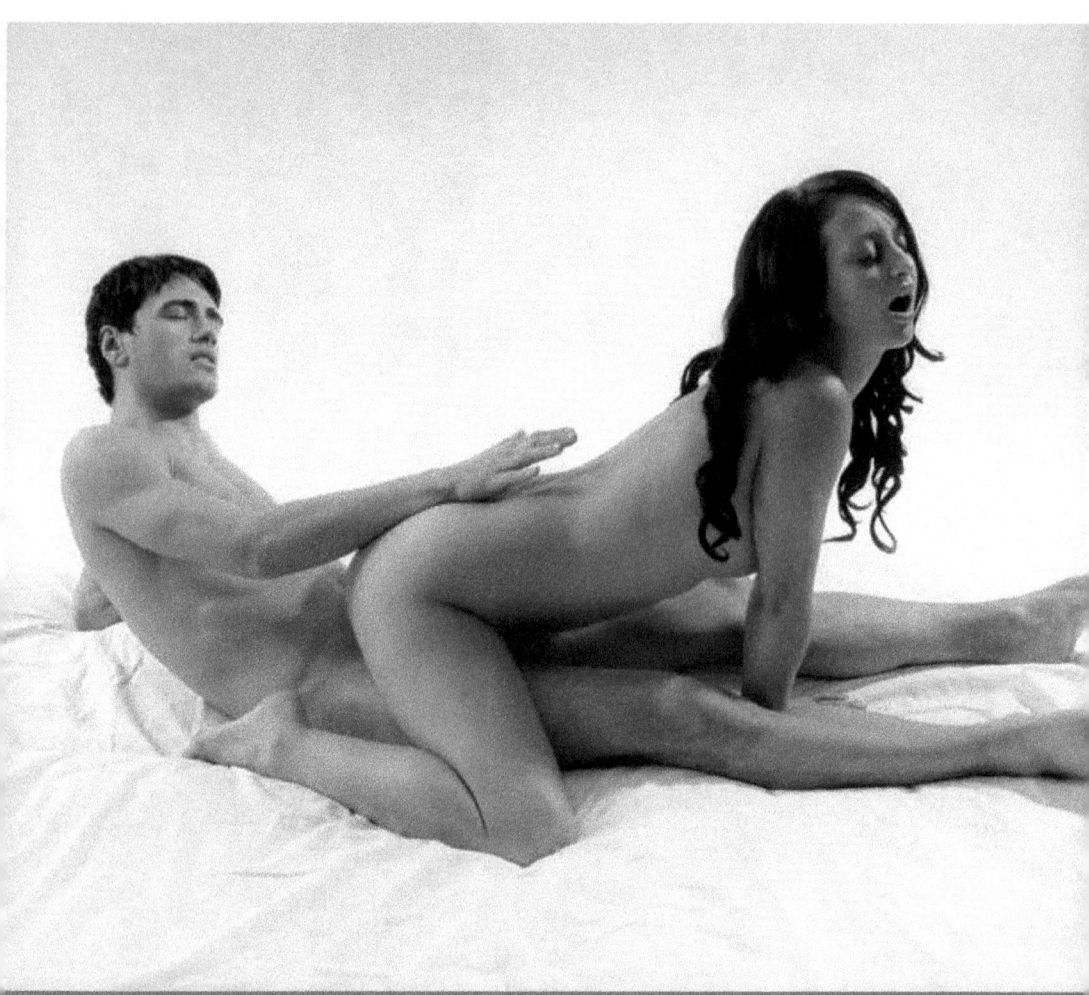

DAY 95

RIDE THE TIGER

The man is on his back as his partner straddles him and faces away. She can rest her hands on his legs or the bed while his are free to explore just about every inch of her body.

DAY 96

FOUR ON THE FLOOR

The woman stands up straight facing away from her lover. She bends at the waist and lowers her palms to the floor. Standing straight up, he penetrates her from behind.

DAY 97

SEXUAL BOOST

The woman gets on a chair and lowers herself into a squatting position with her hands grabbing the chair's back. Her lover bends his knees slightly and enters her from behind. It's best not to get too carried away with the thrusting here.

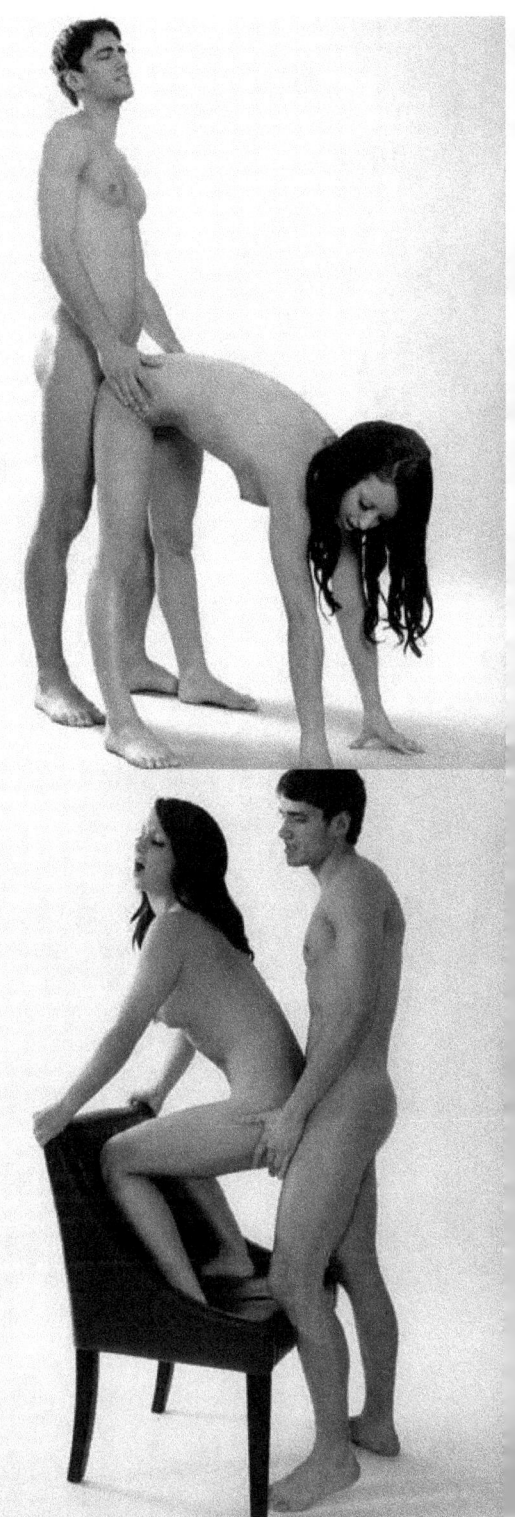

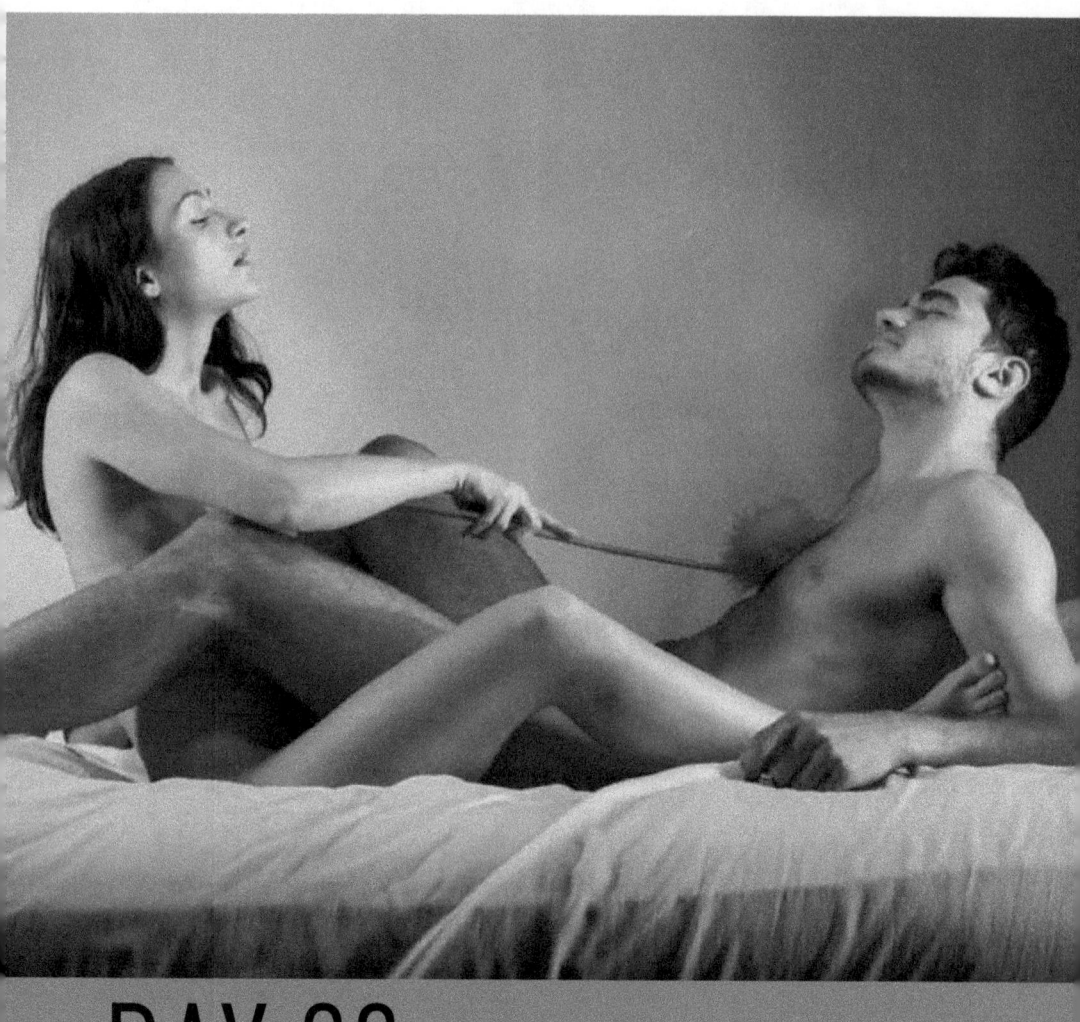

DAY 98

COOCHIE, COOCHIE, COO

The lovers position themselves on the bed facing each other with legs overlapping. They move closer so that he can penetrate her vagina. As he enters her, she trails a feather wand over his chest, arms, and ribs. If he's at all ticklish his convulsions will only add to the pleasure.

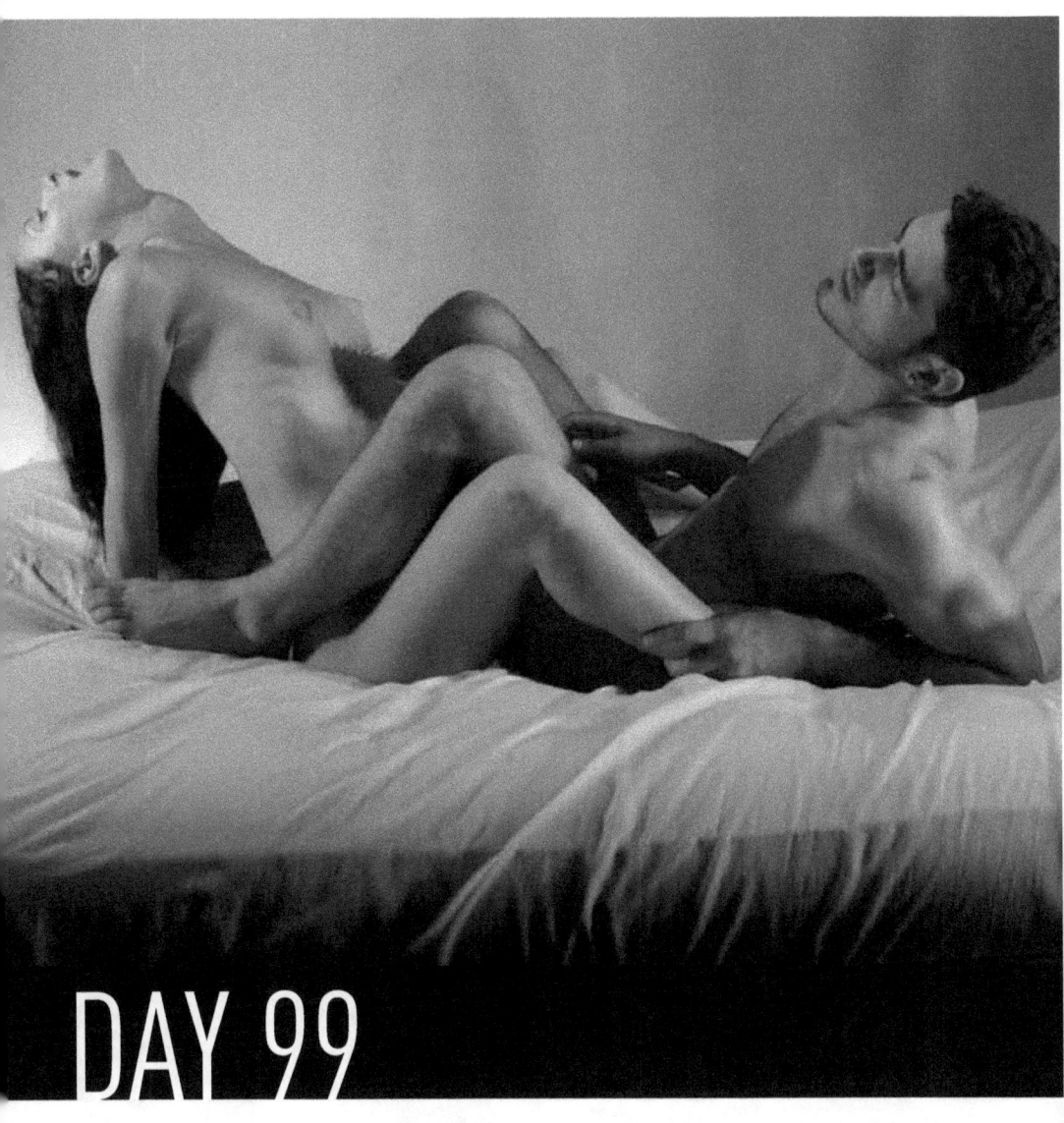

DAY 99

COOCHIE COO TO YOU, TOO

The man and woman once again get into a position on the bed where they are interlocked and facing one and other. This time he's got the feather wand, and she's at his mercy. Each successful tickle will surely be felt by both of them.

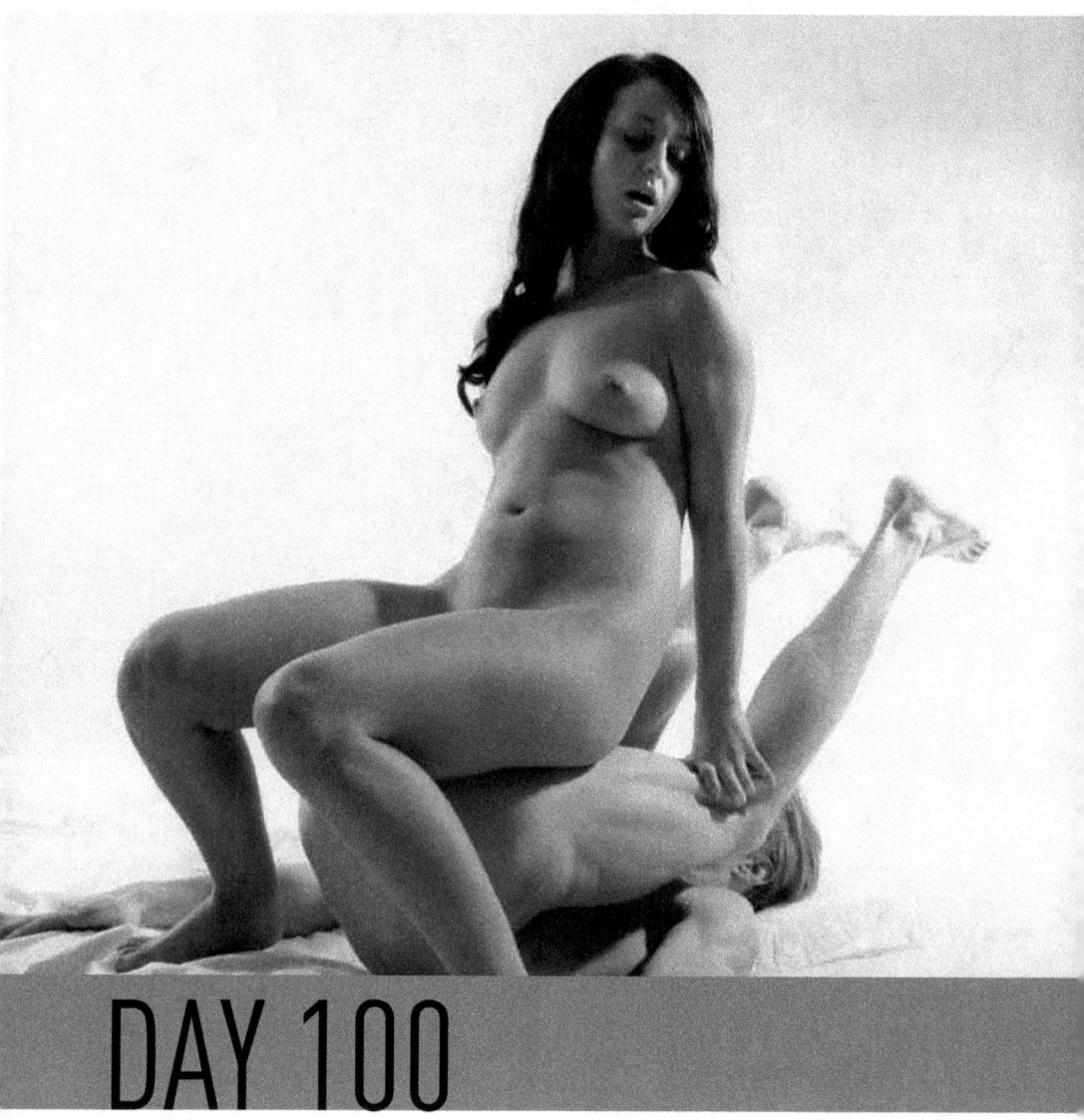

DAY 100

THE QUEEN'S THRONE

This one takes some coordination and a lot of flexibility. He's on his back with his knees pulled in toward his chest and legs at a 45-degree angle. She mounts him by lowering herself onto his thighs in a sitting position.

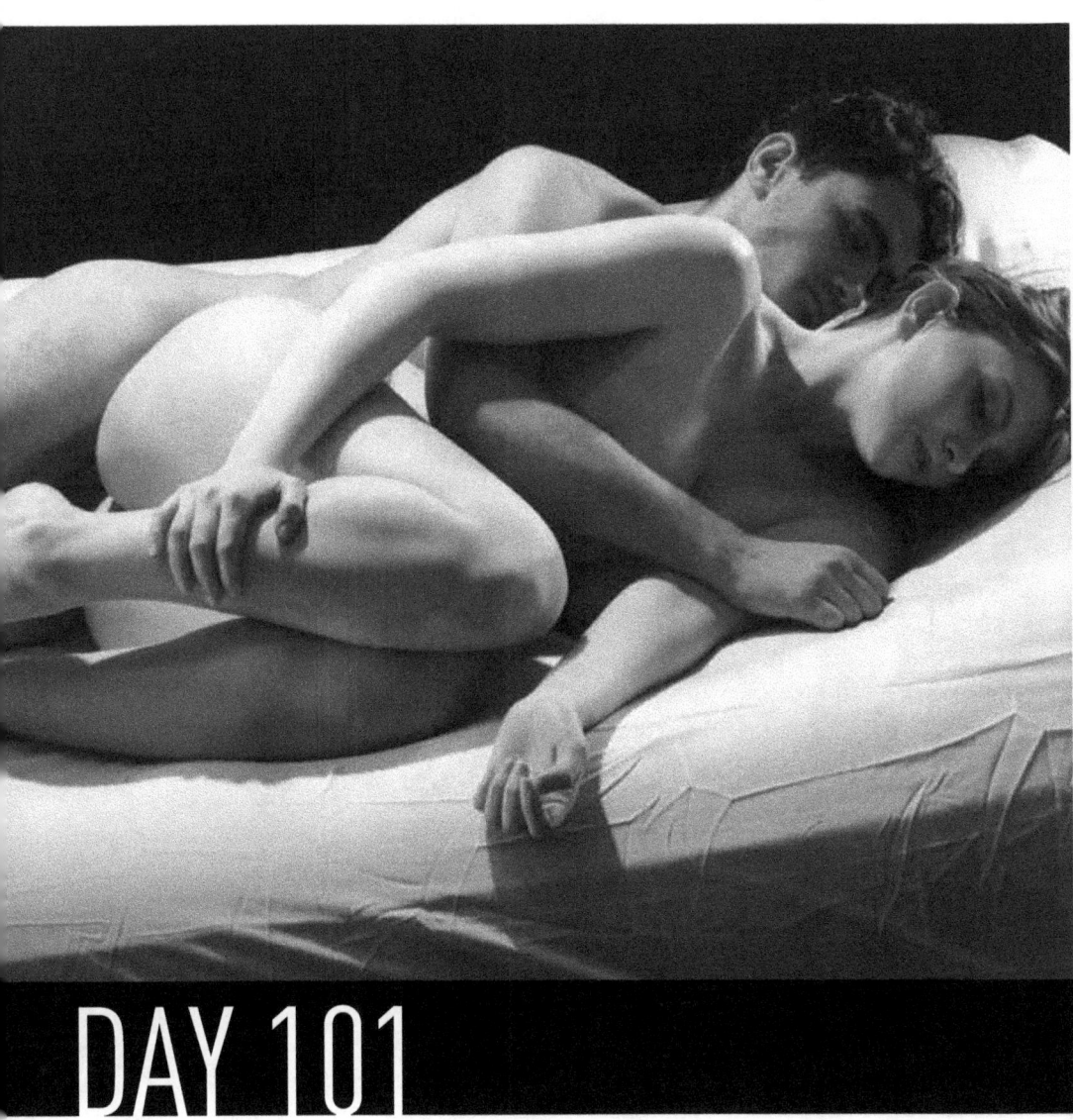

DAY 101

ROLL PLAY

She curls up on her side on the bed. Her lover positions himself behind her. As he enters her he brings his hand around to caress her breasts.

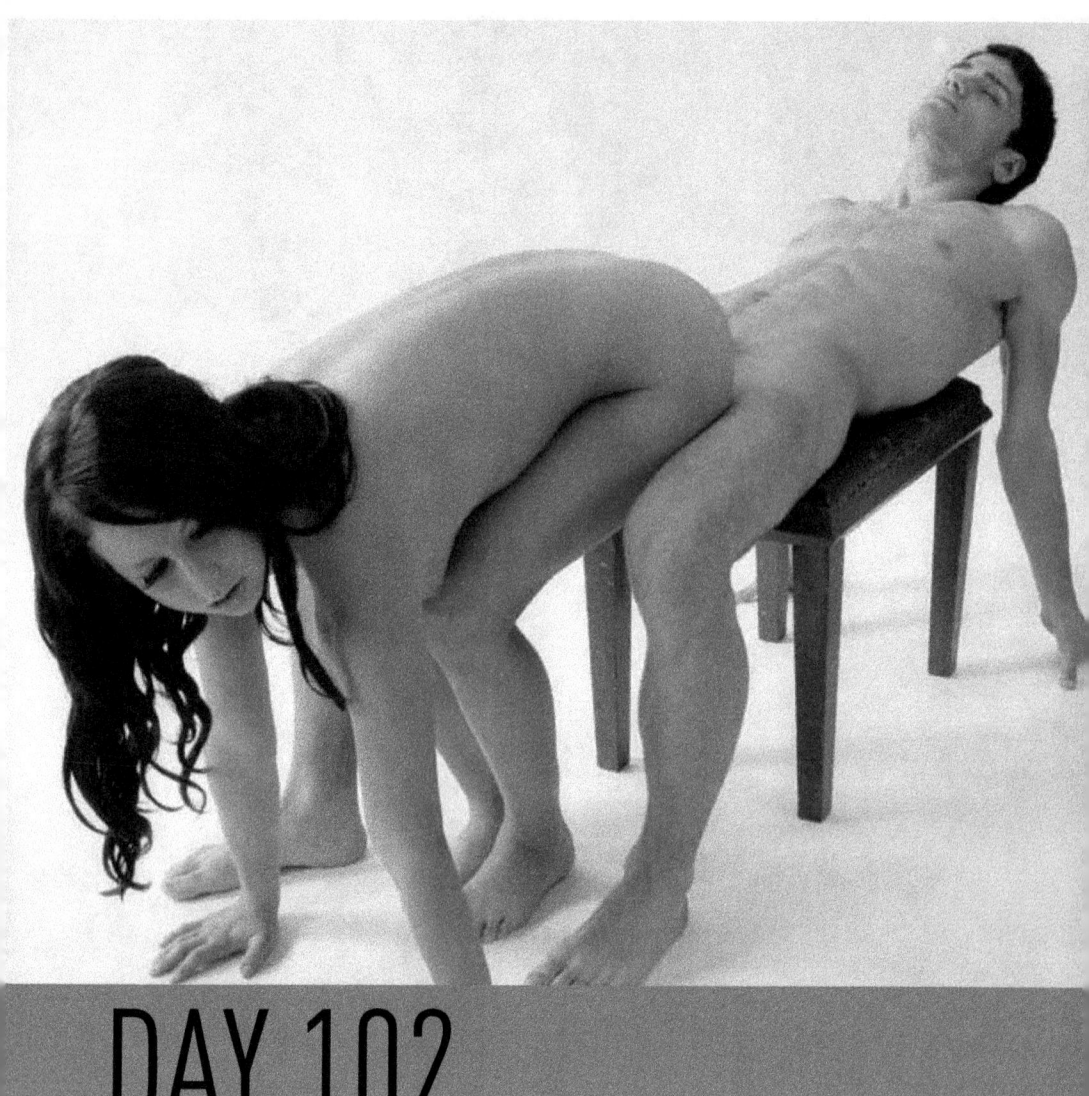

DAY 102

THE LAID-BACK LAP DANCE

He positions himself across a stool so that his feet are on the floor with his knees bent. She climbs on top with her back turned. He's in for the lap dance of his life.

DAY 103

GIVE HER A HAND

The man starts from a standing posture with his knees slightly bent. She places one hand on the floor for support as he lifts her lower half up to his penis. Her other hand is free to massage her clitoris.

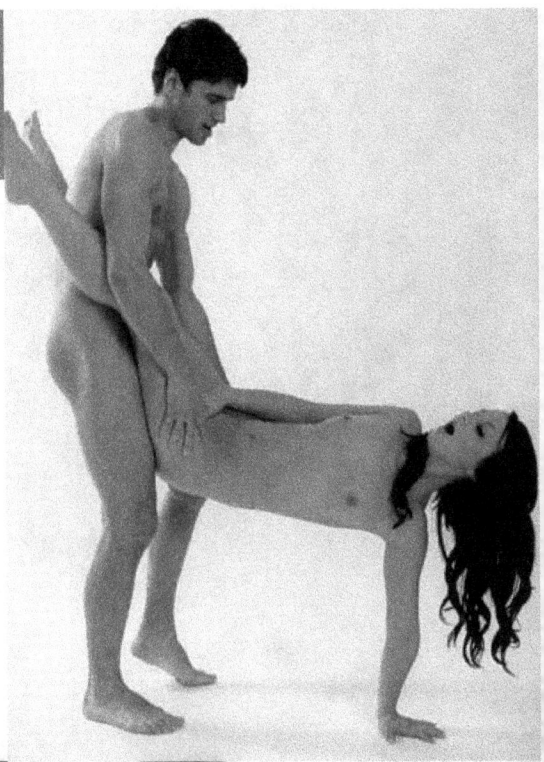

DAY 104

COME AS YOU ARE

He stands up straight as his lover gets on her knees and orally pleasures his penis. His hands are free to stroke and tousle her hair. Sometimes you just can't beat the classic blow job.

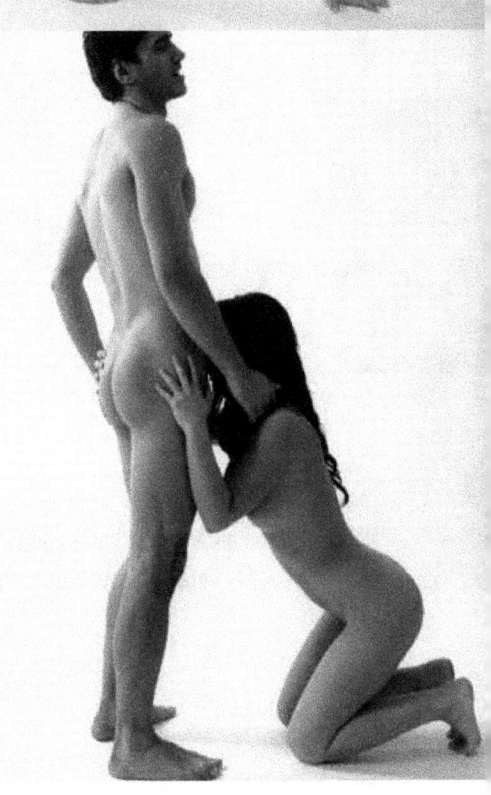

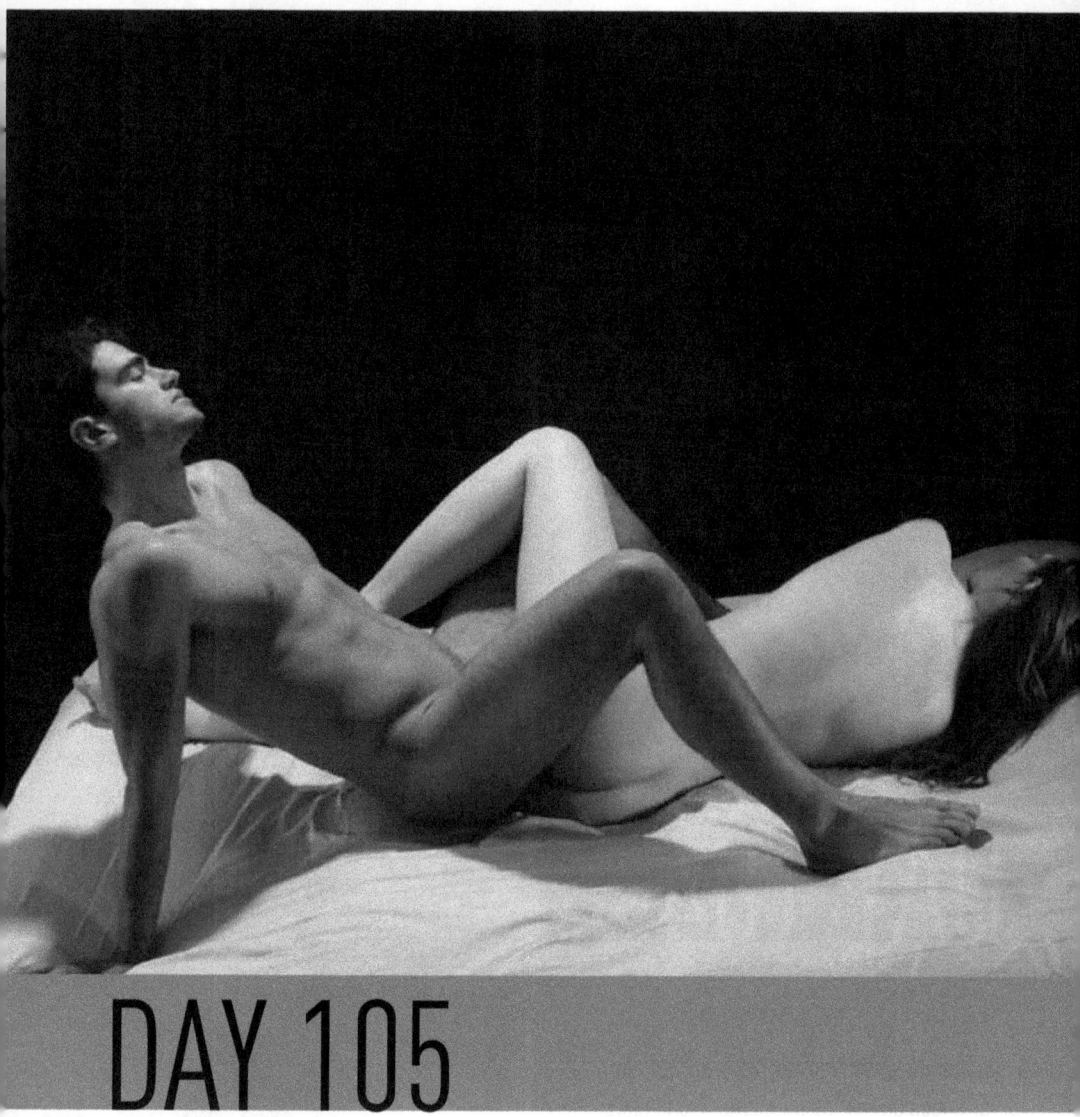

DAY 105

SLIP SERVICE

The woman lies on her side on the bed and swings her top leg upward to open herself wide. The man leans back on his hands and slides his erect penis into her vagina. There's lots of wonderful body contact between the lovers.

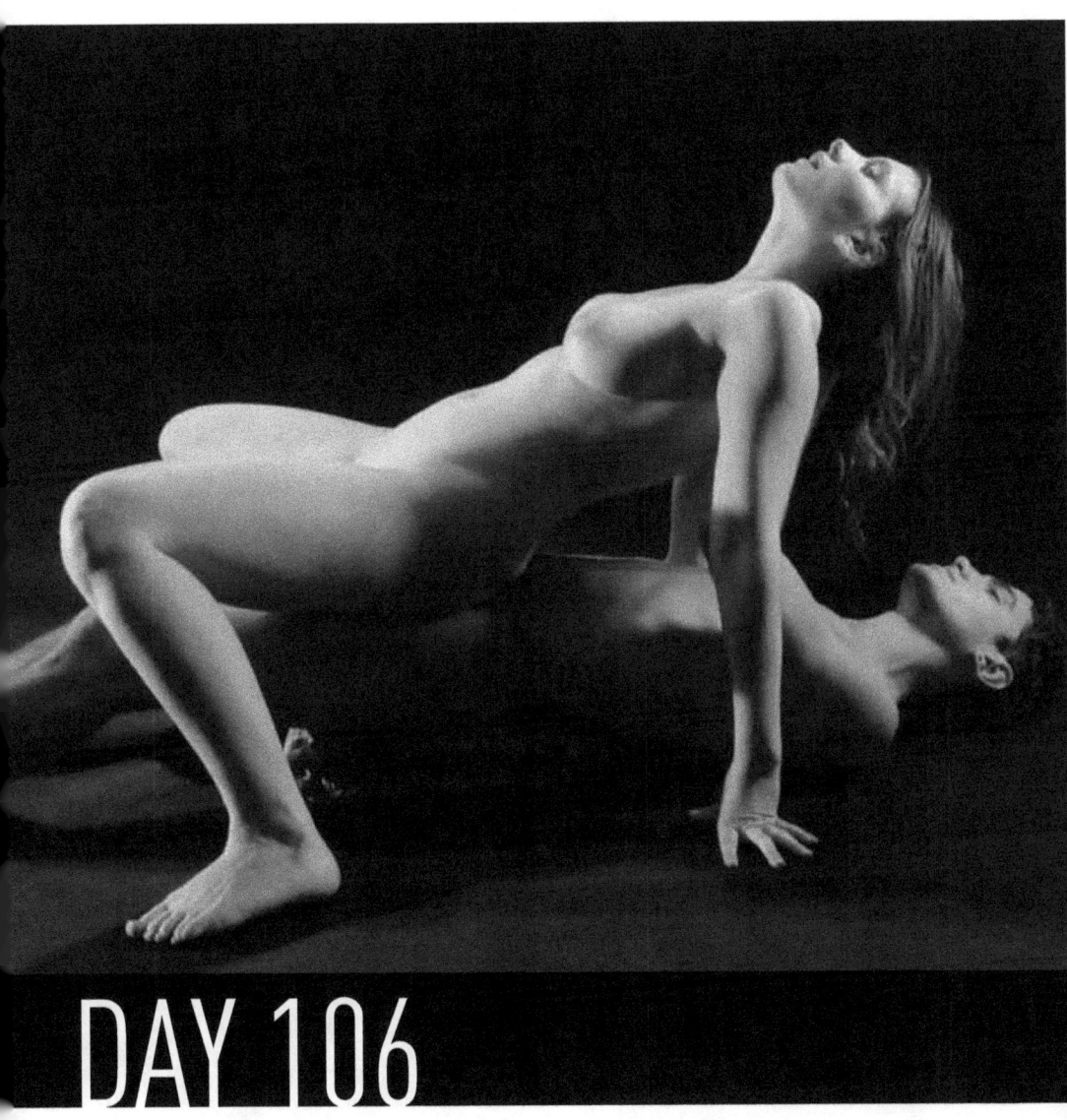

DAY 106

CELESTIAL BODIES

The man places a cushion under his buttocks as he stretches out on the floor. His partner mounts him from the top with her back facing him. It's as if they're both elevated and floating.

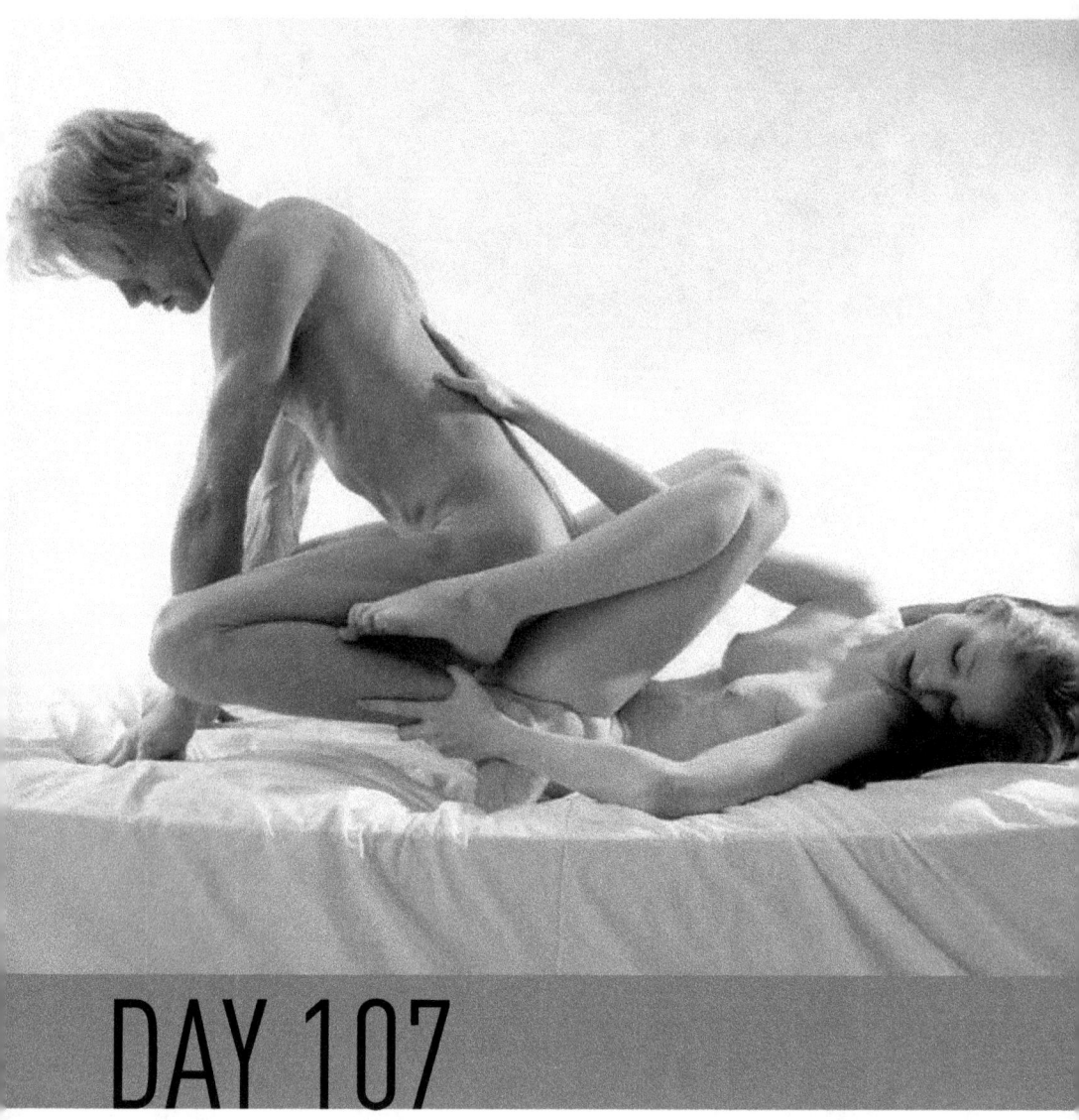

DAY 107

THE DRILL PRESS

The woman lies back on the bed with her legs up and open. Her partner bends forward, backs in against her thighs, and penetrates her in a downward fashion. His hands rest on the bed for support. A bit awkward, but amazing.

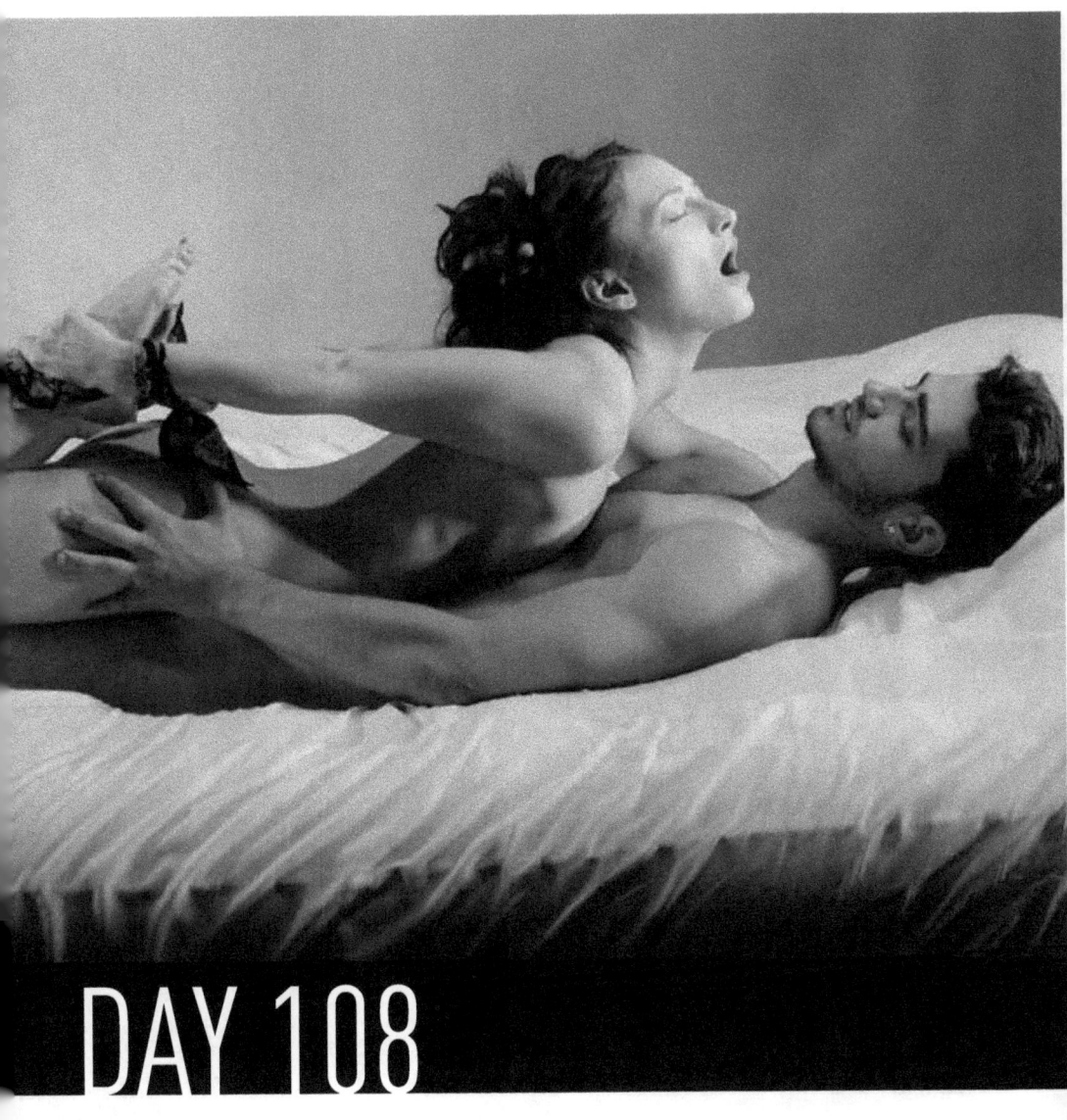

DAY 108

HOG-TIE HEAVEN

This one takes some doing, but it's fun once you get there. She lies flat on her stomach and brings both her hands and feet back so that her lover can tie them together with a silk scarf. Once she's secured, he carefully rolls her to the side and positions himself under her. She gives in to his control as he penetrates.

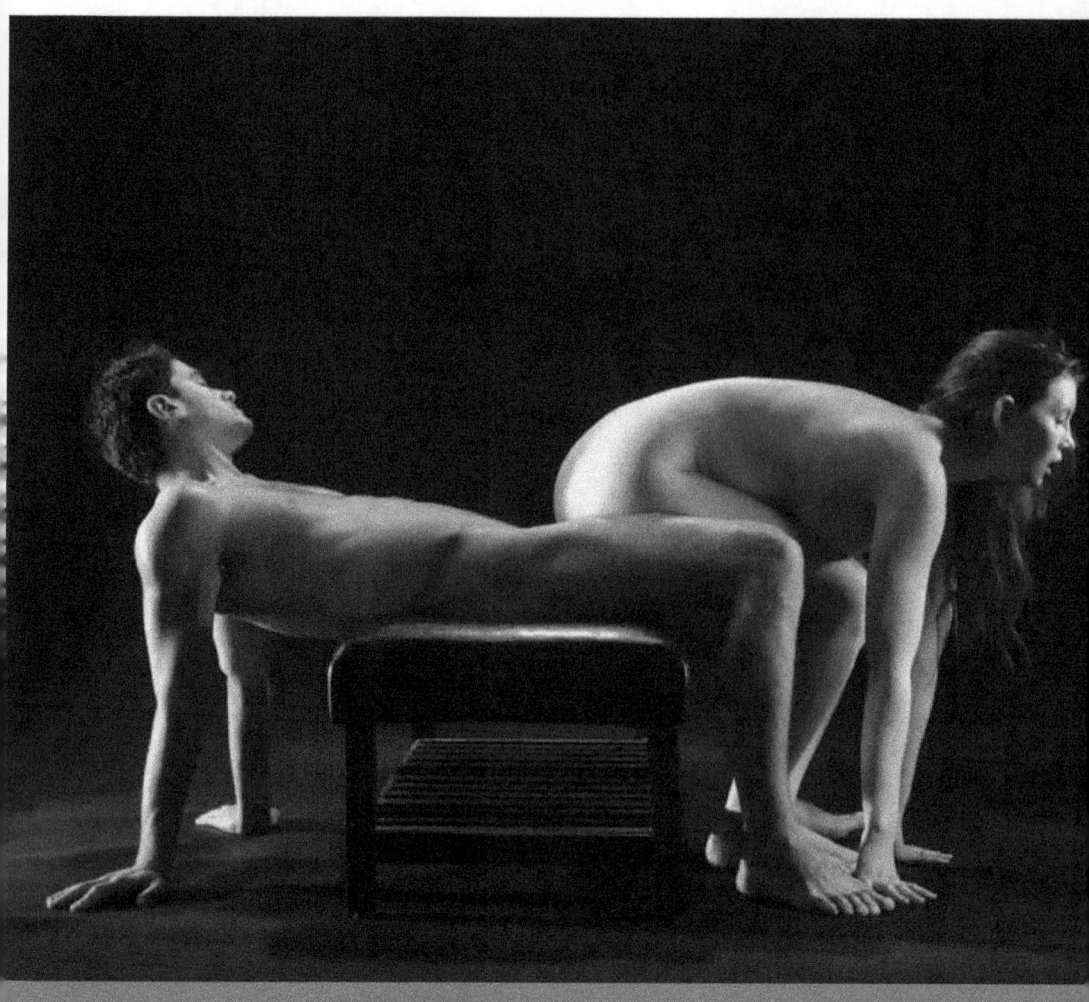

DAY 109

TWIN BENCHES

He lies back across a bench bringing his hands and feet to the floor so that he resembles a bench himself. His partner is more than happy to take a seat on his erect penis as she lowers her hands to the floor, opening herself up to possible G-spot stimulation.

DAY 110

THE HELPING HAND

She bends over and places her hands on the floor, getting into something resembling a downward-dog yoga pose. Her lover enters her from behind offering the support of his hands around her waist.

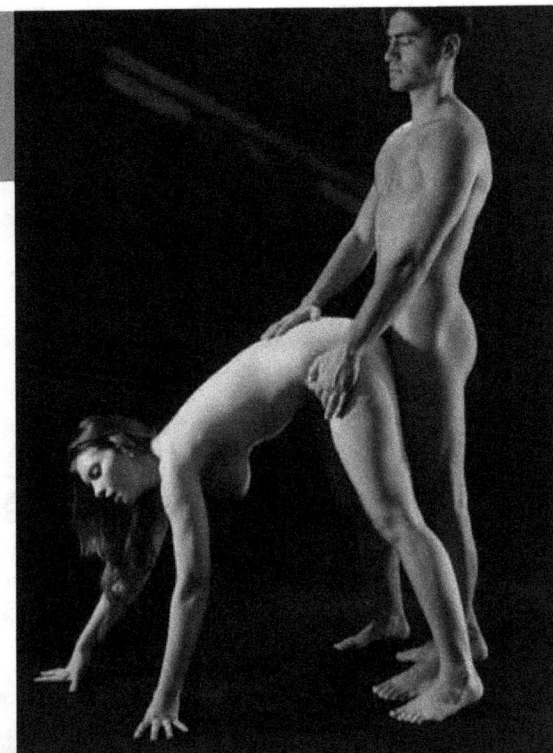

DAY 111

THE HOT SPOT

He's in a chair with his feet up on an ottoman. She finds the perfect spot for herself in her lover's lap. They're practically fused together as he enters her. It doesn't get much steamier than this.

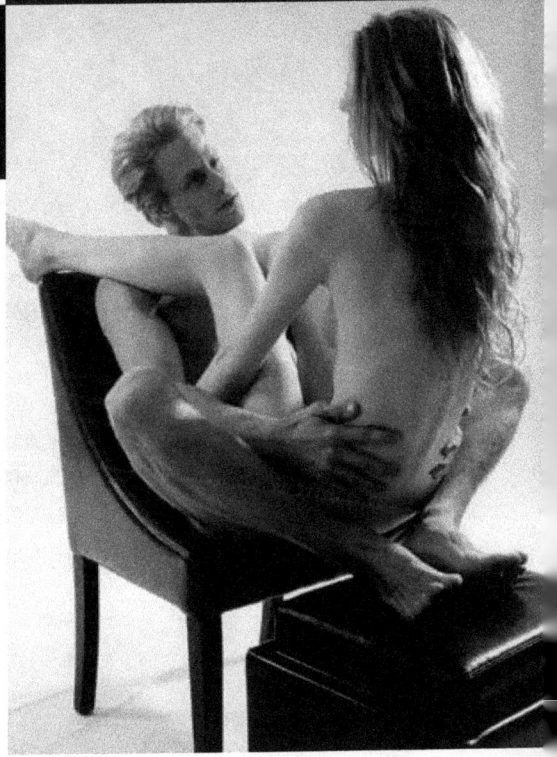

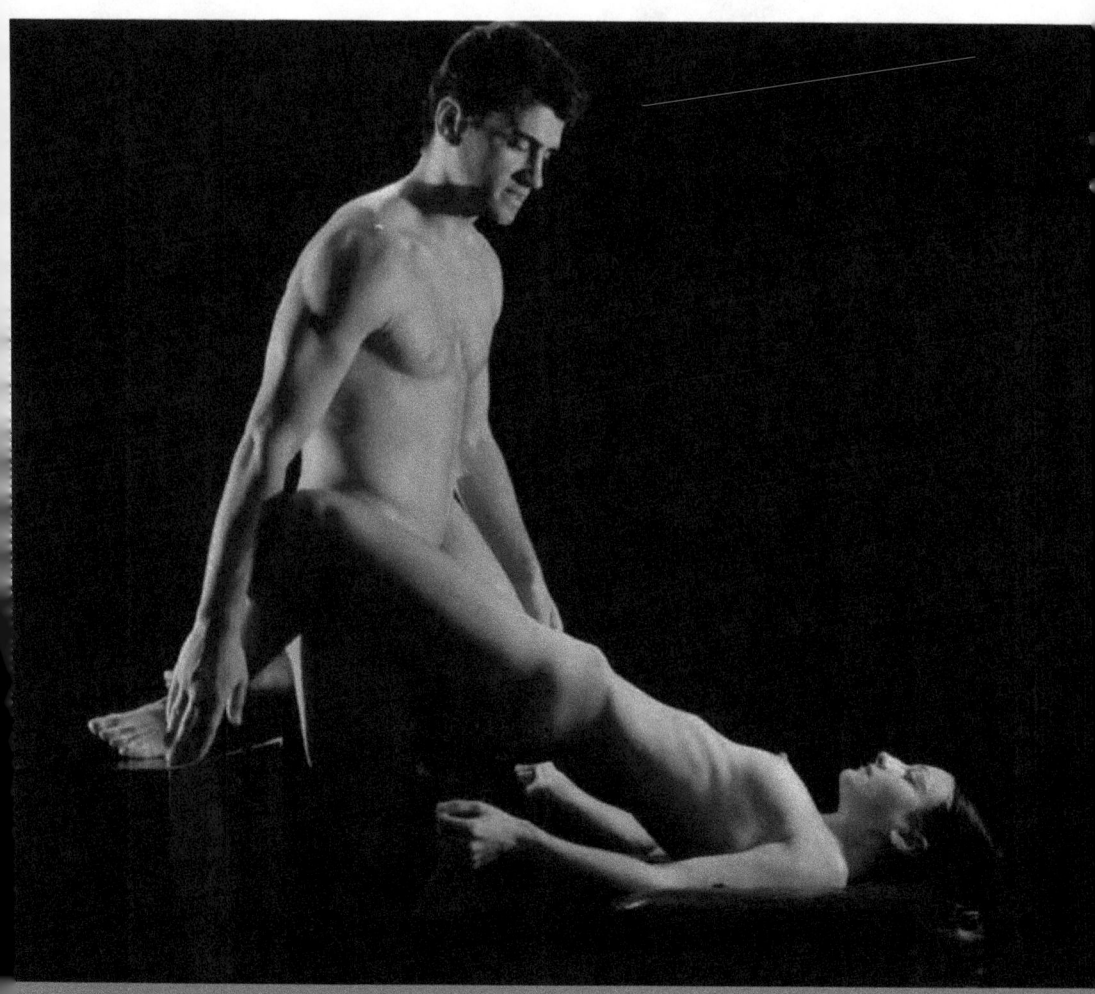

DAY 112

THE MINER

Arching her back, she places her head and shoulders on an ottoman and rests her feet on a slightly taller piece. Her lover positions himself between her legs and enters her at a downward angle. He can grab her hips for support and movement.

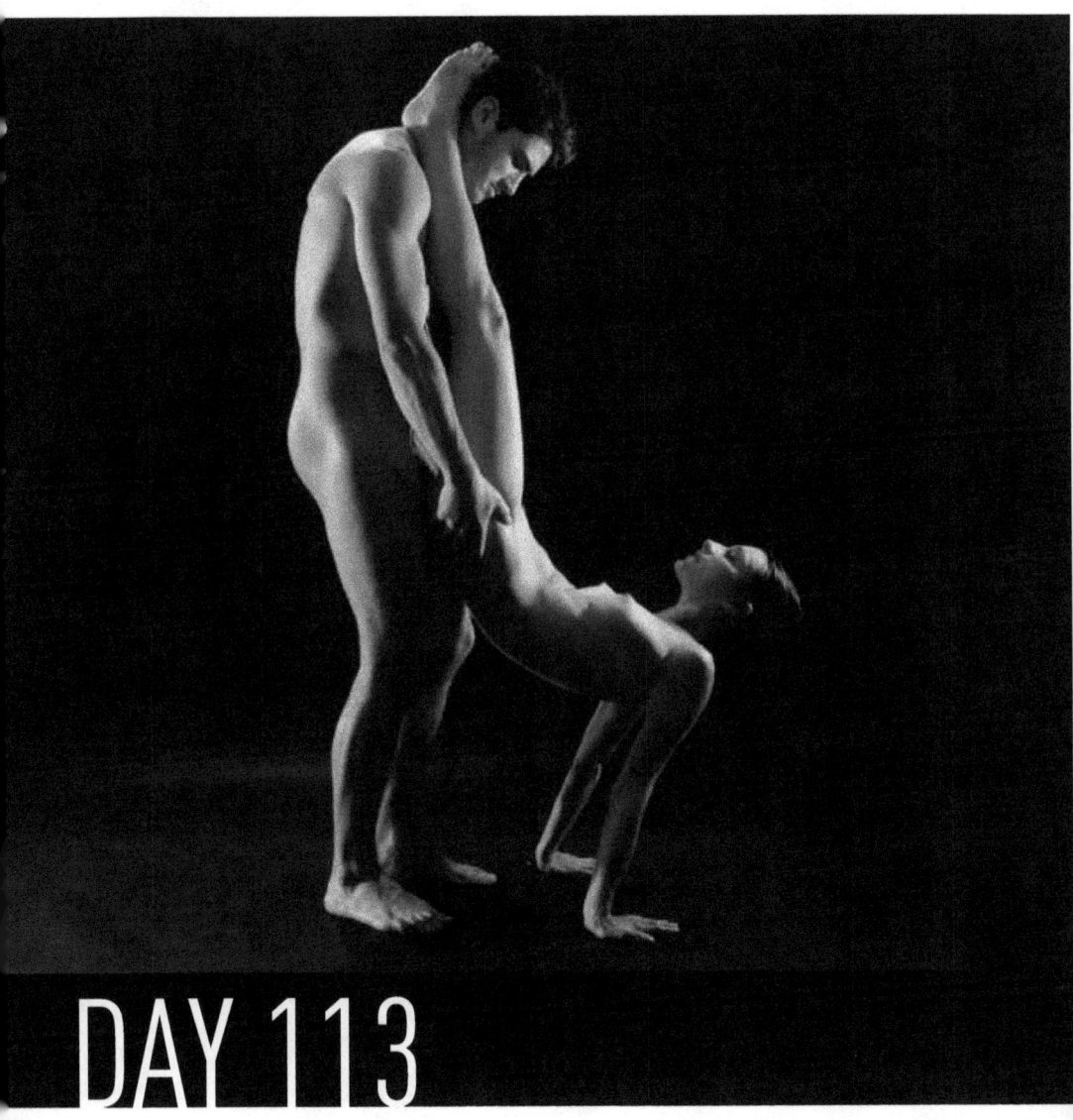

DAY 113

THE FALLBACK

The man stands up straight, supporting his lover around her buttocks as she reaches her hands back to the floor. As he penetrates her, she brings her feet up to his neck. Talk about a great reason to stay in shape.

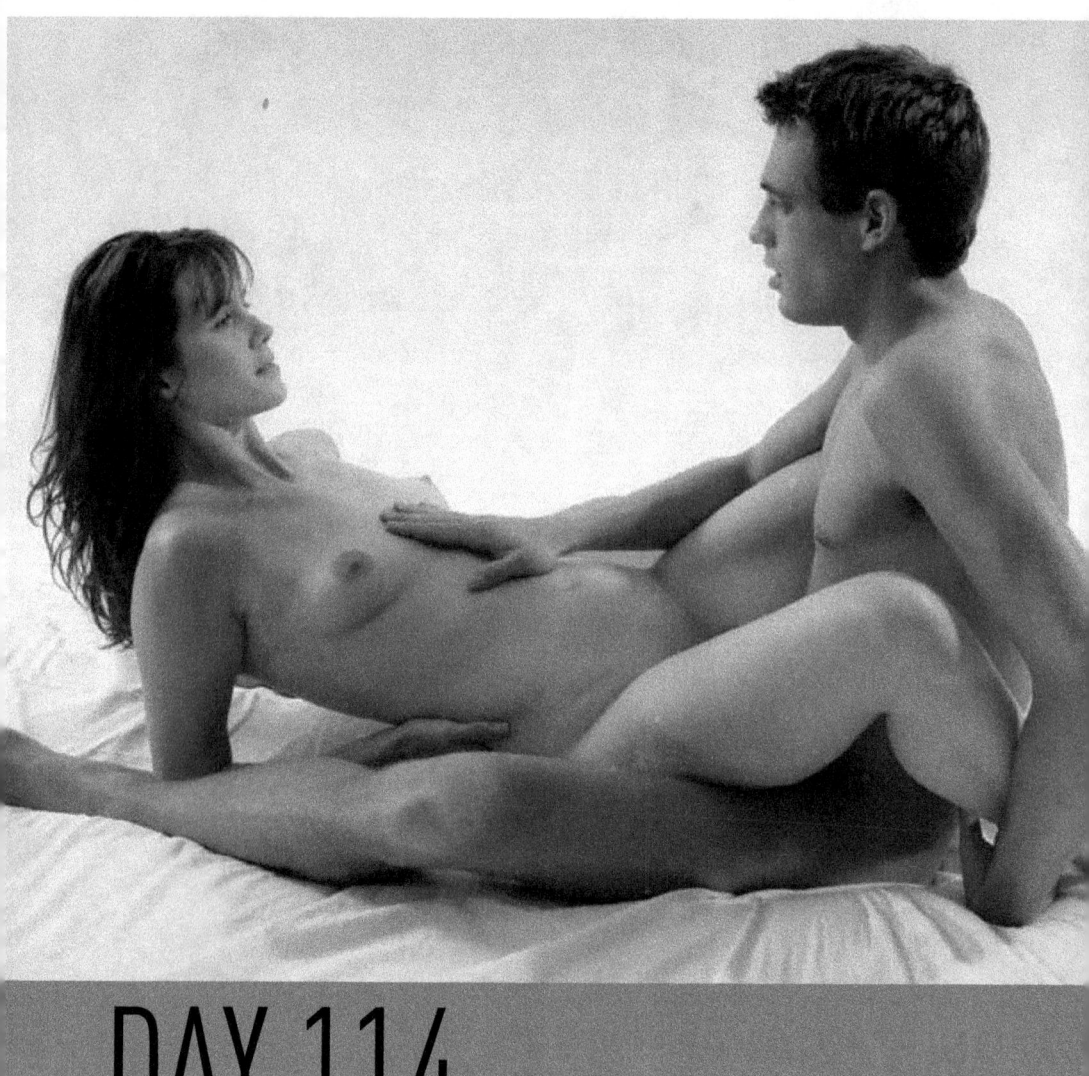

DAY 114

NIRVANA'S EDGE

The woman rests back on her elbows and lifts her pelvis. He enters her from a sitting position with his legs extended. She wraps her legs around his waist and pulls him in.

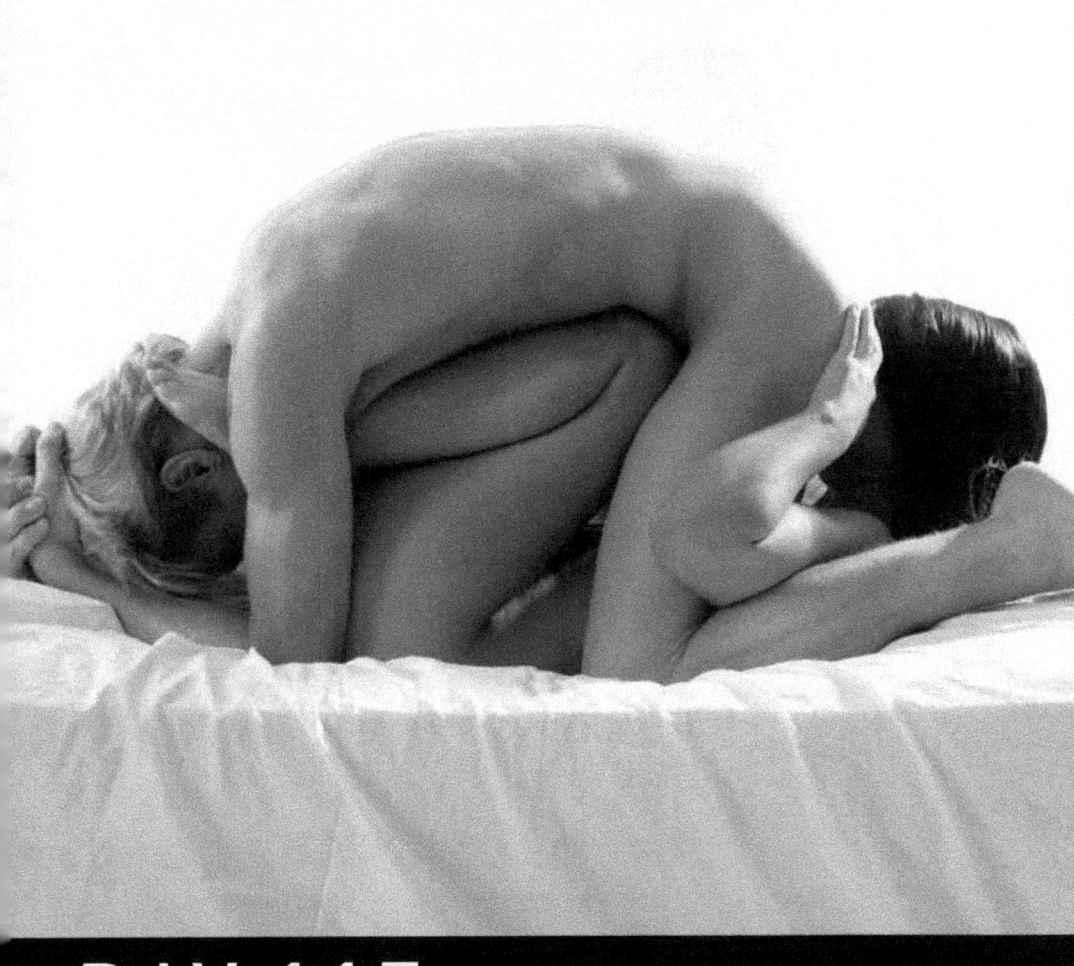

DAY 115

THE HOT PRETZEL

A variation on the classic 69 position, the woman lies on her back, bringing her knees up toward her chest. Her partner straddles her, lowering his genitals to her mouth as he leans forward to administer a thorough licking of his own.

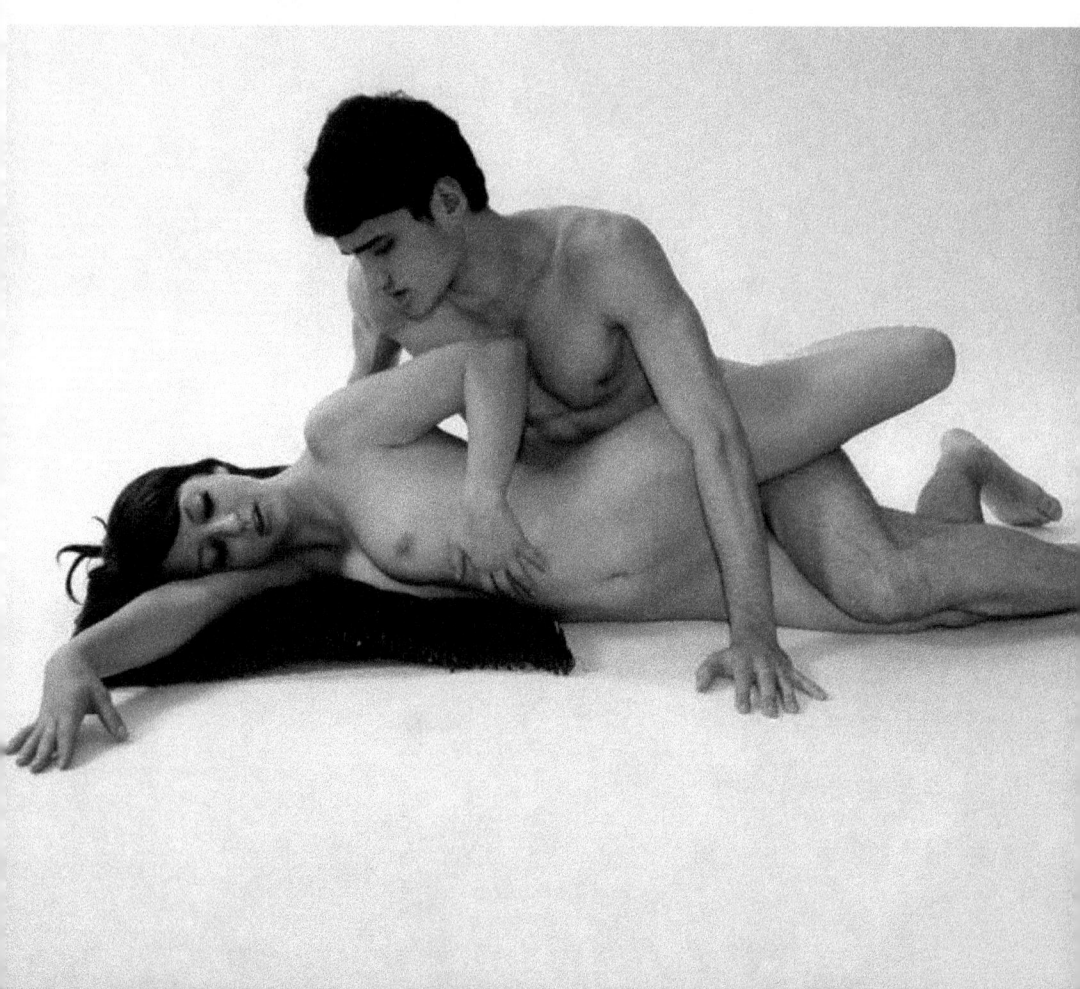

DAY 116

DOWN AND DIRTY

The woman is on her side and as her partner slides up between her legs, keeping his torso perpendicular to hers. As he penetrates her, she curls her top leg over his thigh so that her calf is resting against his buttocks.

DAY 117

BLOW ME DOWN

The man climbs atop a stool or coffee table as the two women let their mouths and tongues linger over his penis and testicles. If he gets weak in the knees, look out below!

DAY 118

STRANGERS IN THE NIGHT

The lovers stand, the woman with her back turned to her partner. She lifts one leg off the floor and bends her knee as he penetrates her. He can help support her leg or run his hands down the length of her body.

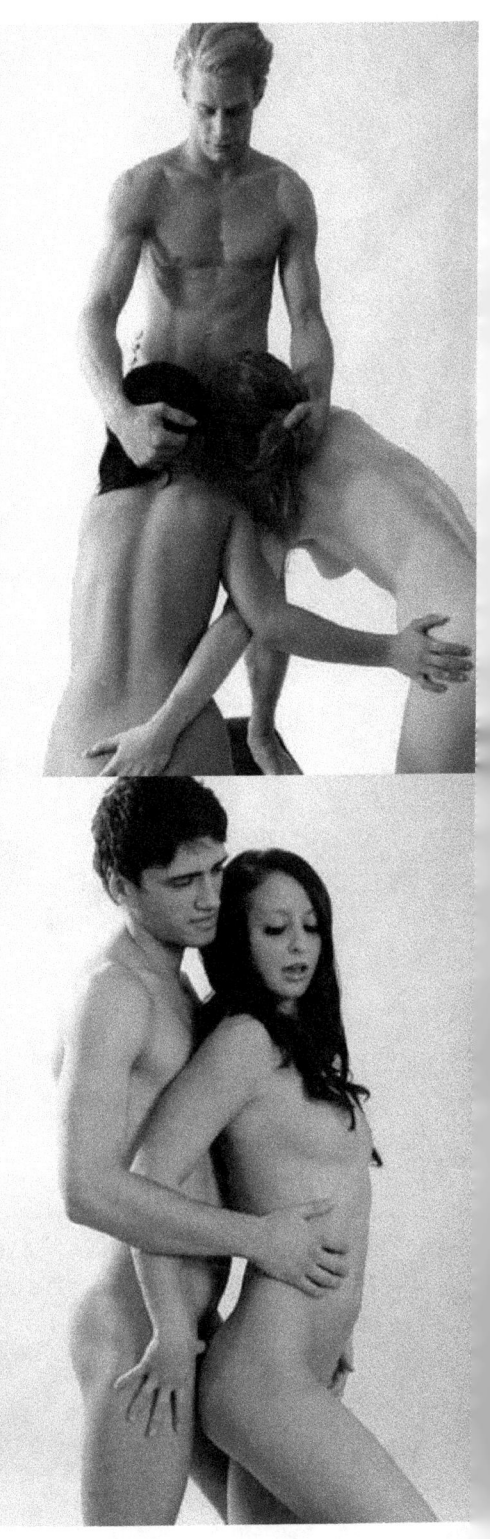

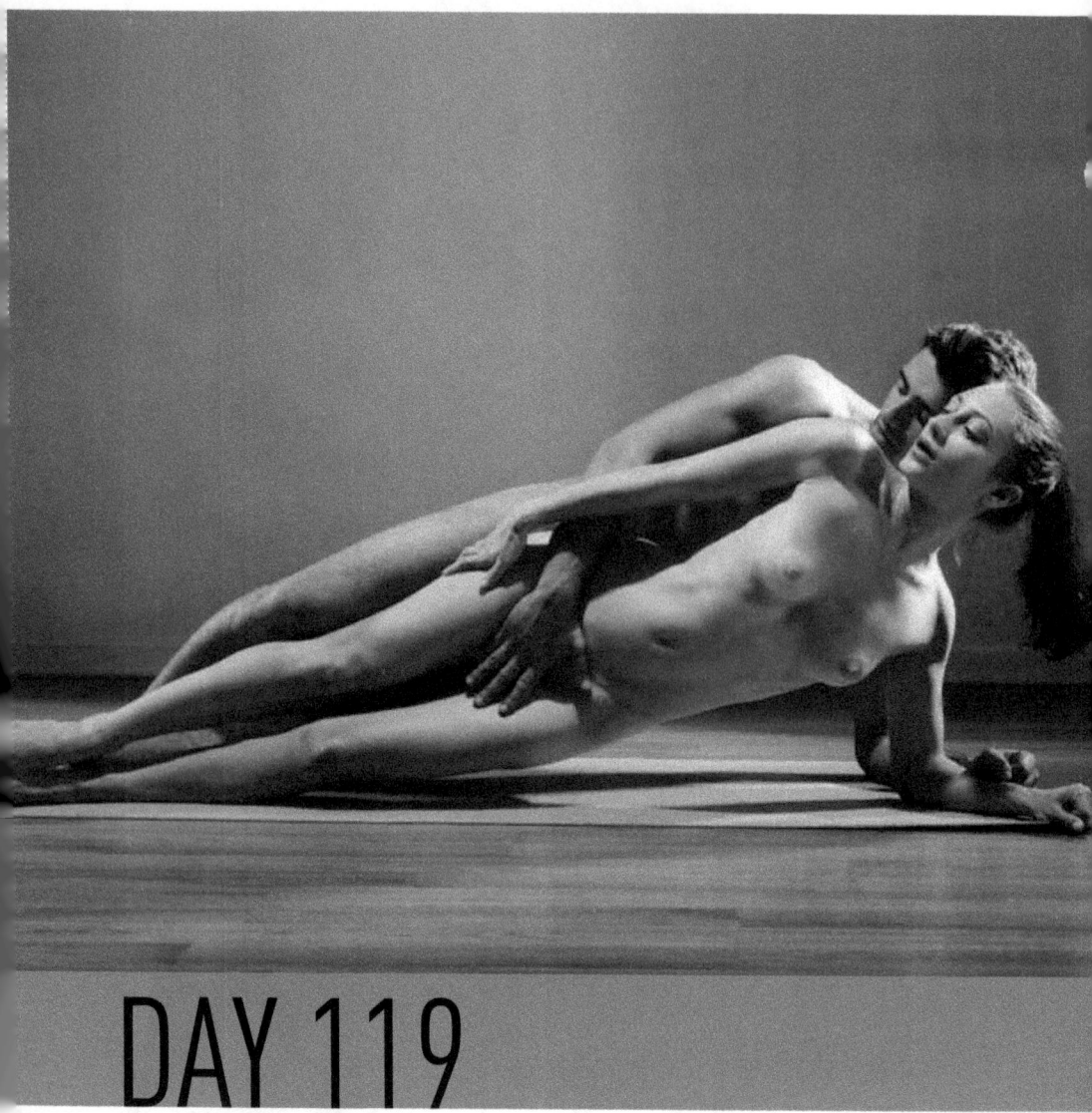

DAY 119

SIDE AND SEEK

The couple position themselves on a yoga mat in a side bridge pose with the man behind the woman. She keeps her body in a straight line as he penetrates her, while he brings his hand around to stroke her clitoris.

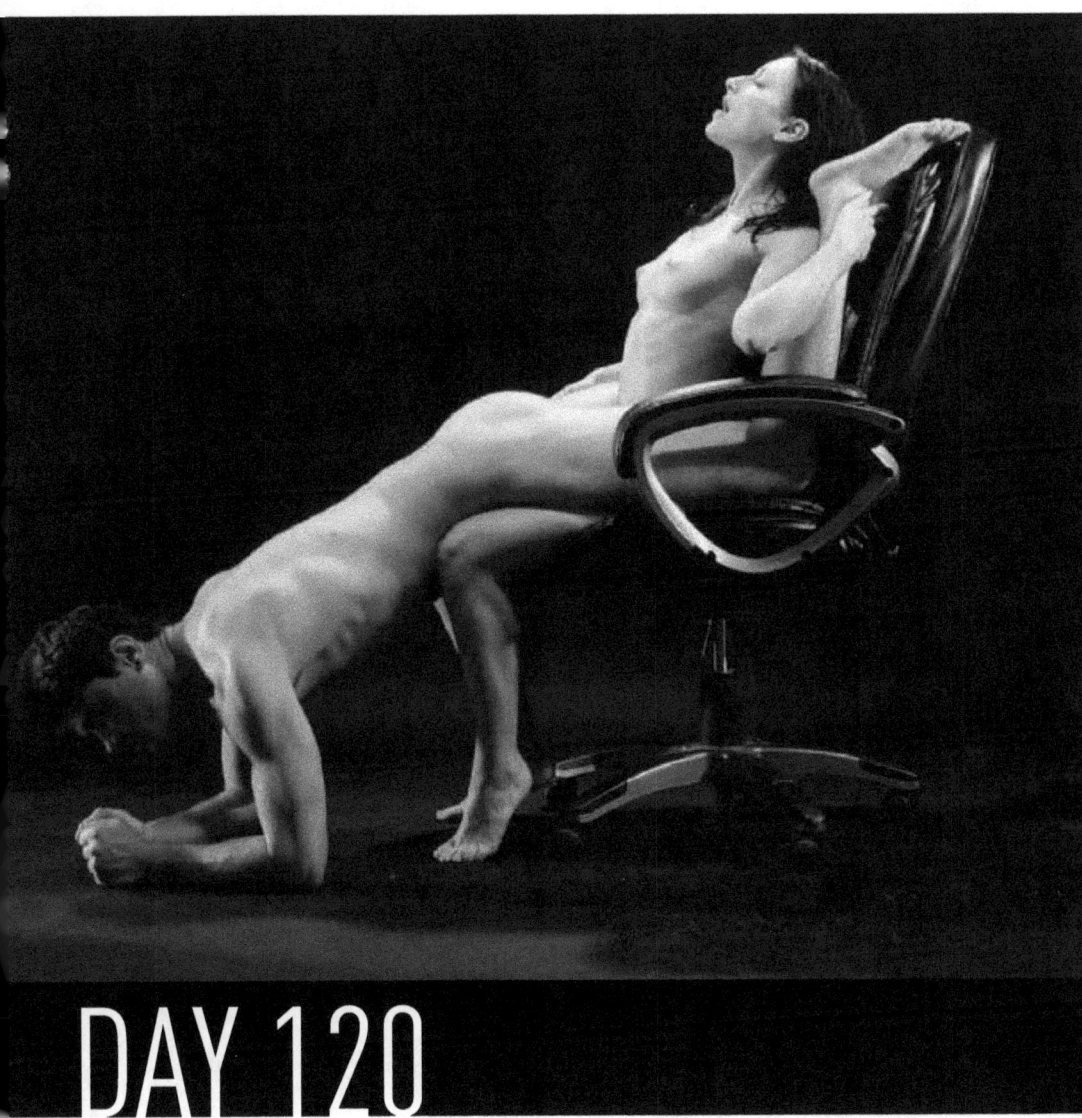

DAY 120

LOST CONTACT

She makes herself comfortable in a chair while her partner rests his forearms on the floor and brings his legs up and back. His butt is at her mercy as they achieve a very interesting angle of penetration.

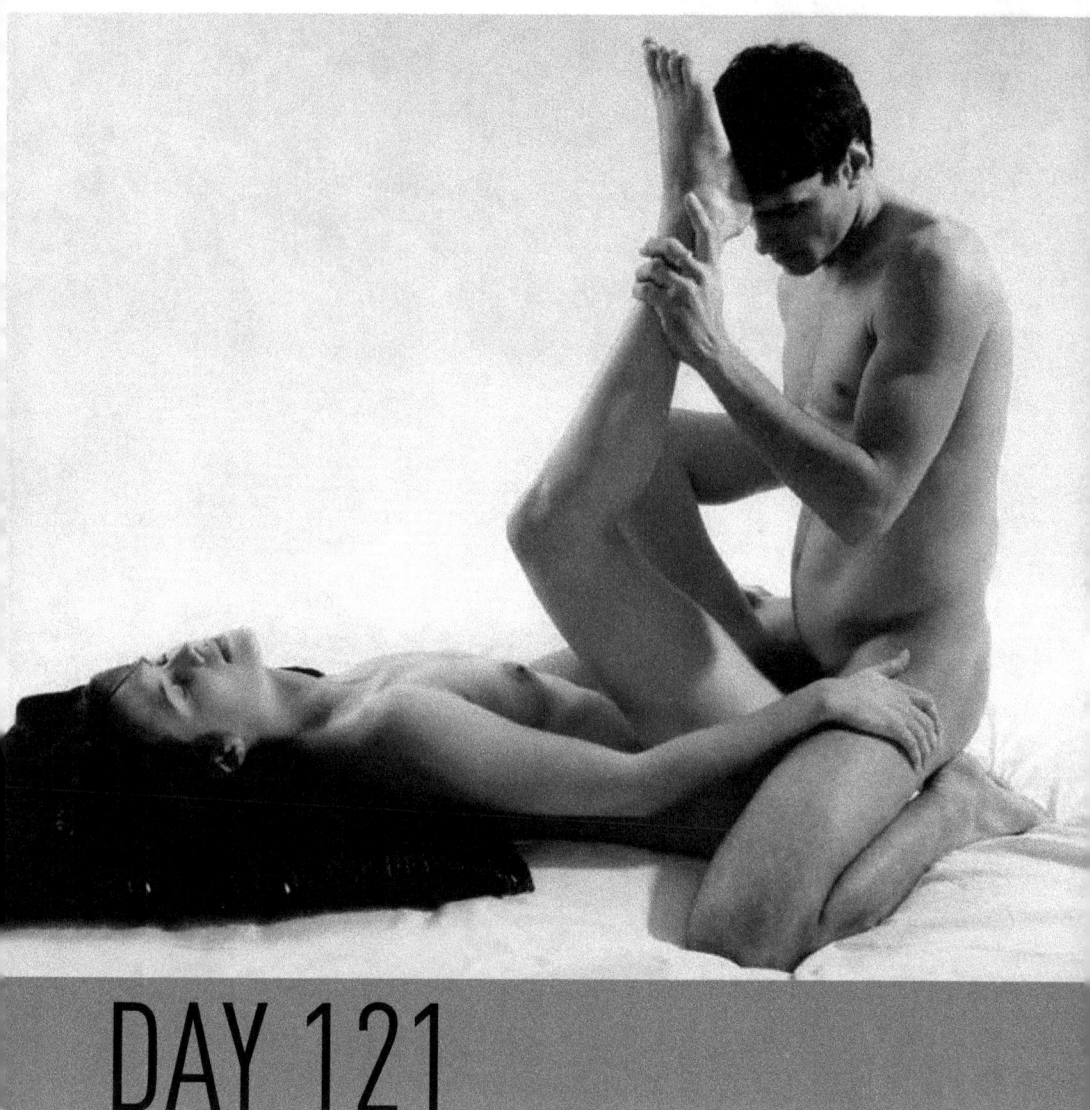

DAY 121

THE HEADLINER

From a kneeling position the man enters the woman while she rests the heel of her foot on his forehead. A position where two heads are indeed better than one.

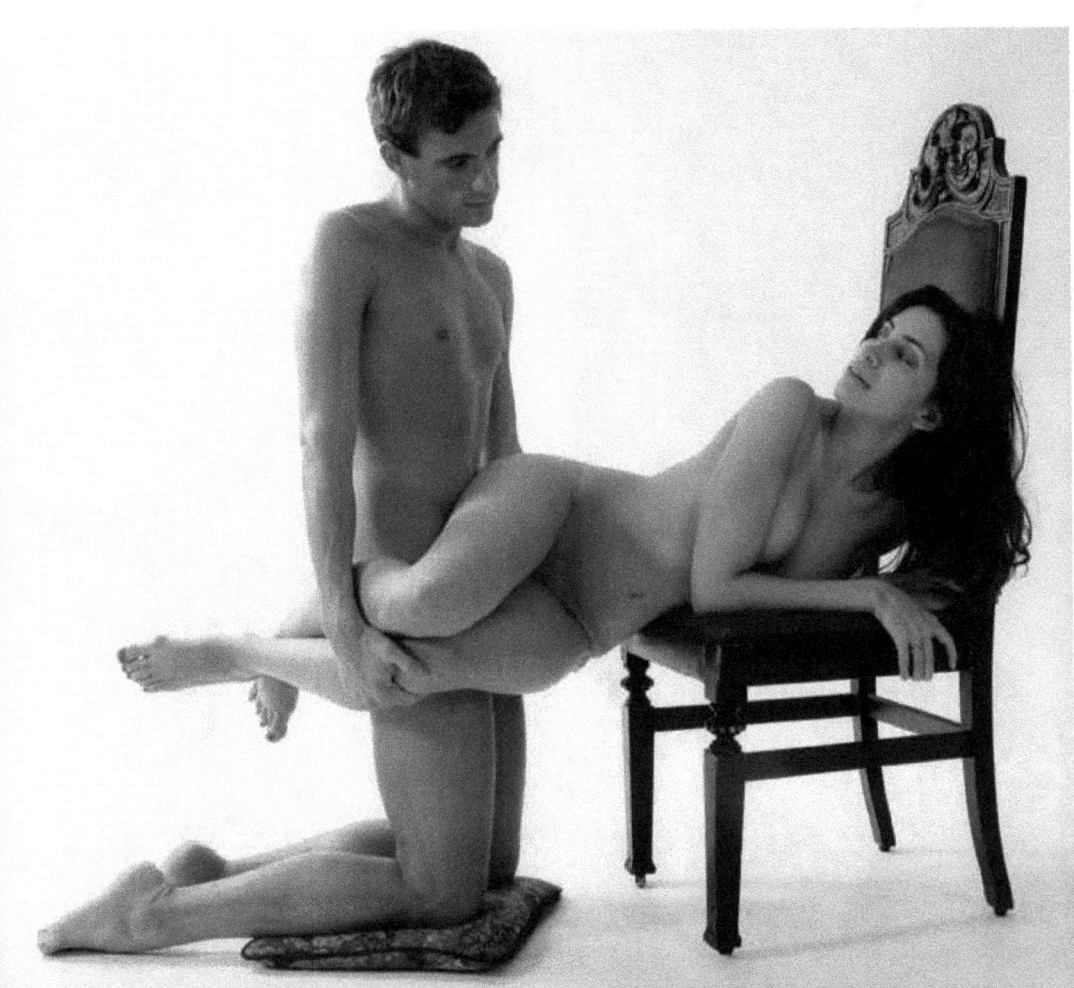

DAY 122

TWIST AND SHOUT

She twists her torso so that it's sideways in a chair. He enters her from a kneeling position as she curls her legs around his thigh. His hands are there to support and caress.

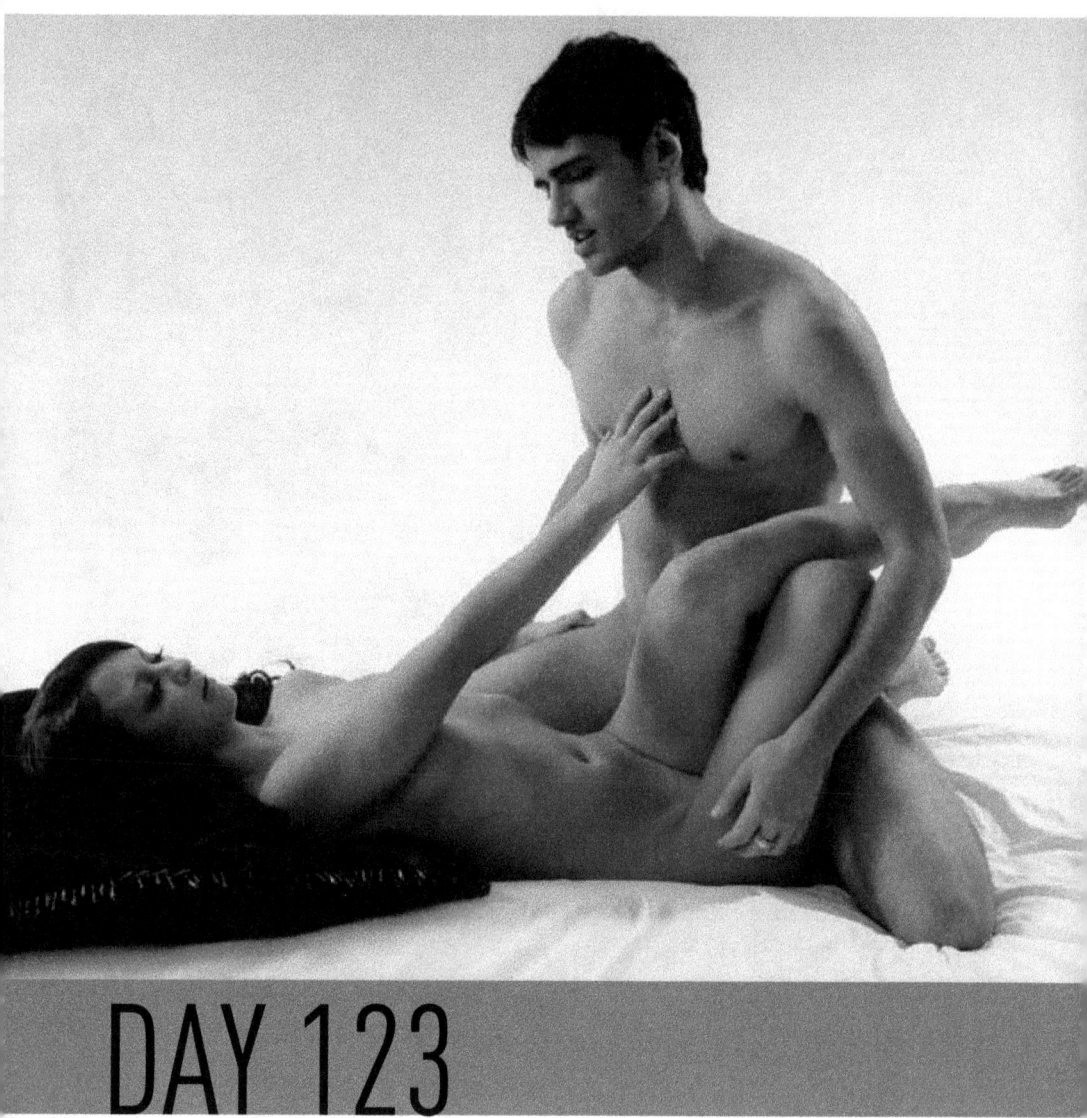

DAY 123

THE SEXY SWAY

The man sits back on his legs and penetrates his lover. She is on her back with her legs hooked around one of his thighs. From this position she moves her legs back and forth alternating sides. A useful technique for locating the G-spot

DAY 124

SPRING FLING

This one is best started on the bed. The woman climbs on top of her lover, facing him with her legs extended toward his head. He grasps her forearms and she holds onto his biceps as he slowly moves into a standing posture. She hooks her feet around his head for more support. It's best to keep this one close to a soft landing spot.

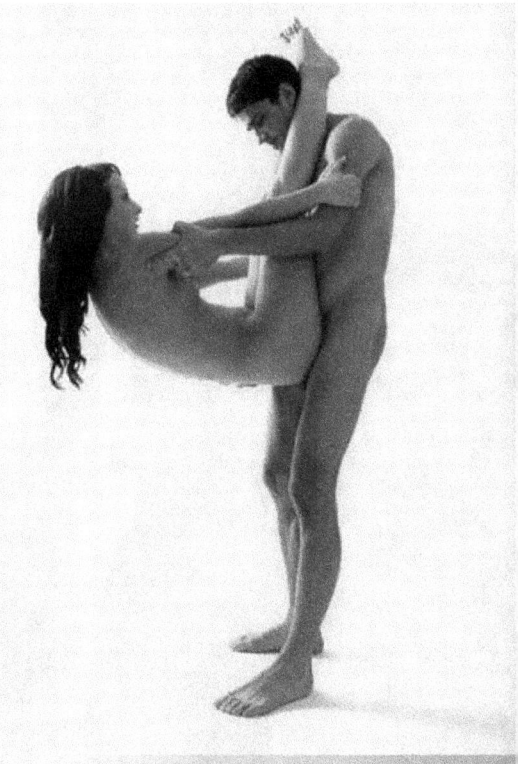

DAY 125

"C" IS FOR CONTROL

The woman starts this position in her lover's arms, lifted off the floor, and facing him. She slowly lets go of him, leans back, and lowers her hands to the floor. Her partner supports her buttocks as her legs remain wrapped around his waist. Not easy, but oh so interesting.

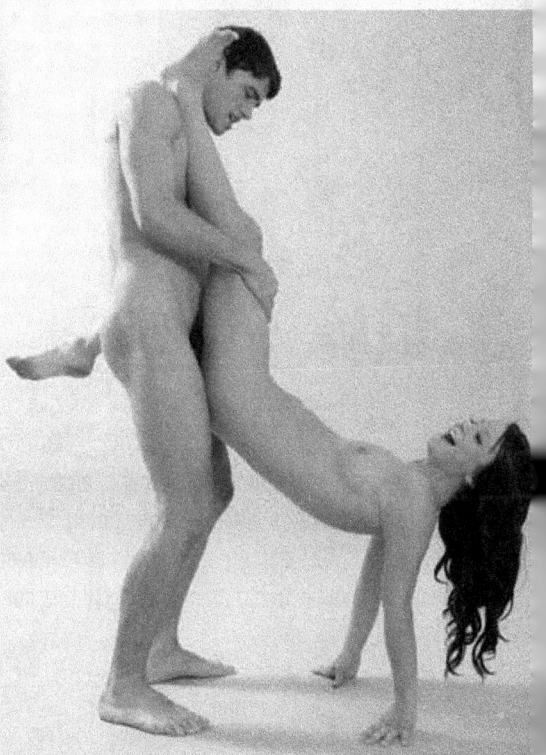

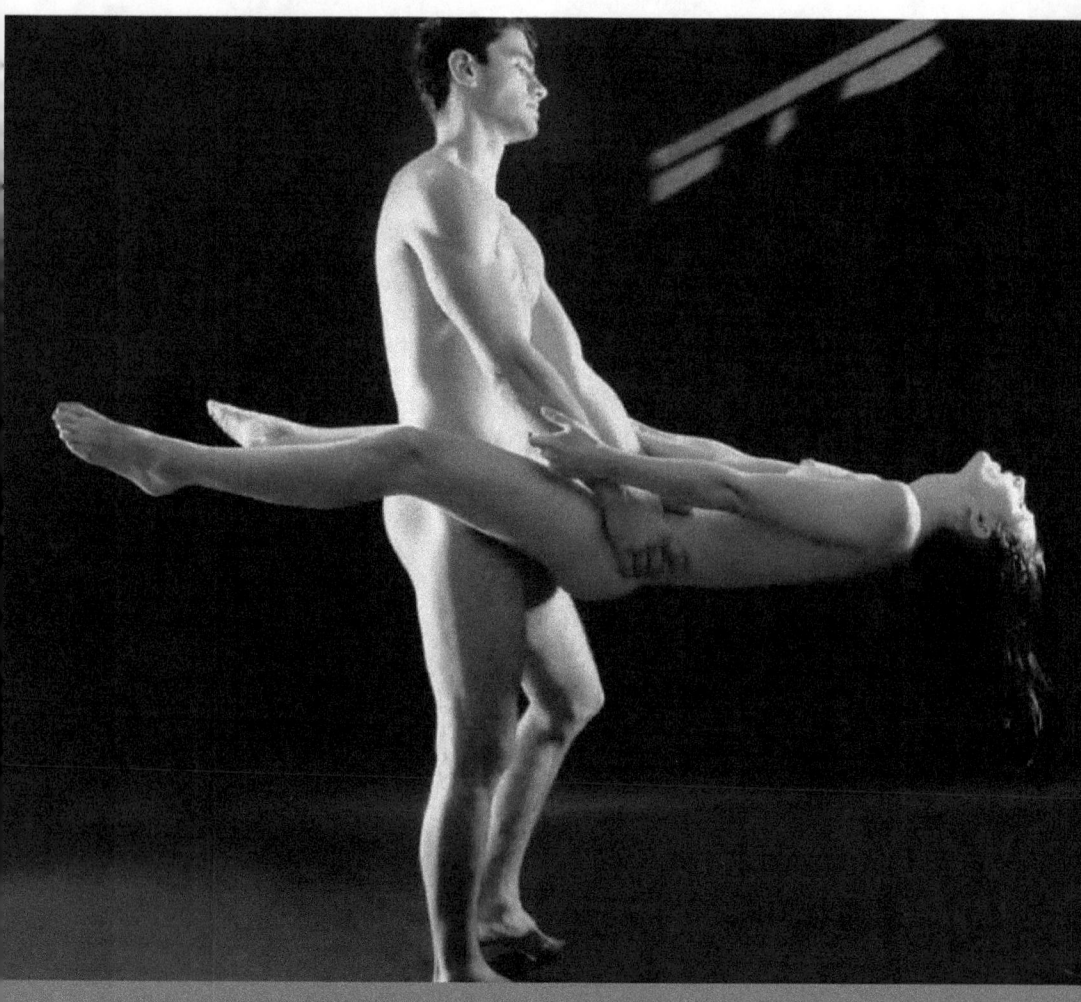

DAY 126

THE LEVITATING LADY

Here's one that takes an enormous amount of skill and strength. The lovers start in a standing position as she climbs onto his penis, wrapping her arms around his shoulders. She slowly lowers herself back until her hands are locked around his wrists and she's completely perpendicular to him. It's best to try this one near the bed until you get the hang of it.

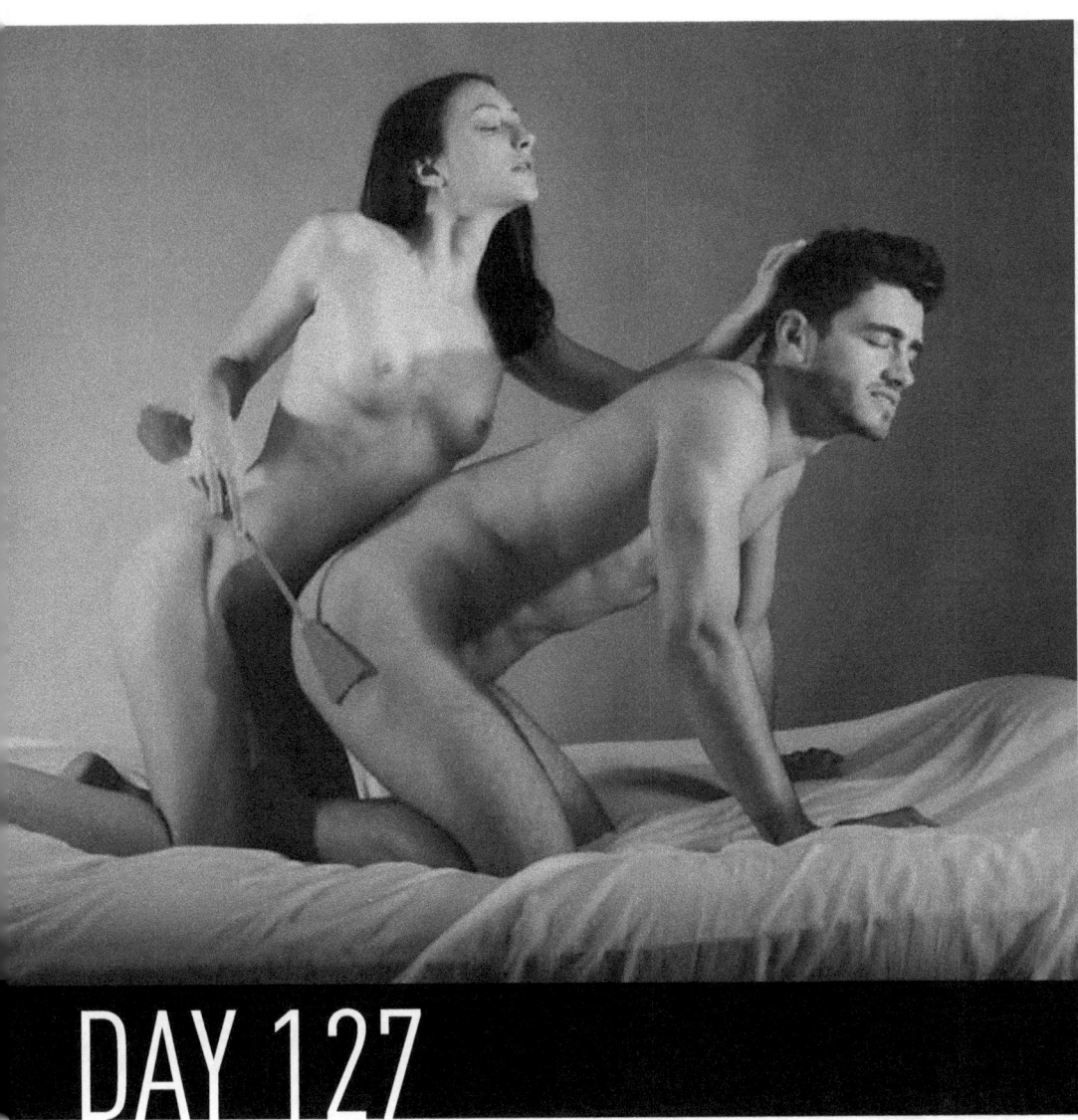

DAY 127

THE WILD MUSTANG

In a little bit of foreplay role reversal, the man assumes a doggie position on the bed while his partner takes her place behind him. She uses one hand to spank his haunches with a riding crop. Her other hand is free to run through his hair or play with his penis and testicles.

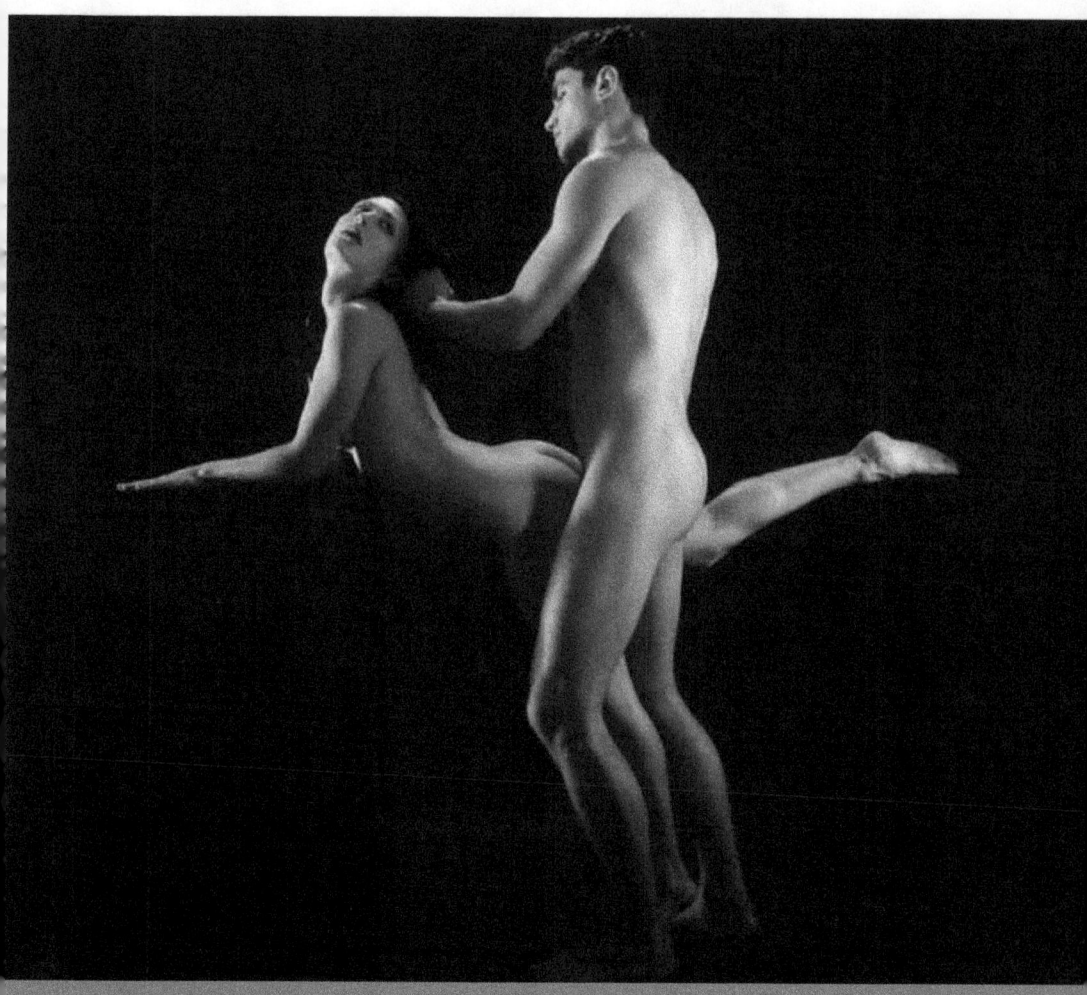

DAY 128

LEG SHOW

You don't have to be a "leg man" to enjoy this position. The woman leans her torso forward, placing her hands on a desk or dresser while bringing one leg straight back and up. Her partner cradles her luscious limb in his hand as he enters her deeply.

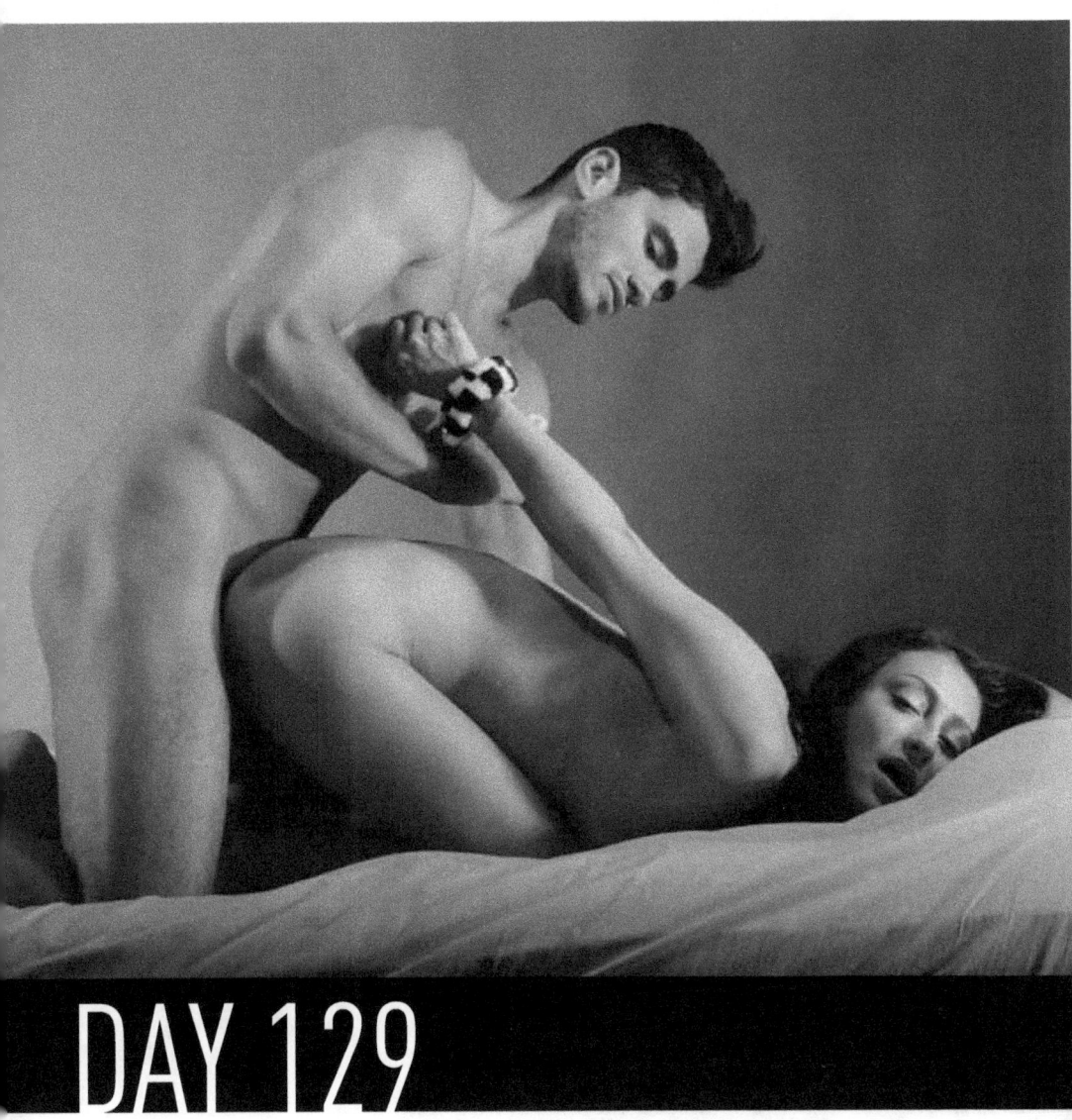

DAY 129

CUFF LOVE

You can use this position for some cop/criminal role play or just for the fun of it. She's on the bed in a prone posture with her head down and hands cuffed behind her back. He enters his lover from behind as she begs him to go easy on her.

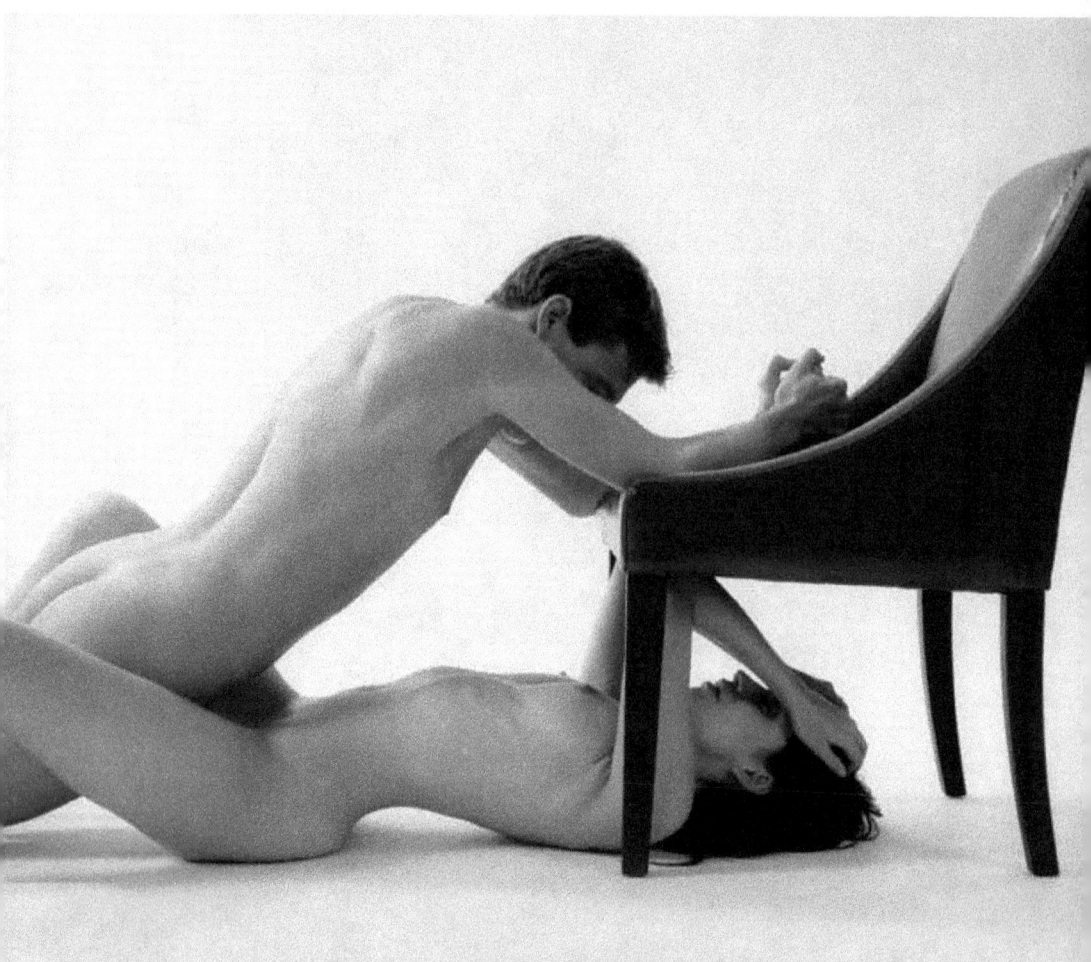

DAY 130

OUTTA SIGHT

Nothing like a little hide and seek to spice things up. In this position, she lies on her back with her head and shoulders beneath a chair. Her lover enters her from a missionary pose as he rests his arms on the chair. As he thrusts away, the two never lay eyes on each other.

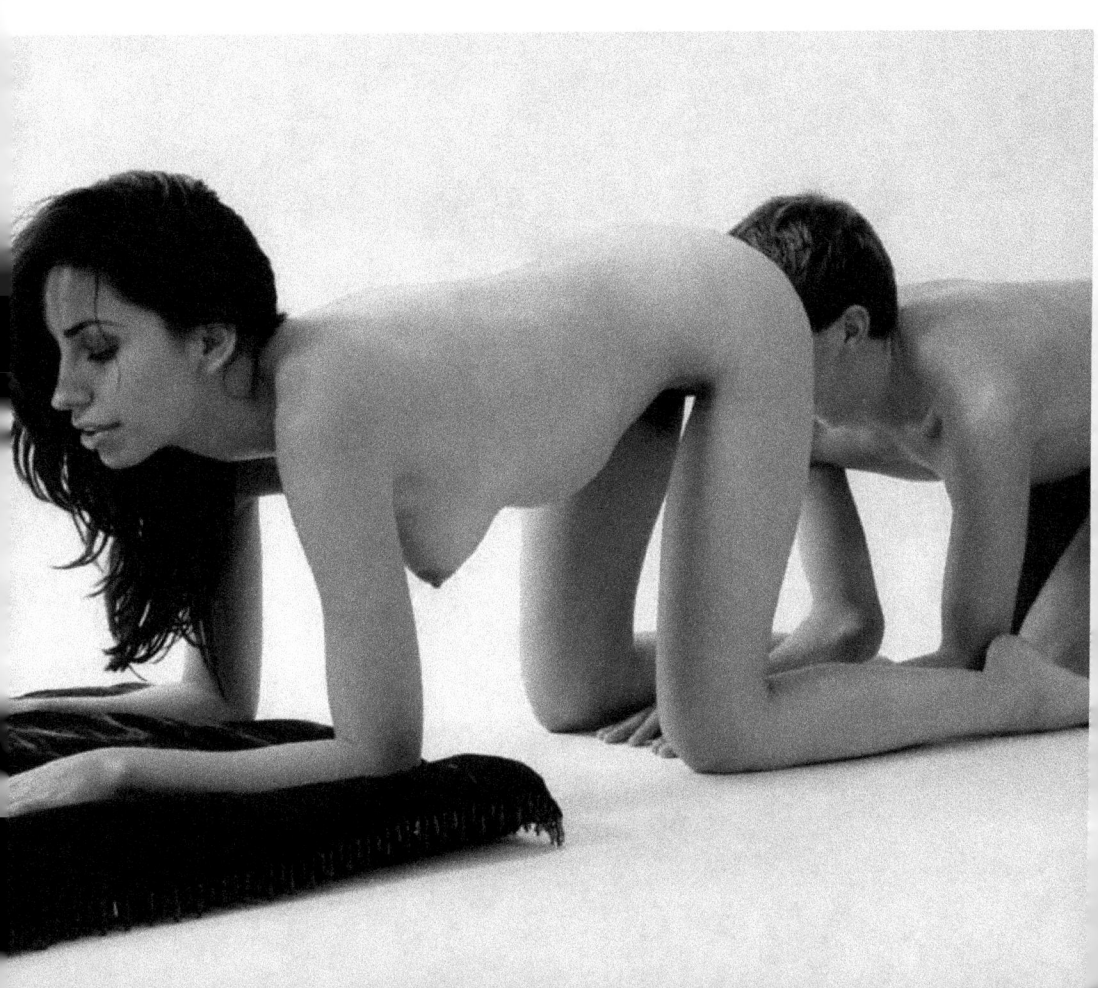

DAY 131

THE CURIOUS CAT

The woman gets down on all fours, her legs slightly parted, and rests forward on her forearms. Her partner playfully crawls in behind her like a cat drawn to a saucer of milk.

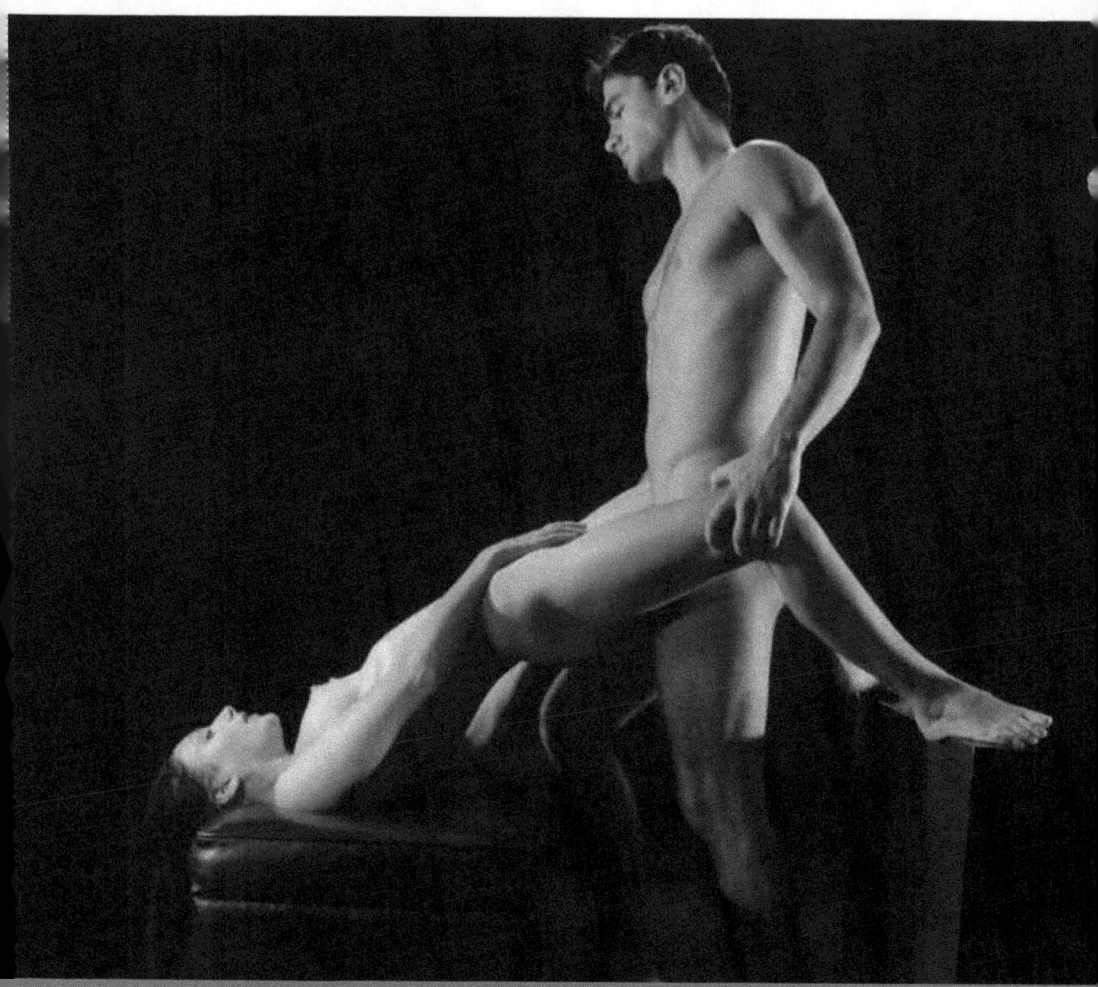

DAY 132

MOVING DAY

It's amazing how many uses you can find for any piece of furniture. The woman lies her head and shoulders back against an ottoman while bending her knees and resting her feet on a slightly taller piece. Her lover positions himself between her open legs and enters her. His hands are there for support and stimulation.

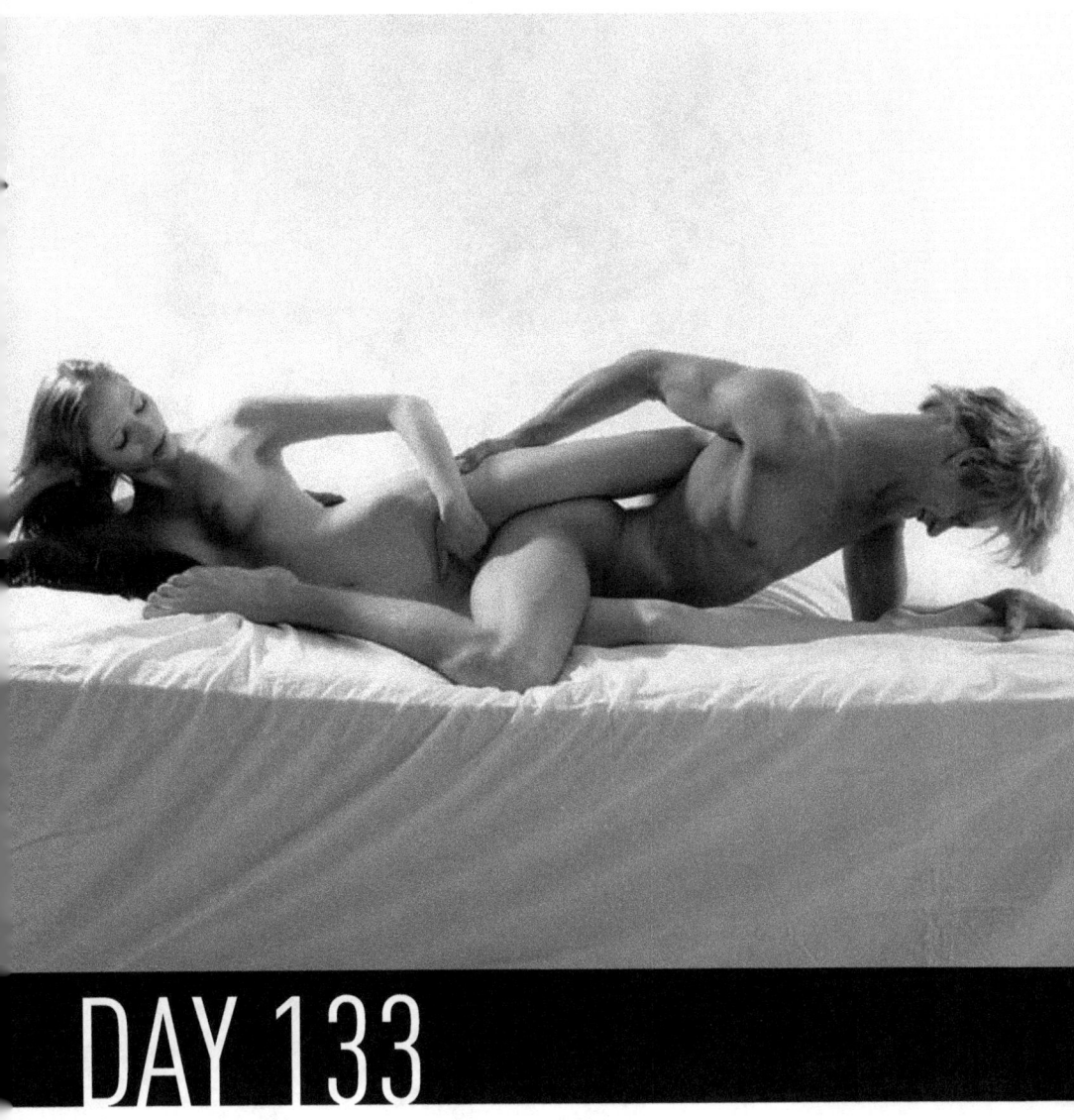

DAY 133

THE FINAL FRONTIER

The lovers stretch out on a bed in opposite directions. She's on her side with her legs parted while he's able to back his way into her vagina. Foot massage, anyone?

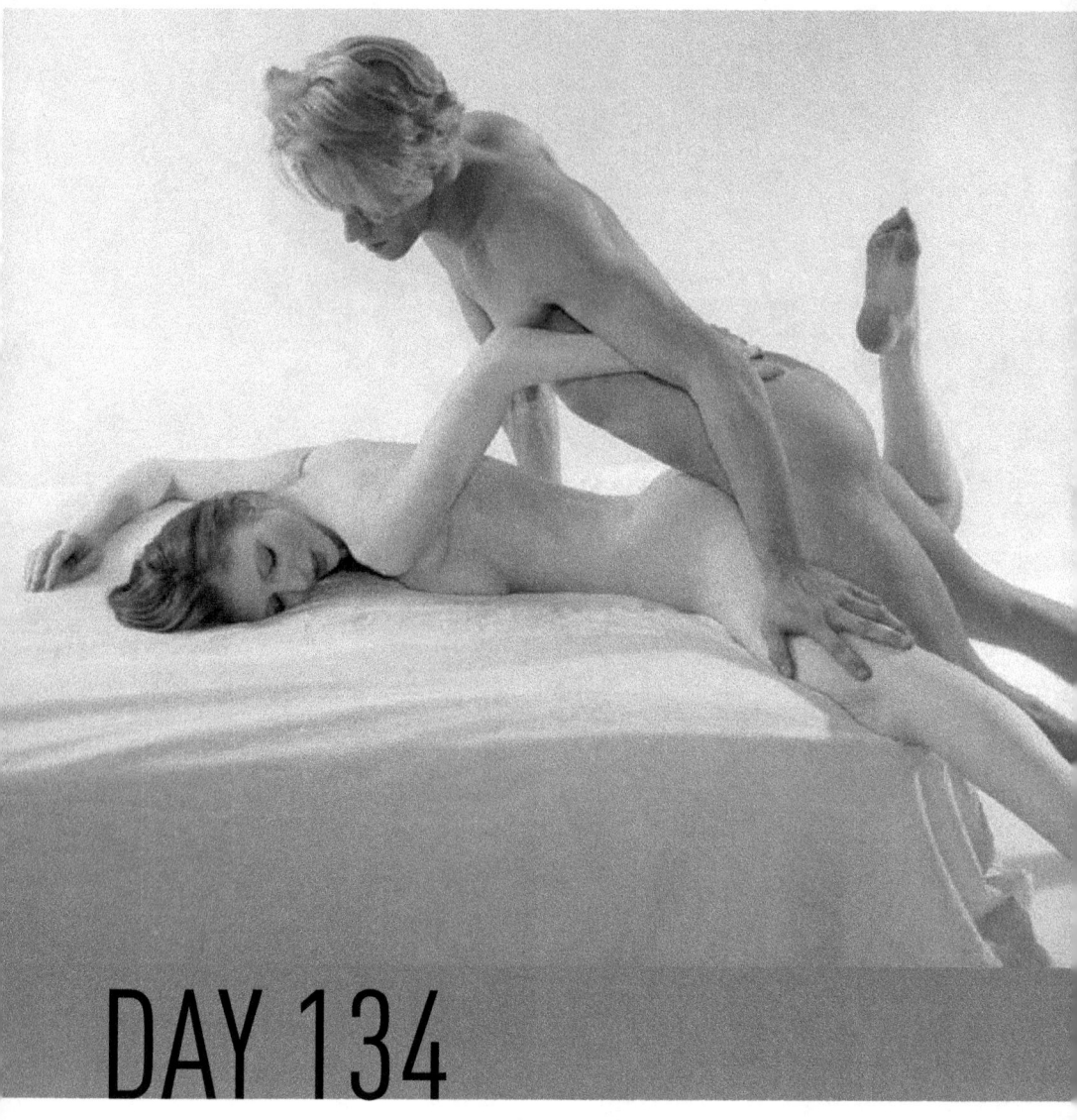

DAY 134

THE HALF AND HALF

She lies across the bed on her stomach with one leg out to the side and the other hanging off the edge. He lover straddles her leg and enters her from behind. As he thrusts she can use her thigh to tease his testicles.

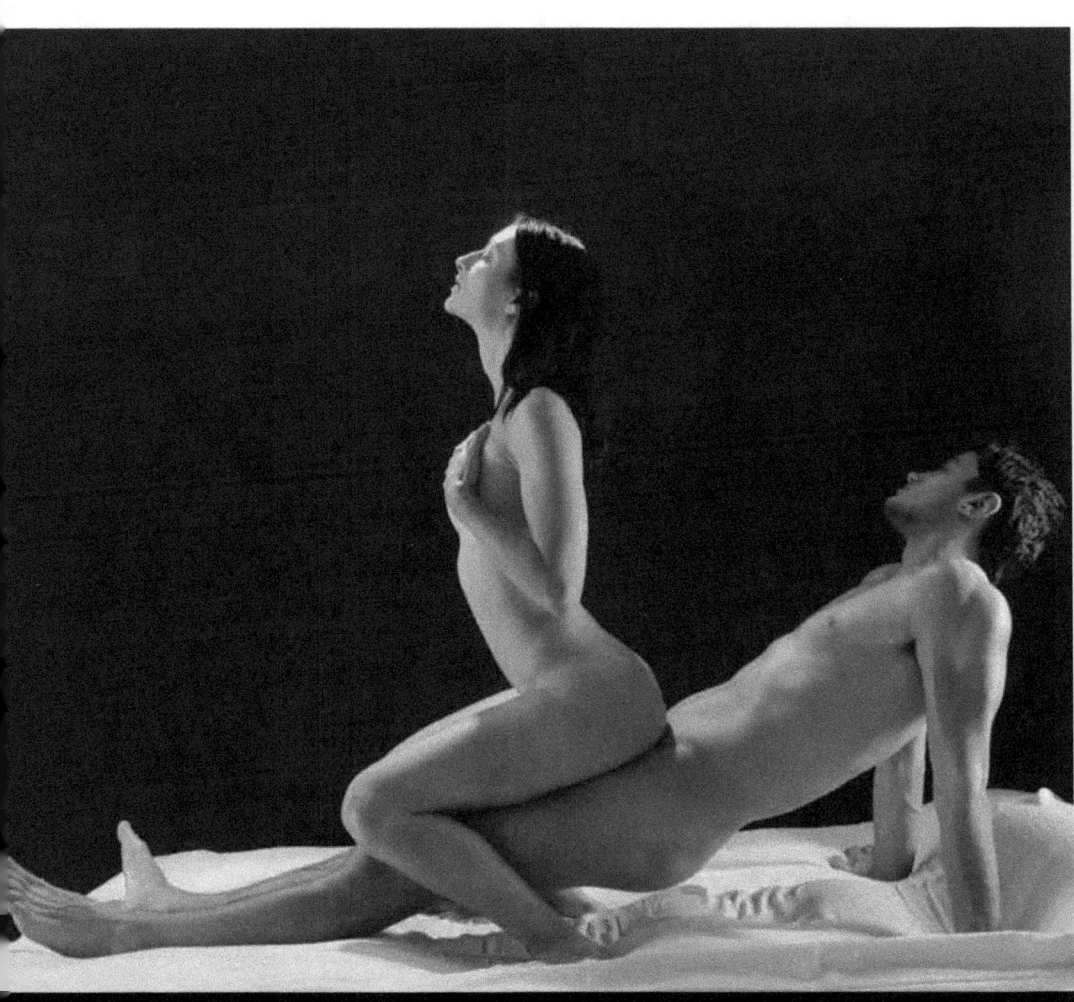

DAY 135

THE PONY RIDE

The man gets himself into a bridge pose facing upward with his legs extended and arms back and down. His lover climbs aboard, placing her feet down to either side. Giddy up!

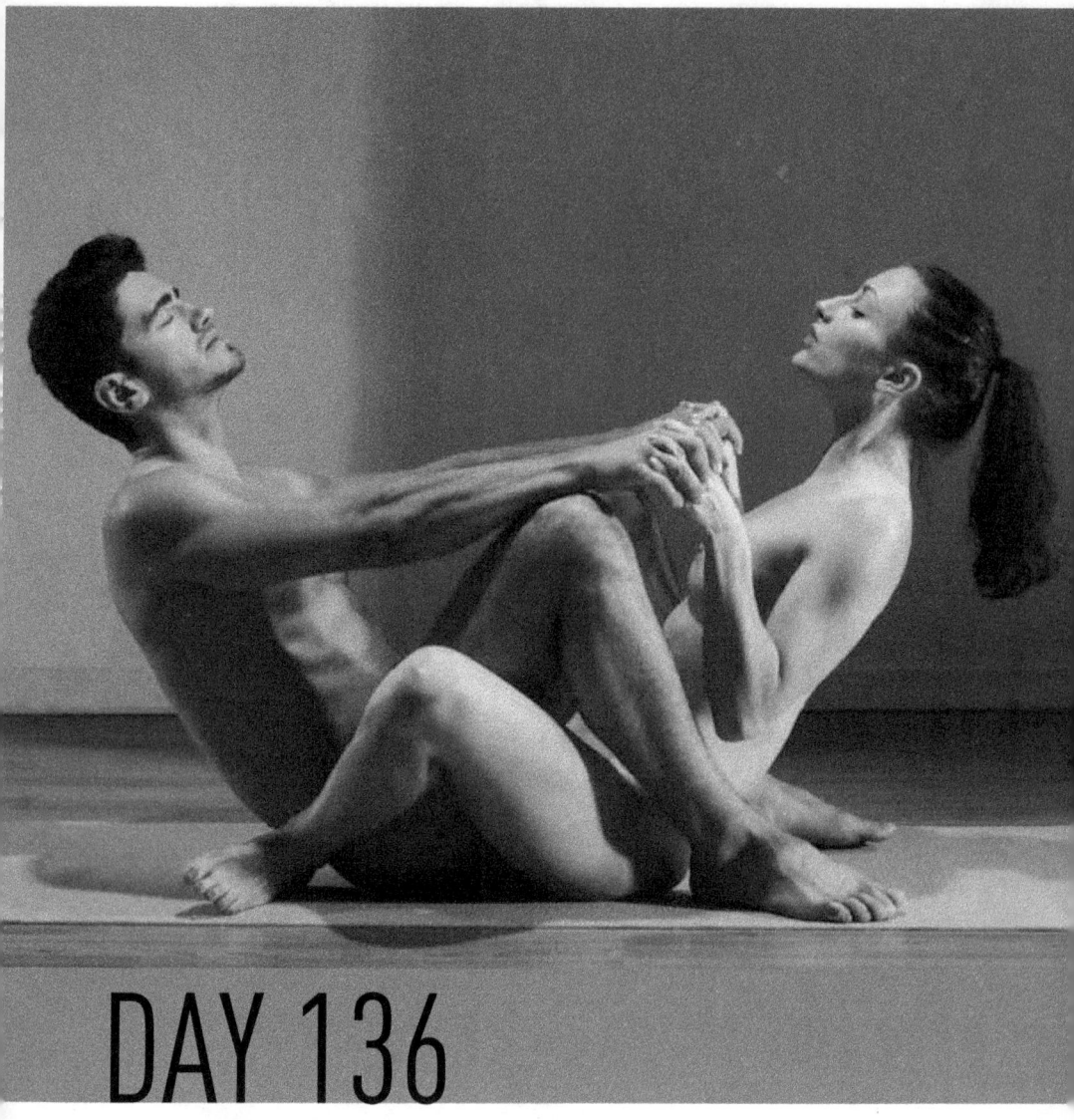

DAY 136

FAB ABS

The couple sit on an exercise mat facing each other with his legs overlapping her thighs. They pull themselves close enough so that he's able to penetrate her vagina. Once inside they lock hands and take turns leaning back and forth while tightening their abdominal muscles.

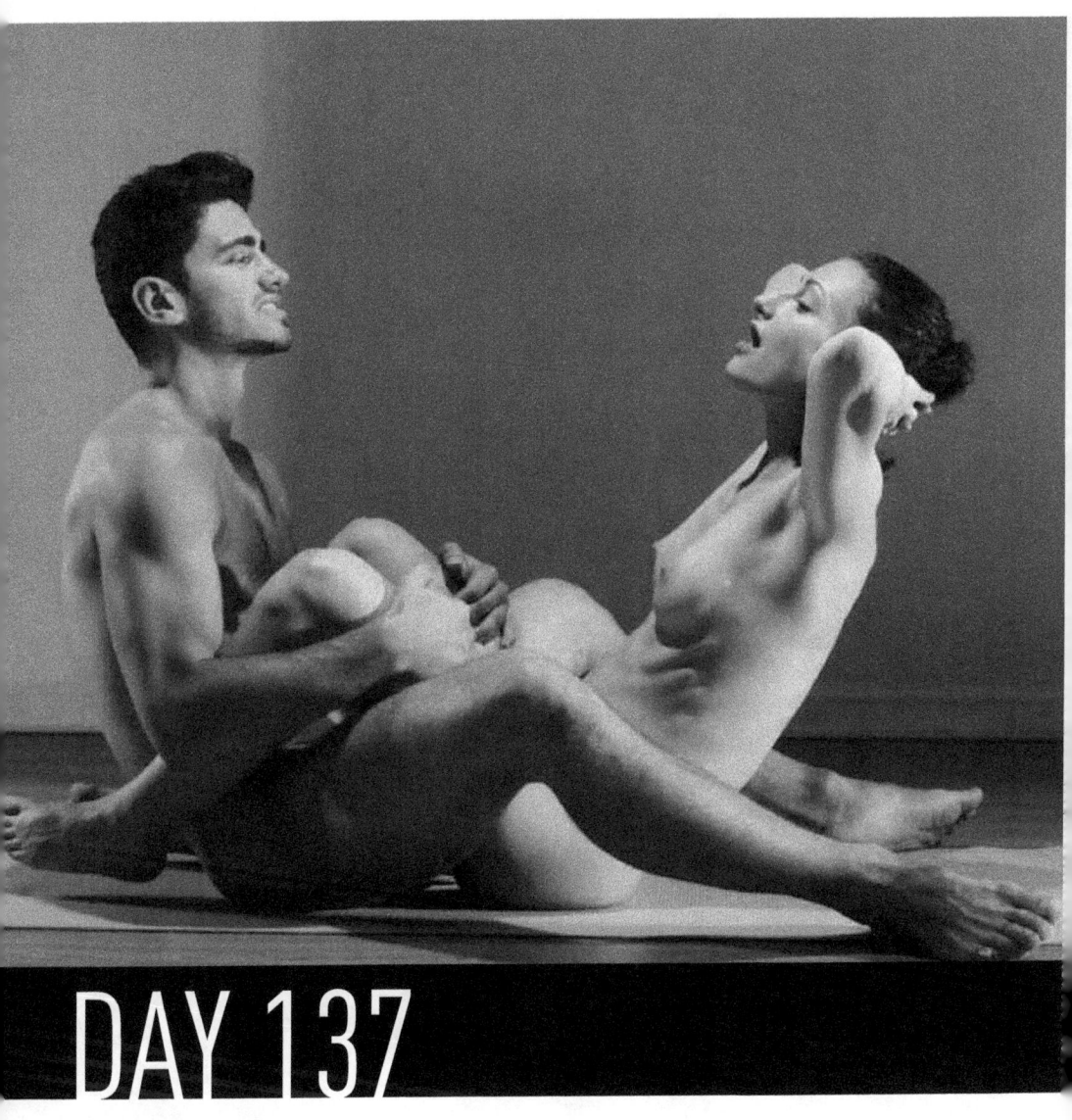

DAY 137

SIT-UP SEX

The couple sit facing each other on a yoga mat. She moves in between his legs allowing him to enter her vaginally. While he's inside her, he grabs her knees, allowing her to perform sit-ups. The sensations created by her movement are pretty intense—they'll both feel the "burn."

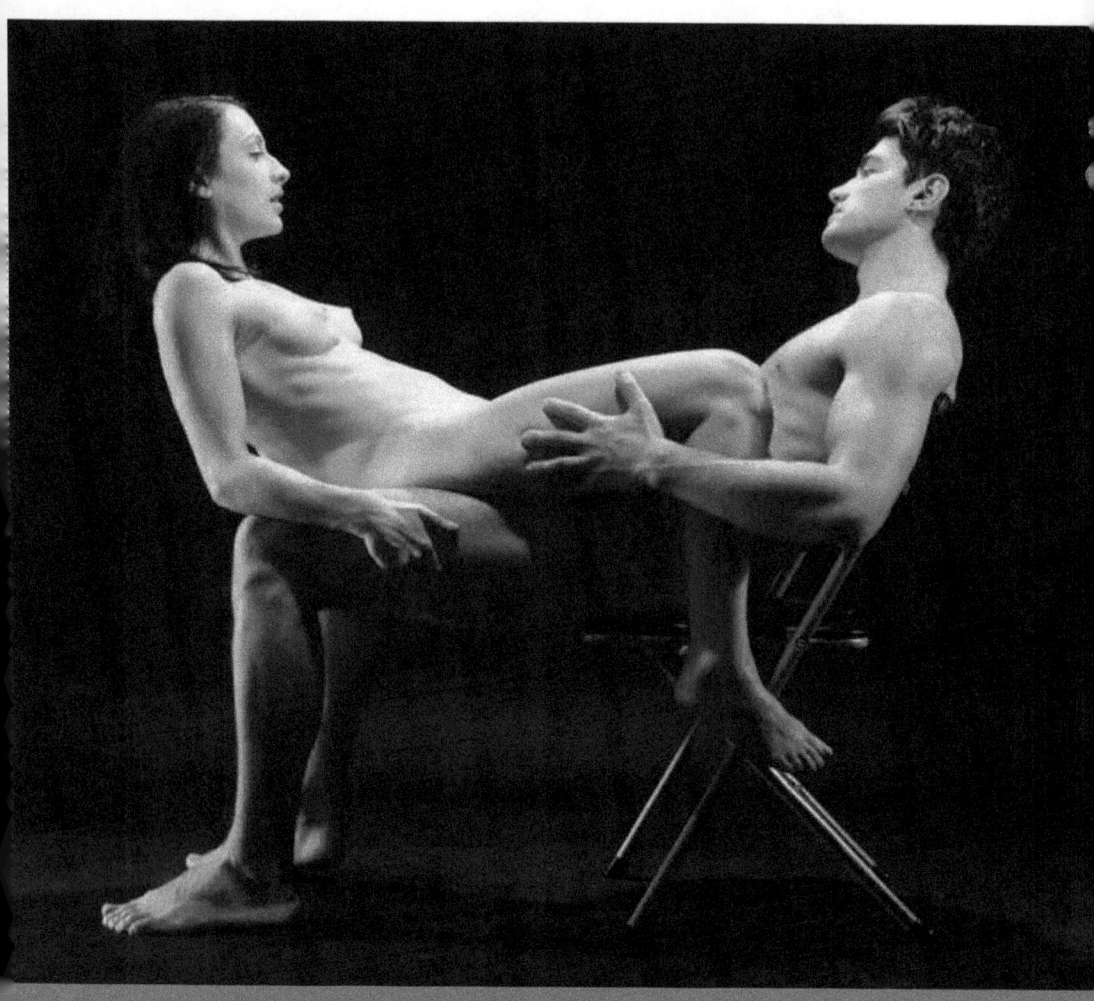

DAY 138

LET'S FACE IT

He sits low in a chair with his legs extended out and down, providing an ample seat for his partner to take. Facing him, she lowers herself onto his penis. She leans back in hopes of getting some G-spot activation.

DAY 139

CUSHIONED CONNECTION

With the help of a chair and a cushion, lovers can experience exciting new angles. She arranges herself sideways in a chair while he gets down on one knee in front of her. She rests her leg over her partner's thigh as he enters her. A cushion or pillow makes things much nicer for the knees.

DAY 140

FORBIDDEN FRUIT

The man and woman face each other as she holds a strawberry in her mouth and moves in to share it with her lover. As he samples her fruit she lifts her leg, allowing him access to her other gift.

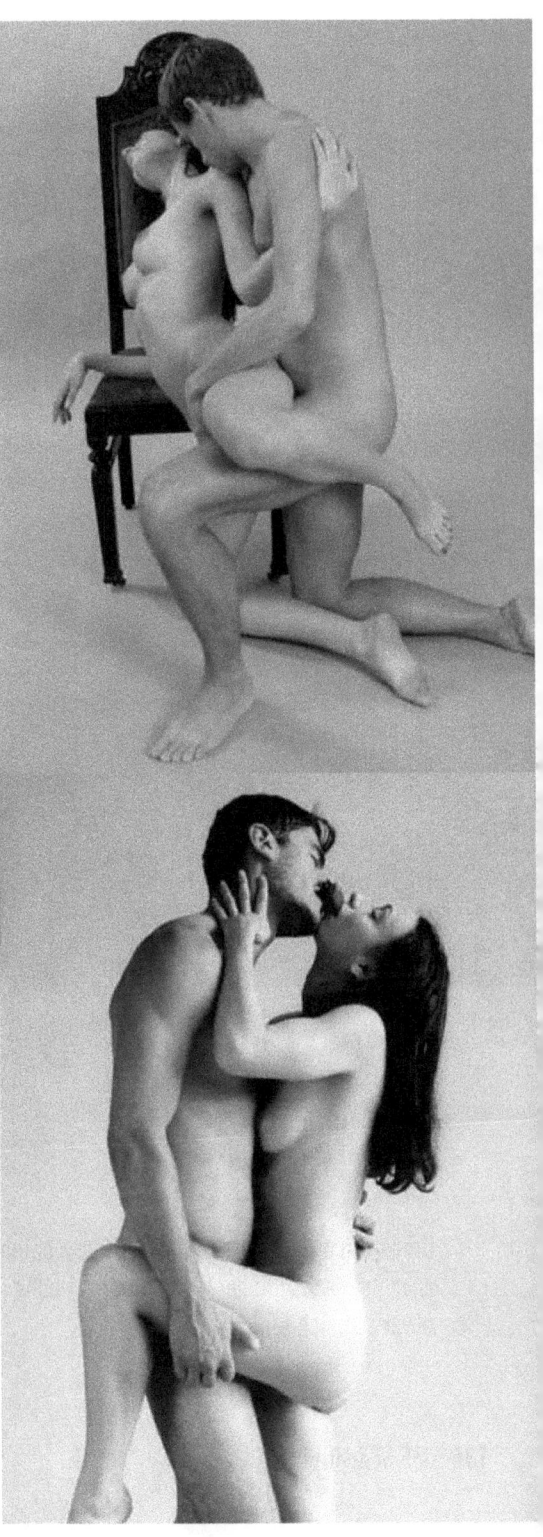

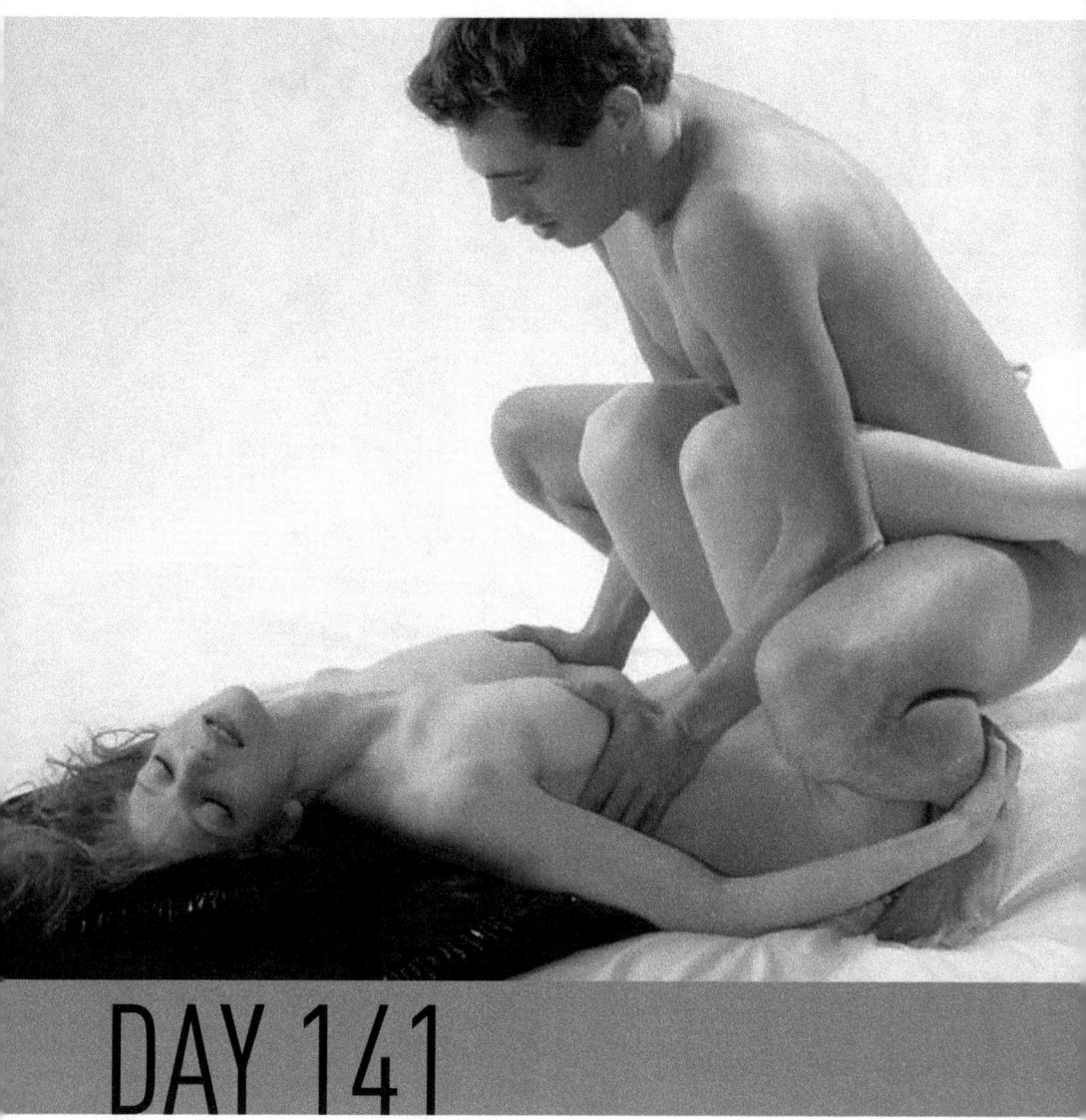

DAY 141

THE LUCKY CATCH

Crouching on the balls of his feet like a catcher, the man penetrates the woman. She is on her back with her legs up on his thighs as though she's sliding into home. Baseball was never so much fun.

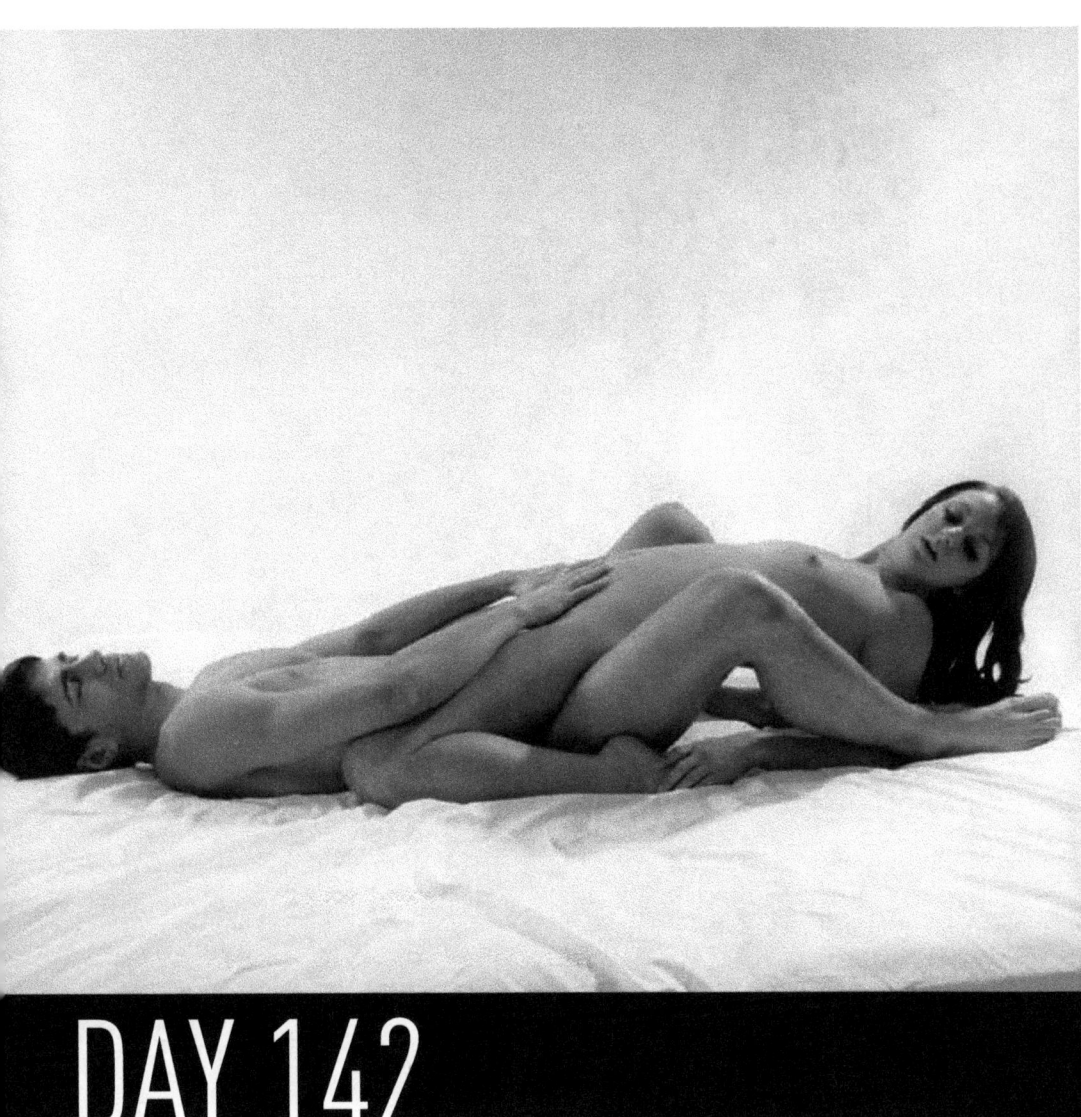

DAY 142

OPEN SESAME

The man is on his back with his legs extended and open. She's on top, facing him, with her legs bent back. As she leans back on her elbows, she opens her clitoris to her lover.

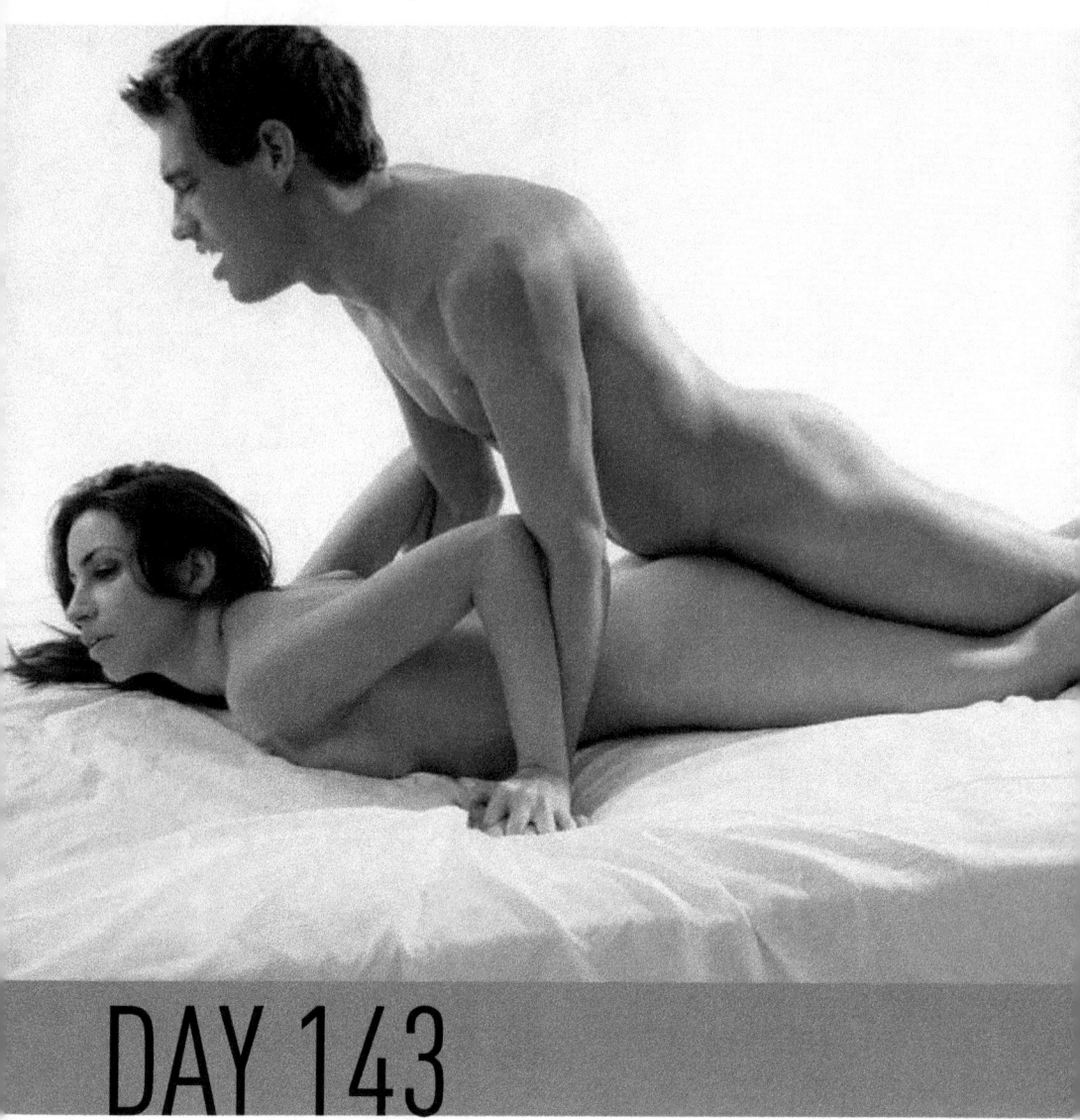

DAY 143

SWEET SKINSATION

The woman stretches out and lies on her stomach. Her partner does likewise on top of her, supporting himself with his arms. As he penetrates her, there is plenty of sensual skin-on-skin contact.

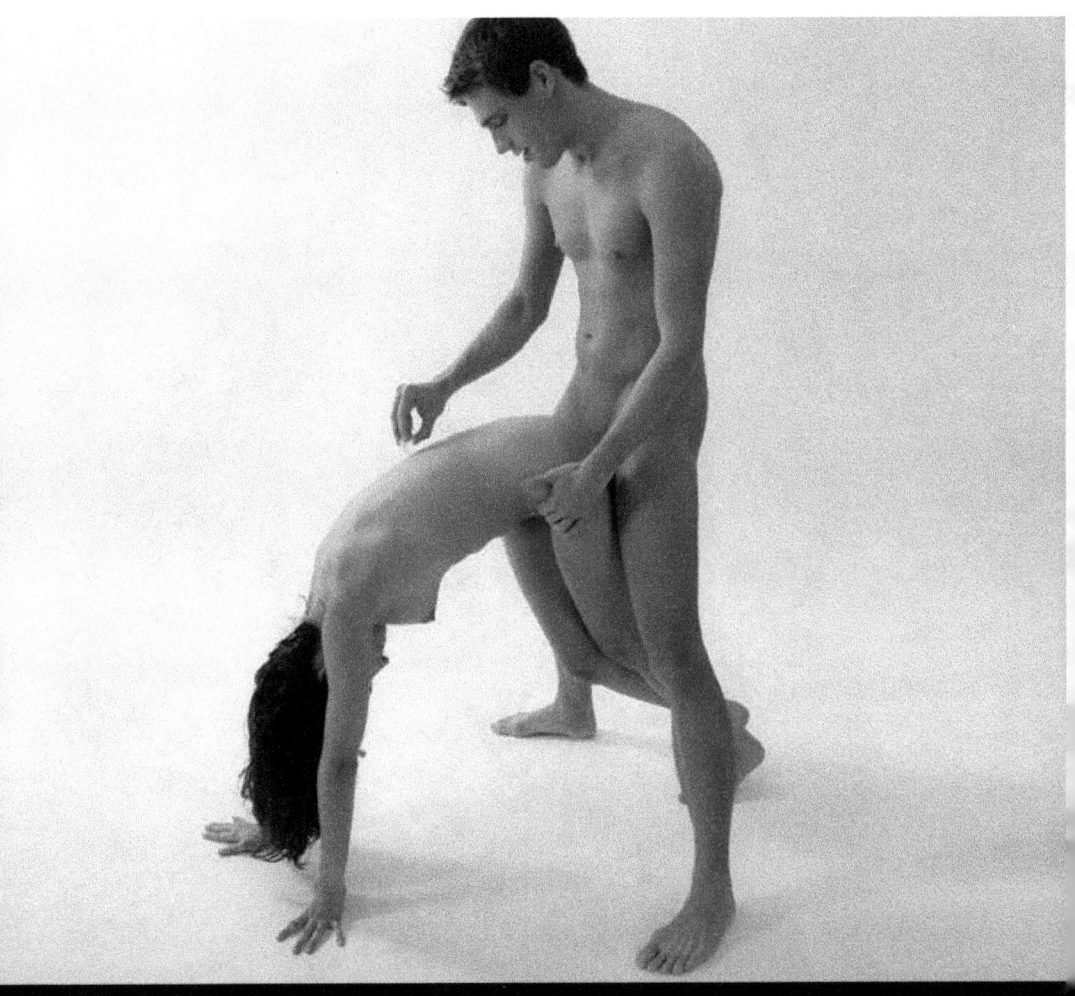

DAY 144

THE ICEMAN COMETH

She stands with her back to her lover as she bends over and reaches her hands toward the floor. As he enters her from behind, he slides an ice cube up and down her elongated spine.

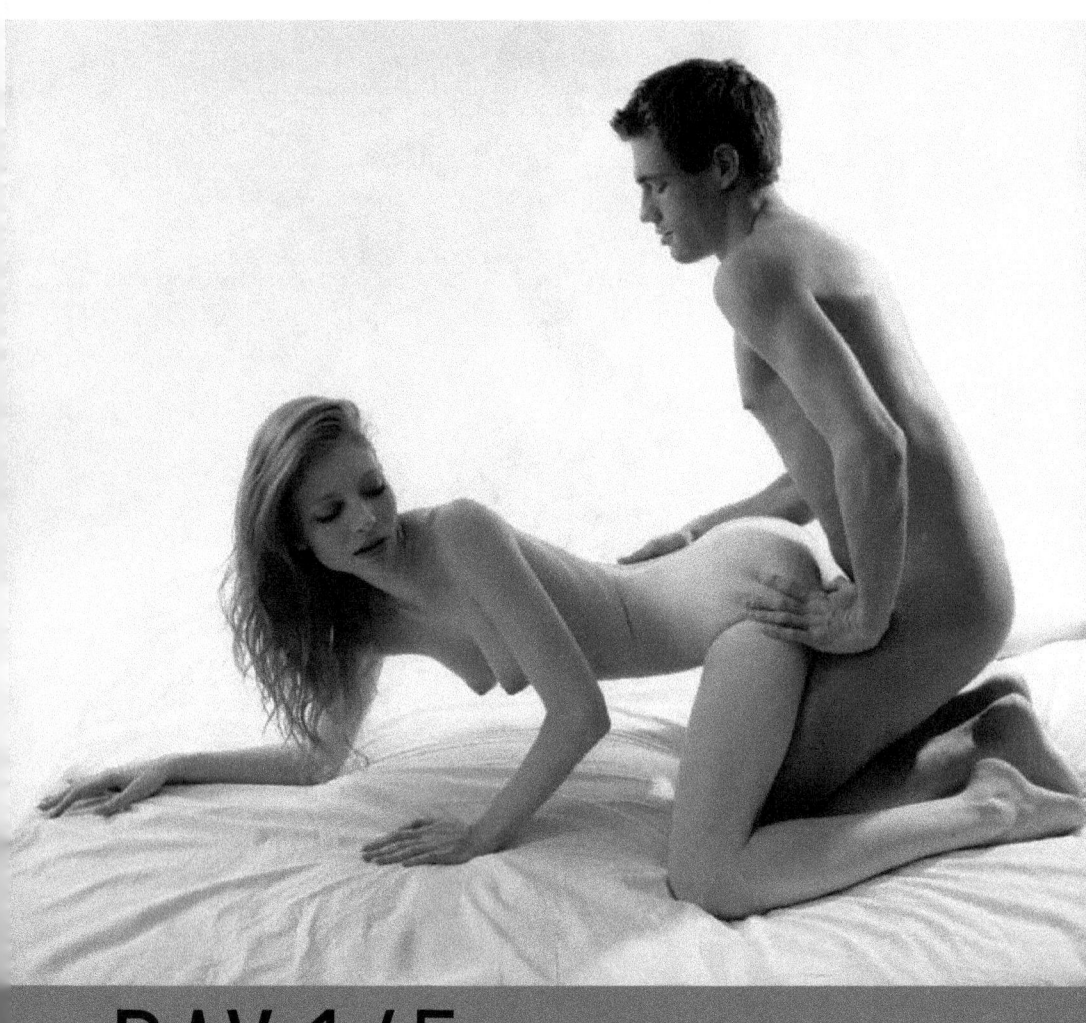

DAY 145

THE WICKED WINDMILL

The woman is on her hands and knees as her lover mounts her from behind. She meets his thrusts by extending one leg back and then the other in a windmill fashion. The angle of entry changes with every motion. Some pillows may be required for extra support.

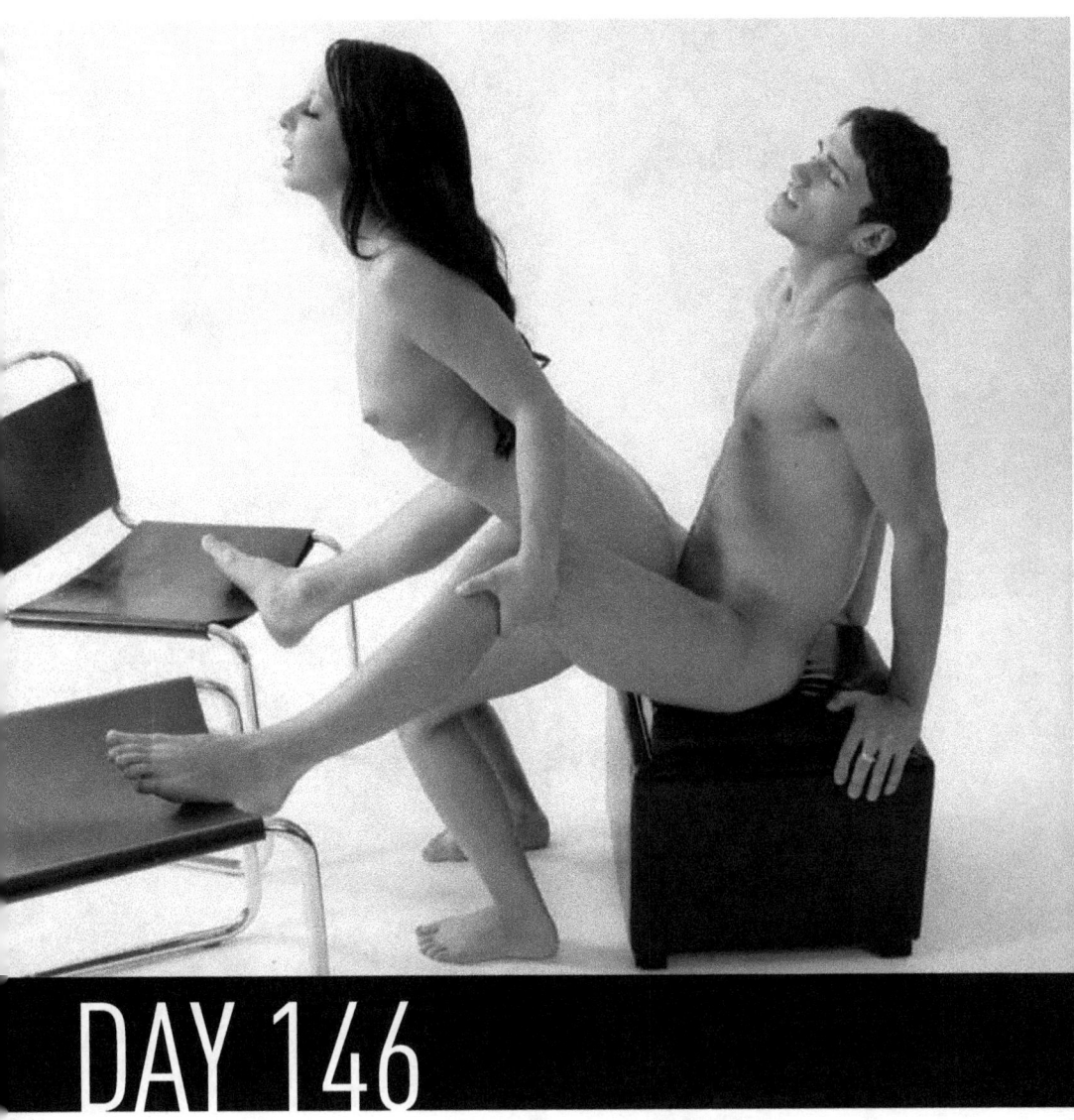

DAY 146

STUCK IN THE MIDDLE WITH YOU

This fun maneuver requires three chairs. He places his hands back against a chair or ottoman while supporting each of his feet on a separate chair. From the middle of the triangle, she lowers herself down onto her lover using his legs for support.

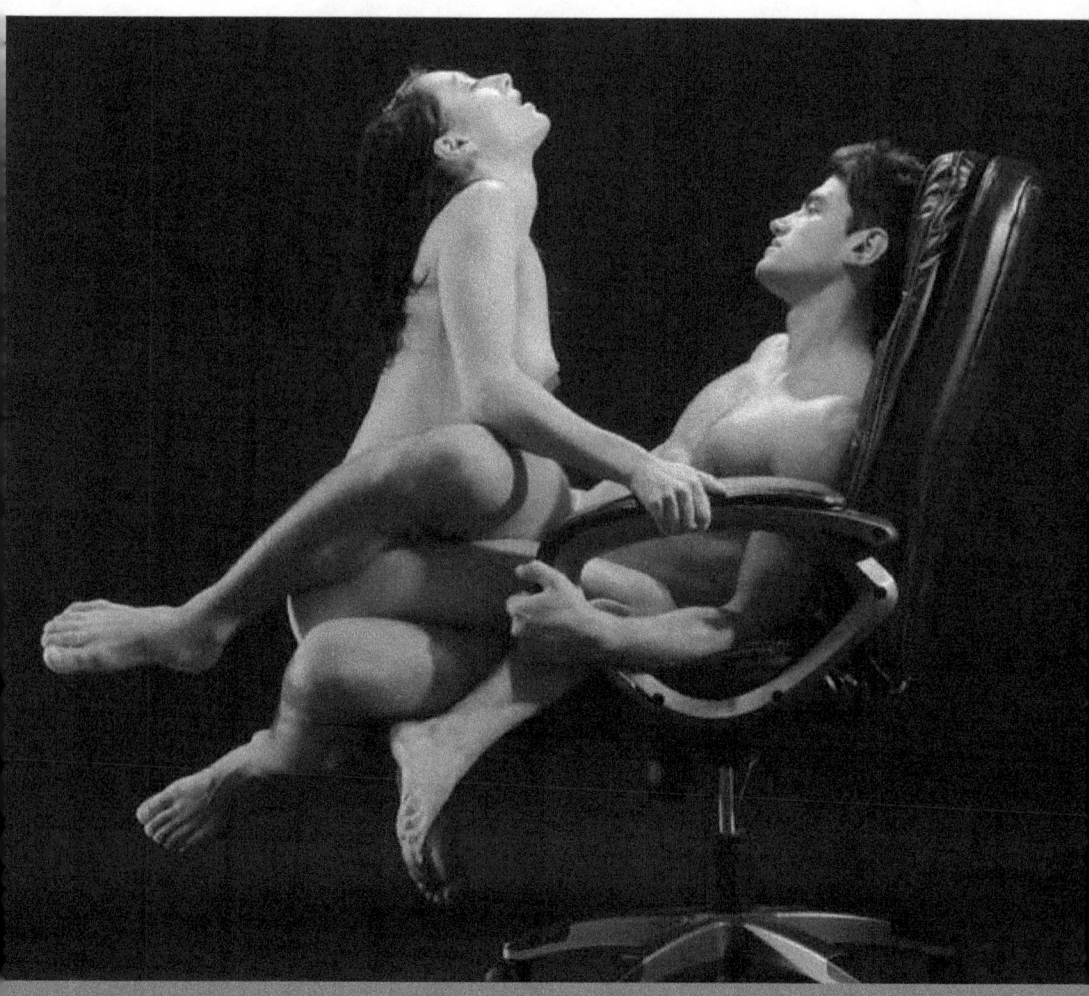

DAY 147

THE HIP SWIVEL SHAKE

He sits in a chair and swivels his hips to the side with his legs bent at the knees. His lover gets in between his legs in a kneeling pose, allowing him to enter her. They move up, down, and all around.

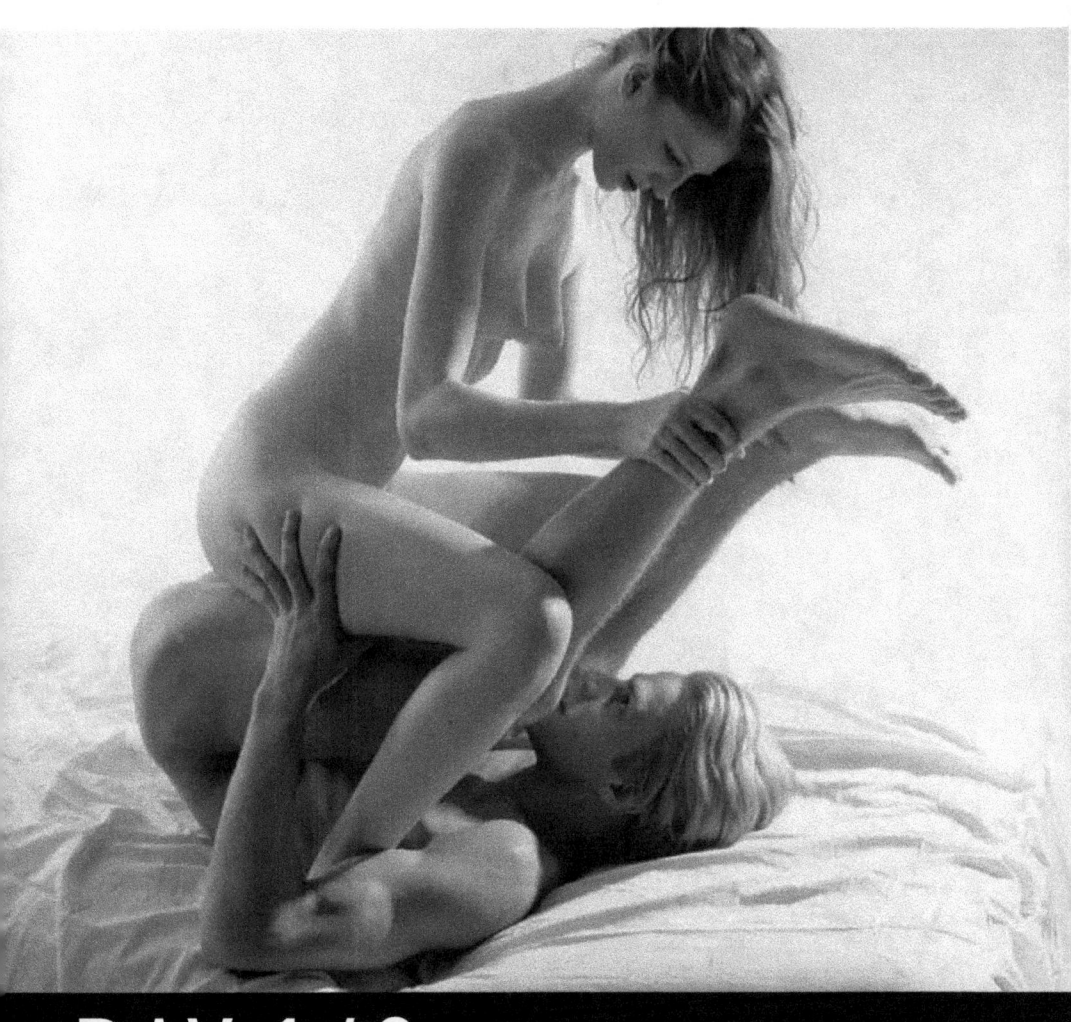

DAY 148

THE RUMBLE SEAT

The man lies back on the bed with his butt raised and knees and legs back in a bicycling pose. His partner maneuvers herself onto his "seat" as he guides his erect penis inside her. Her feet and legs can make this ride as bumpy as she wants.

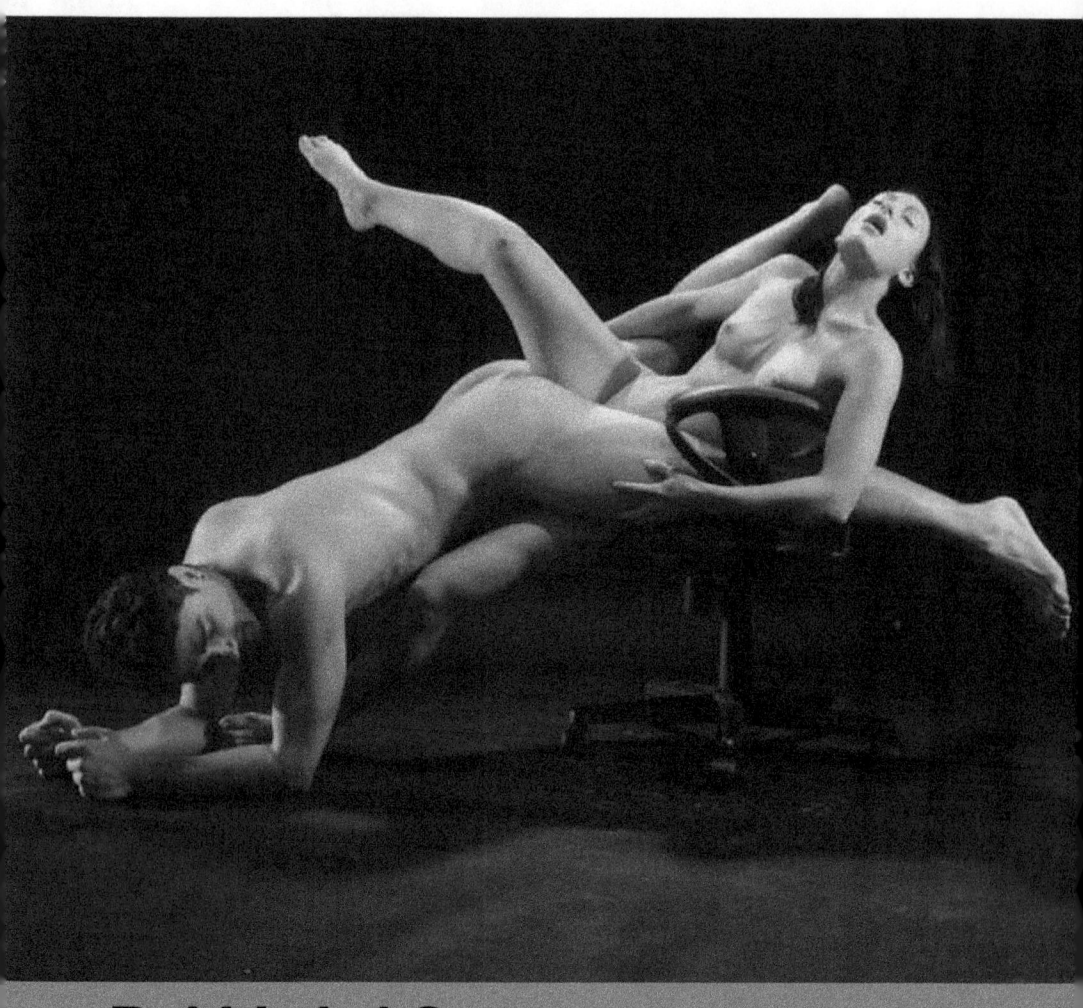

DAY 149

ROCK, SCISSORS, PLEASURE

The woman leans back in a chair and scissors her legs out to either side. On his forearms and facing away from his lover, the man guides his rock-hard penis into her vagina.

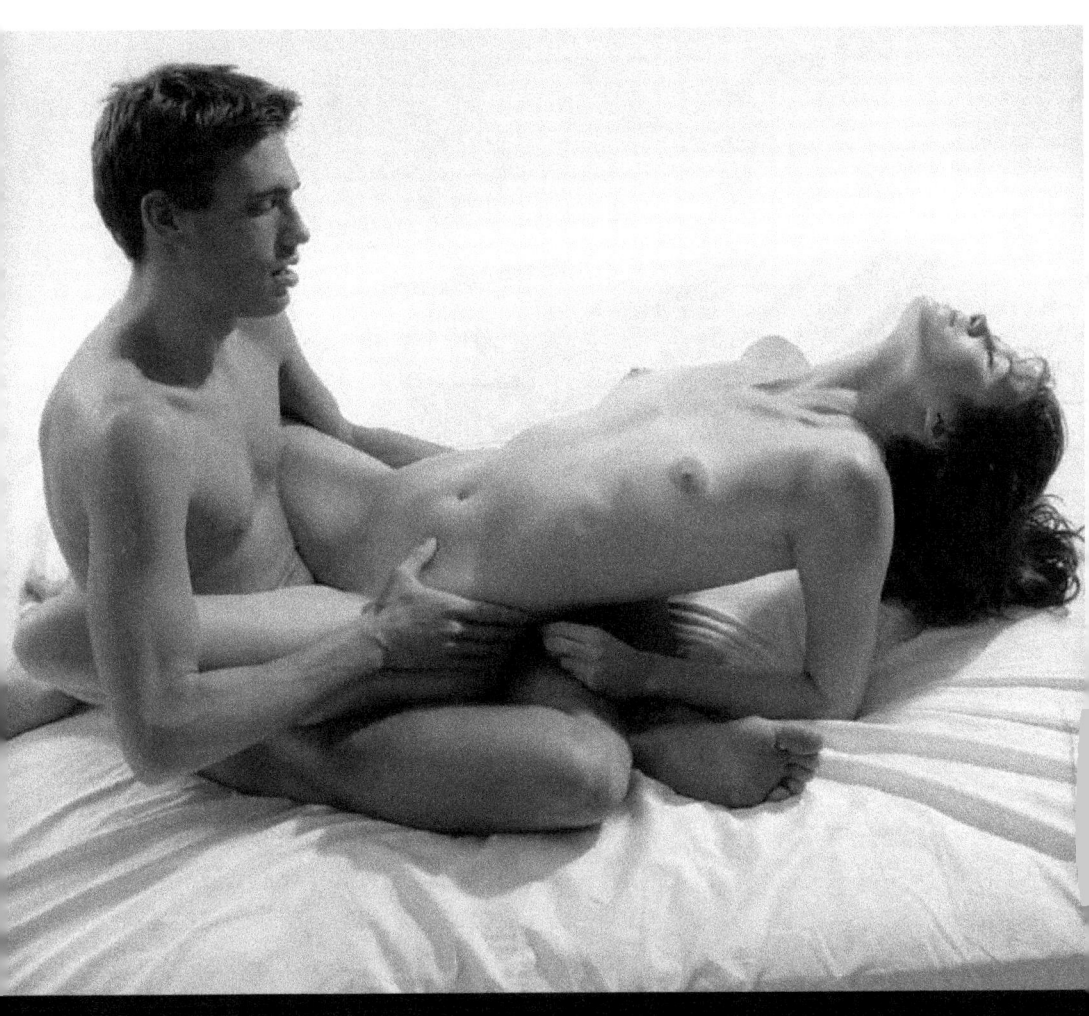

DAY 150

THE LOVE LOCKER

The woman thrusts her pelvis up toward her partner. As he enters her, she wraps her legs around his waist and locks her feet. A terrific position for clitoral contact.

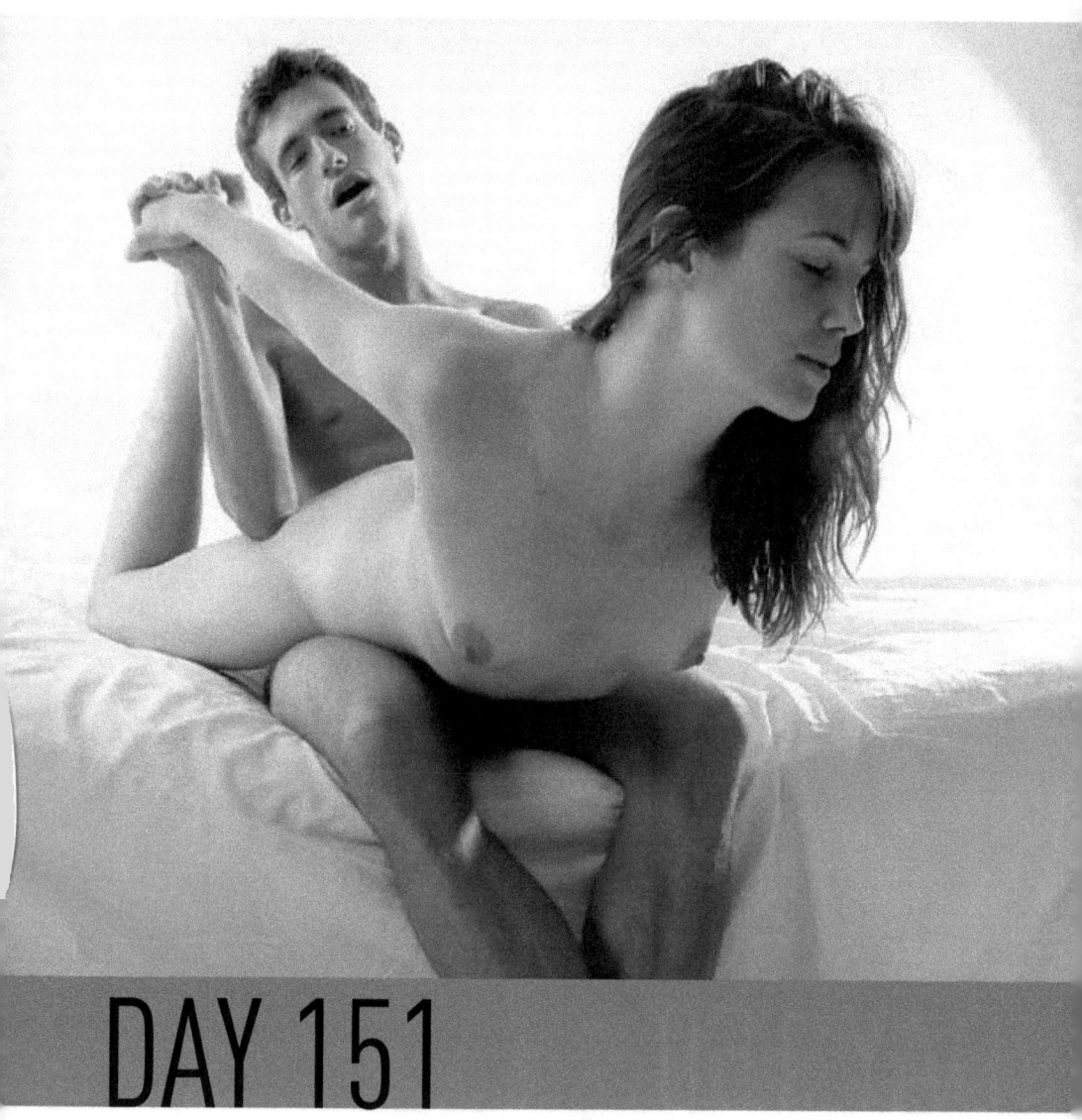

DAY 151

WANG BENEATH MY WINGS

The woman positions herself in her lover's lap, facing away from him. She brings her arms and legs straight back as they both prepare for takeoff.

DAY 152

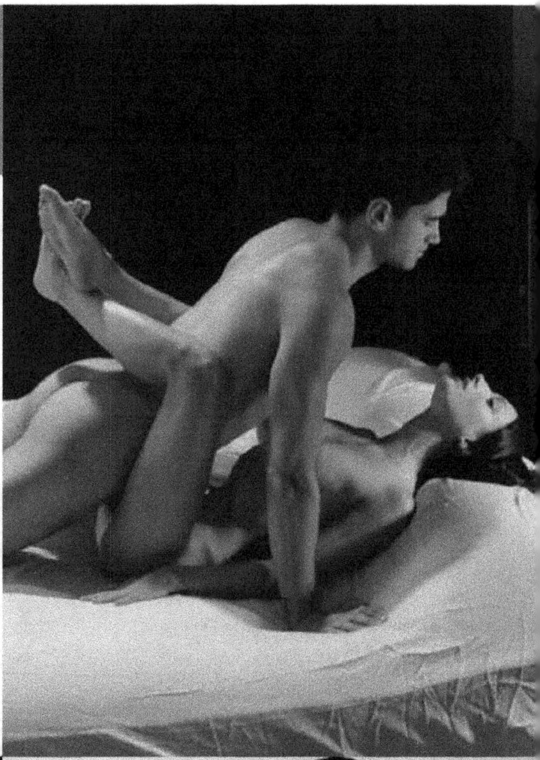

THE ROCKET LOCKET

The woman lies back on the bed as her partner enters her from a missionary position. She locks her legs around the small of his back, pulling him closer as he penetrates her deeply.

DAY 153

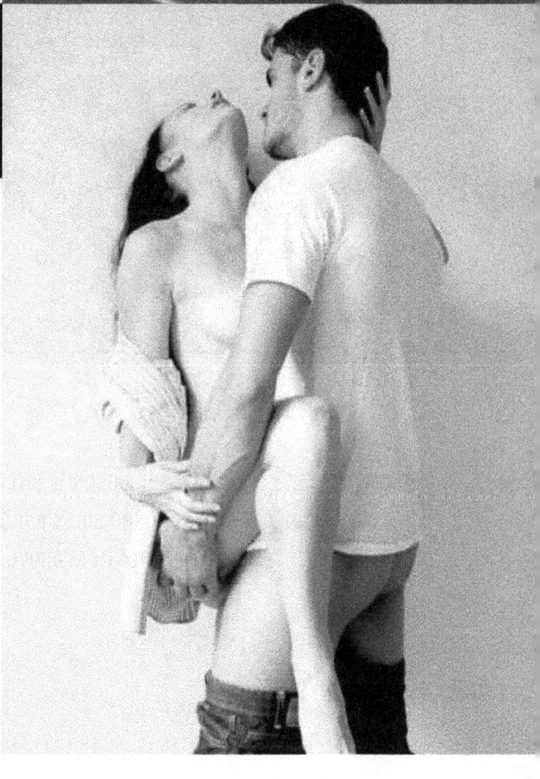

CLOTHES ENCOUNTER

There's a certain eroticism that comes with leaving some clothes on during sex. For some, the feeling of fabric against skin only heightens the level of arousal. She puts on one of his favorite shirts and leans seductively against the wall. He lowers his jeans and takes her right there.

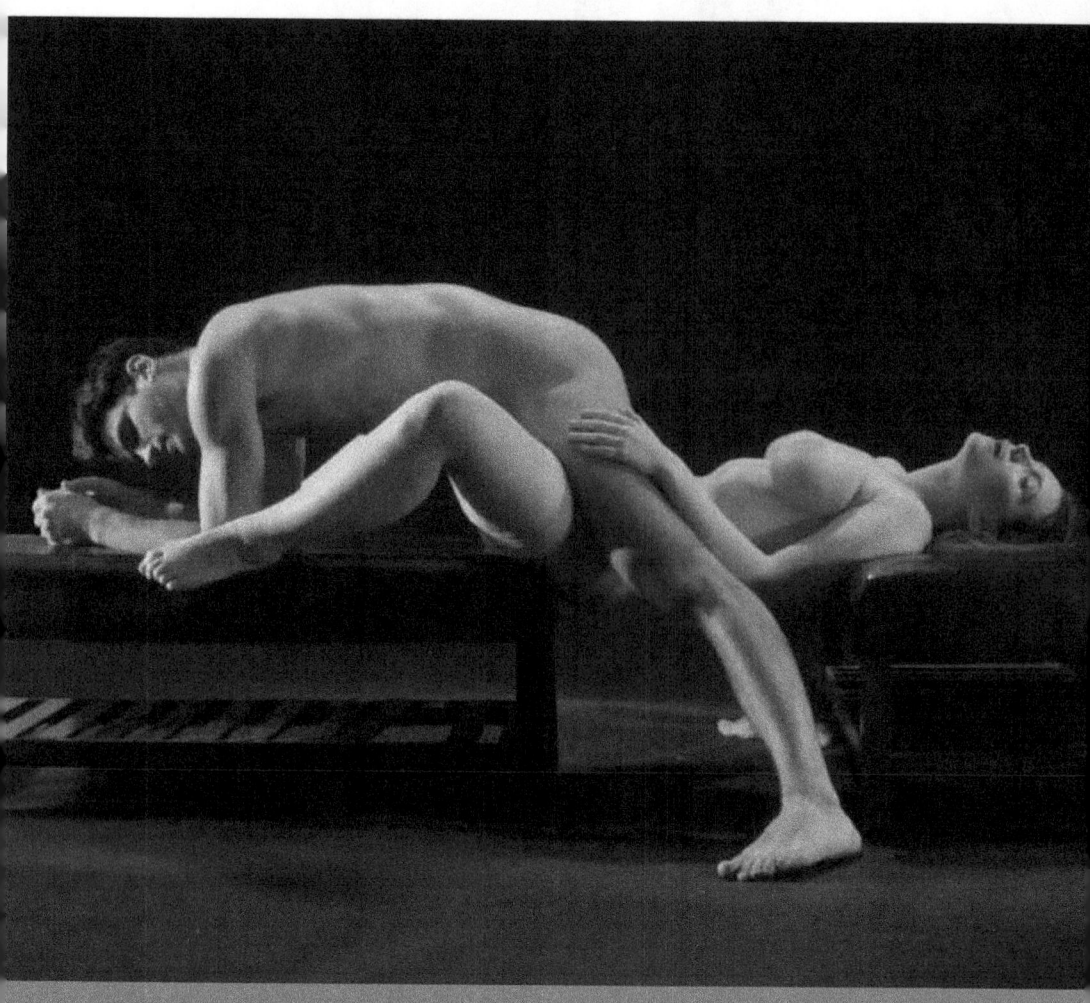

DAY 154

STAR-CROSSED LOVERS

The couple place themselves in opposite directions between two pieces of low-lying furniture. She's on the bottom with her head and shoulders resting on one piece and her feet on the other. Her partner penetrates her from above as he stretches out away from her.

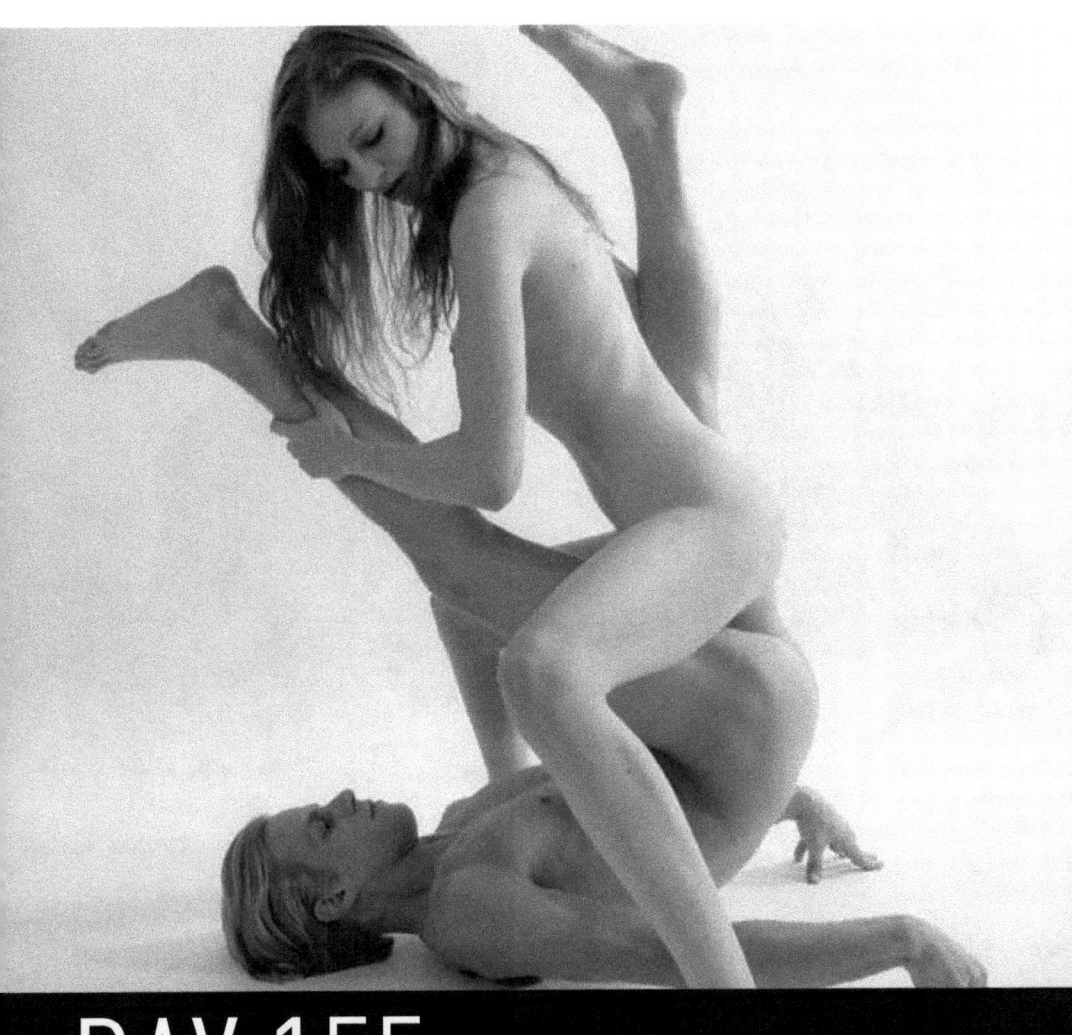

DAY 155

COMMAND CENTRAL

Starting on his back, the man lifts his legs up into a shoulder stand and then scissors one of them back. His partner positions herself between his legs and lowers herself down so that he can penetrate her. From this point on, she's the one calling all the shots.

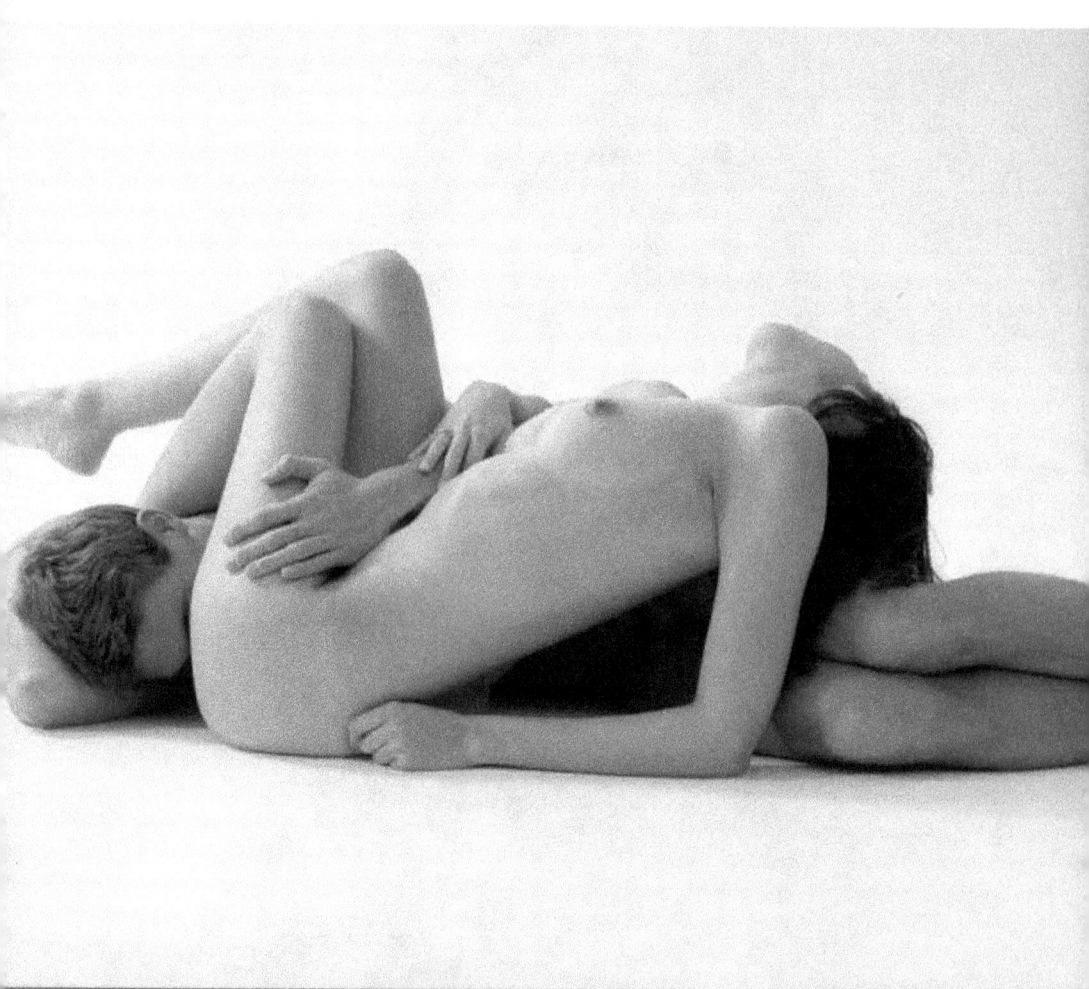

DAY 156

SOUTHERN EXPOSURE

The woman is curled up comfortably as her lover moves in to orally explore her nether regions. Her hands are free to do some exploring of their own.

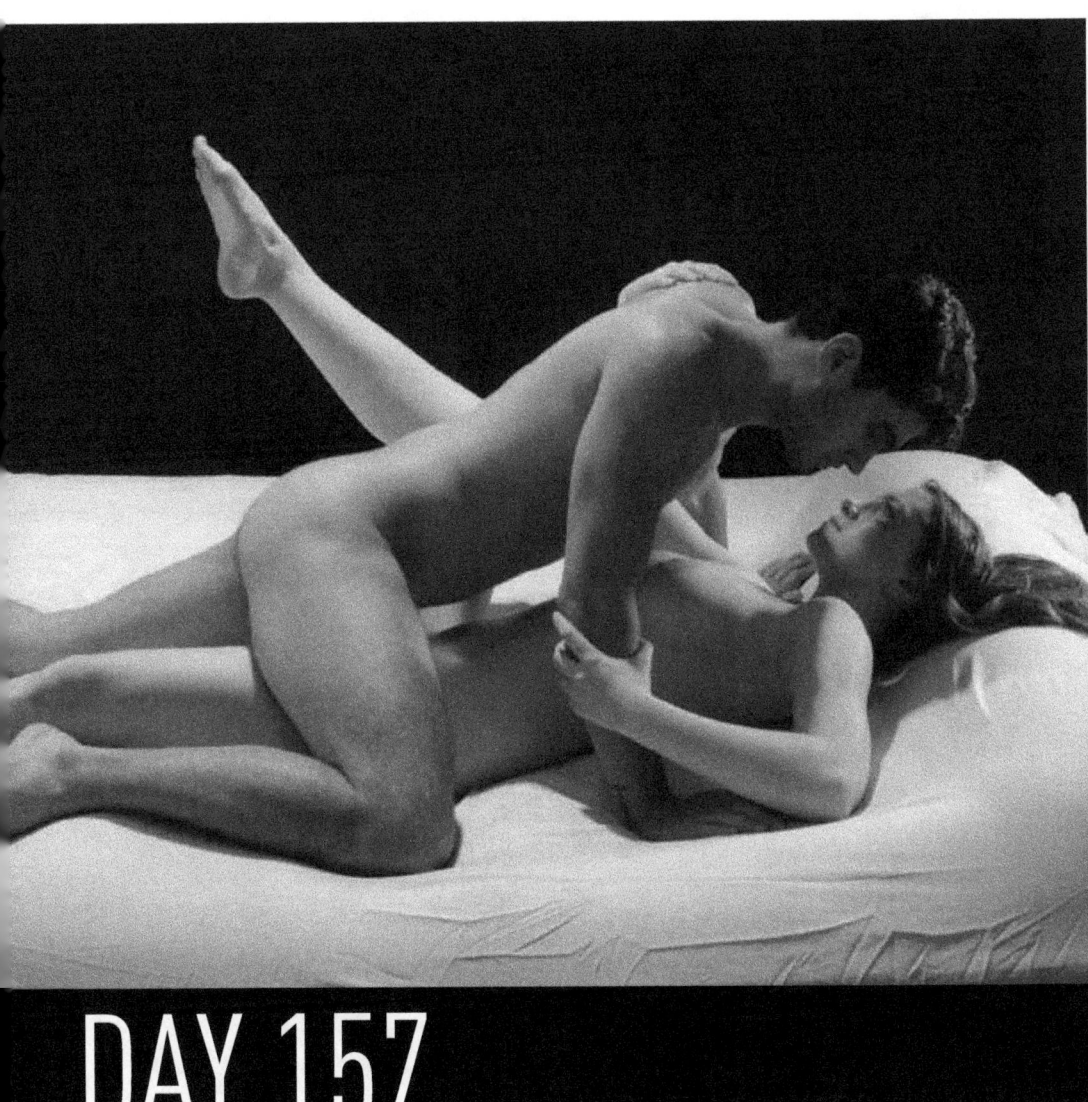

DAY 157

SHE'S GOTTA HAVE IT

She stretches out on the bed and opens her legs as an invitation to her partner. He takes up the offer and straddles one of her legs and enters her. She's not about to let him go anywhere as she pulls him closer and deeper.

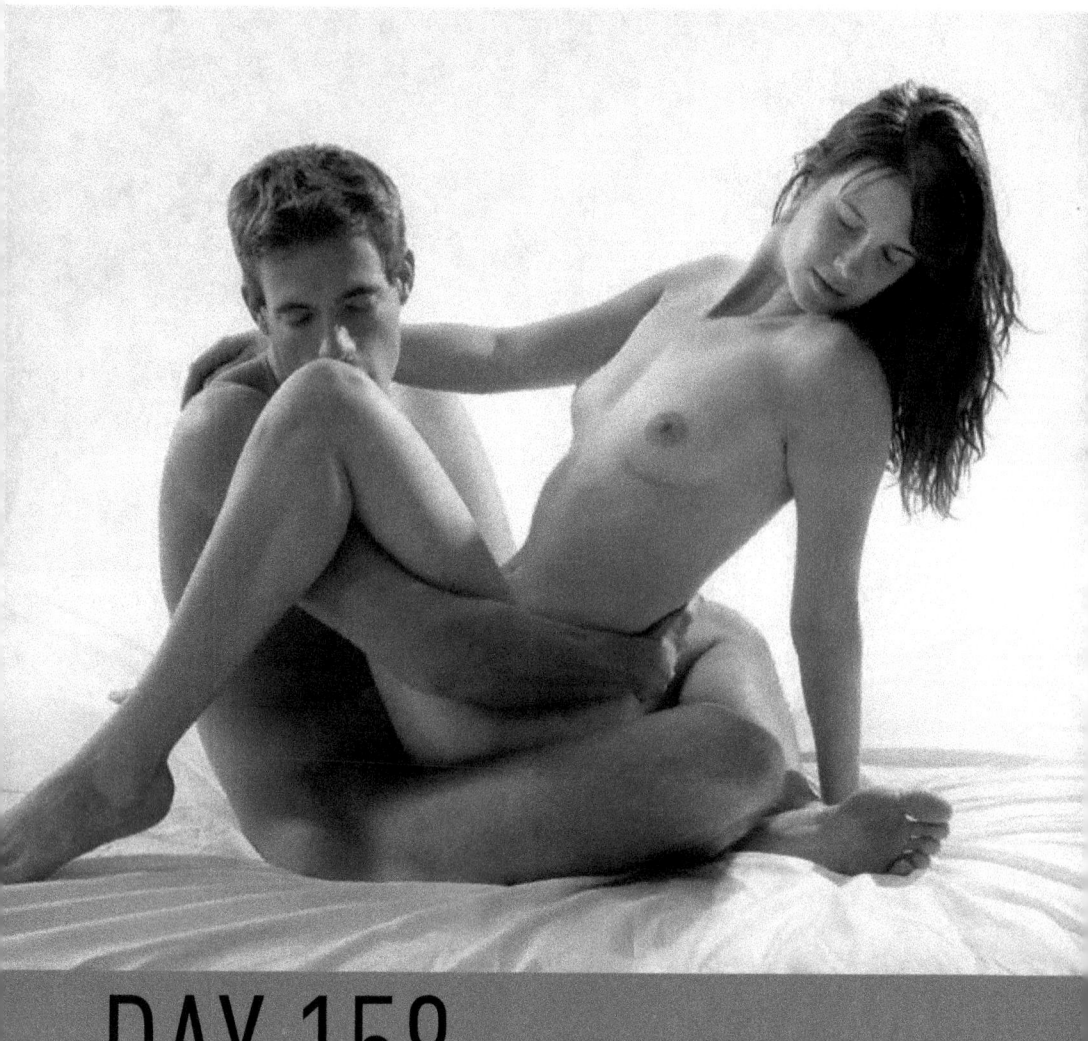

DAY 158

CARNAL CAPTURE

The lovers face each other. The man sits cross-legged as the woman mounts him. Once she's atop home, he threads his arms under her knees. From this position, he can move her any which way he pleases. If the need arises, she can also lean back on her hands a bit to take on some of the weight.

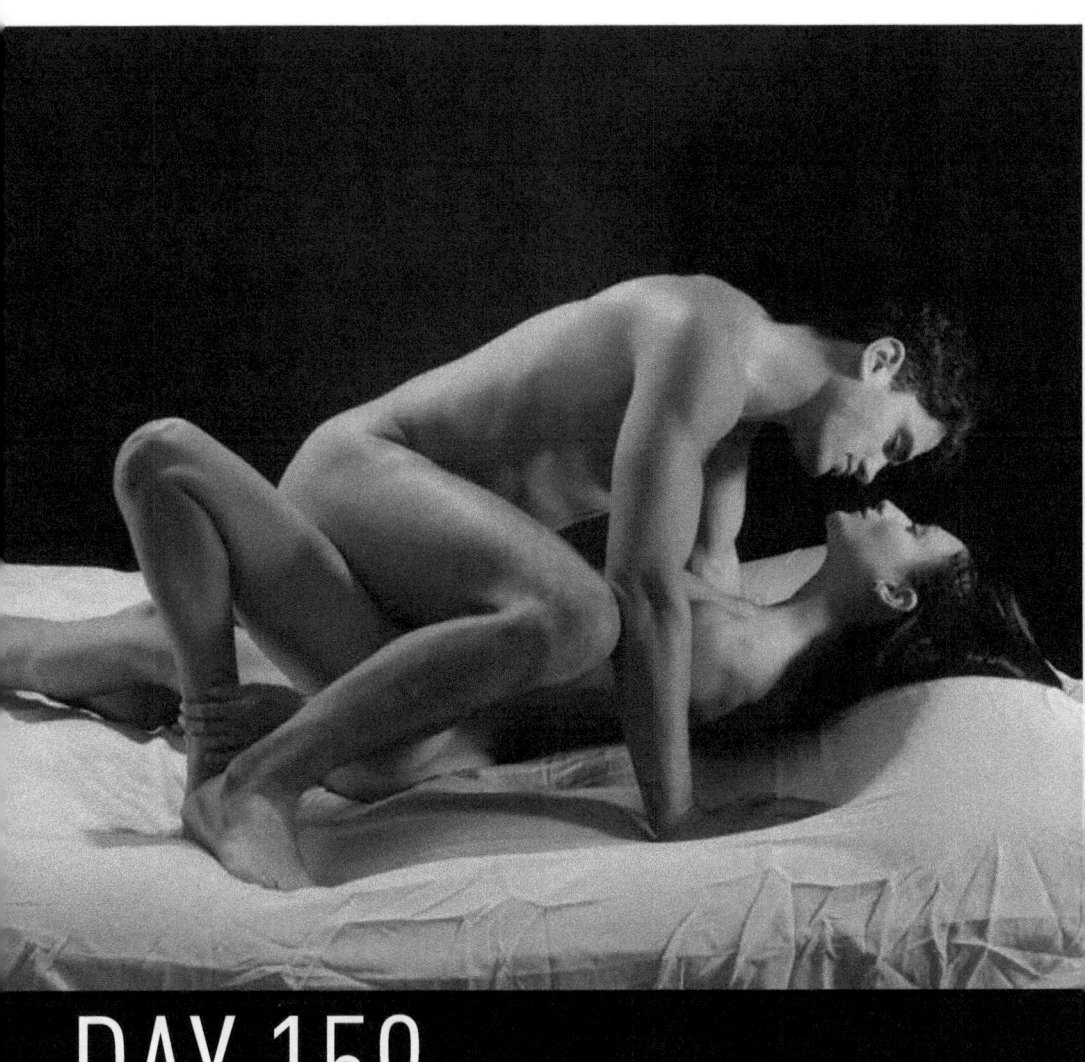

DAY 159

THE DROP ZONE

She lies back on the bed with one leg extended and the other bent at the knee and resting on the ball of her foot. Her partner squats over her, penetrating deeply while providing a good deal of clitoral contact.

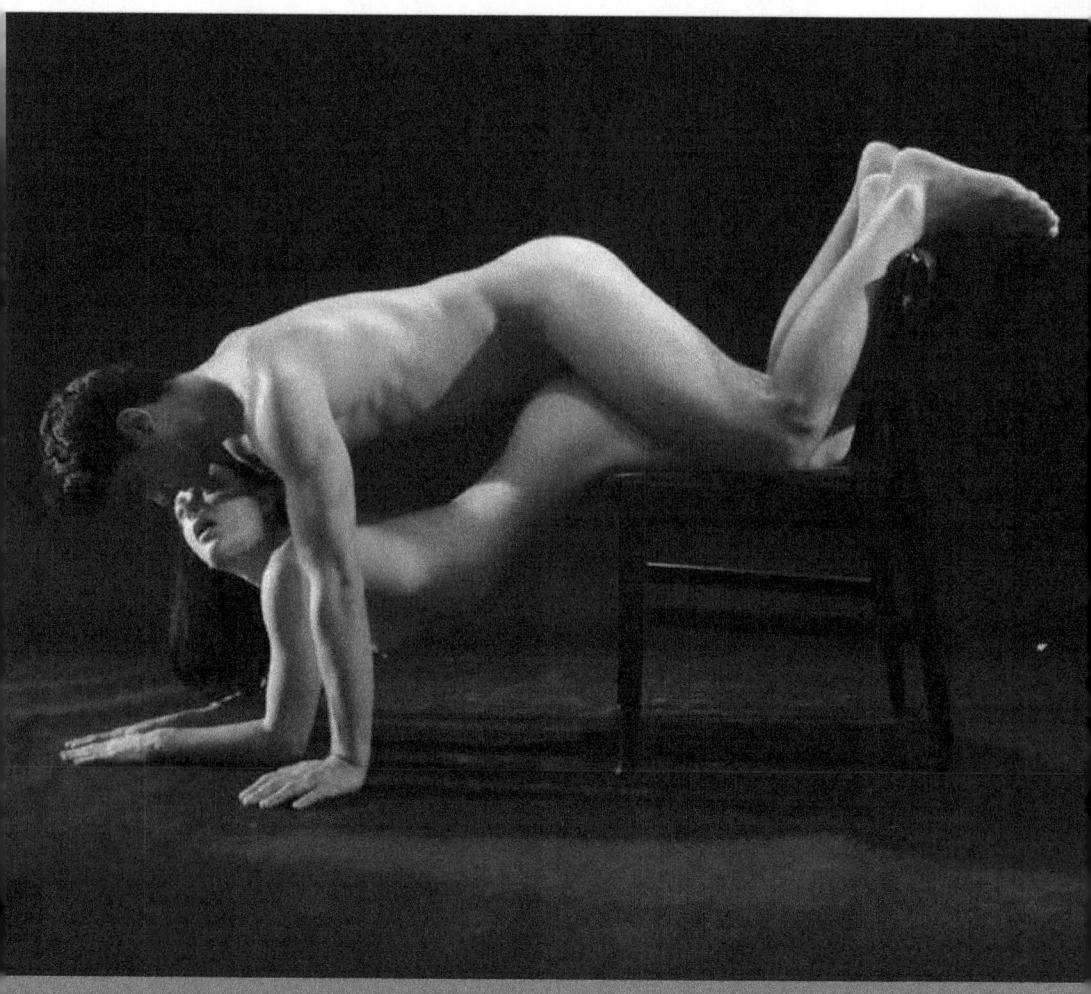

DAY 160

GET DOWN

There's no falling in love without a little falling. The woman places her thighs on a chair as she extends her forearms down to the floor. Her limber lover assumes a similar position as he enters her from behind.

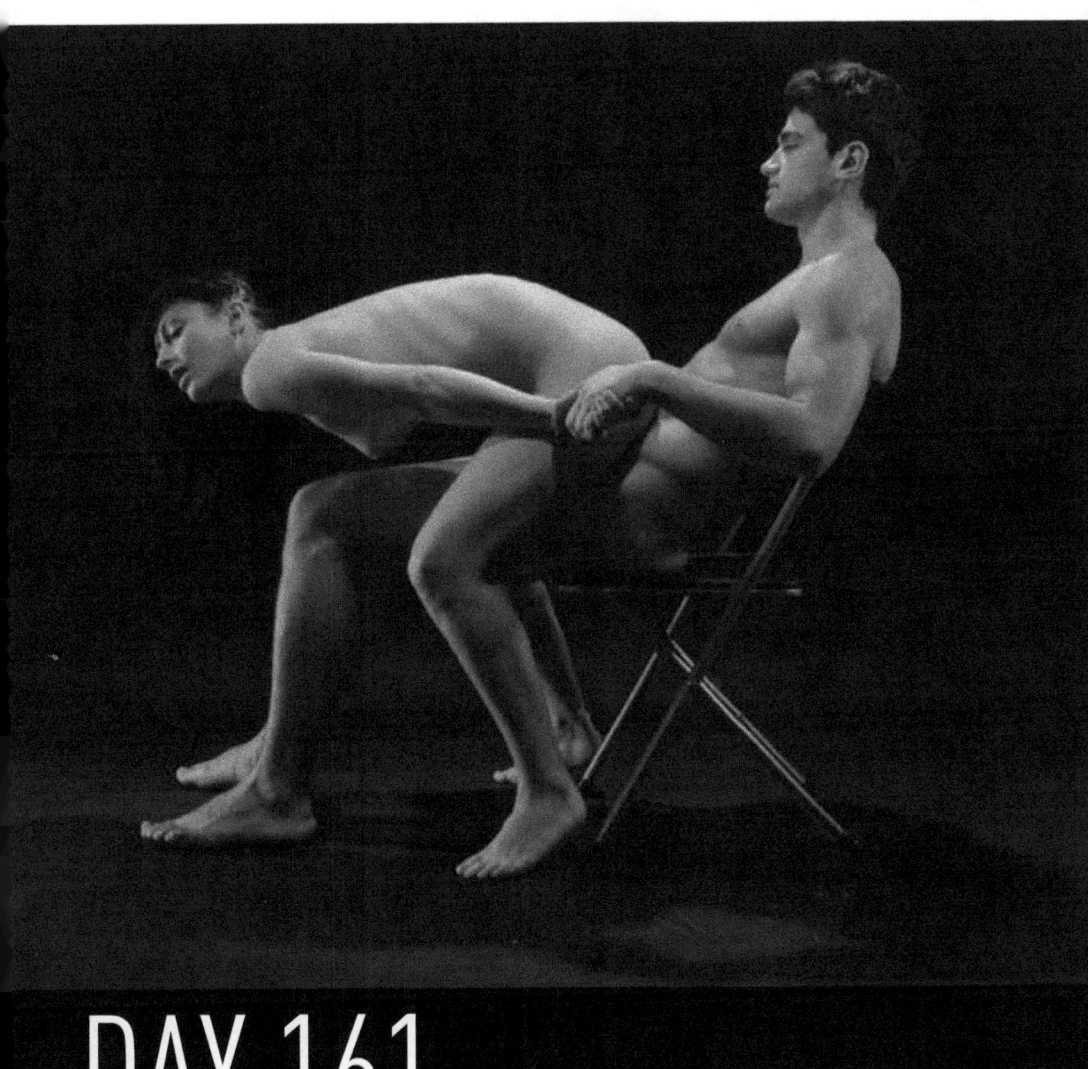

DAY 161

THE LAST GRASP

He's comfortably seated as his lover mounts him facing outward. As they hold onto each other, she undulates her hips and torso to increase the penetration sensation.

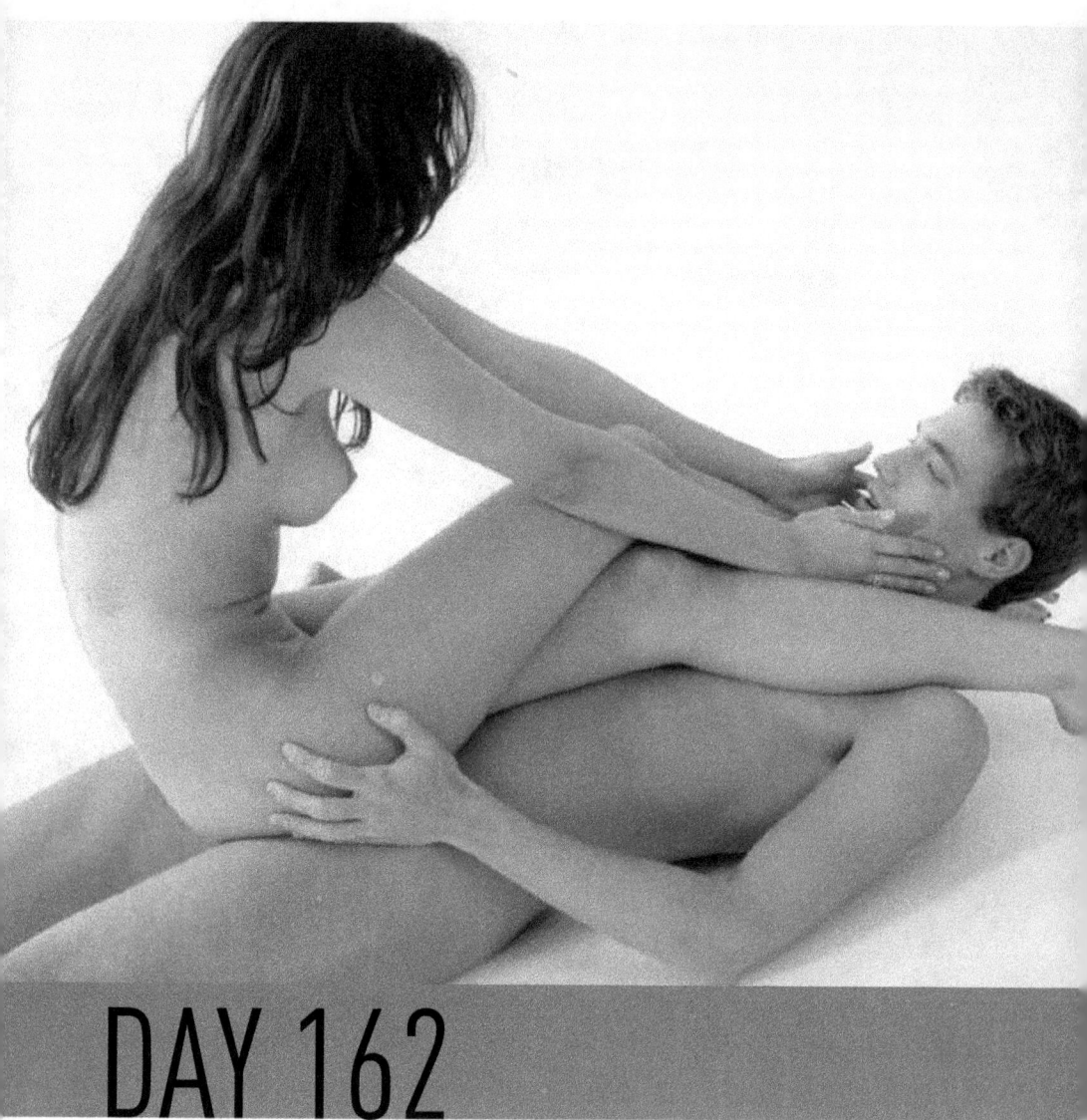

DAY 162

THE CROSSROADS

The man stretches out on the floor with his hands out to his sides. His lover mounts his penis and crosses her legs, which heightens the sensation of penetration for both of them. She uses her hands to gently stroke his face.

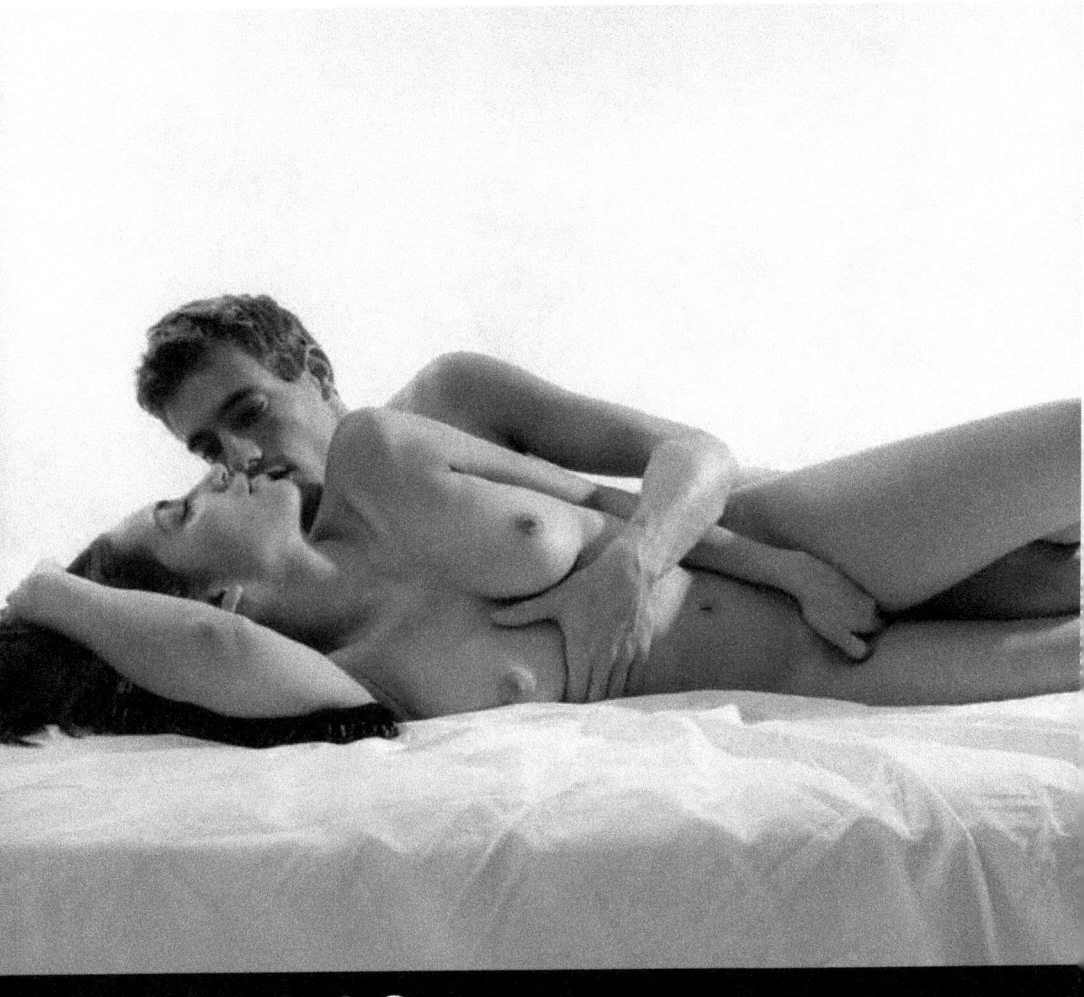

DAY 163

FEEL THE HEAT

The lovers position themselves on their sides. The woman lifts her leg as her partner enters her from behind. They both can enjoy stimulating her breasts and clitoris.

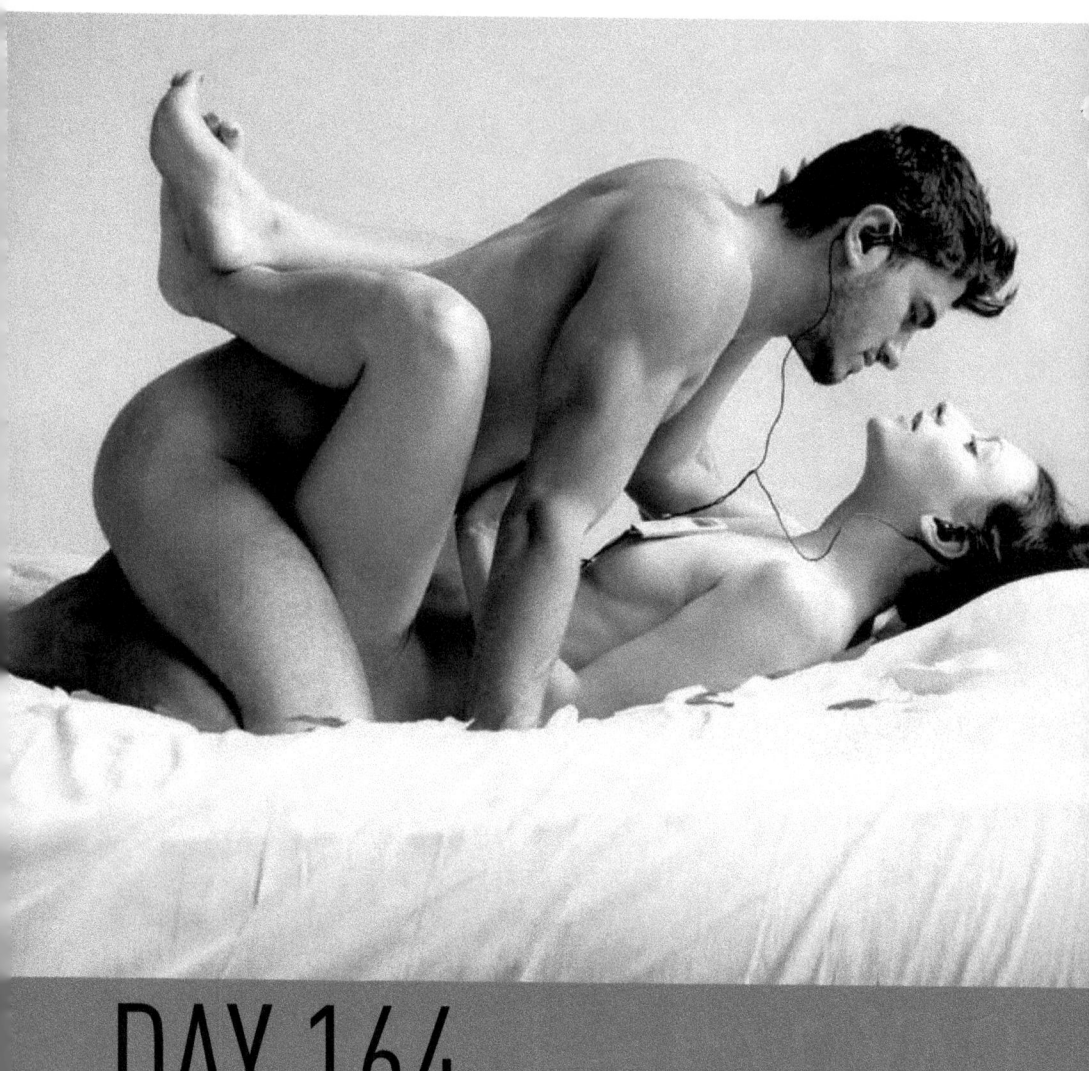

DAY 164

TUNED IN AND TURNED ON

The woman lies back on the bed and lifts her legs, allowing her partner to enter her. They each place an earpiece in one ear and move in concert to the music in their ears.

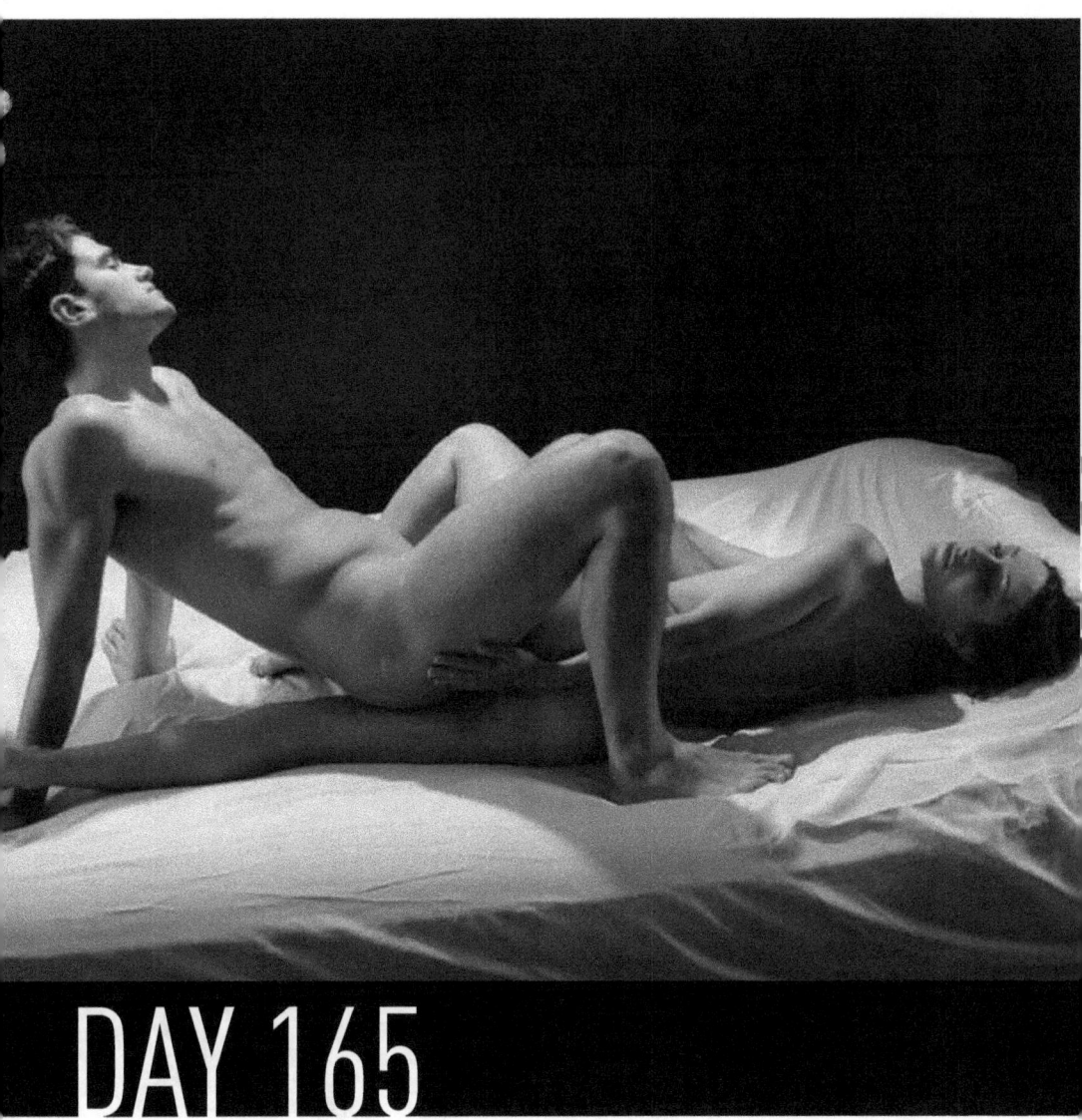

DAY 165

ROCK AROUND THE CLOCK

As the woman lies on the bed, she slightly twists herself to the side, creating a point of entry for her partner. He leans back on his hands and slides his pelvis forward until his penis penetrates her vagina. Though they're locked together like the hands on a clock, their ecstasy knows no time limit.

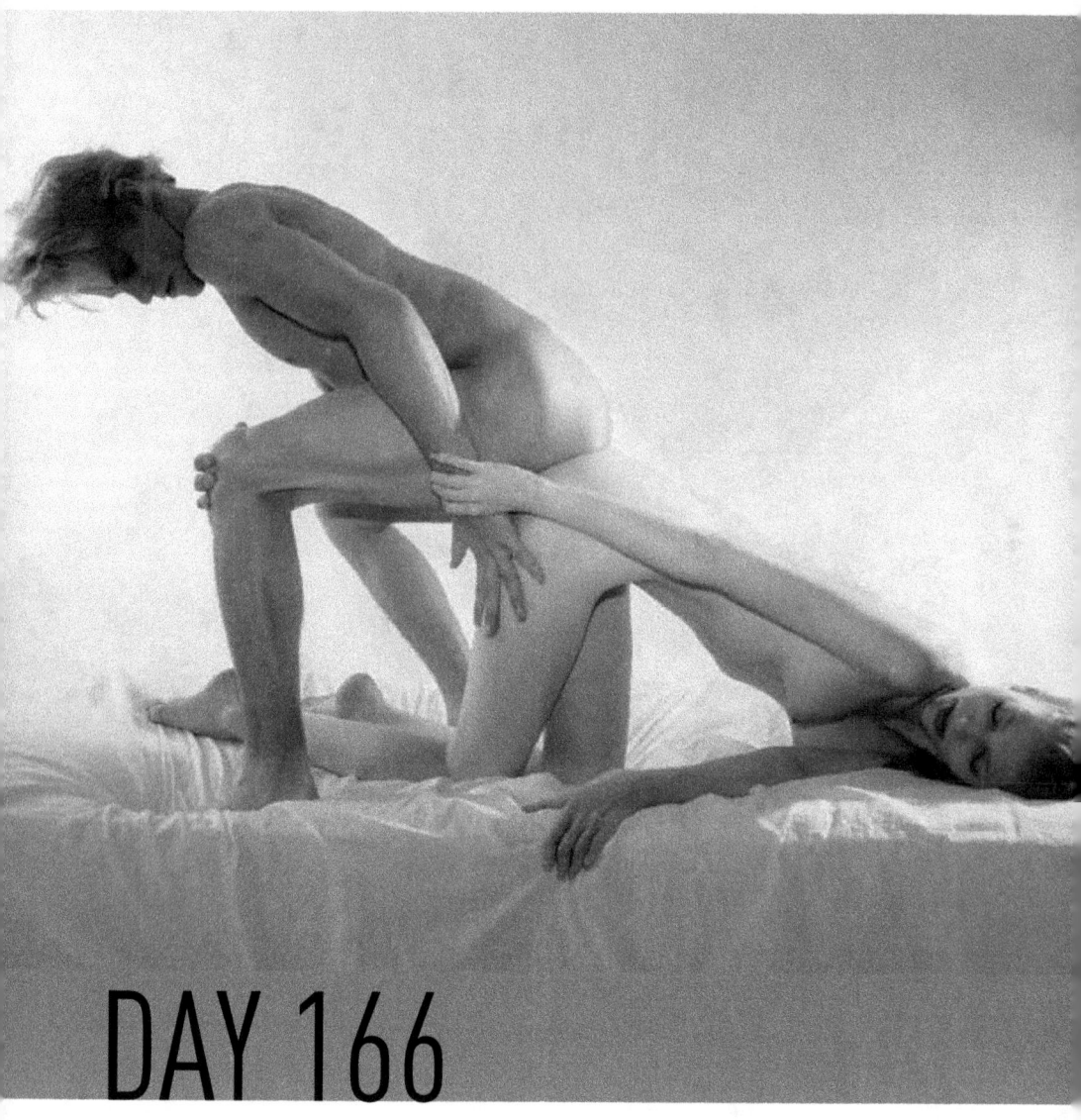

DAY 166

CHEEK TO CHEEK

She's on her knees with her head resting down against the bed. Her partner is facing away as he squats down and enters her from above. They hold each other for support.

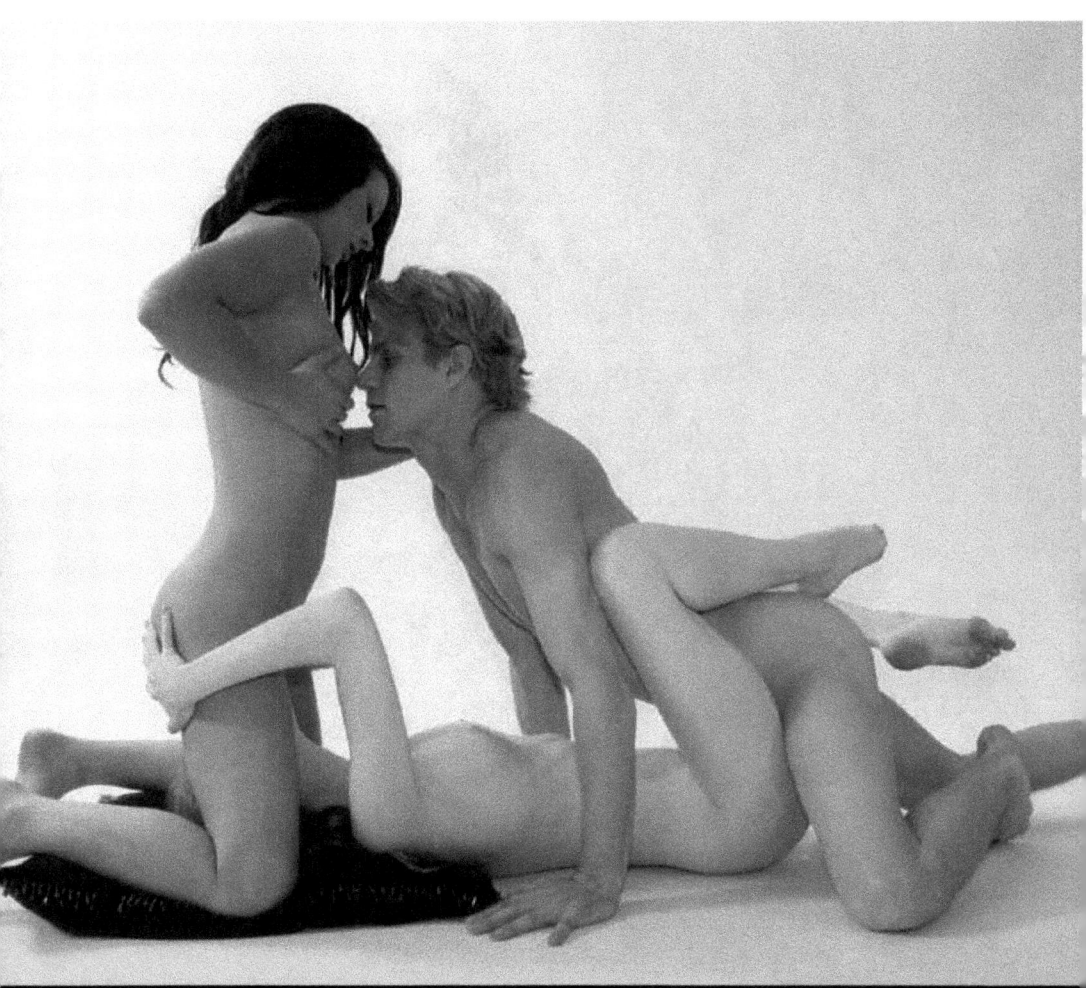

DAY 167

MISSIONARY MAN

The man enters his prone partner from the missionary position as she lies on her back with her head and shoulders resting on a pillow. Her girlfriend kneels over her face and offers her vagina for oral gratification, as he leans forward to sample her tempting breasts.

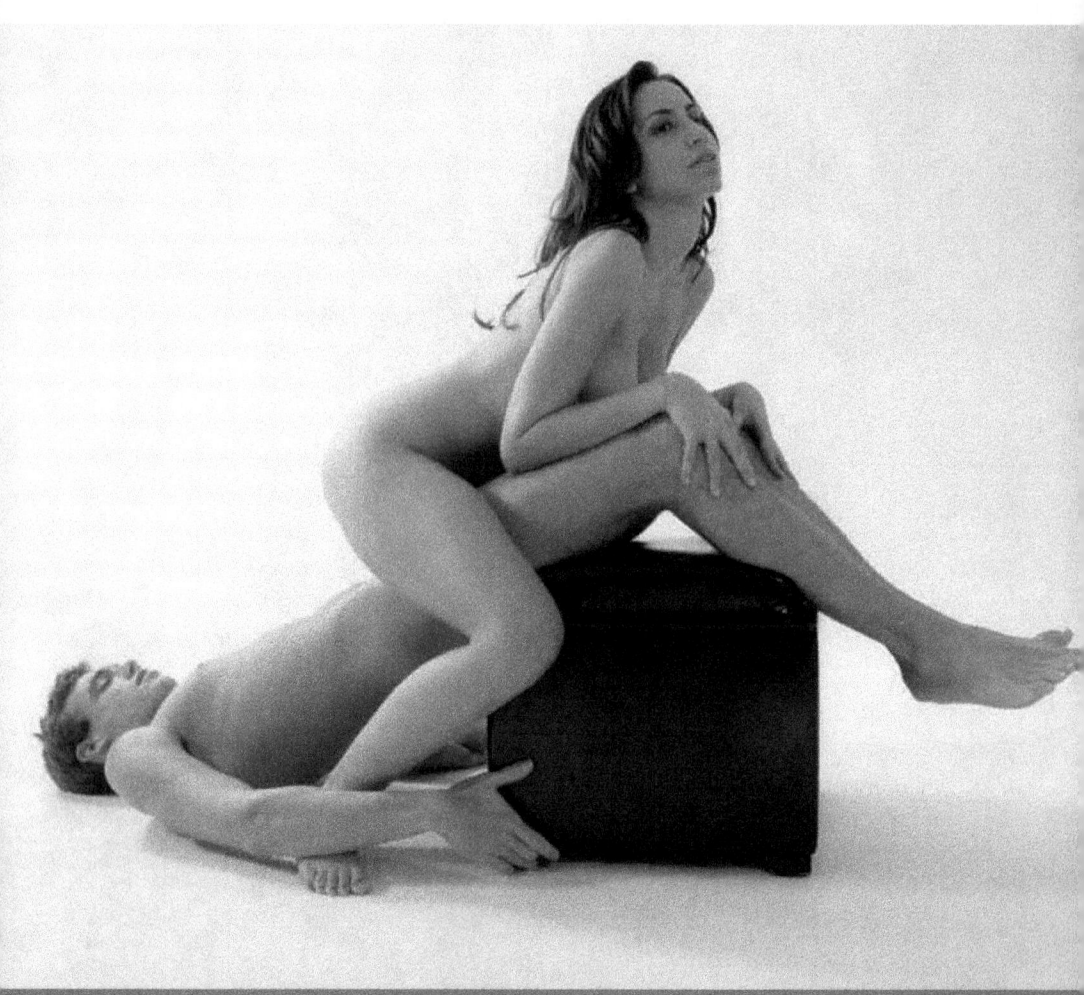

DAY 168

THE EROTIC ESCALATOR

The man places the edge of his butt and upper thighs against an ottoman and his head and shoulders back toward the floor. His willing partner is more than happy to climb on board. Going up?

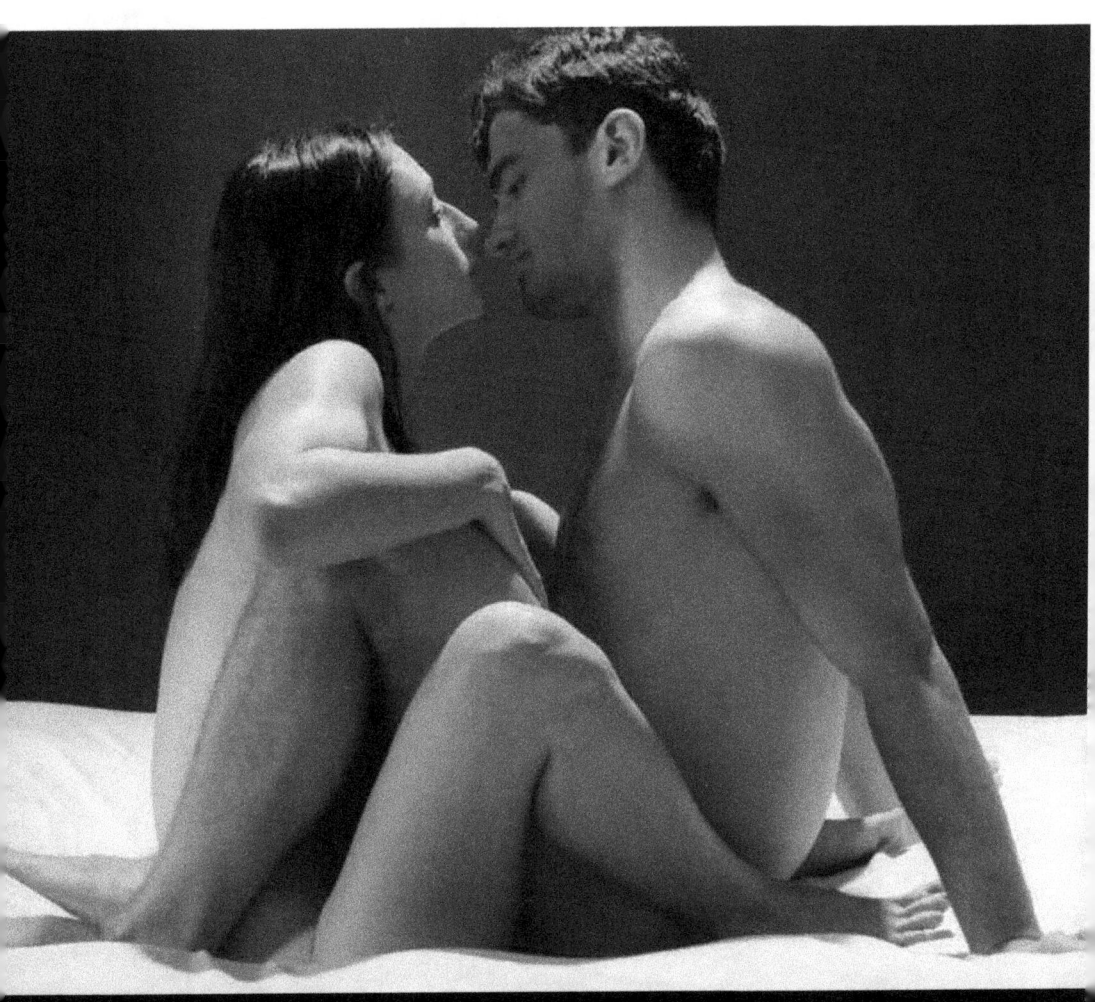

DAY 169

THE KINKY COIL

Feeling a little salty? In this position the lovers sit on their buttocks facing each other. As they bring their knees up it opens their respective genitals for penetration. The more they tangle themselves together like a pretzel, the better.

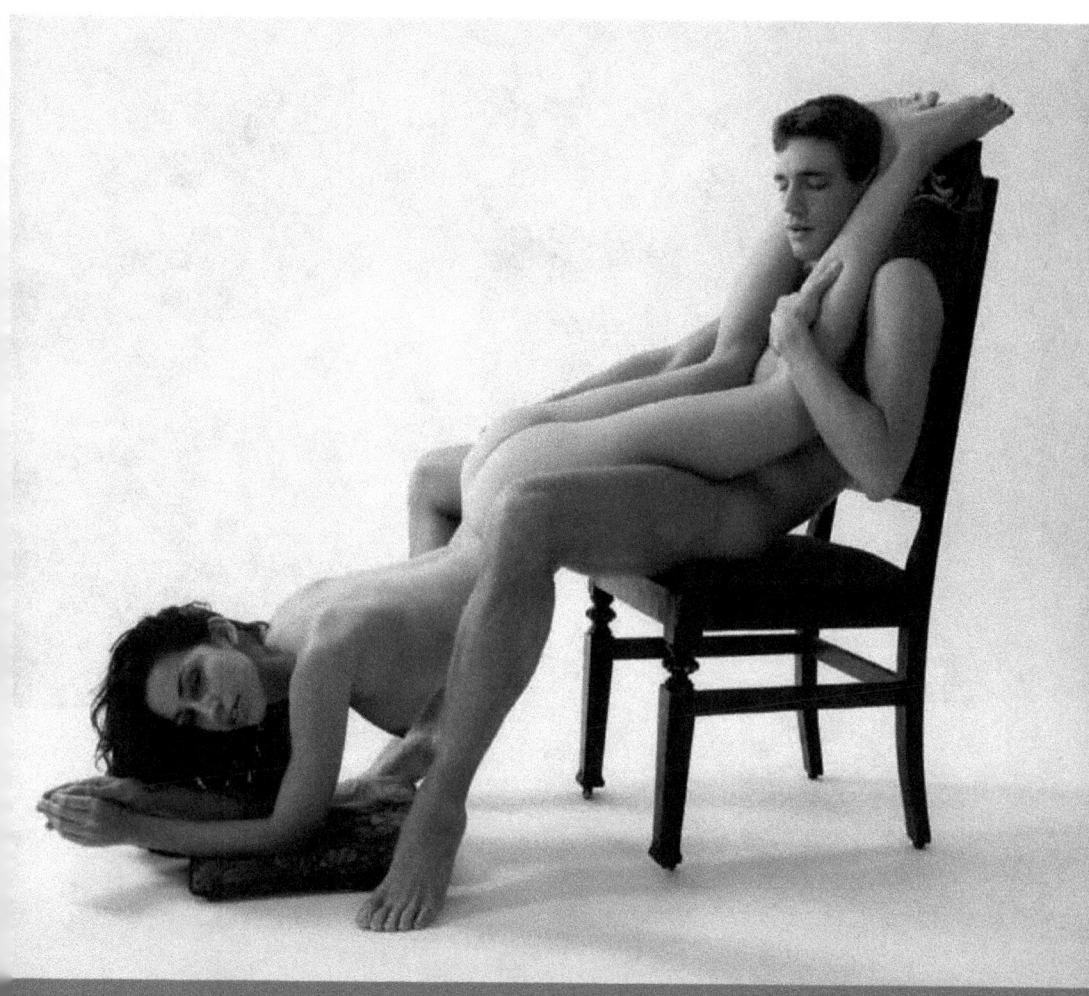

DAY 170

ELECTRIC OUTLET

The man reclines in a comfortable chair with his legs open and feet on the floor. His partner connects with him by resting her arms on the floor and bringing her legs up over his shoulders. His hands can explore her buttocks. The partners may also switch positions for an entirely different experience.

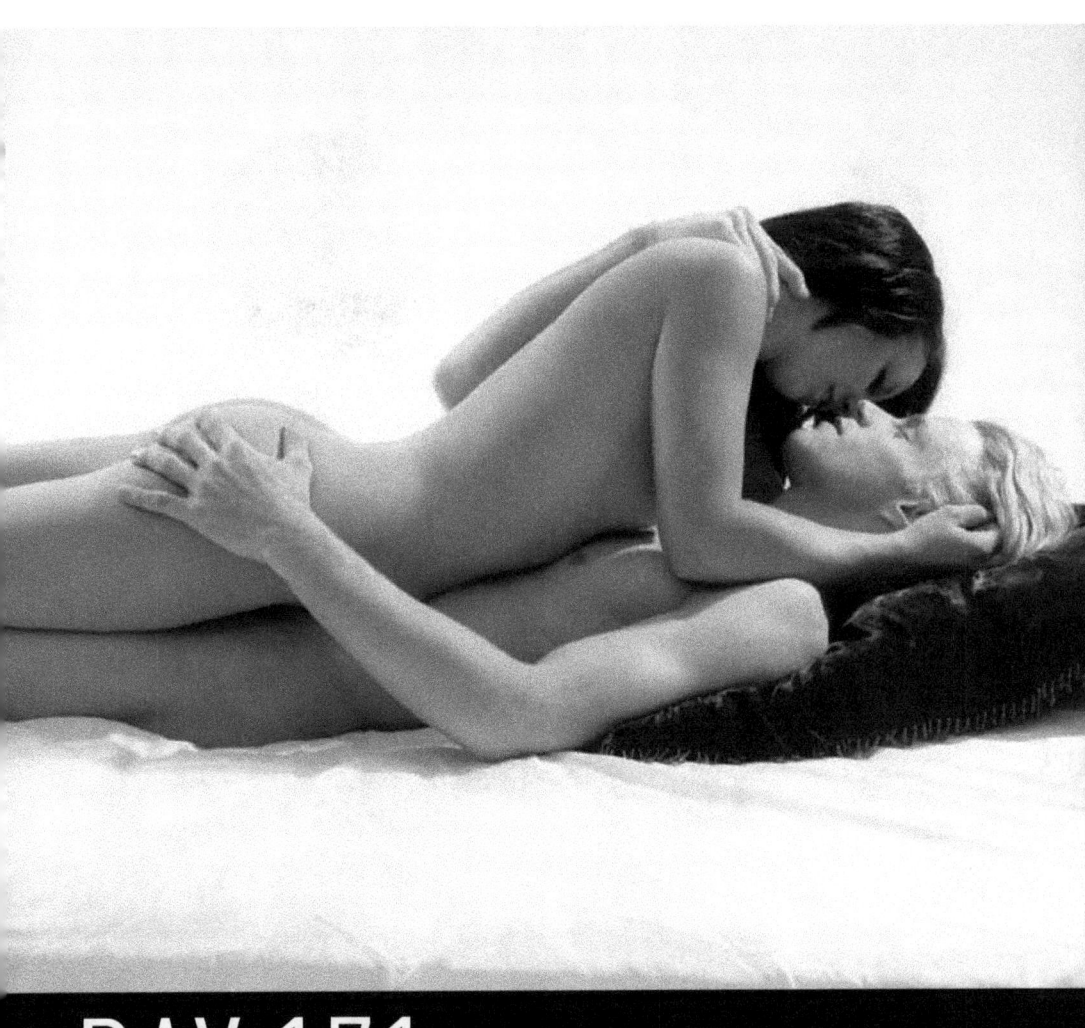

DAY 171

THE TIGHT TWOSOME

He lies back on the bed with his legs extended and only slightly apart. His lover takes a similar position on top of him as he enters her. They each close their legs, allowing the tightness of the penetration to guide their movements.

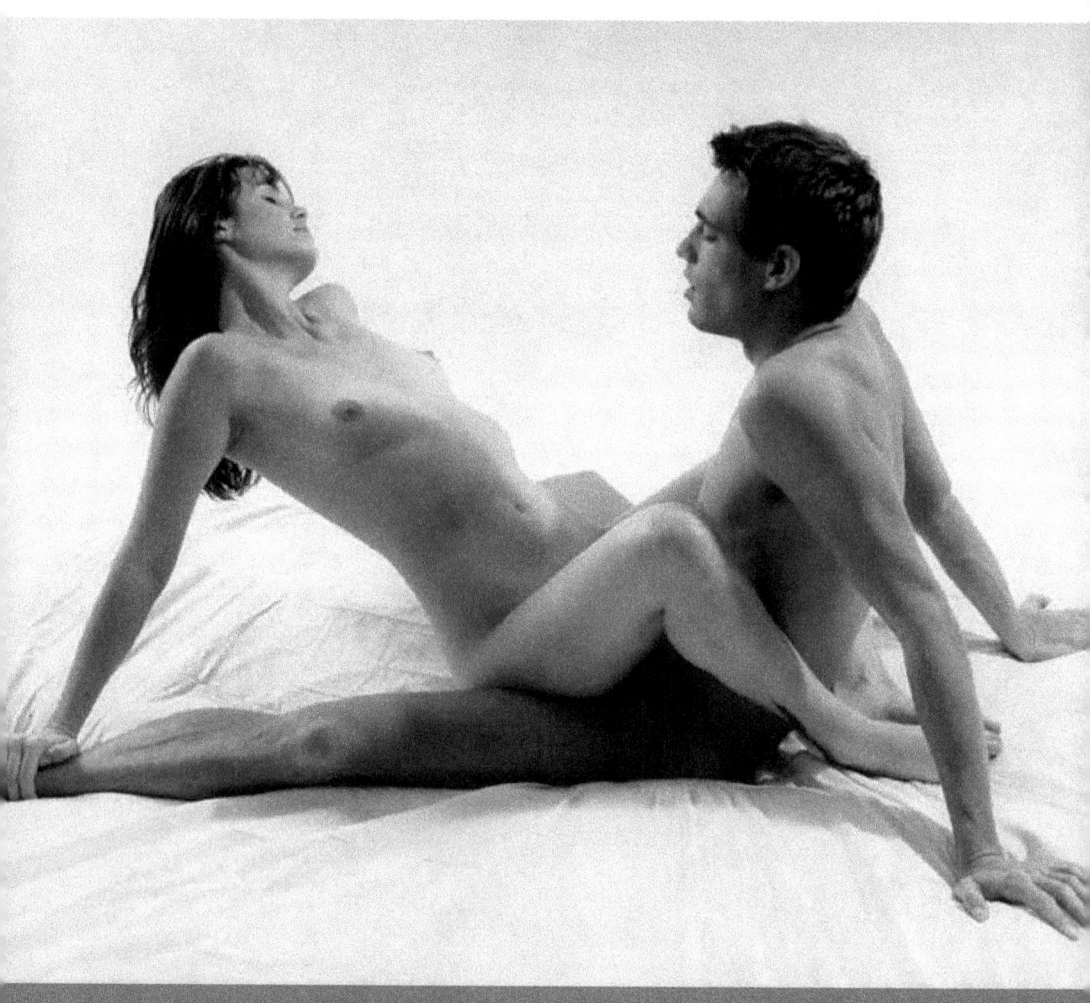

DAY 172

FLESH DANCE

The woman is seated in her lover's lap facing him. As she leans back and grabs his ankles she tightens her pelvic muscles. Some gentle rocking is more than enough movement for this pleasurable position.

DAY 173

LEOPARD'S LAIR

This easy doggy pose is a good one for anal penetration. She gets on all fours and stretches out across a padded bench. Her lover slowly enters her lubed behind, being sure not to force the issue.

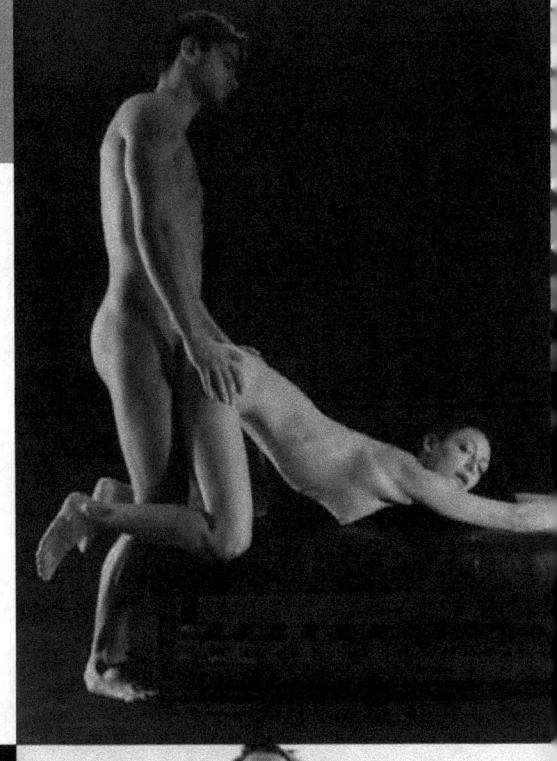

DAY 174

SUMMER SENSATION

The woman lies back near the edge of the bed. Her lover straddles her with his feet on the bed and arms and hands extended down to the floor. As he penetrates her she curls one leg up his back toward his shoulder.

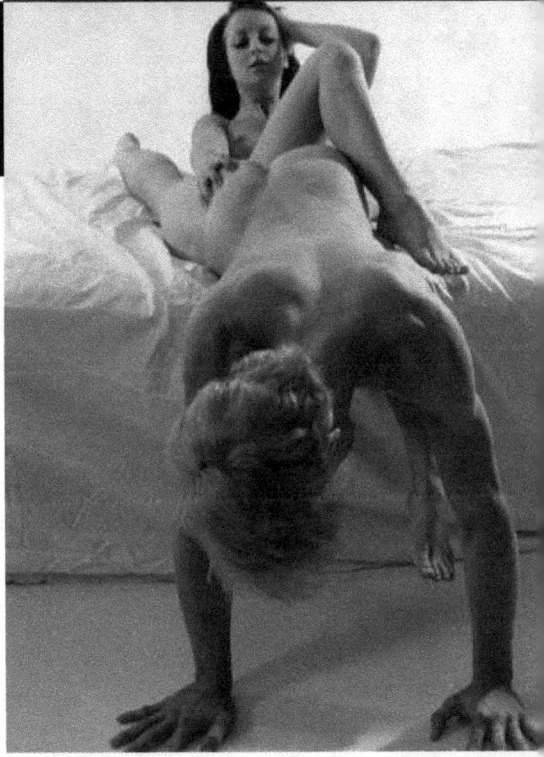

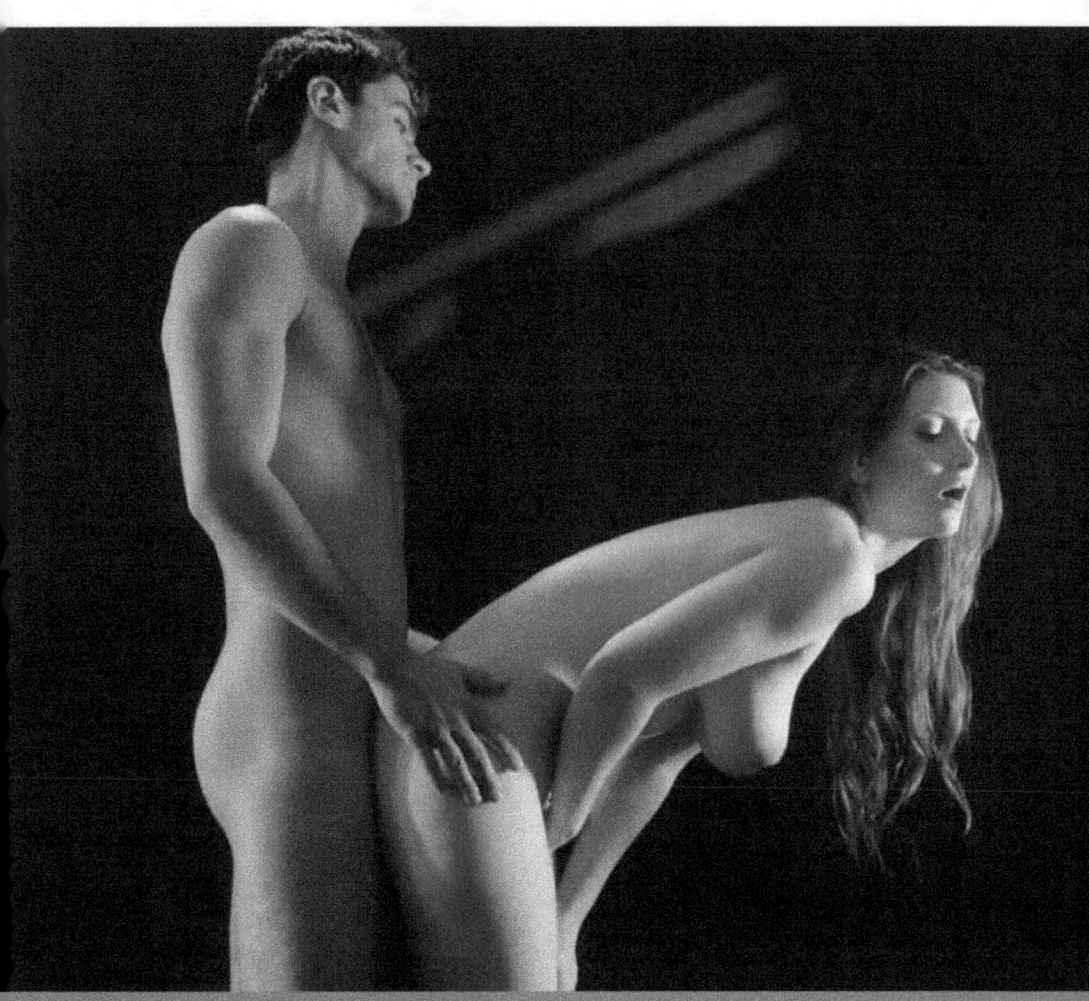

DAY 175

LET'S GET NUTS

The lovers start in a standing position with the woman in front of the man. She bends over and allows him to enter her. As he thrusts she reaches her hand back to fondle his testicles.

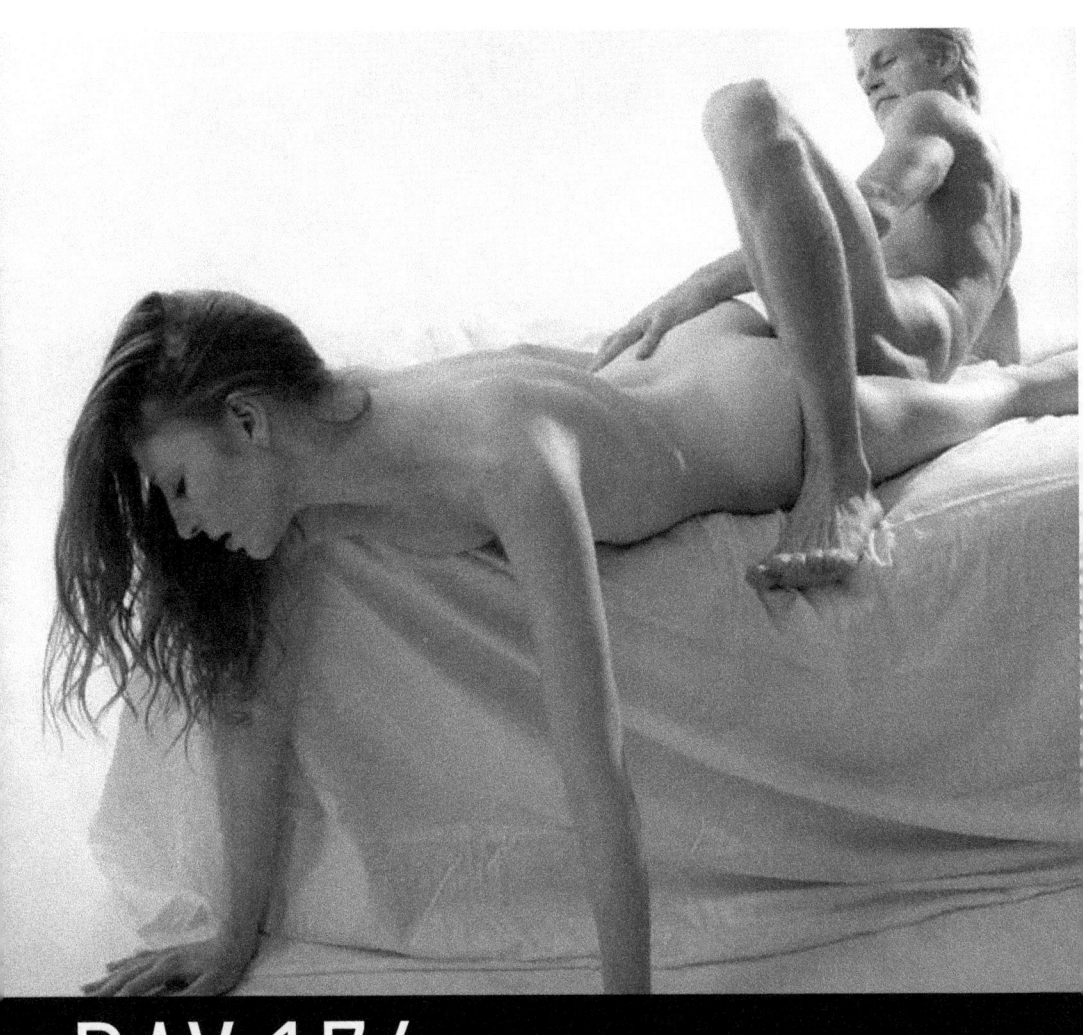

DAY 176

LINKED IN

The woman stretches across the bed on her stomach bringing her hands to the floor. Her partner gets on his side and moves in between her legs so that he's straddling one as he enters her. They're locked together but loving every minute of it.

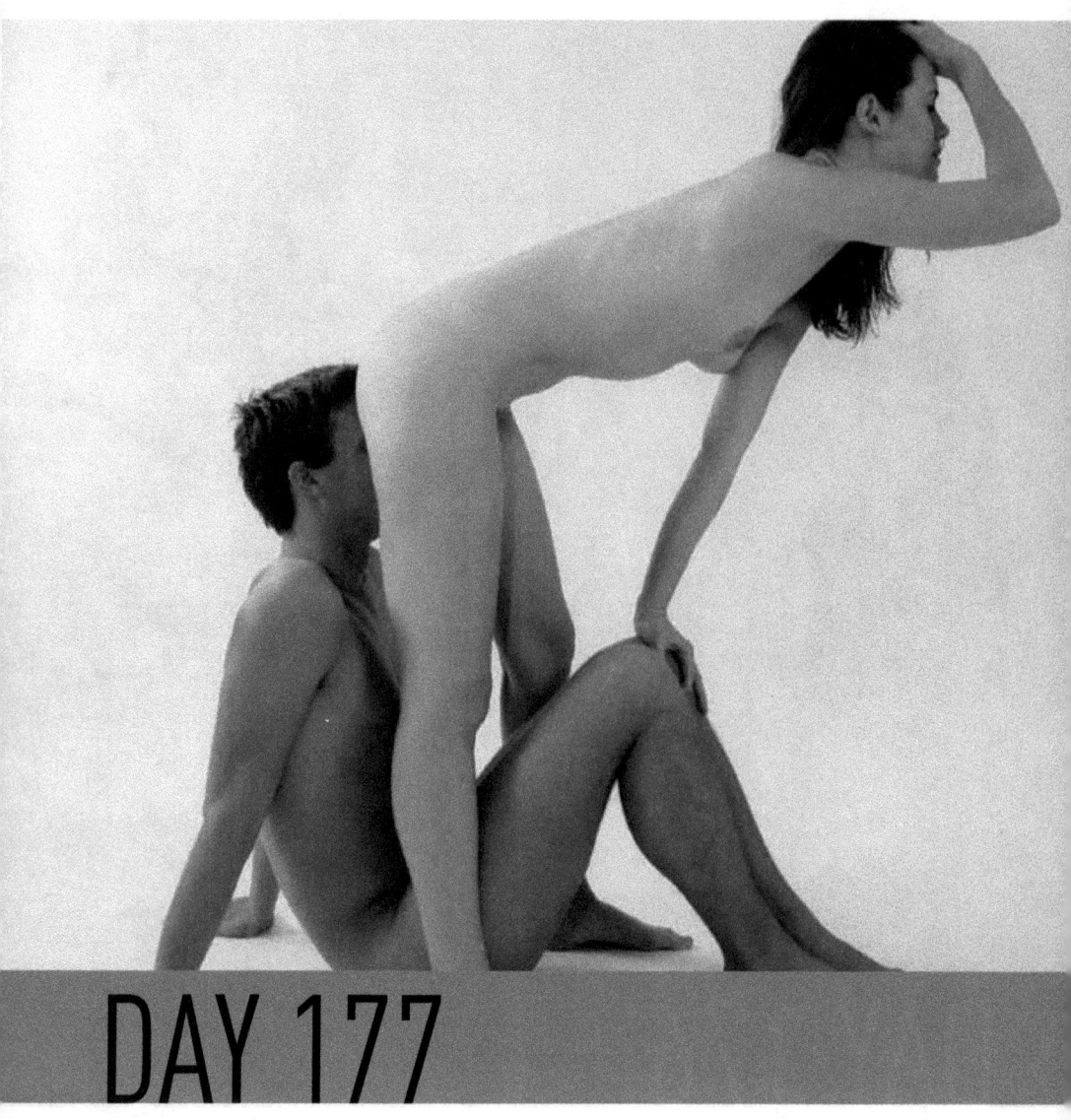

DAY 177

LICKETY SPLIT

The woman bends at the waist and places her palms on the floor. Her lover slides underneath her vagina and takes a seated position. From here he can perform cunnilingus until she can no longer catch her breath.

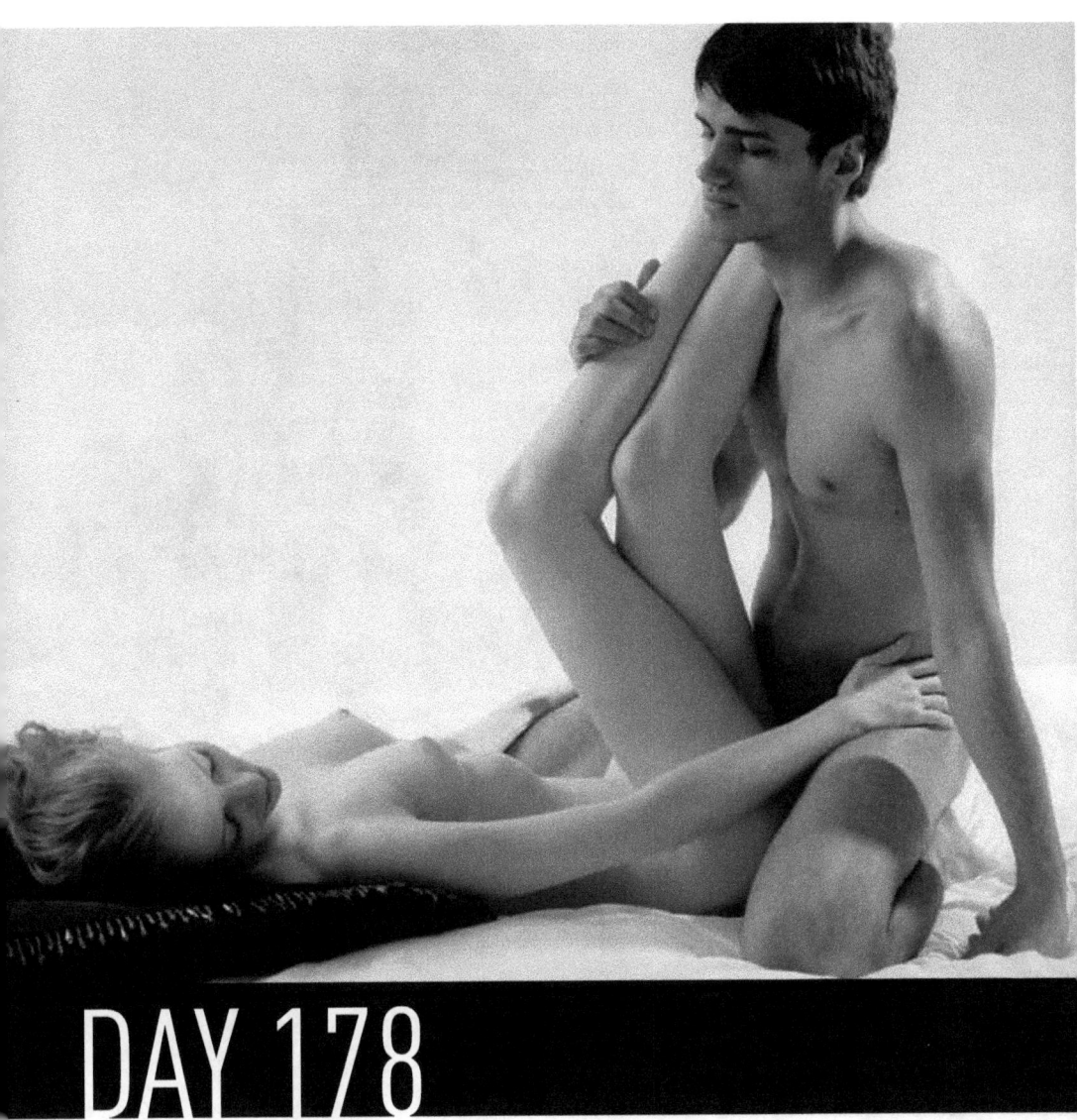

DAY 178

THE MECHANIC

He kneels on the bed, while she has both legs propped on one of his shoulders. From this starting position, he's free to maneuver her legs from side to side as he penetrates her. The constant motion creates all sorts of interesting angles and sensations for both partners.

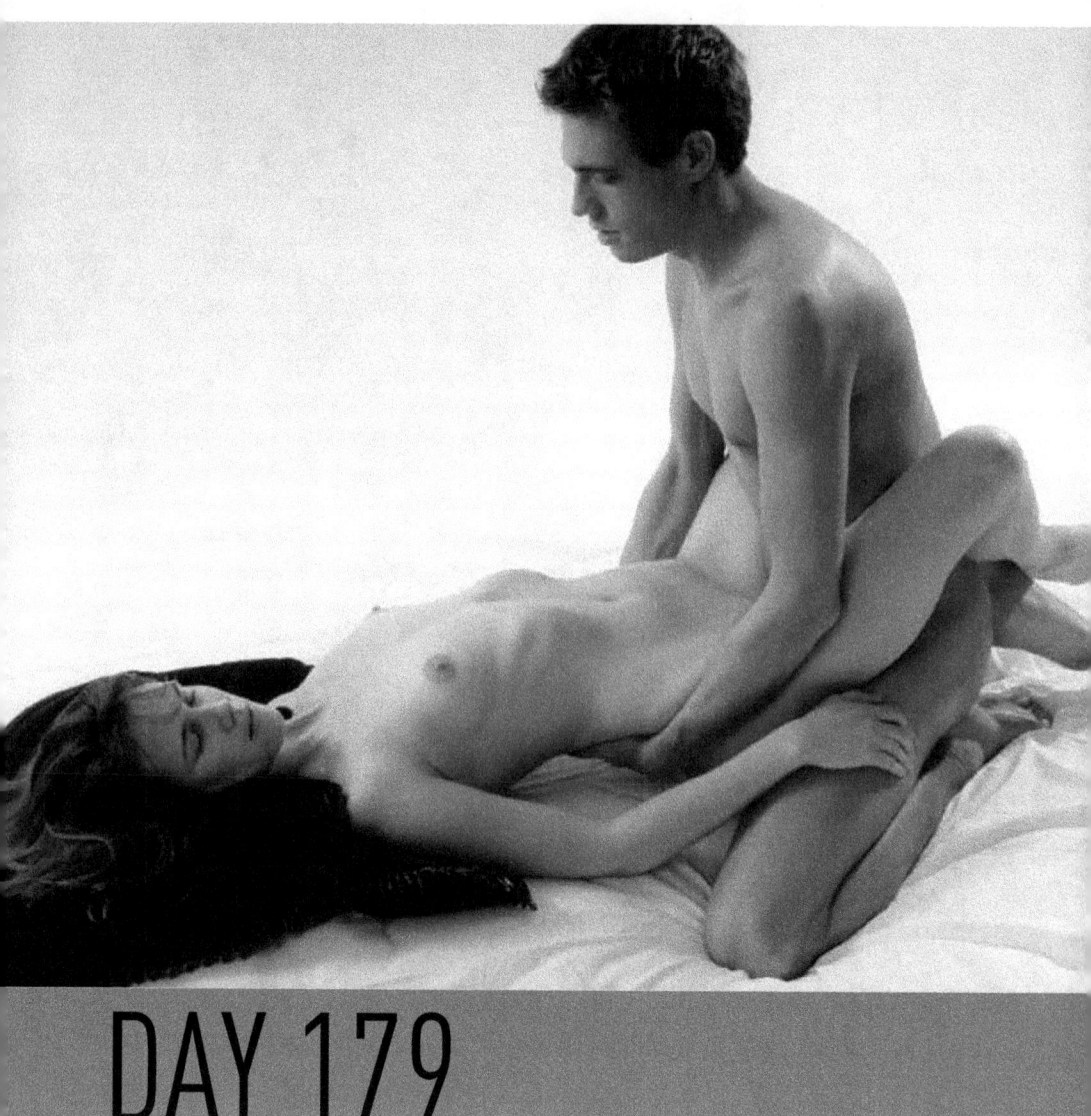

DAY 179

THE PELVIC PULSE

The woman is on her back and facing her lover. She arches her spine and lifts her pelvis up. The man slides in underneath her, sitting back on his legs, so that she can rest her buttocks on his thighs. They move together in stimulating harmony.

DAY 180

BENT FRIENDS

The couple places a pillow on the floor as the woman bends over and assumes a modified headstand position. Her hands are on either side of her head for support and her legs are back with knees bent. He lover enters her from behind, careful not to get too carried away with his thrusts.

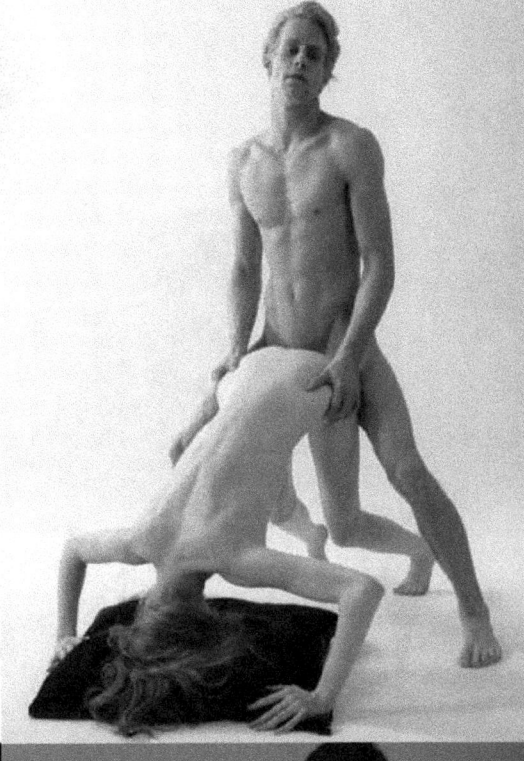

DAY 181

THE STRIP SEARCH

A little role playing always adds some fun. She's been caught red-handed and assumes the position with her legs spread and hands against the wall. He penetrates her from behind while giving the rest of her body a thorough search.

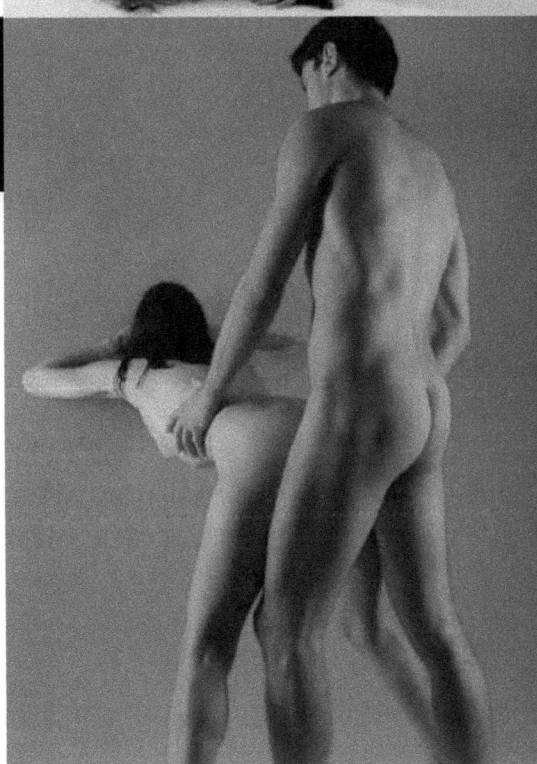

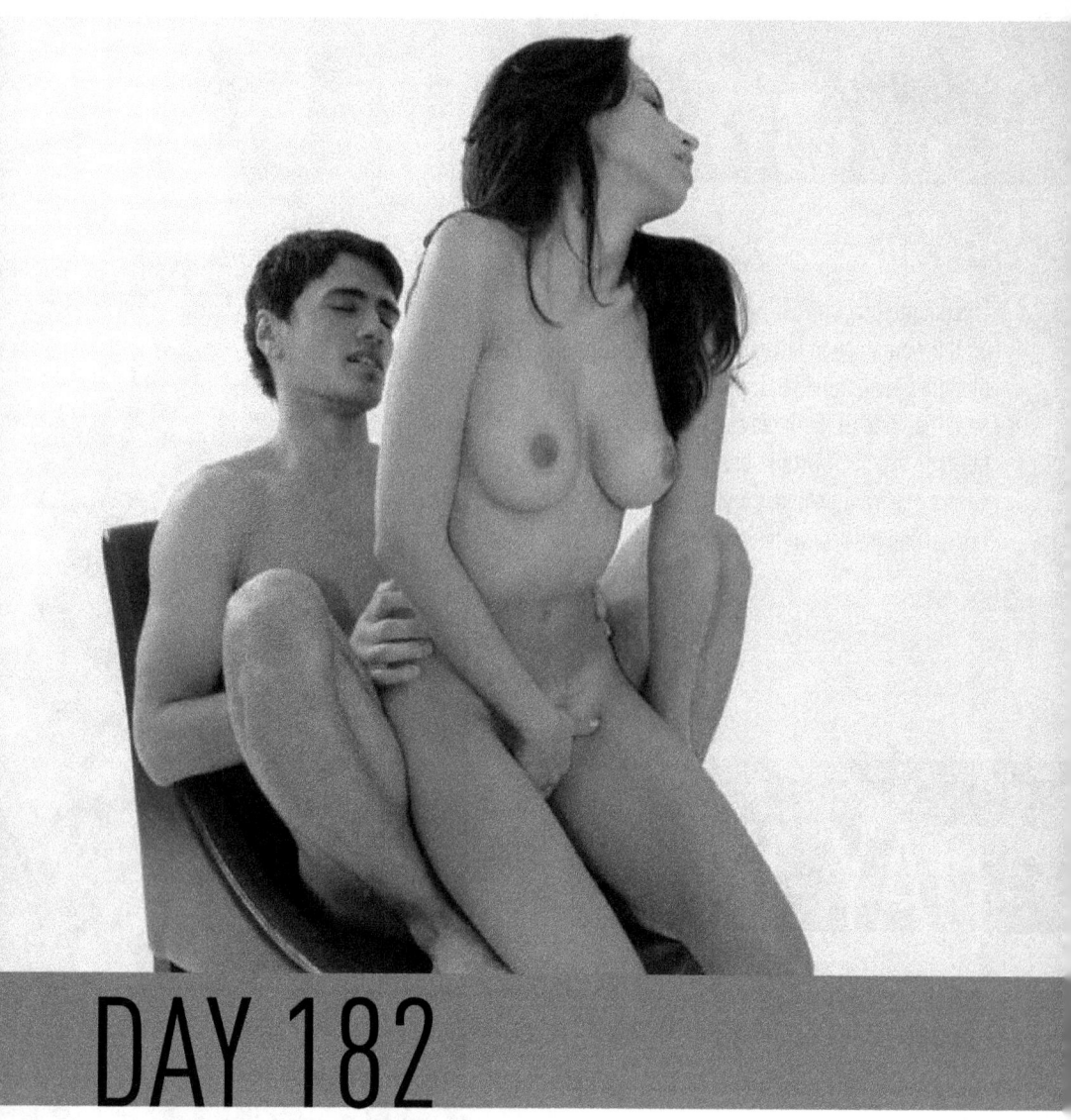

DAY 182

THE CHAIR ESSENTIALS

The man is in a chair with his knees pulled up and legs spread open. His lover mounts him, facing outward. She can play with his feet while he focuses on her breasts and clitoris.

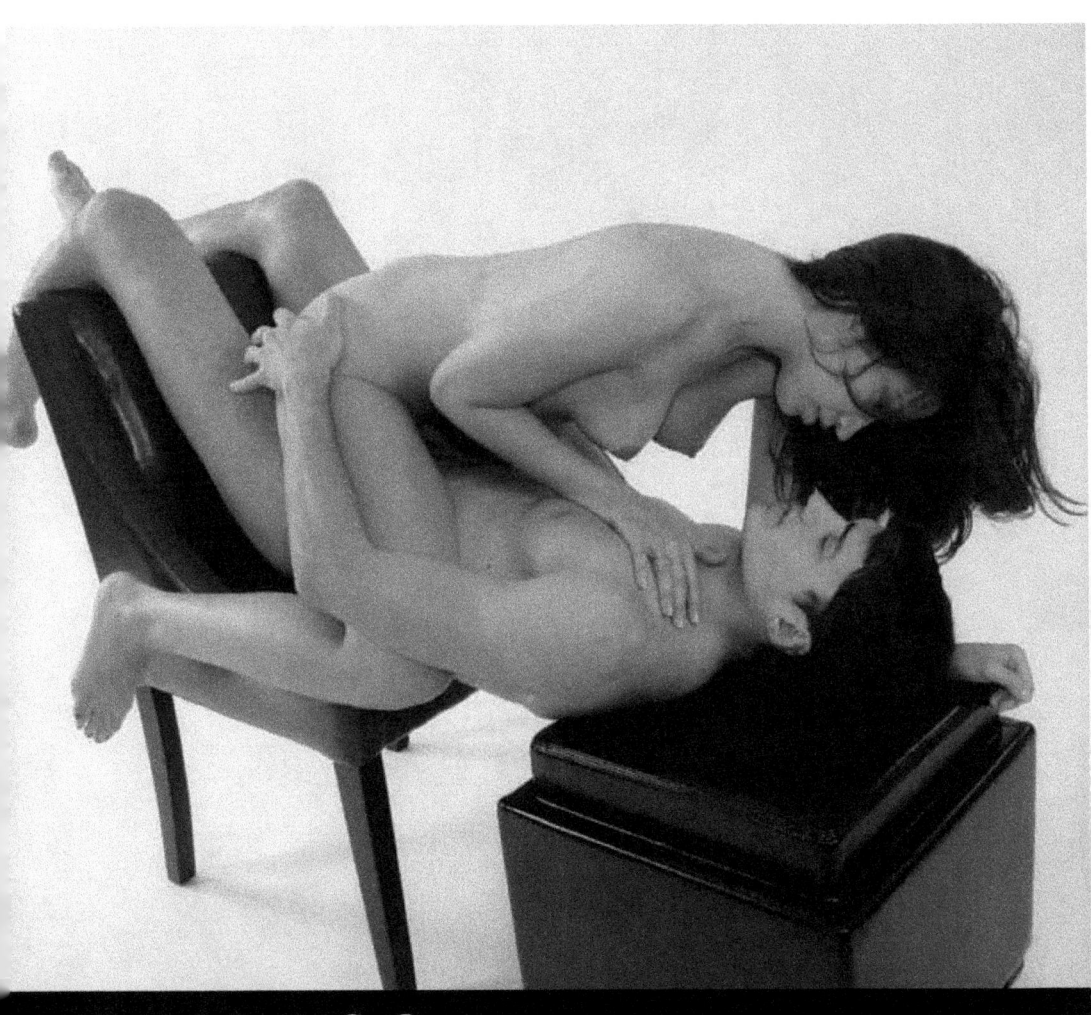

DAY 183

THE HAPPY HOSTAGE

He's resting back on an ottoman his legs draped over the back of a chair. His lover climbs on top and mounts him. He may be trapped, but he's not complaining.

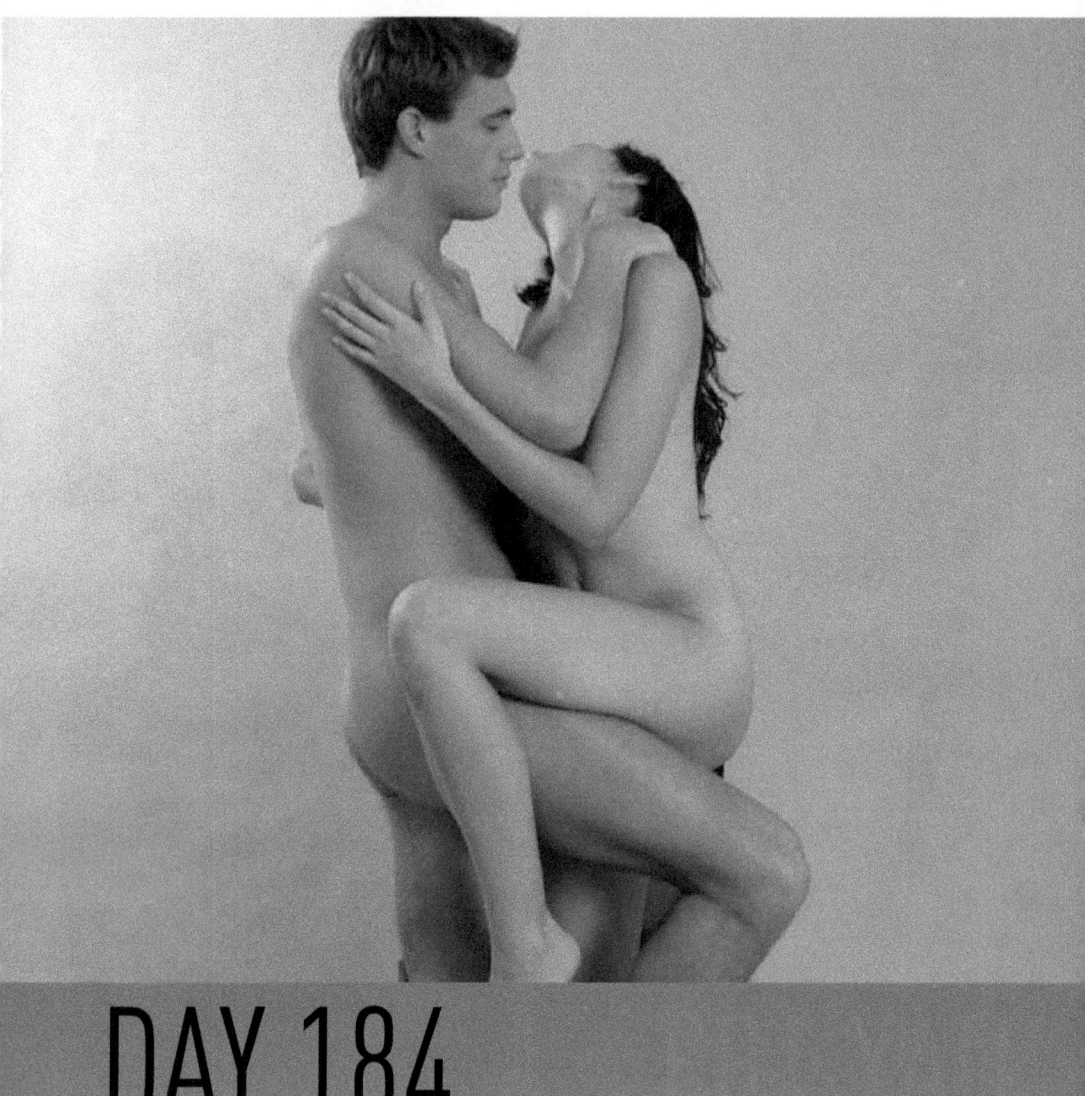

DAY 184

THE BALANCING ACT

The lovers stand facing each other as both raise a leg. She positions her leg over his and holds on to the underside of her partner's thigh. He steadies them both by resting his hand on a chair or dresser.

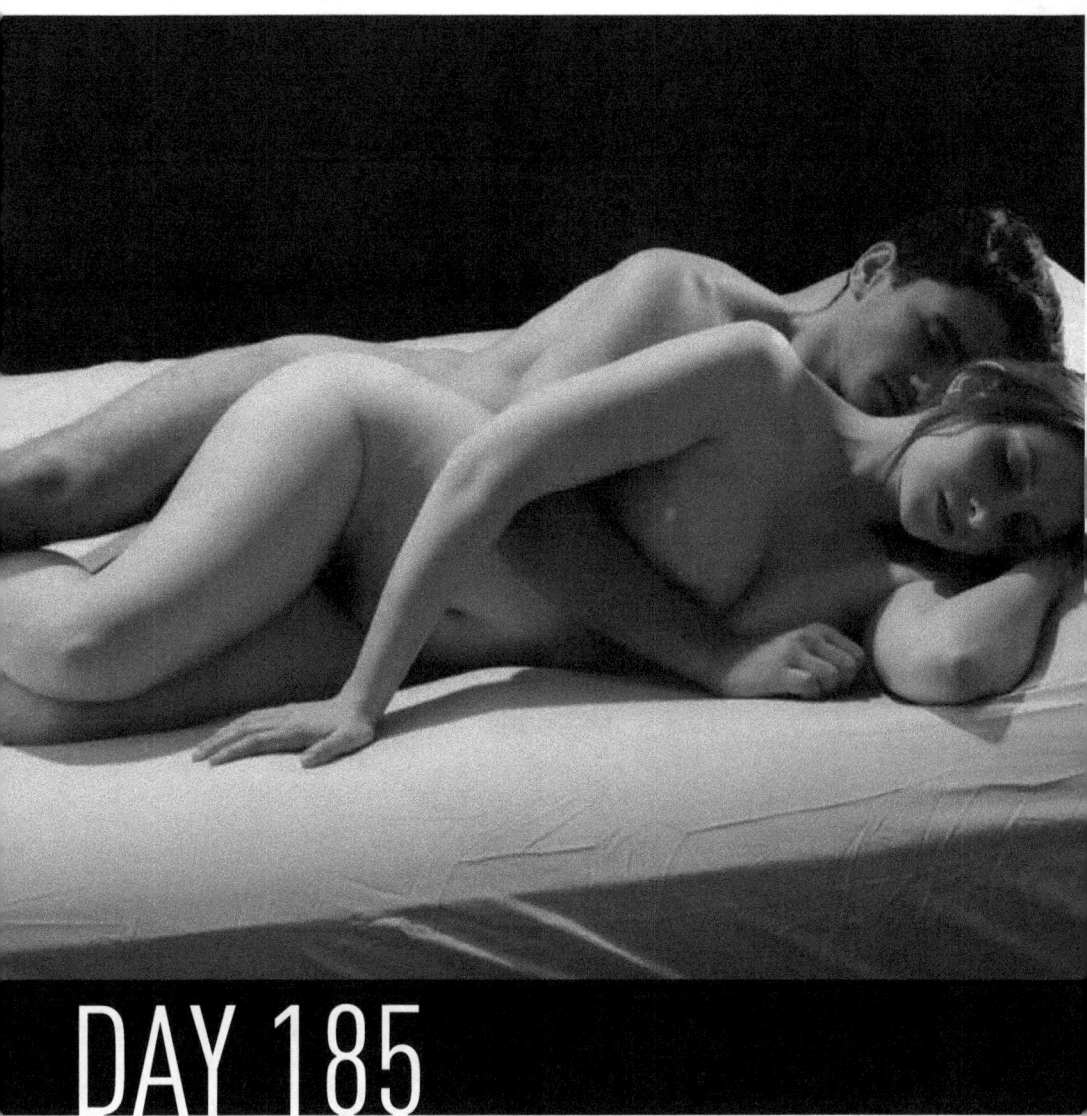

DAY 185

GOOD-NIGHT SPOON

The man and woman place themselves on their sides in a classic spooning pose. As he penetrates her from behind he can continue to embrace his lover or move his hand down to stroke her clitoris.

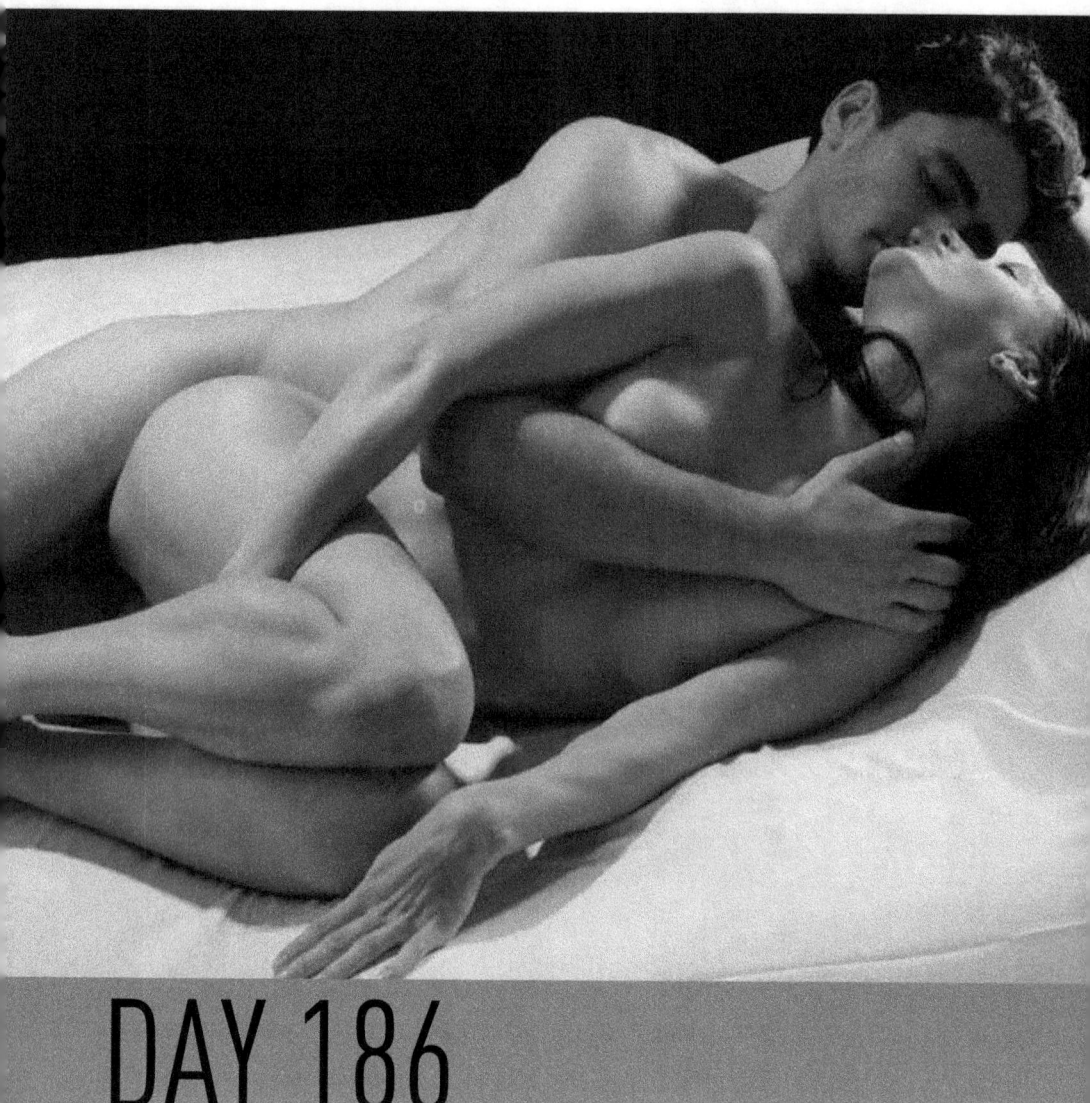

DAY 186

CHOOSING UP SIDES

The lovers position themselves on their sides with the man behind the woman. She tucks her knees up as he enters her from behind. She can turn her head for deep kisses as he runs his free hand over her entire body.

DAY 187

BENDING BEAUTY

Bending over backward for someone doesn't always have to be a chore. In this position, the woman sits in her lover's lap and reclines backward until her hands hit the floor. He's free to caress every inch of her.

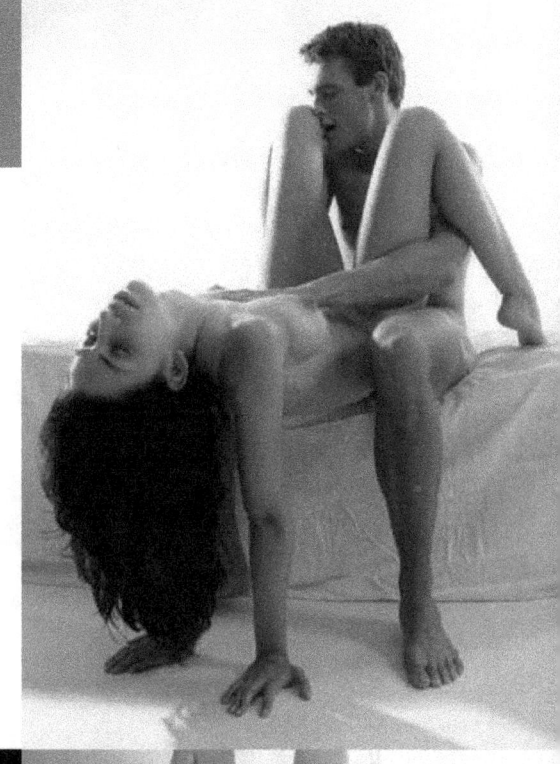

DAY 188

THE HANG GLIDER

He hangs off a bar as his lover wraps herself around him. As he penetrates her they swing back and forth. She might even try to release one of her hands and play with his testicles.

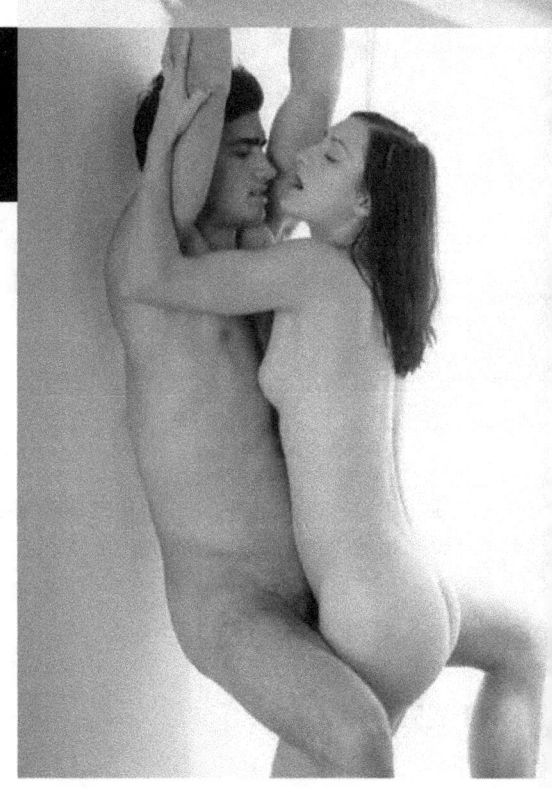

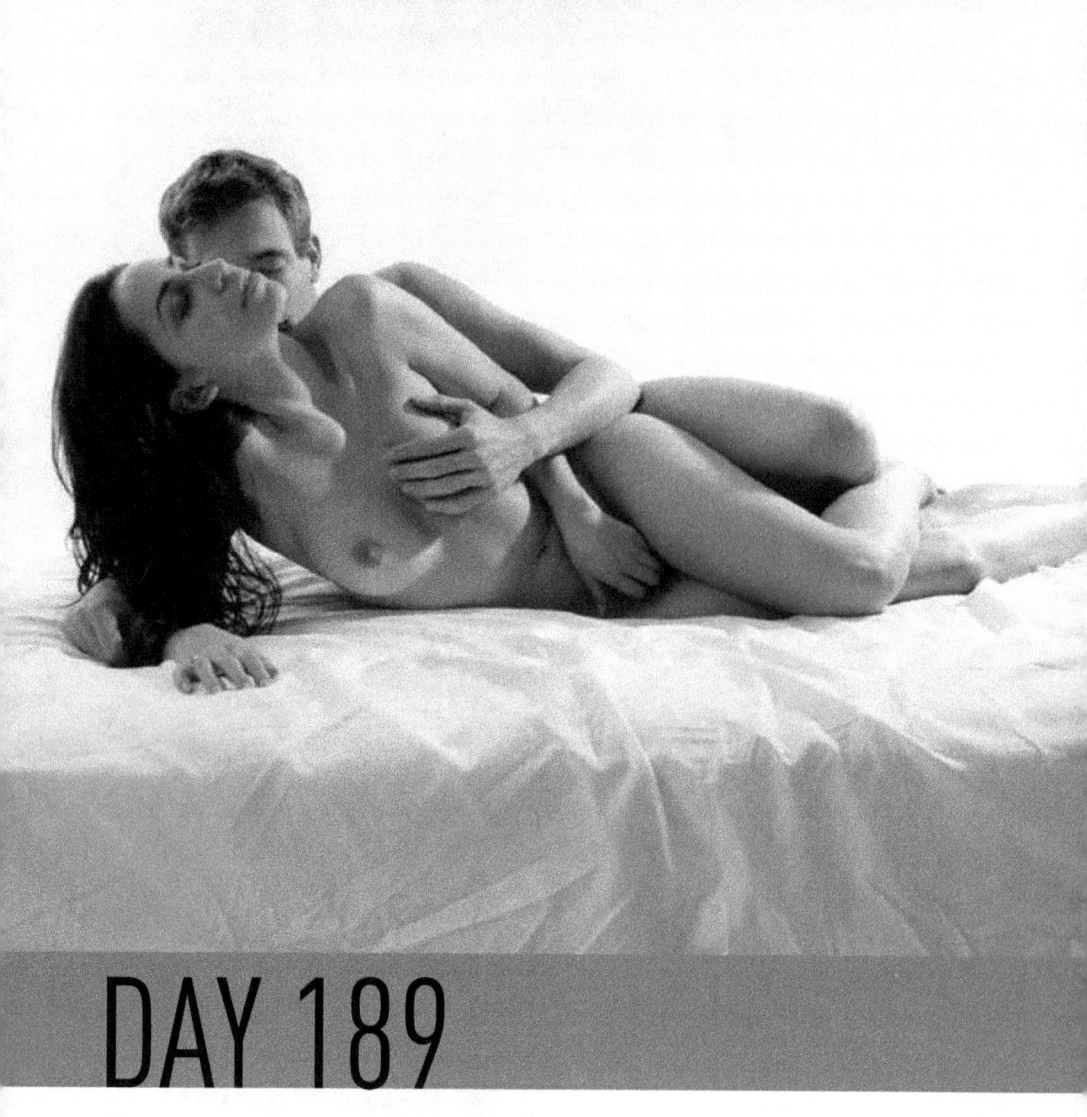

DAY 189

THE STIMULUS PACKAGE

Both lovers are stretched out on their sides with the man behind the woman. As he penetrates his partner anally, the man hands are free to stimulate her clitoris and breasts.

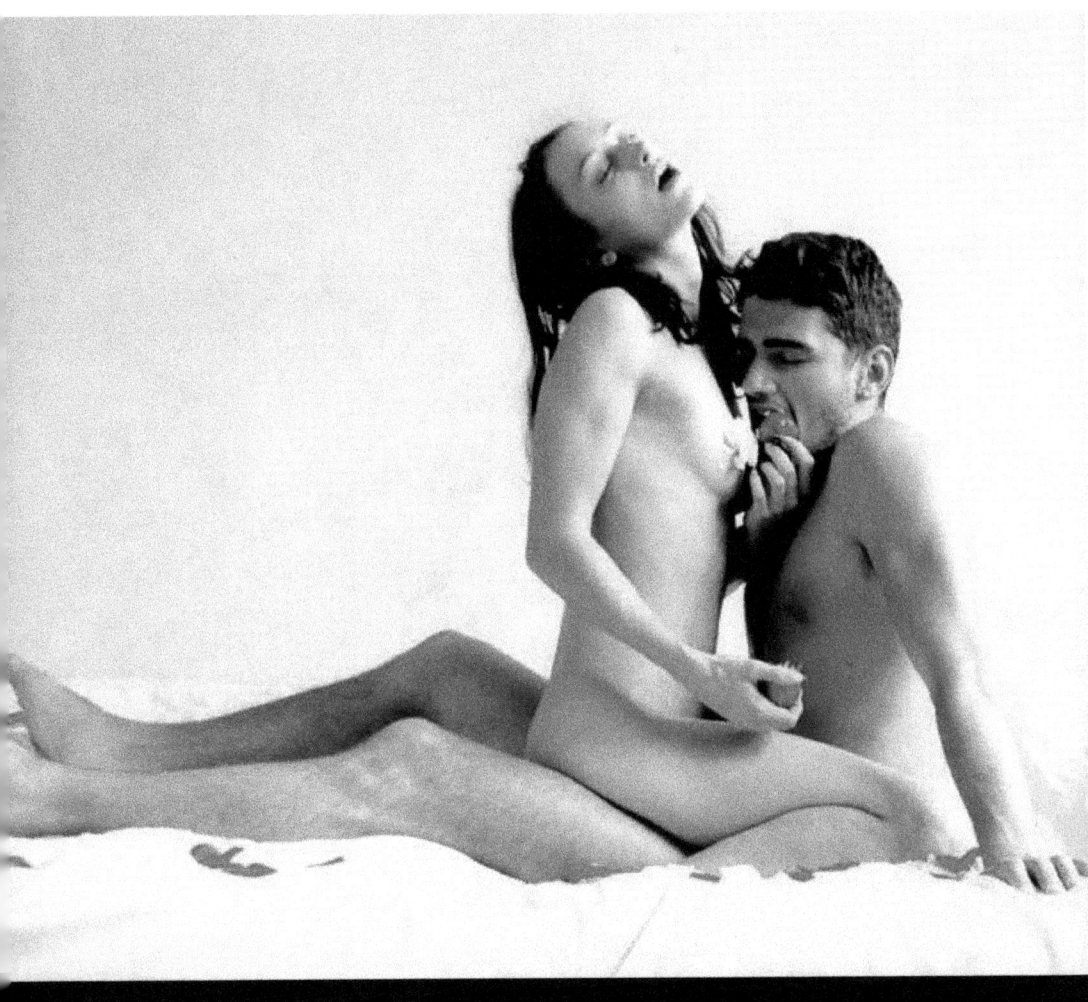

DAY 190

THE WIMBLEDON

Here's a fun spin on the signature treat at the world's most famous lawn tennis tournament. The man sits up on the bed with his legs extended while his partner straddles him. As he penetrates her she offers up a ripe strawberry as well as a whipped cream–covered nipple.

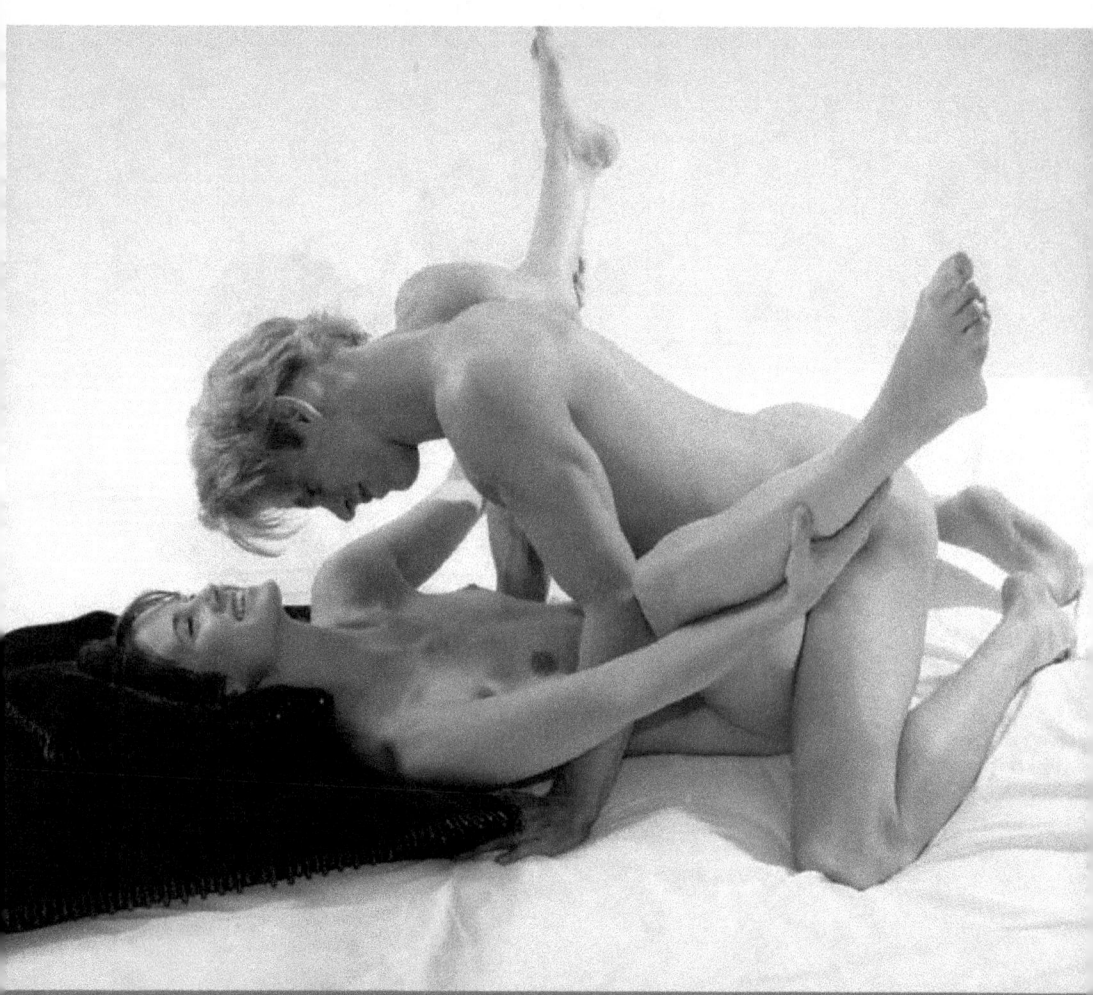

DAY 191

OPEN ALL NIGHT

Resting on her back, the woman pulls her legs halfway up toward her chest and then wide out to the sides. Her vagina is invitingly open for her partner to enter her deeply.

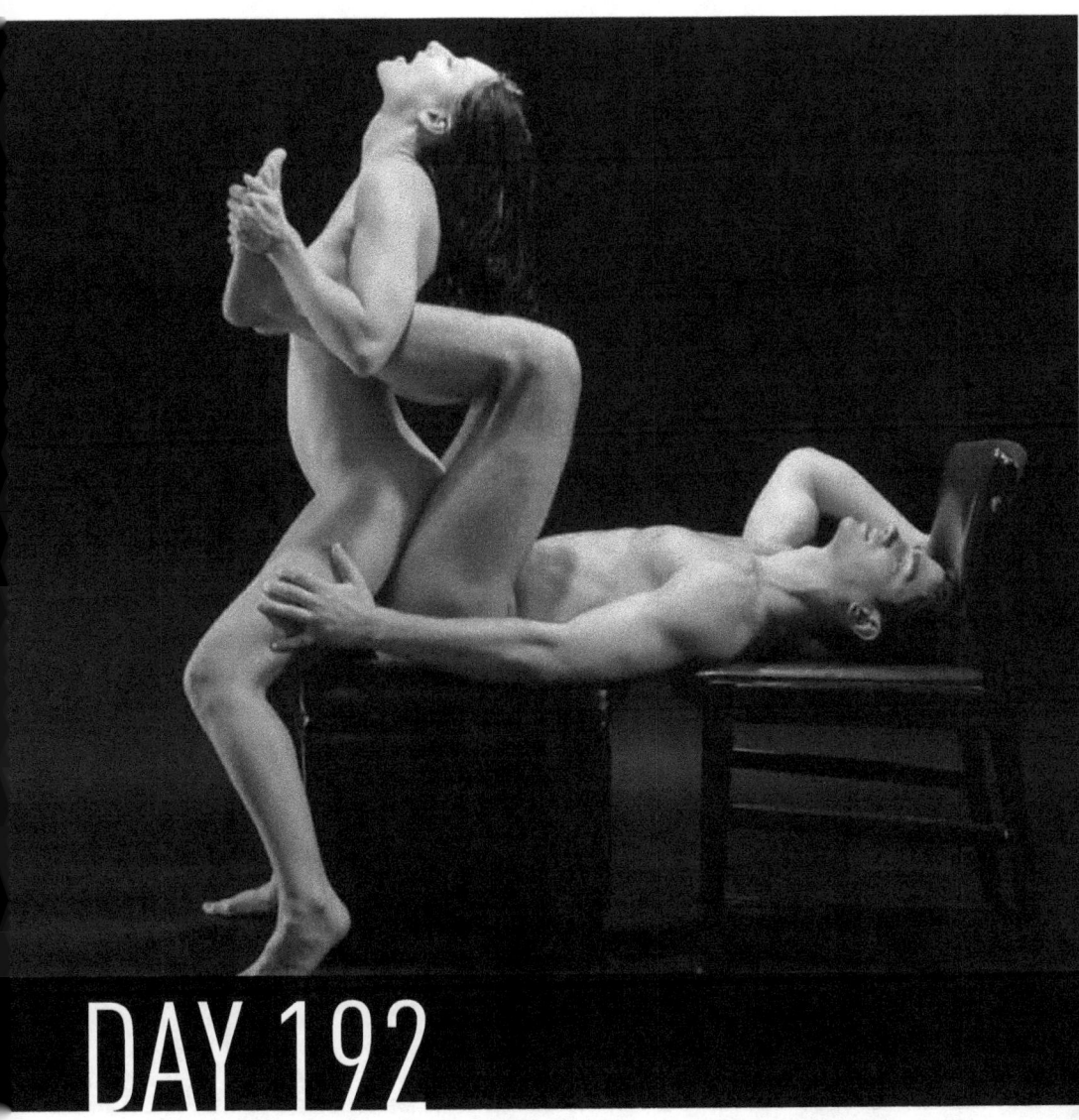

DAY 192

BACKDOOR MAN

He places his head on a chair and his butt on an ottoman as he brings his legs up and bends them. She lubes her anus up and then lowers herself onto his penis. She grabs his legs and controls the penetration and pace.

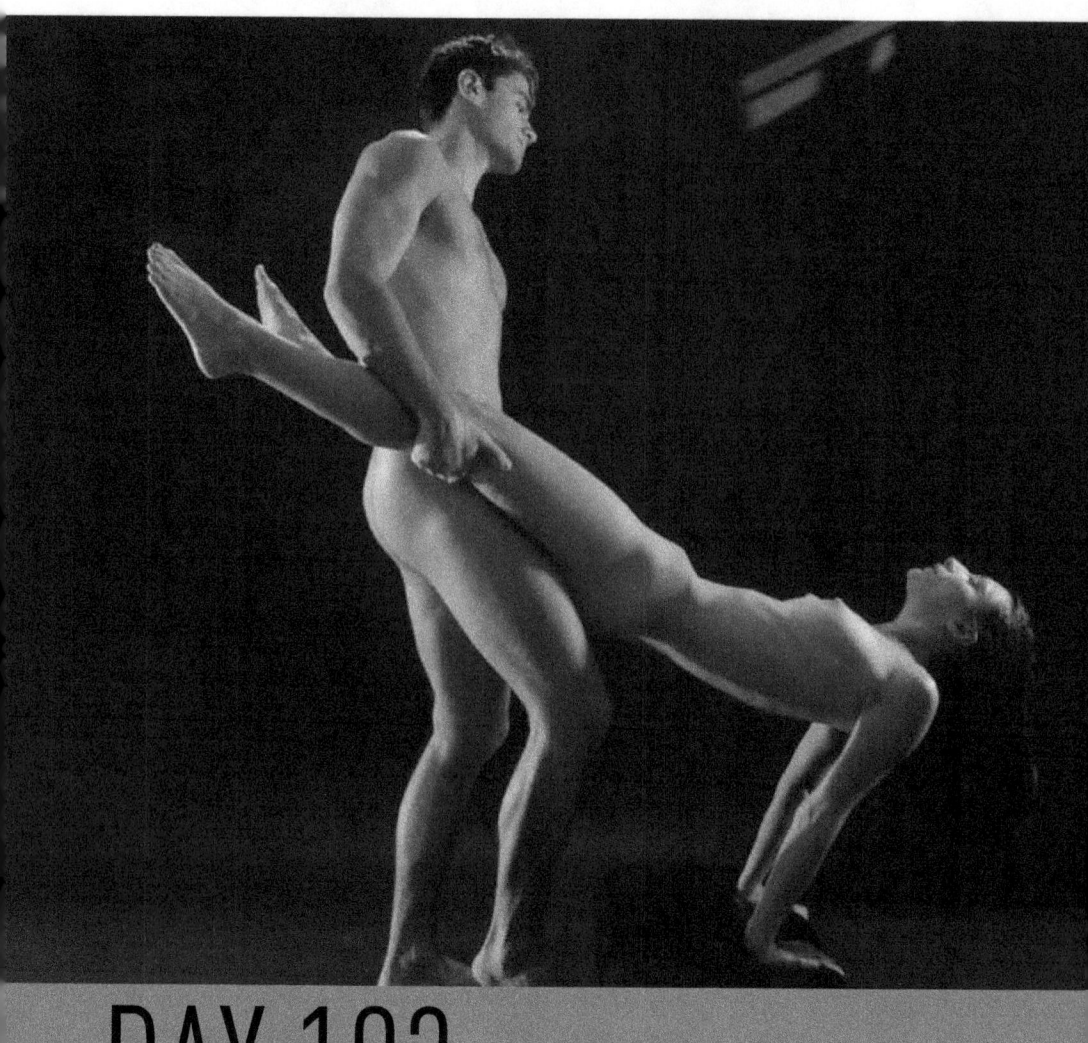

DAY 193

LOVE LIFT US UP

This one requires great strength and concentration from both partners. The man penetrates the woman from a standing position as she tilts her body backward and places her hands on the floor. He needs to offer ample support in order to maintain penetration.

DAY 194

HOP IN THE SACK

In a kneeling position, he sits back on his heels and brings his hands behind his body. She lowers herself onto his erect penis, keeping some weight on the balls of her feet. From here the lovers can bounce and hop until they drop.

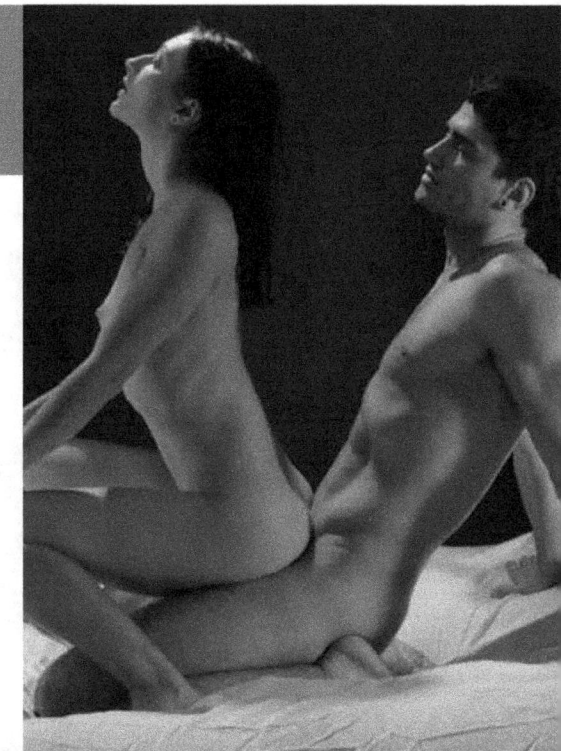

DAY 195

YOU SCRATCH MY BACK...

The woman starts on all fours while her lover is on a single bended knee behind her. As he enters her, she lifts up her leg and brings it around to rest on his back.

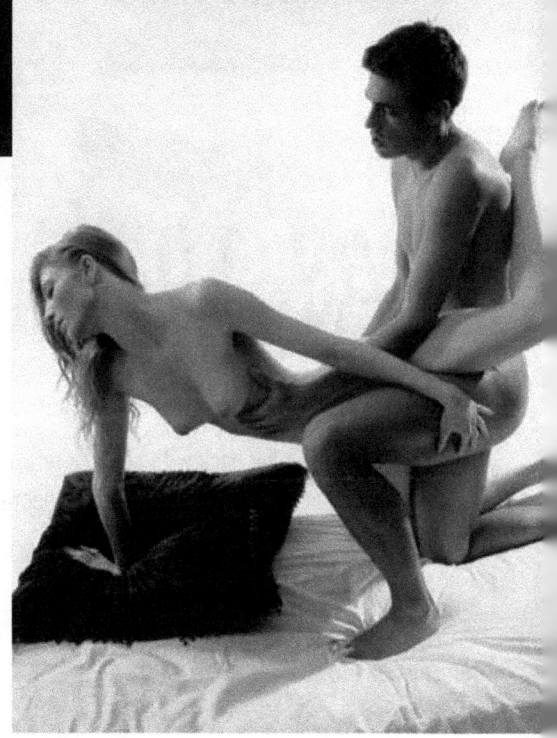

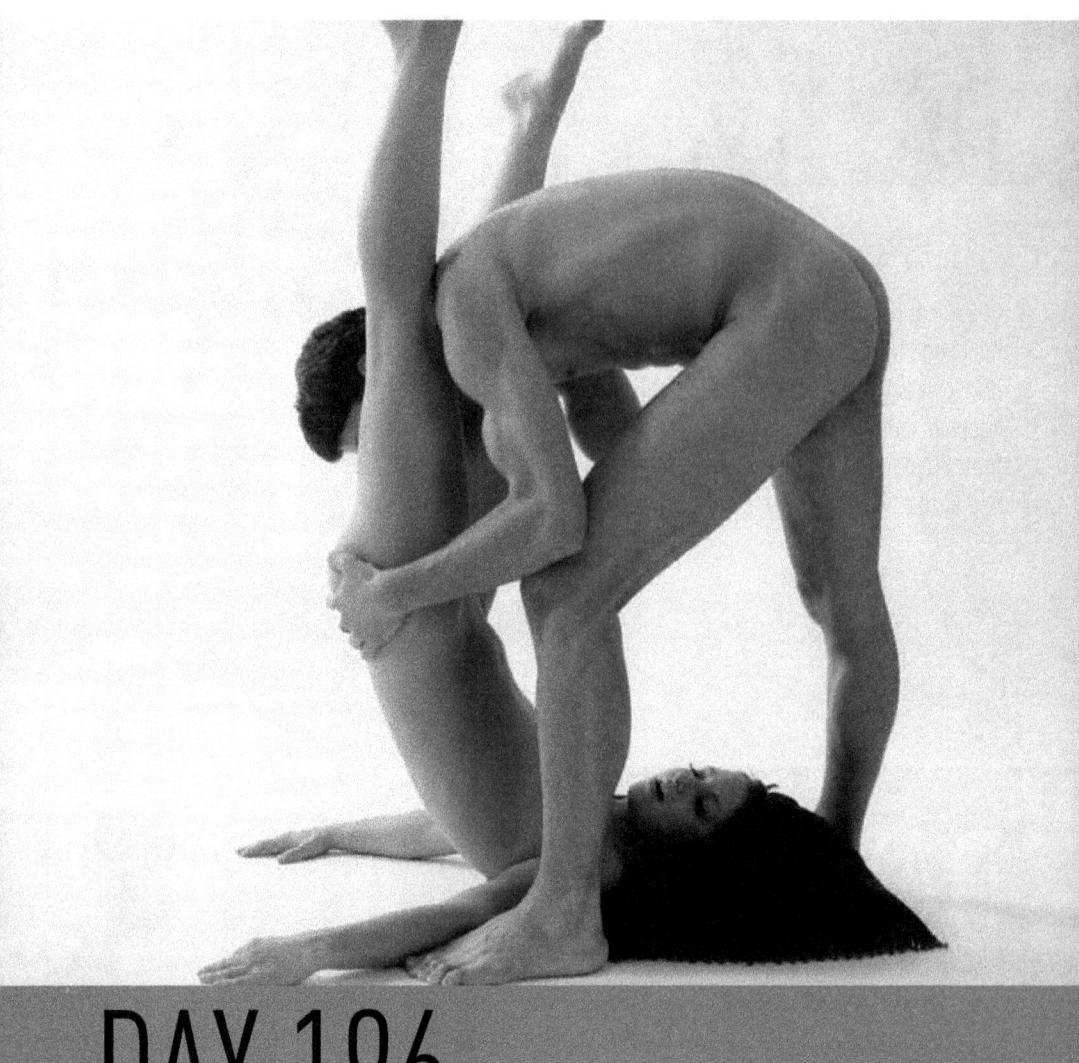

DAY 196

THE BUSY BEE

The woman is on her back with her legs relaxed and open. Her lover lifts her from the waist and lowers his head down to sample her nectar.

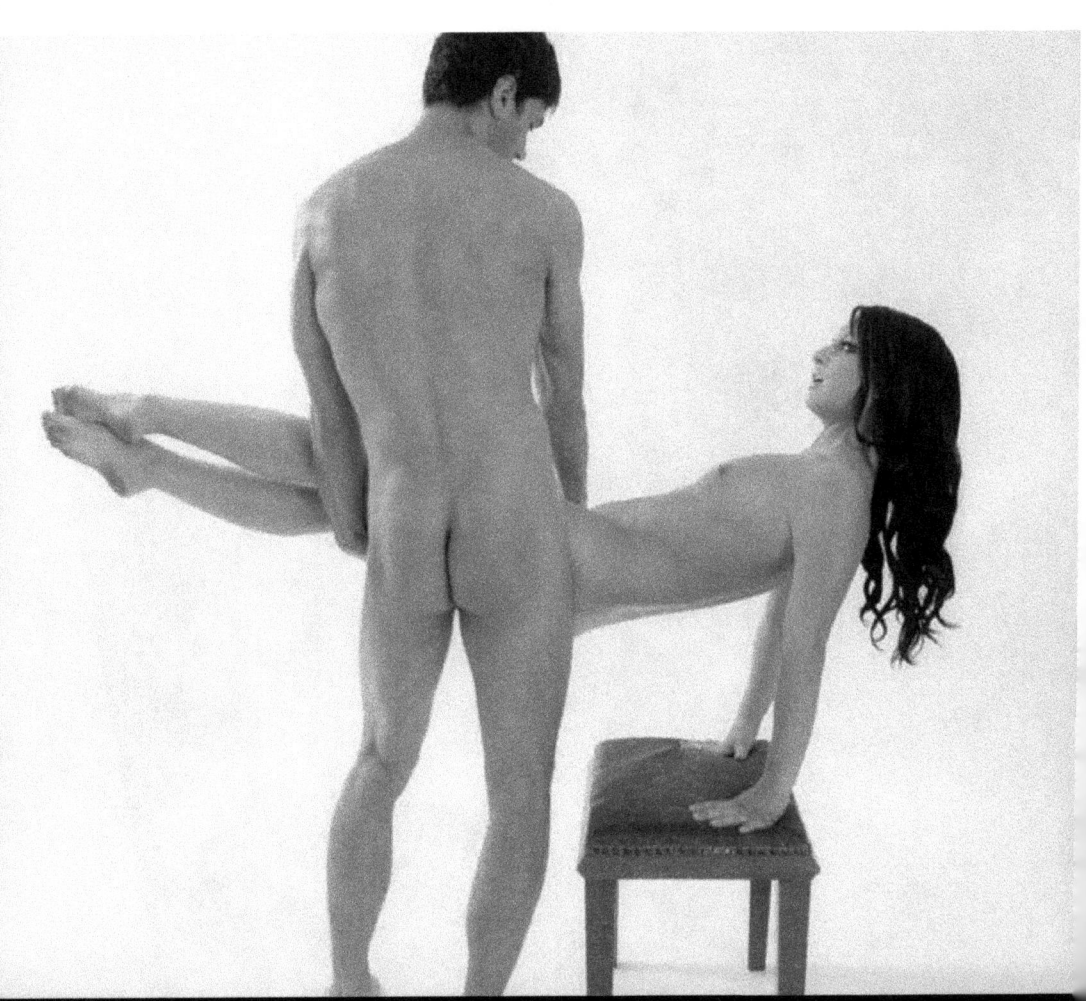

DAY 197

SIDEWAYS SATISFACTION

She places her hands on a bench or stool for support as her lover lifts her lower body up. Once she is perpendicular to his penis, she swivels her hips sideways allowing him to enter her.

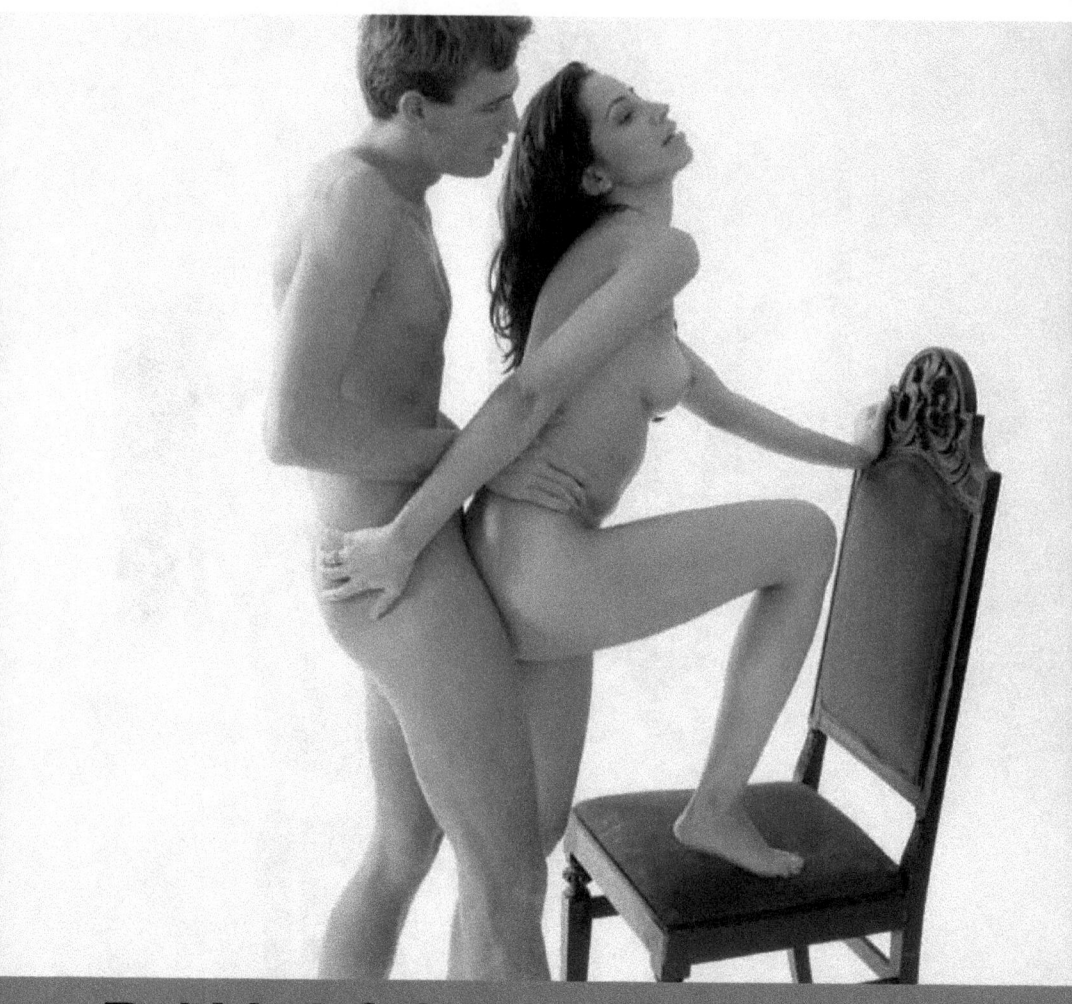

DAY 198

THE NEXT STEP

Sometimes you need to take your lovemaking to another level. In this position, the woman steps one foot up onto a chair as her partner enters her from behind. They both have the freedom to let their hands explore the other's pleasure points.

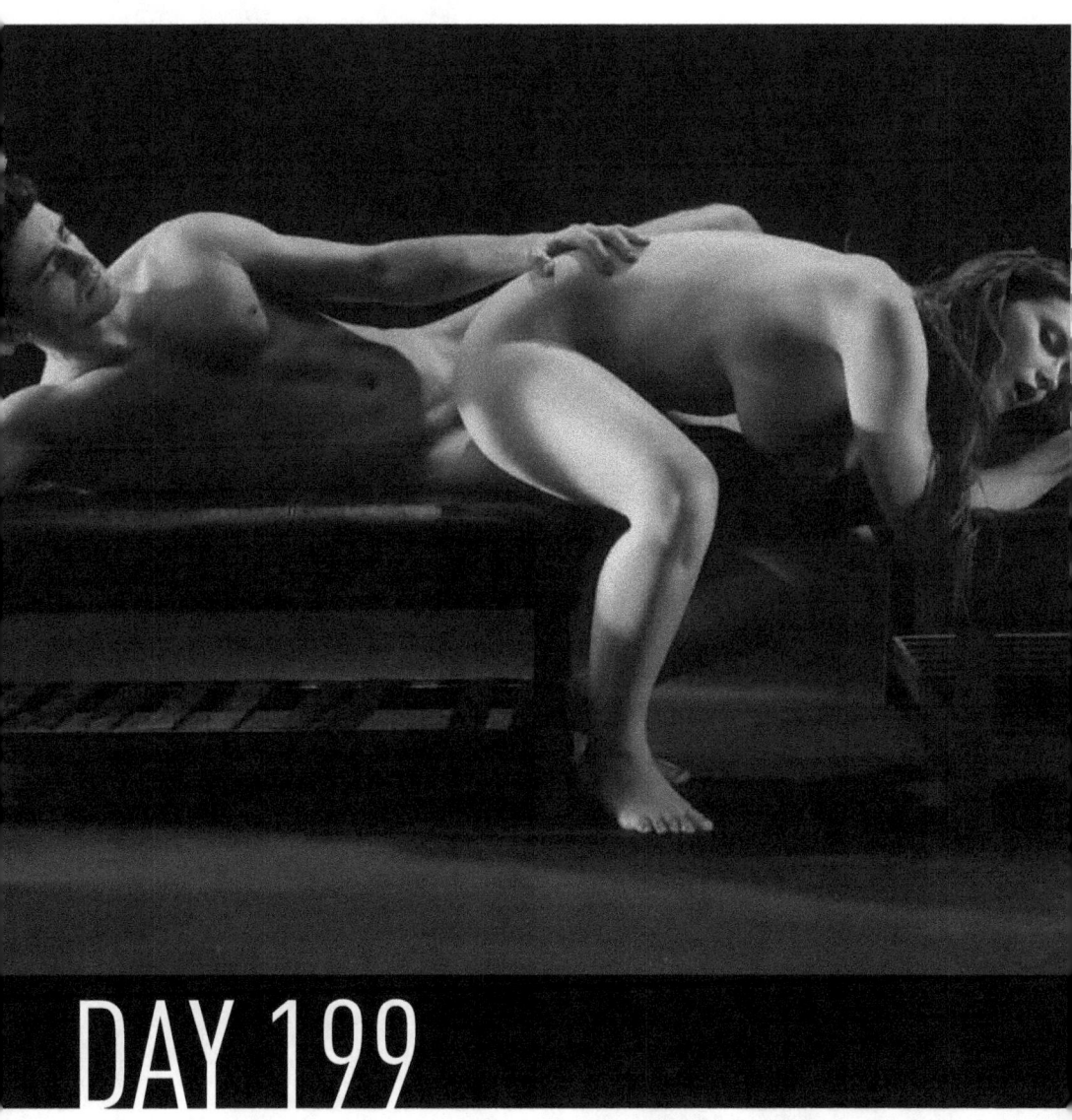

DAY 199

THE CASUAL LOVERS

The man stretches out on his side, leaning his elbow on one piece of furniture and his feet on another. The woman straddles his lower leg, allowing him to enter her. Her clitoris gets a lot of contact once things really get going.

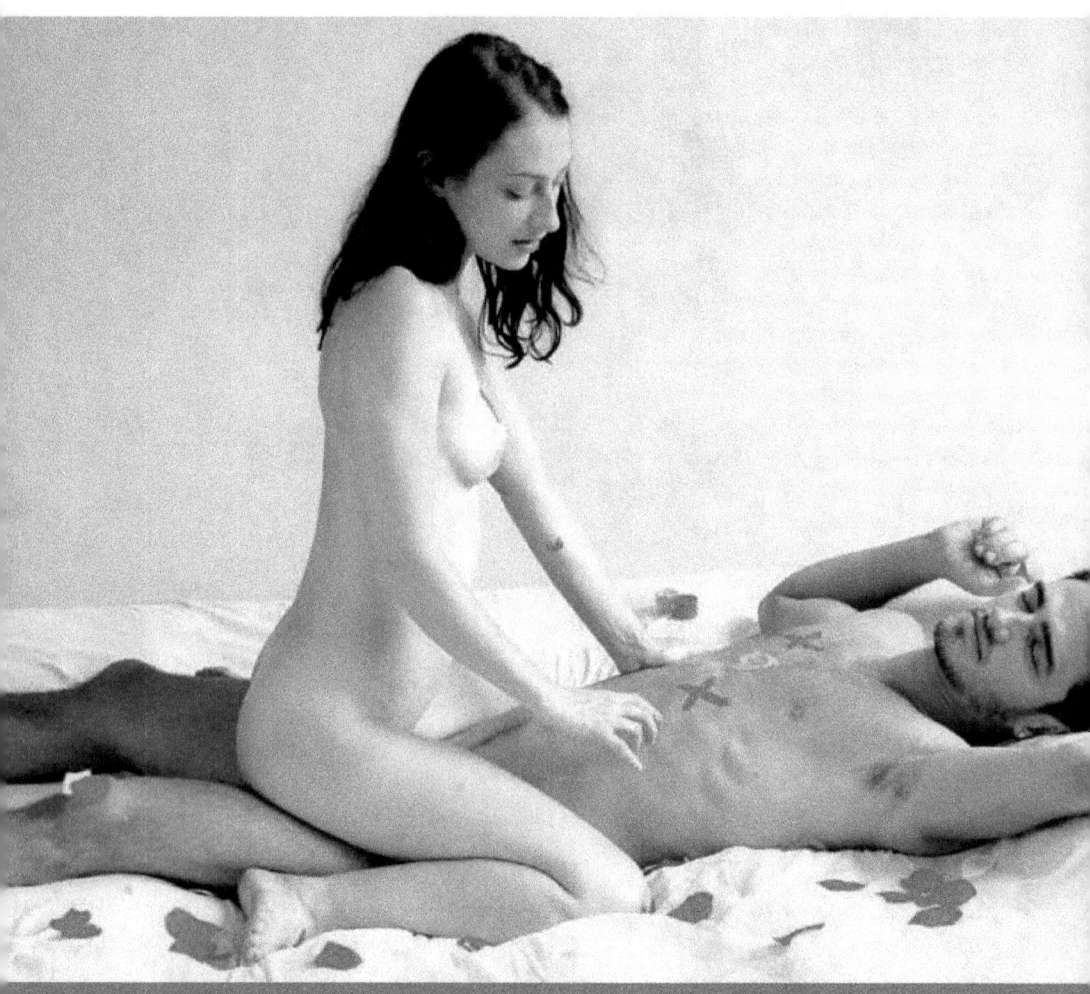

DAY 200

LOVE LETTERS

The man lies back across his bed as his partner mounts him. Using edible body paint, she turns his torso into a canvas as he penetrates, keeping his thrusts shallow and languid.

DAY 201

THE HOLDING COMPANY

Here's a good argument for having a striptease pole installed in your house. The woman reaches up and grabs hold of a pole or column. Her lover penetrates her from behind and grabs the pole himself. From here they can spin themselves into a 360-degree orgasm.

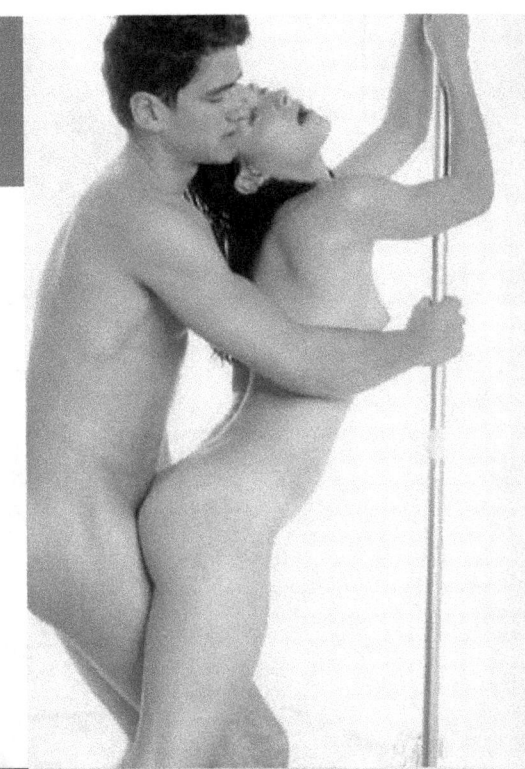

DAY 202

THE STANDING SPONGE BATH

Who says cleaning up has to be a chore? After a night of wonderfully messy body painting and lovemaking, she sponges him down while lifting her leg and allowing him to penetrate her once more.

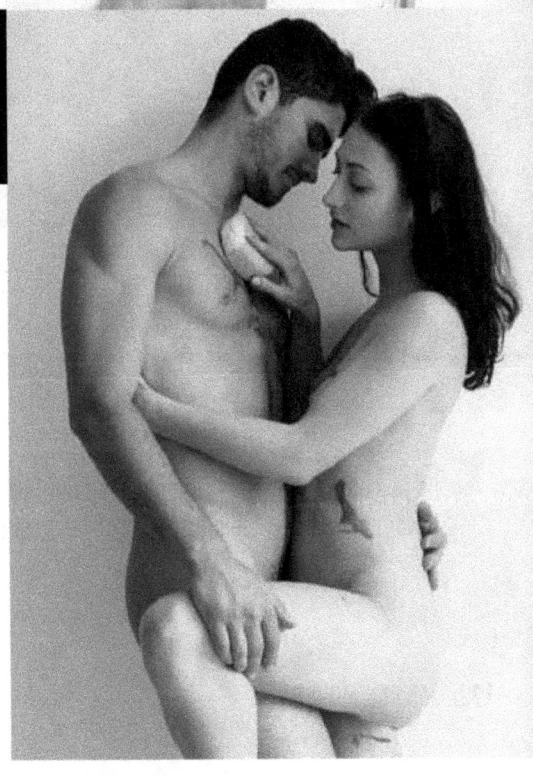

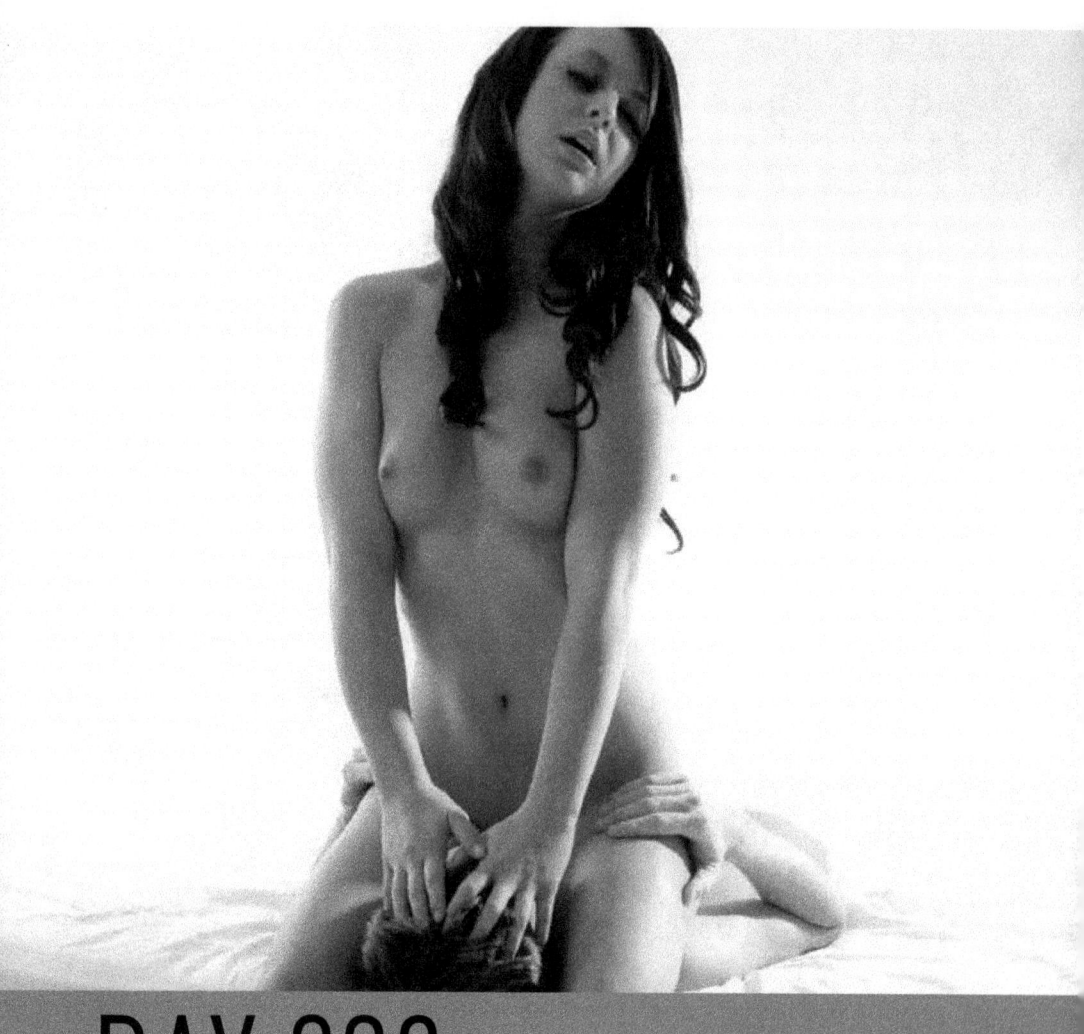

DAY 203

BOX SEAT

He lies back on the bed with his head right up against the edge. His lover lowers herself down toward his waiting tongue. She's got the best seat in the house as he brings her to climax.

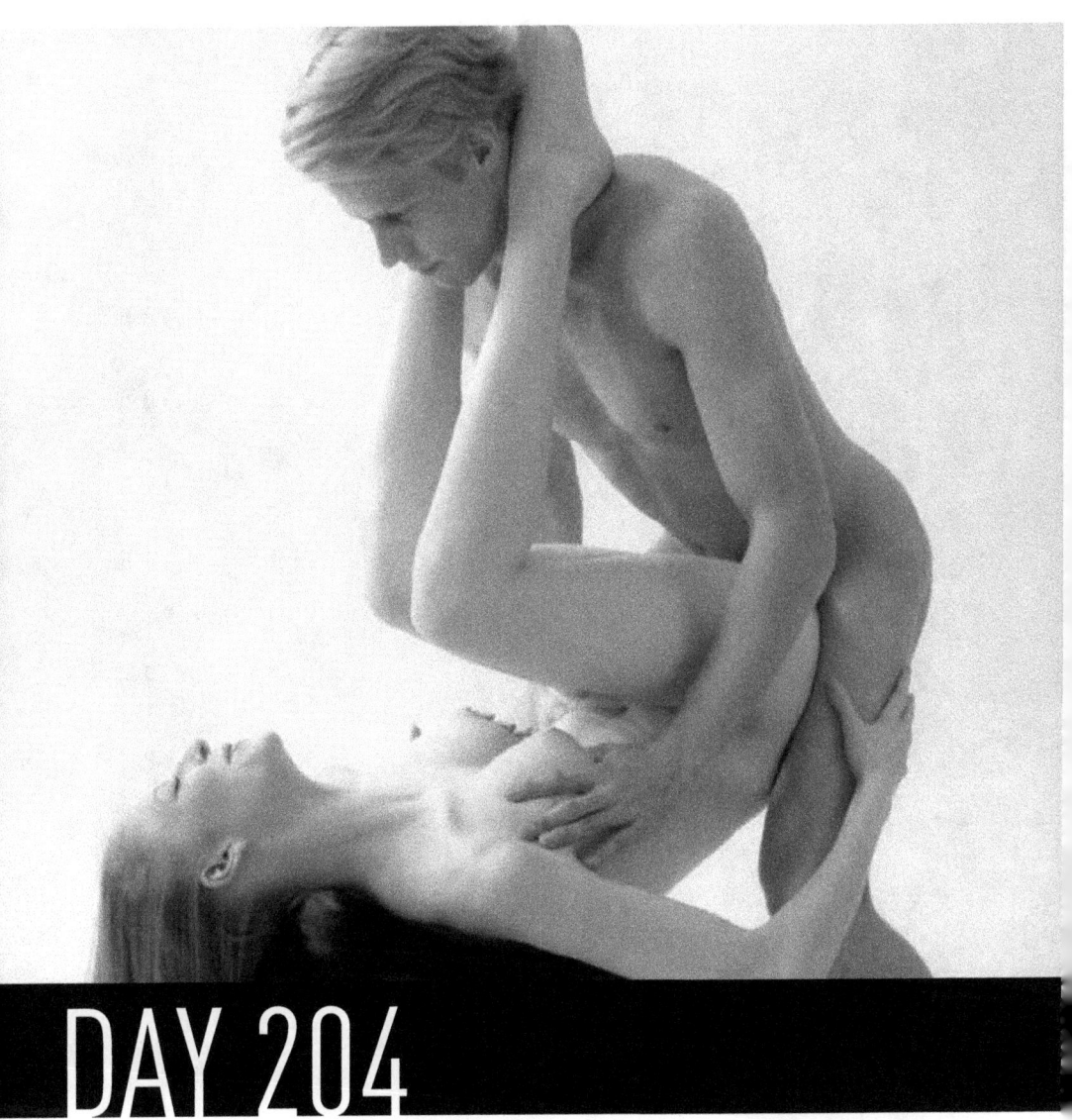

DAY 204

TAKING CHARGE

The woman rests her head and shoulders on a padded stool as her lover lifts her hips and enters her. She wraps her feet around his neck as he controls the pace.

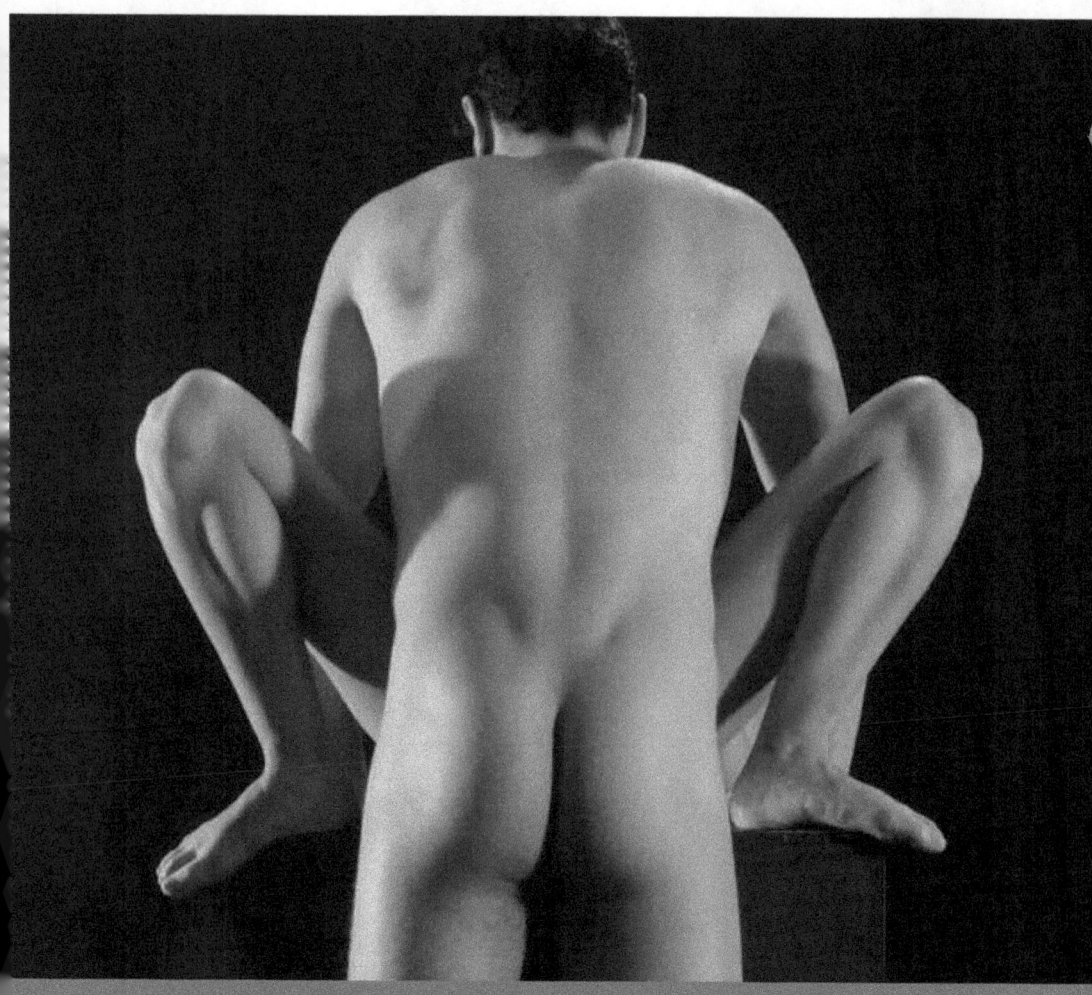

DAY 205

HIGHER POWER

The woman lies back on a dresser or other high piece of furniture with her legs open and knees bent. Her lover may have to get up on his toes to get there, but when he enters her it will all be worth it.

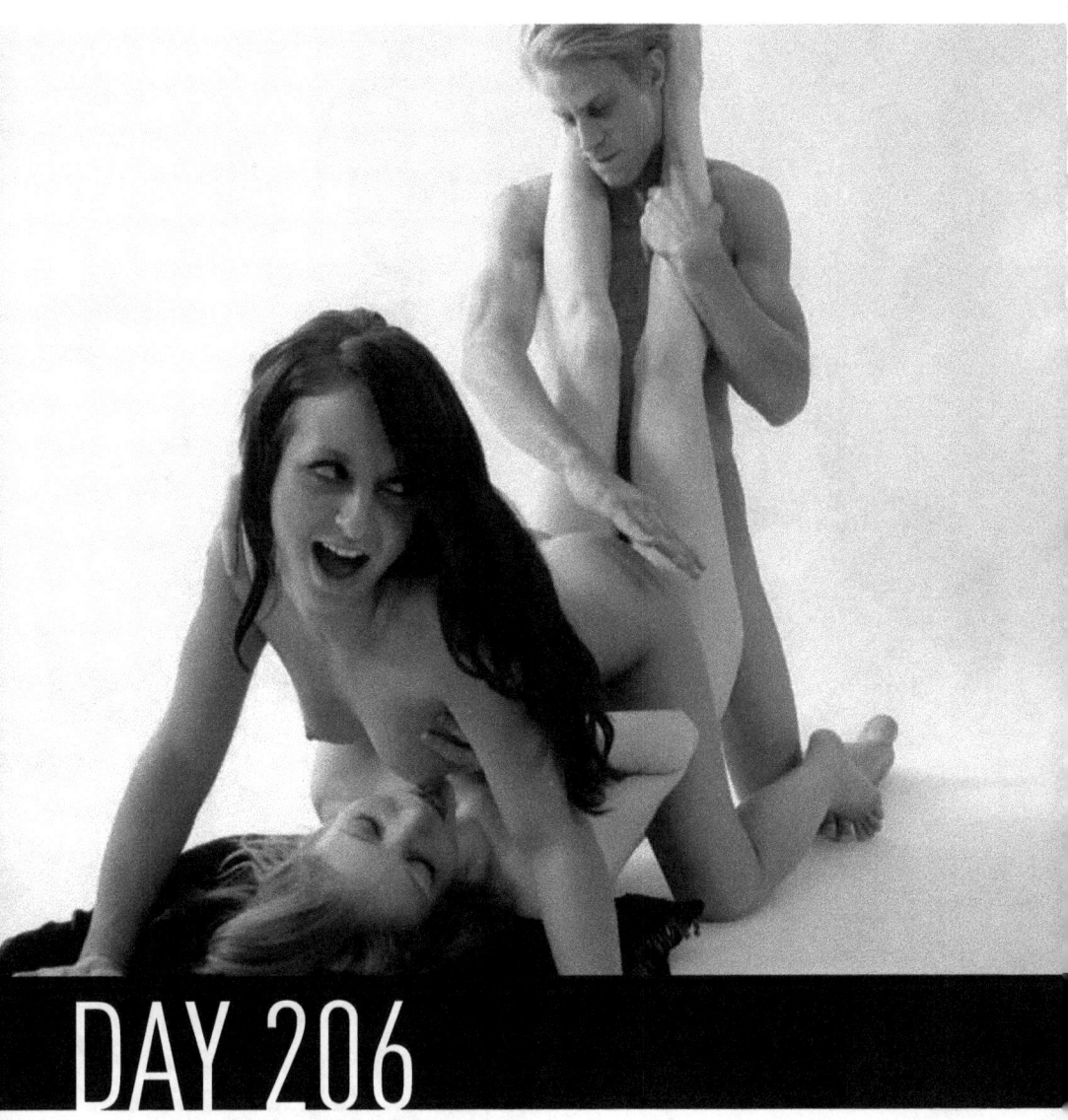

DAY 206

THE CHEEKY MONKEY

Here's another position for a trio of lovers. One woman lies on the floor and snakes her legs up past the man's shoulders as he slides himself inside of her. The other woman straddles her girlfriend who licks her breasts and strokes her clitoris. The man can join the fun by lightly spanking her buttocks.

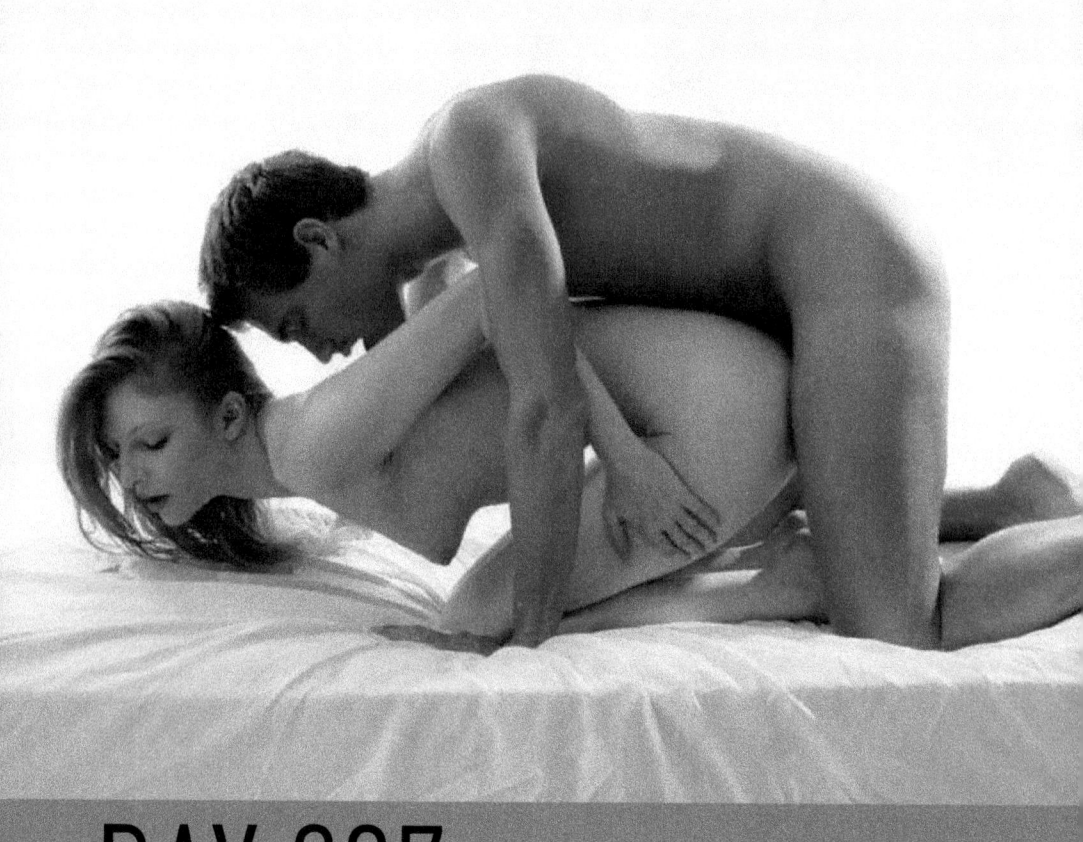

DAY 207

TUCK BUDDIES

The woman tucks her legs underneath her and leans forward. He gets on his knees and enters her from behind. Her back is open for soft strokes and gentle kissing.

DAY 208

FALLING FOR YOU

From a position wrapped around her lover's torso, she falls back into a handstand, never allowing his penis to slip from inside her as he supports her buttocks from underneath. With her body fully exposed to him, he uses his fingers to stimulate her clitoris. Being light-headed never felt so good.

DAY 209

THE CANNOLI

Just because you skipped dessert at the restaurant doesn't mean you still can't find time for something sweet. He stands up straight as his ravenous lover applies whipped cream to his penis and devours him.

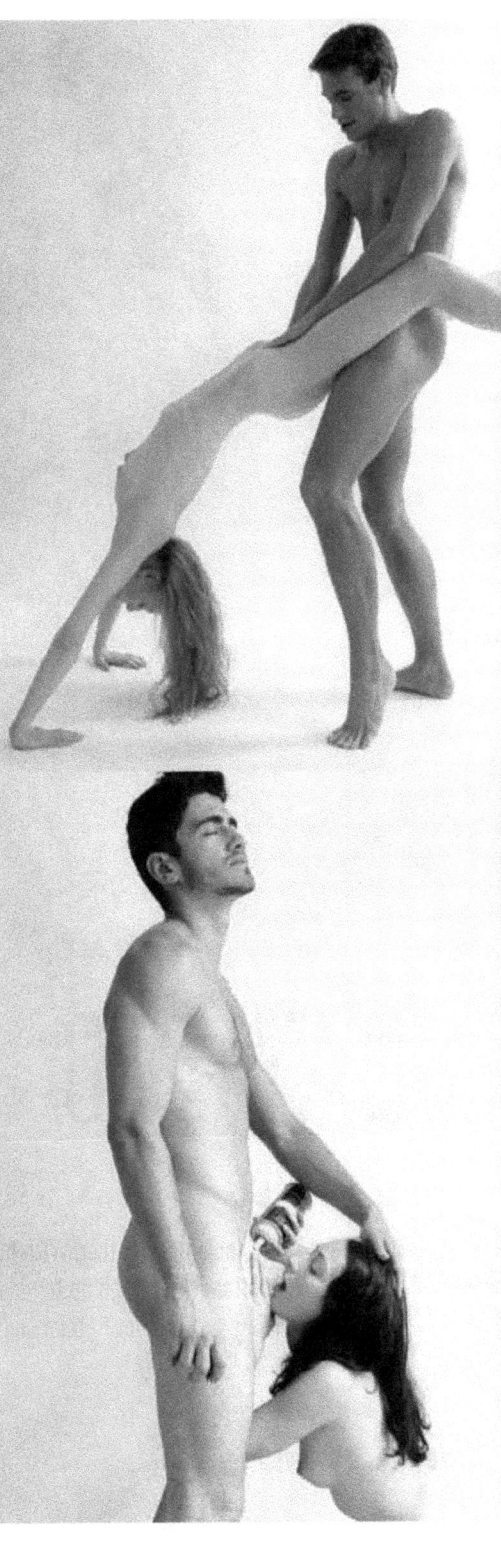

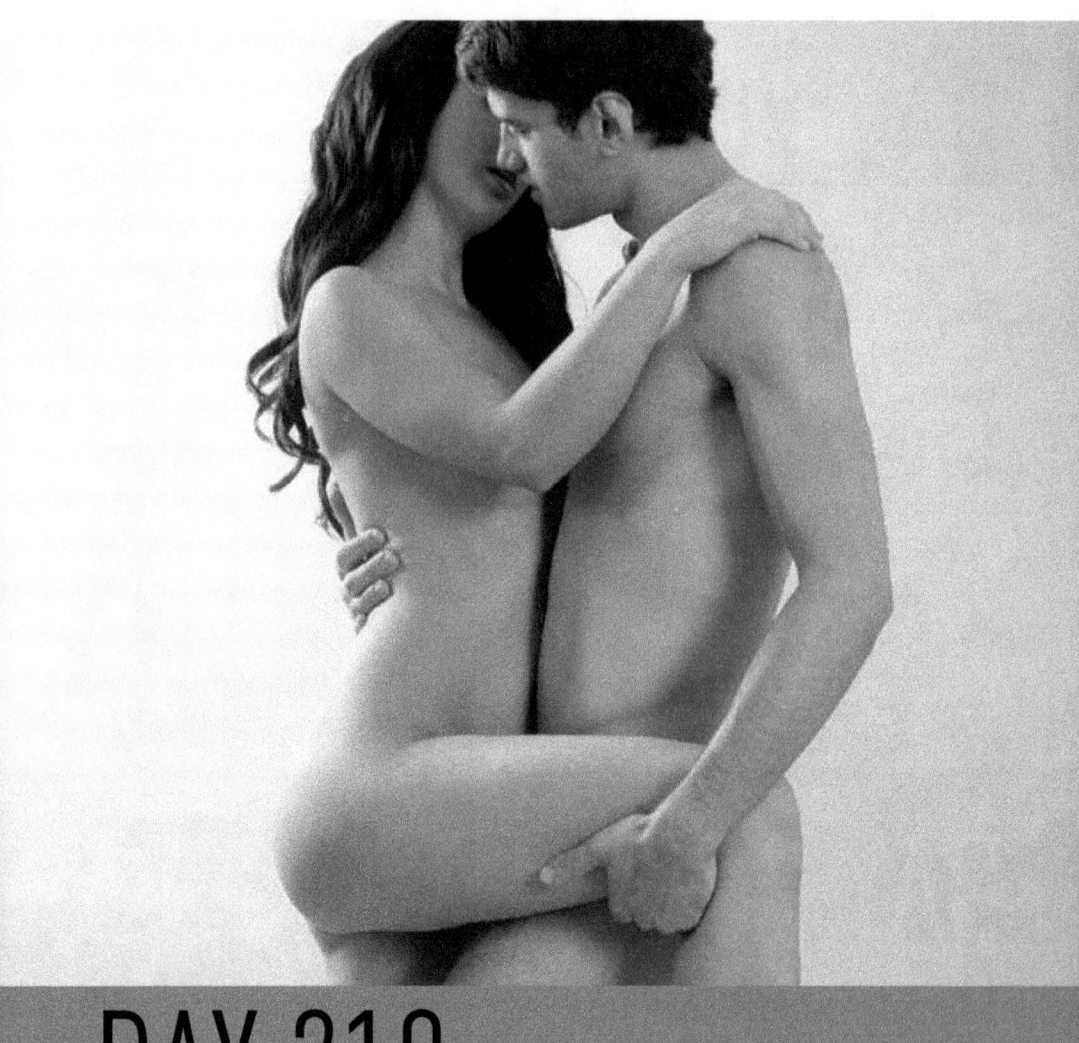

DAY 210

ELEVATED EXPECTATIONS

The lovers stand facing each other. With his feet shoulder-width apart, the man lifts his partner as she hitches her thigh up to his waist to glide herself down onto his penis. As with any lifting, be sure not to take on more than you can handle.

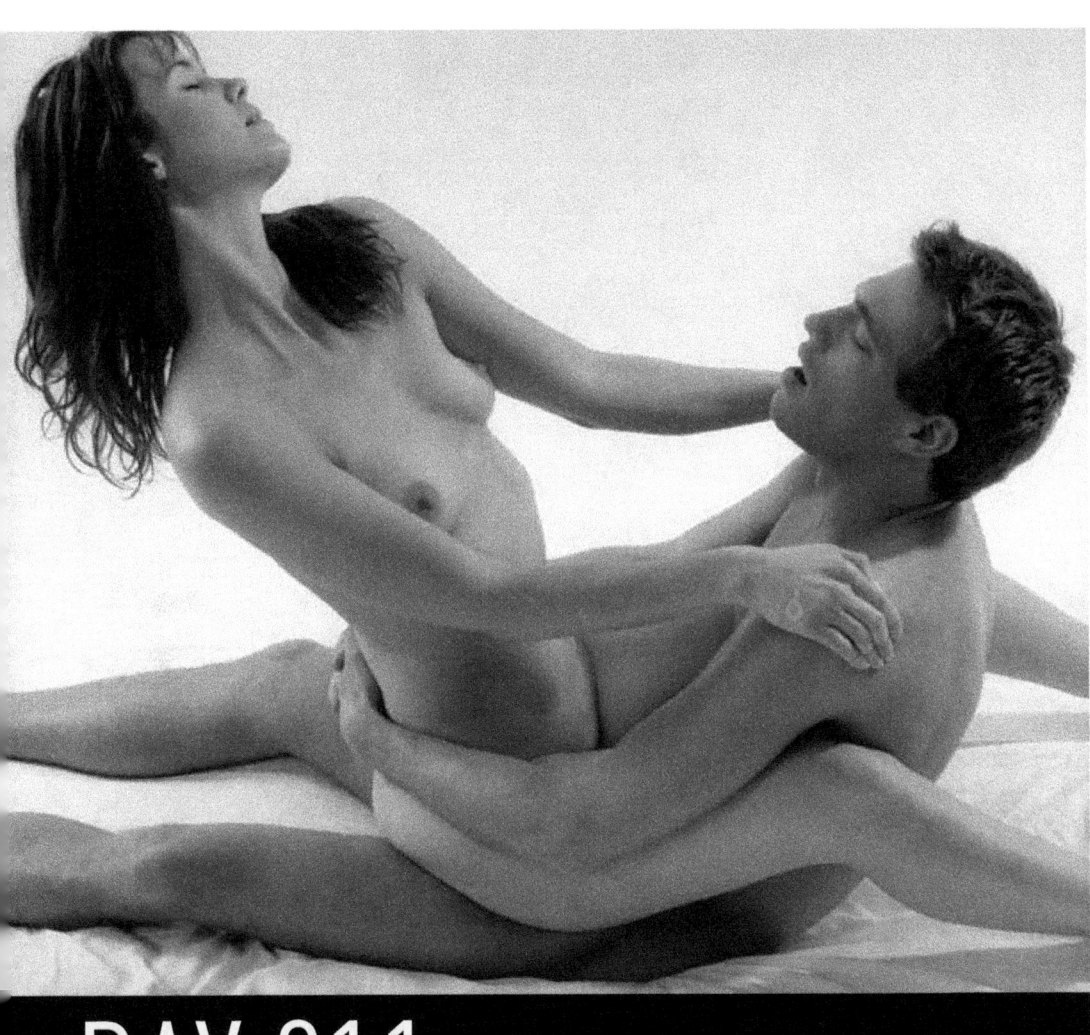

DAY 211

MIRROR, MIRROR

She's in her lover's lap, facing him. They strike identical poses with their legs stretched out and open. They make a perfect pair.

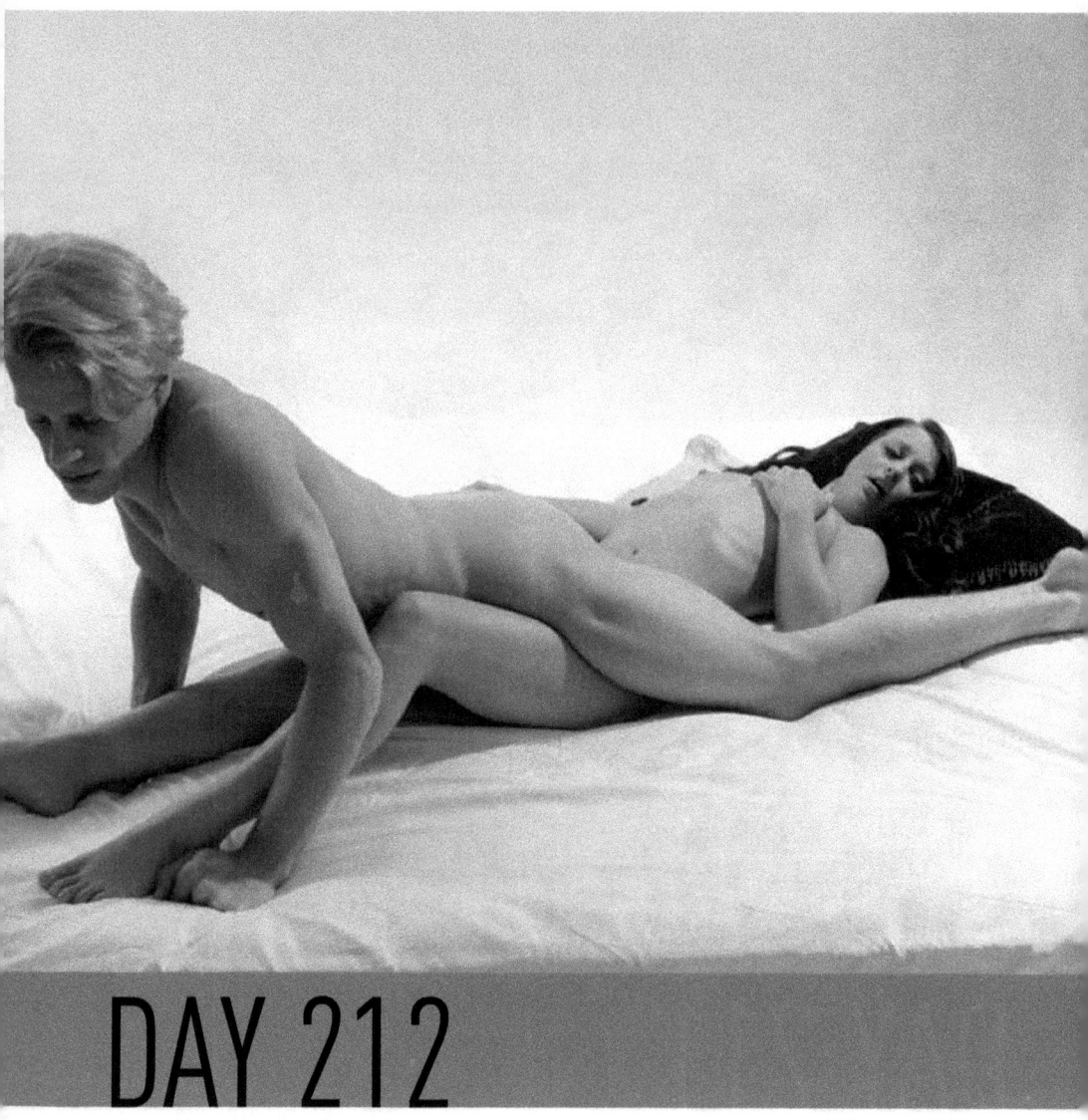

DAY 212

PLANTING SEASON

The lovers stretch out across the bed. She's on her back and he's on top facing in the opposite direction. They move toward each other until he's able to penetrate her vagina with his penis. If she's feeling naughty, she can give him some spanks across his butt.

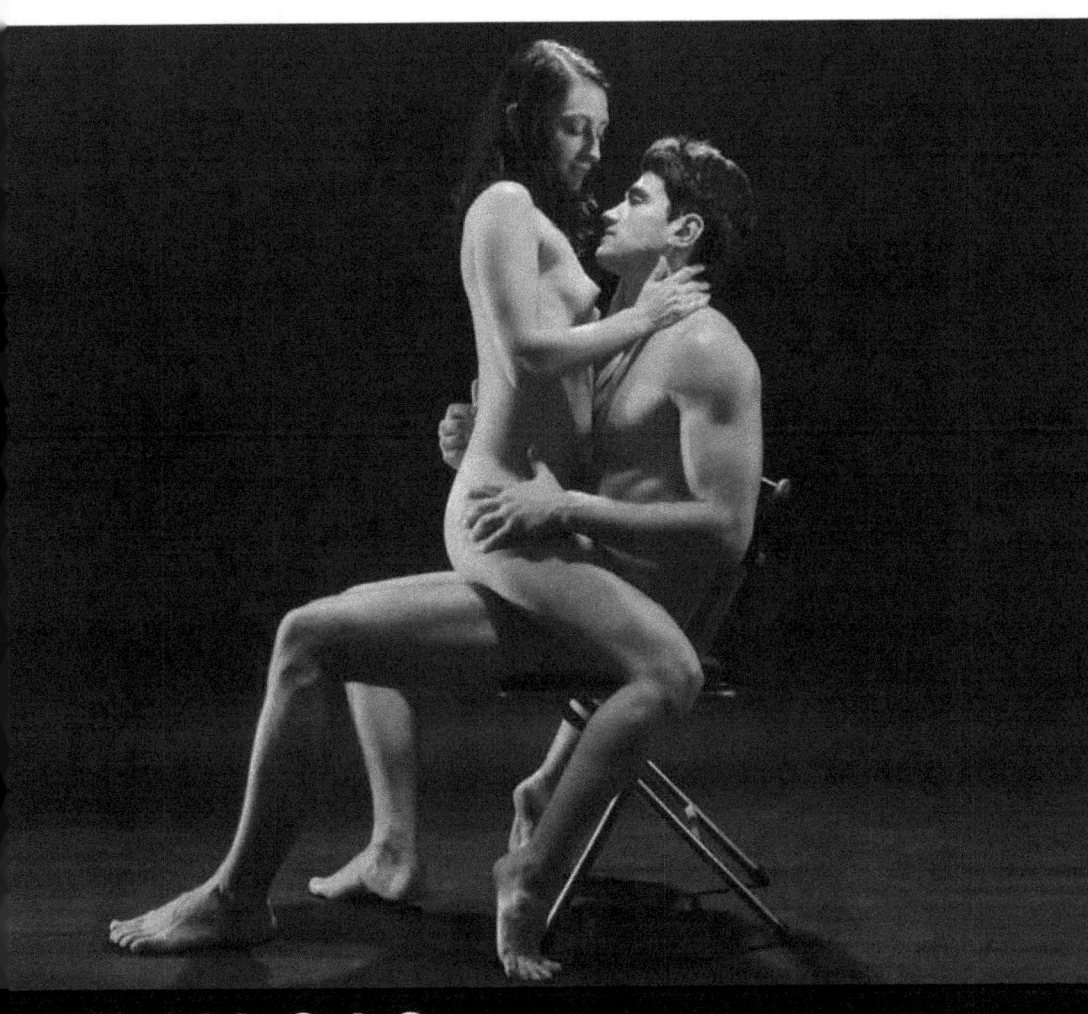

DAY 213

SEATED SEDUCTION

The man sits back in chair with his legs shoulder-width apart. His lover straddles him and pushes herself down, allowing the full length of his penis to enter her. She can either bounce up and down or stay right where she is and let her hips do the talking.

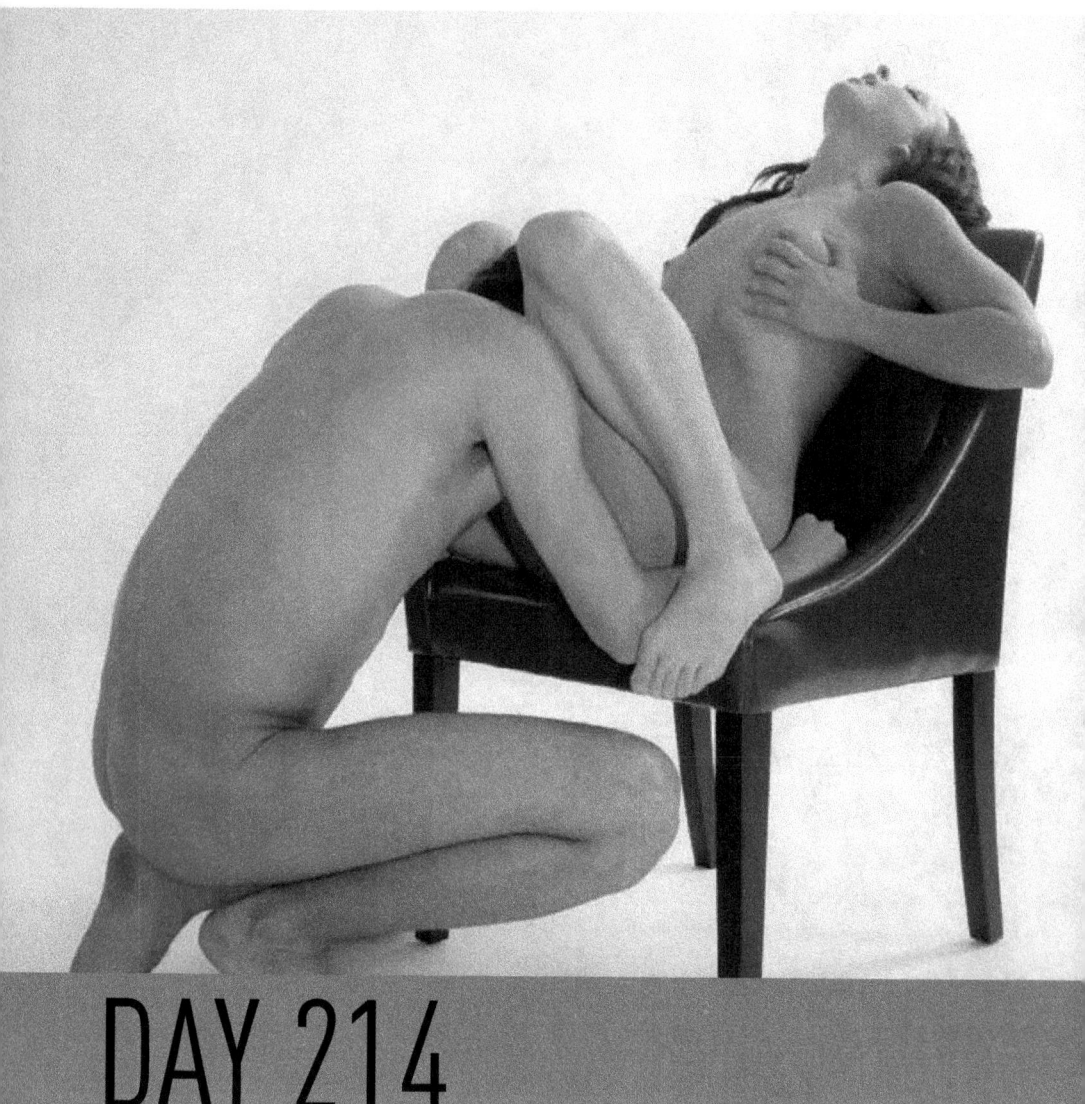

DAY 214

LADY AND THE CLAMP

The woman is in a chair with her knees bent and feet against the edge. As her partner licks her vagina she clamps her legs around is head.

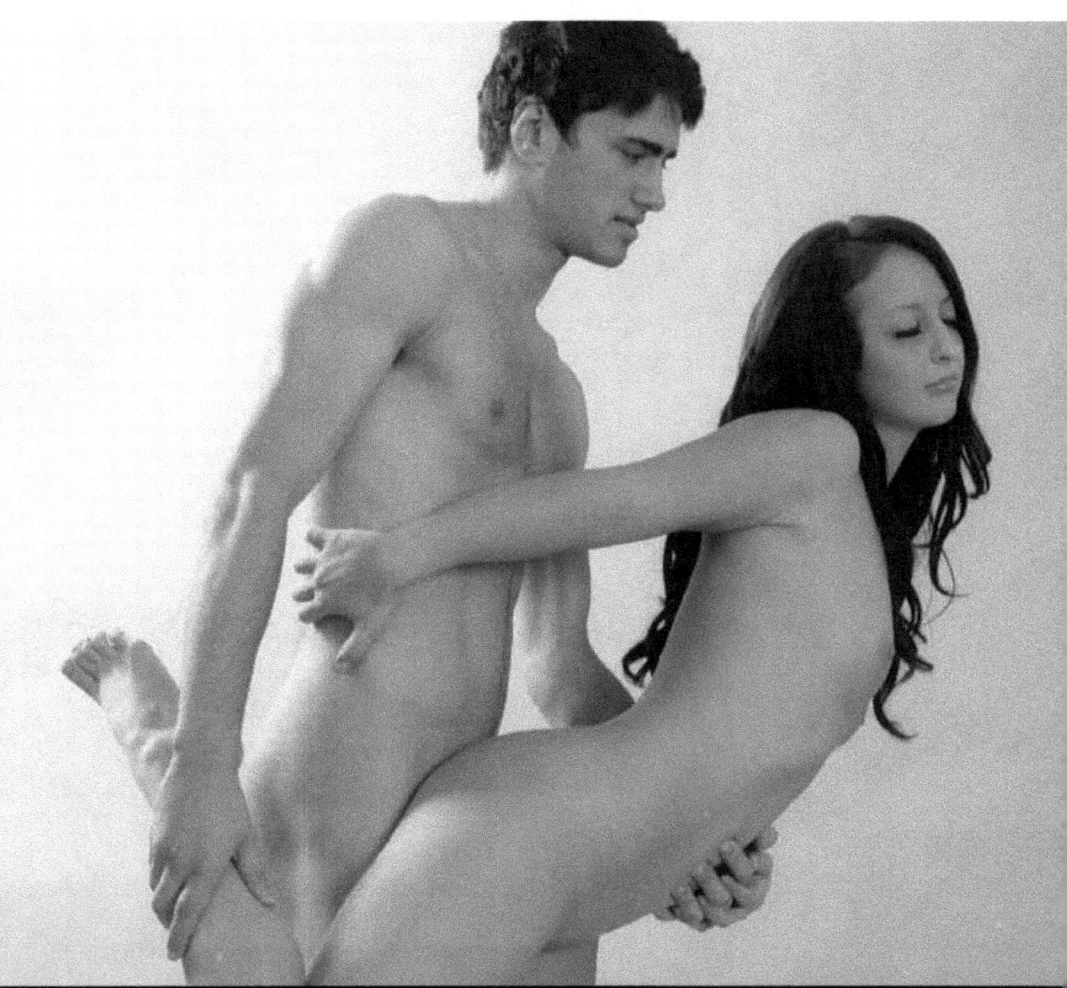

DAY 215

THE SWAN

Standing with her back to her lover the woman leans forward and hooks one leg around his back. He holds her for support. A graceful yet gratifying position.

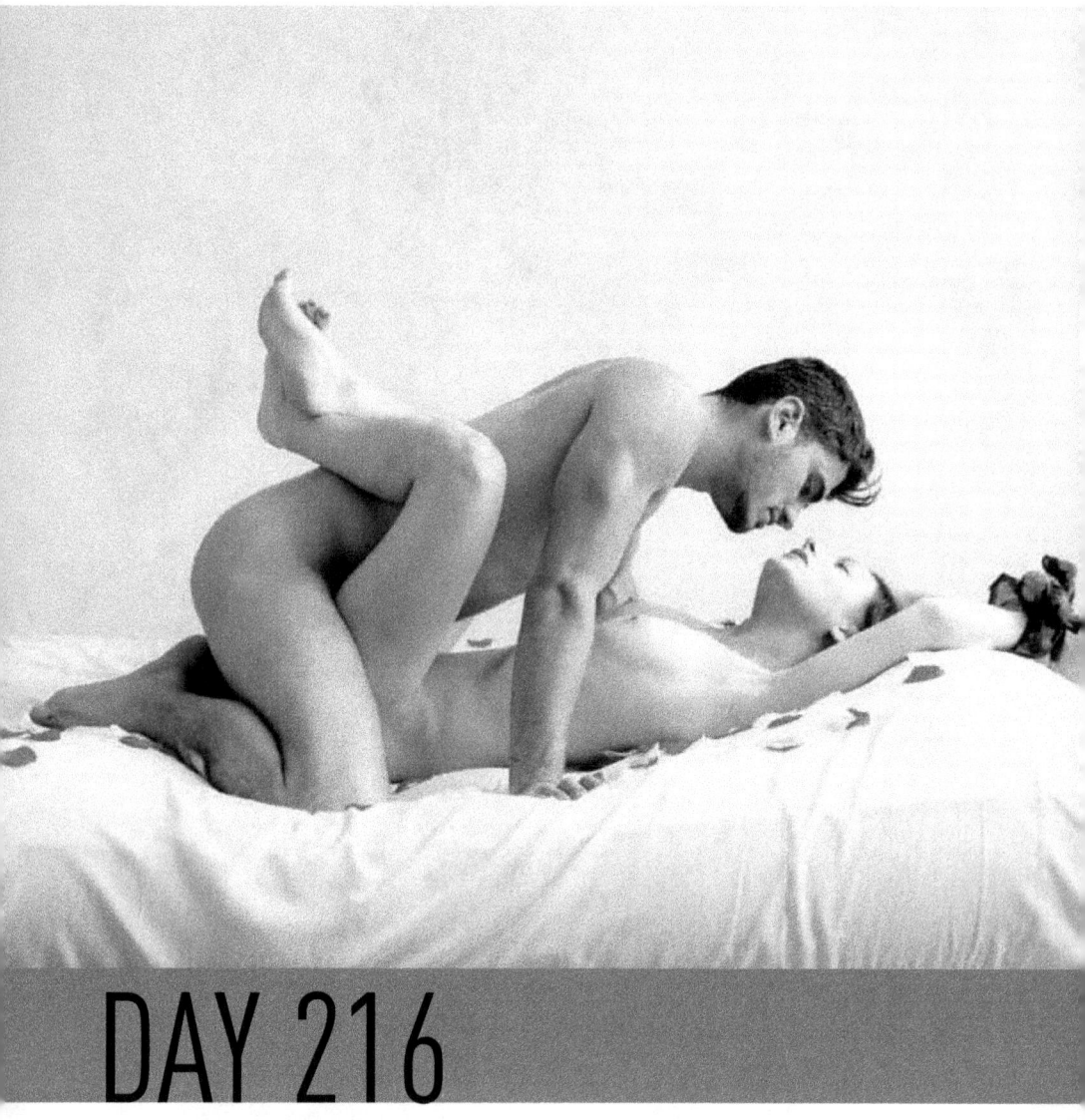

DAY 216

TIE FOR TWO

The man binds his lover's hands together with a silk scarf while she lies back on the bed. As he enters her from a kneeling position, she returns the favor by clasping her legs around his back and pulling him closer. They're prisoners of passion.

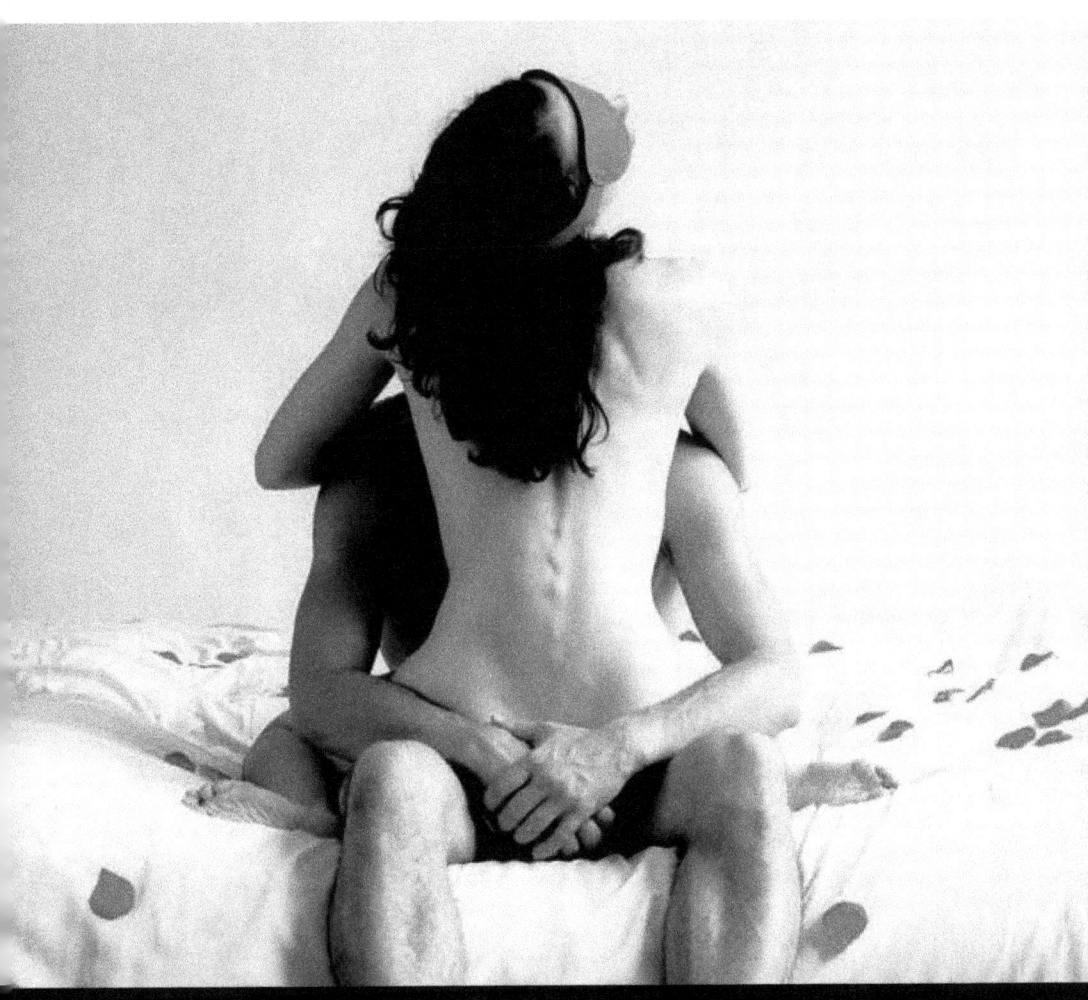

DAY 217

HIDDEN DESIRE

It's a good idea to clear the floor for this position. She starts blindfolded across the room from her partner. Dropping clues for her other senses, he can help her find him by leaving a path of flower petals or occasionally whispering naughty directions. Once he's located, she mounts him and the game really begins.

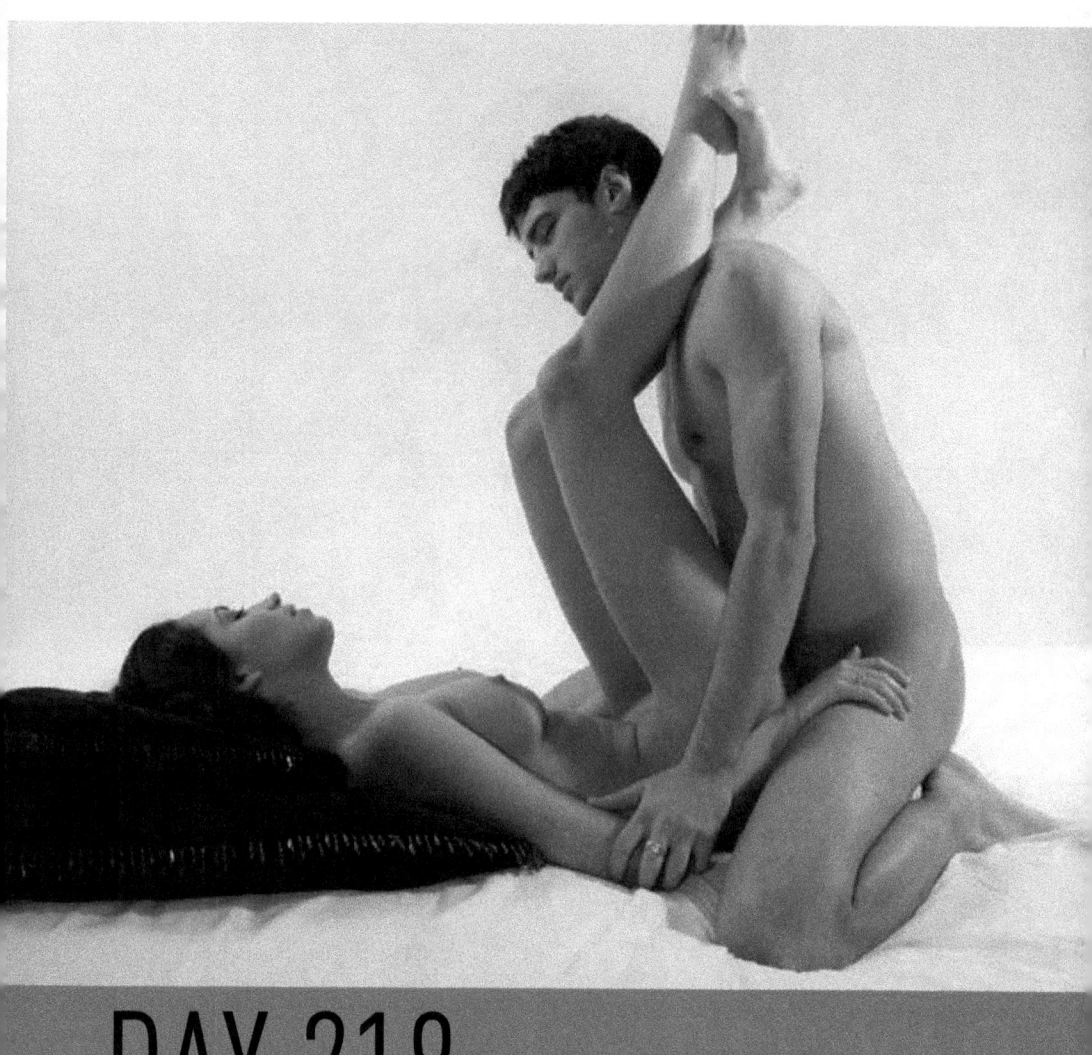

DAY 218

THE SILK SCARF

There's no shortage of skin-on-skin sensation here as the man kneels and faces his lover while she snakes her legs up and around his neck. His hands are free to caress her thighs as he penetrates her while she can let her fingers wander wherever they please.

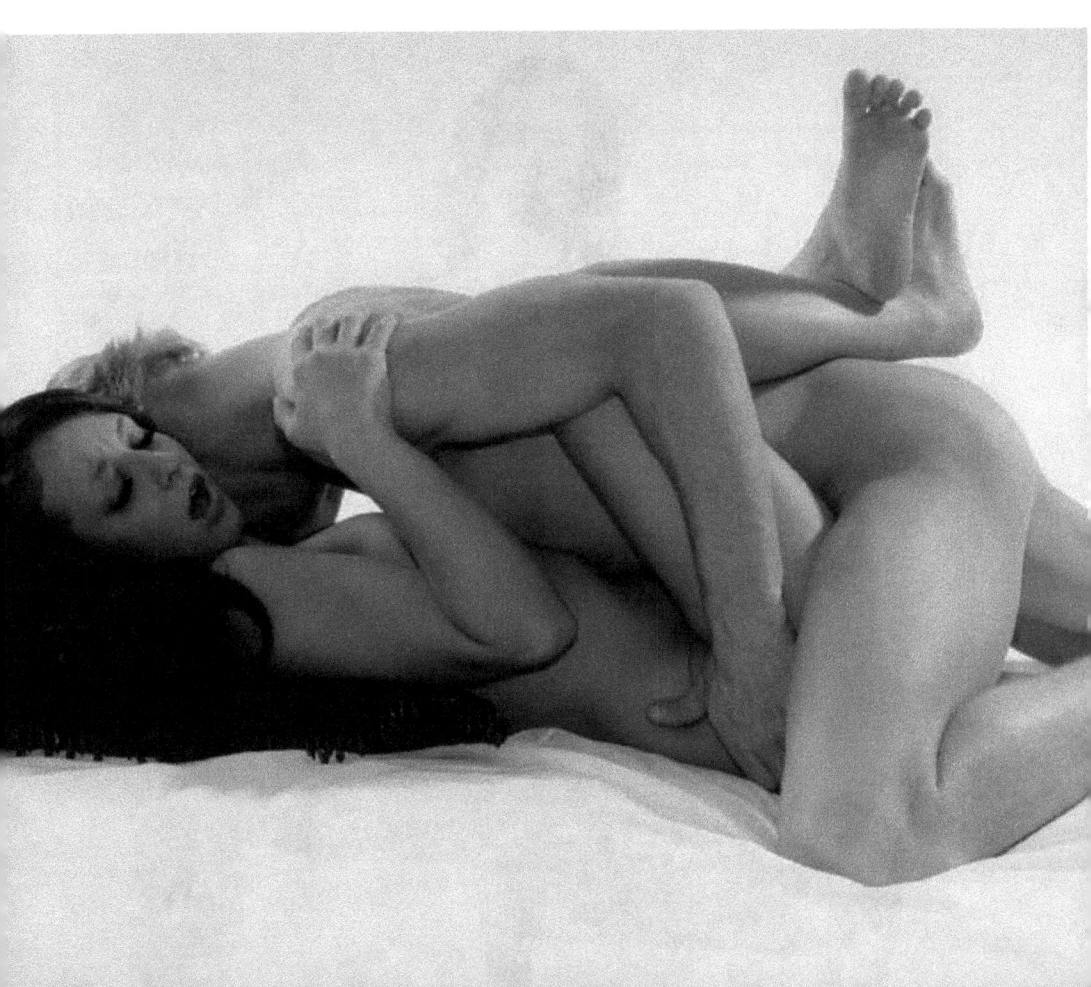

DAY 219

THE LEG LOCK

She lies on her back with her legs open as her partner penetrates her from a kneeling position. She then brings her knees back and wraps her legs around him tightly, pulling him down to her. They can feel each other's breath as they approach orgasm.

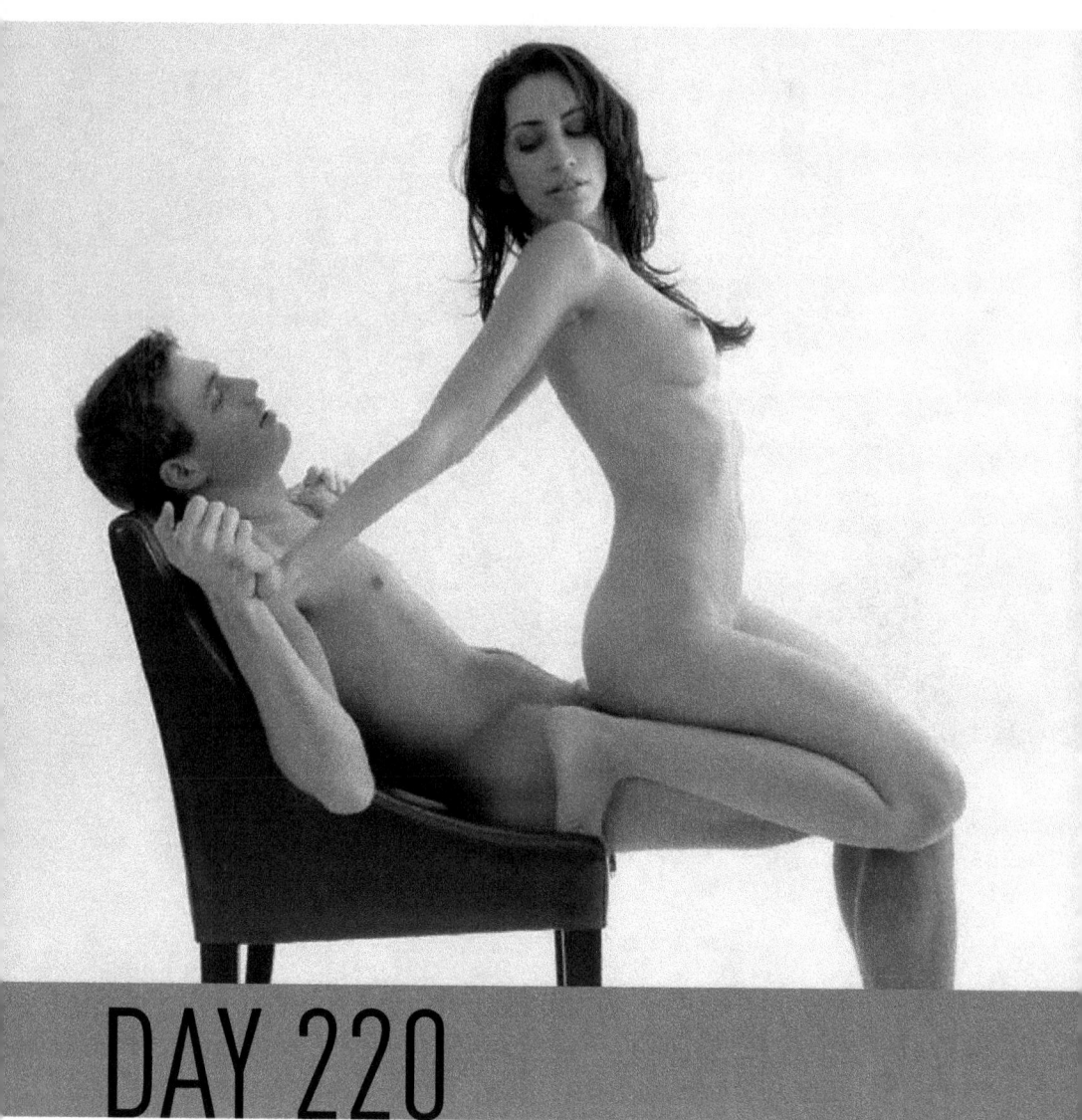

DAY 220

THE LOOKOUT

The man sits low in a chair as his lover straddles him facing outward. He grasps her hands as she rotates her hips, fast and slow.

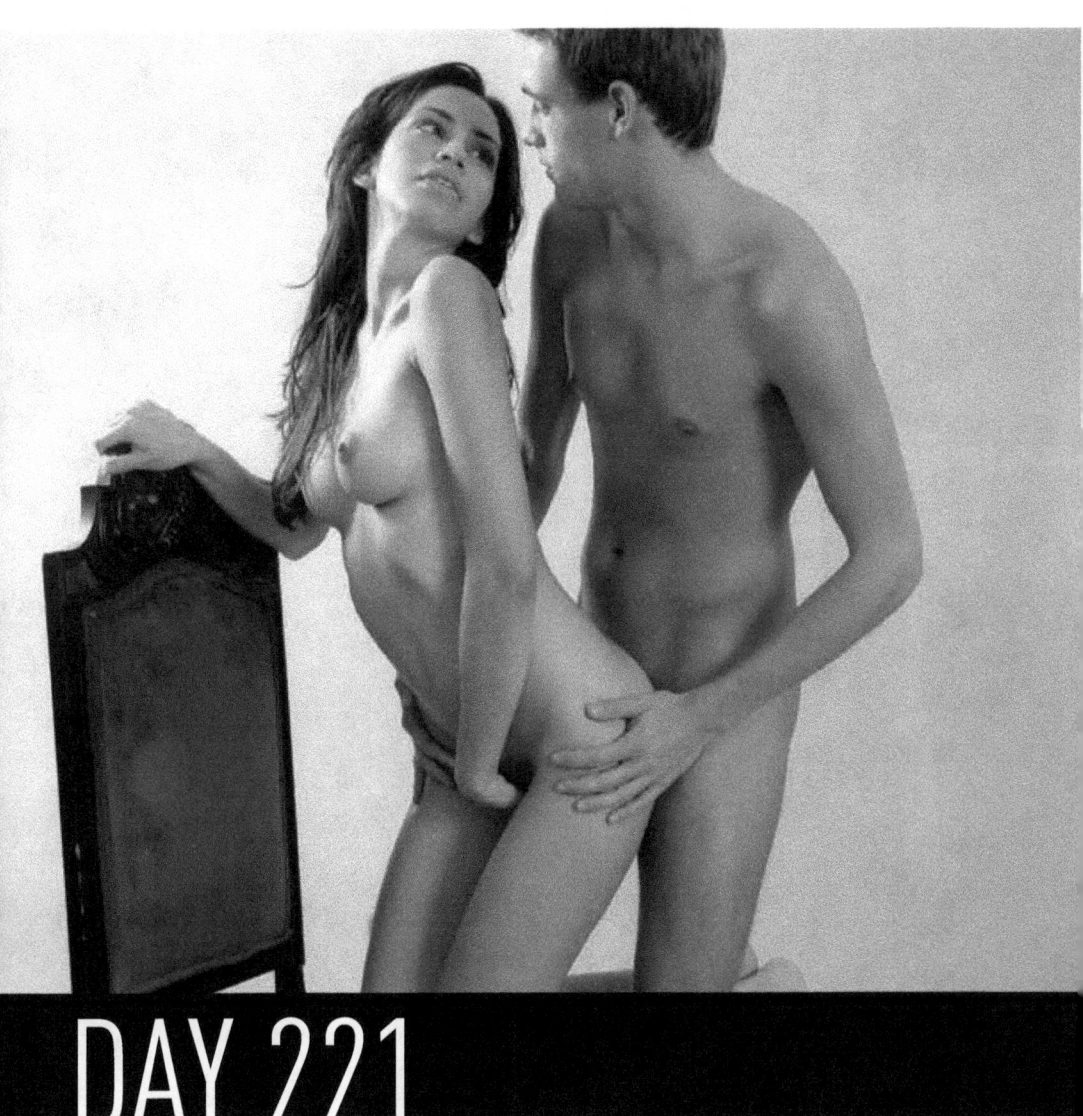

DAY 221

BAD KITTY

The woman positions herself up on a chair with her back to her lover. She can hold onto the chair's back as he enters her from behind. Just *purr*fect.

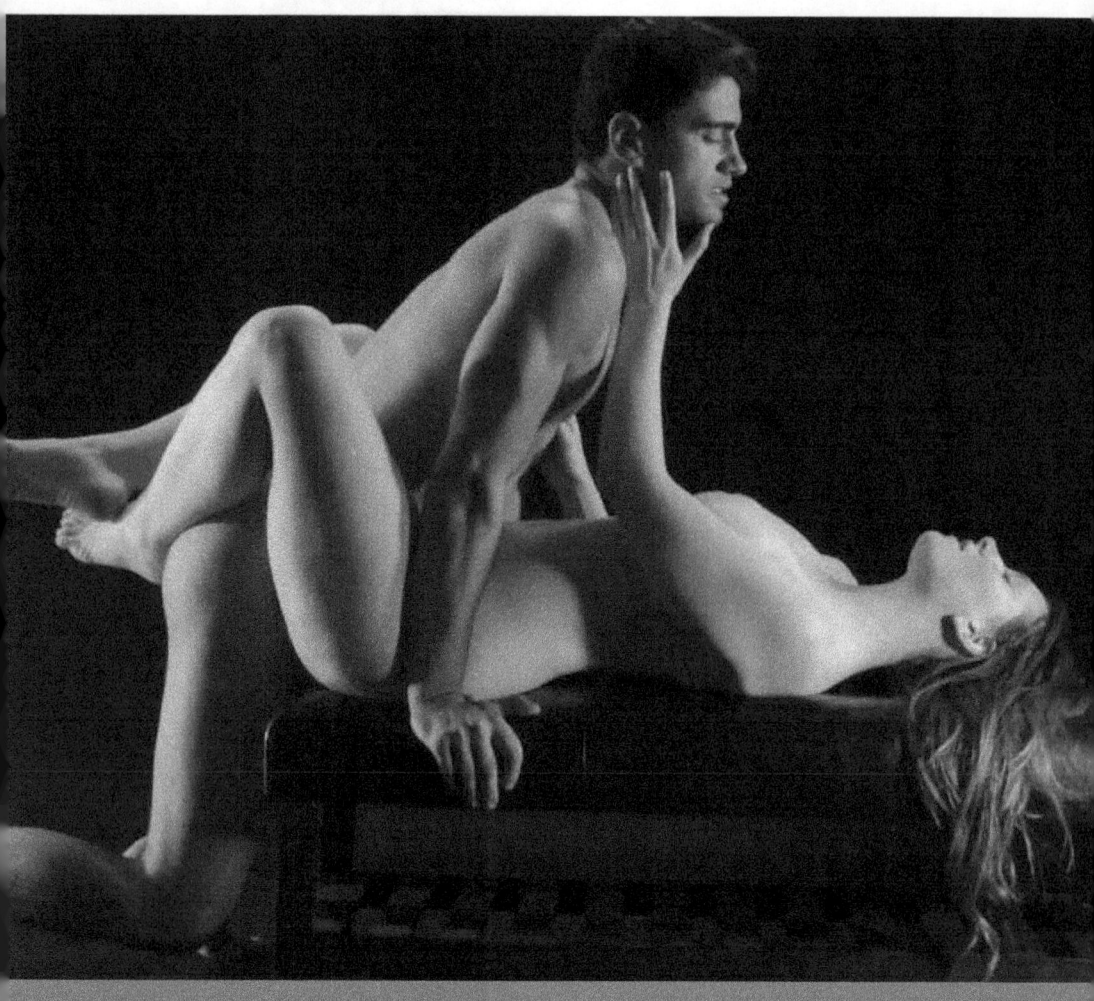

DAY 222

THE SILENT PARTNER

Sometimes silence truly is golden. She lies back across an ottoman or padded bench, letting her open legs dangle off the side. As her partner penetrates her she remains quiet, instead letting her hands relay her feelings.

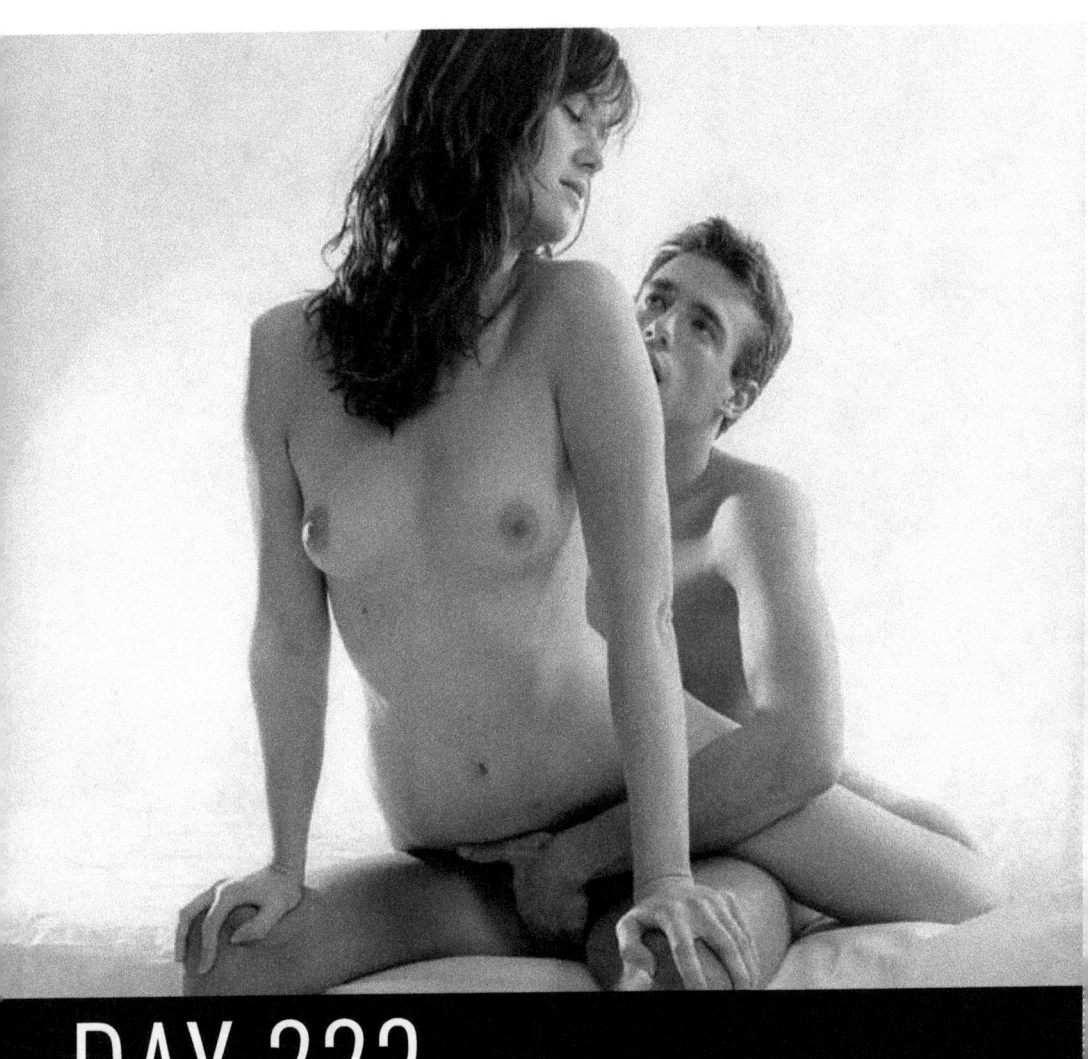

DAY 223

THE SERPENT

He's sitting up straight while his partner straddles his legs and mounts him. She places her hands on his knees and arches her back, and grinds downward into his lap.

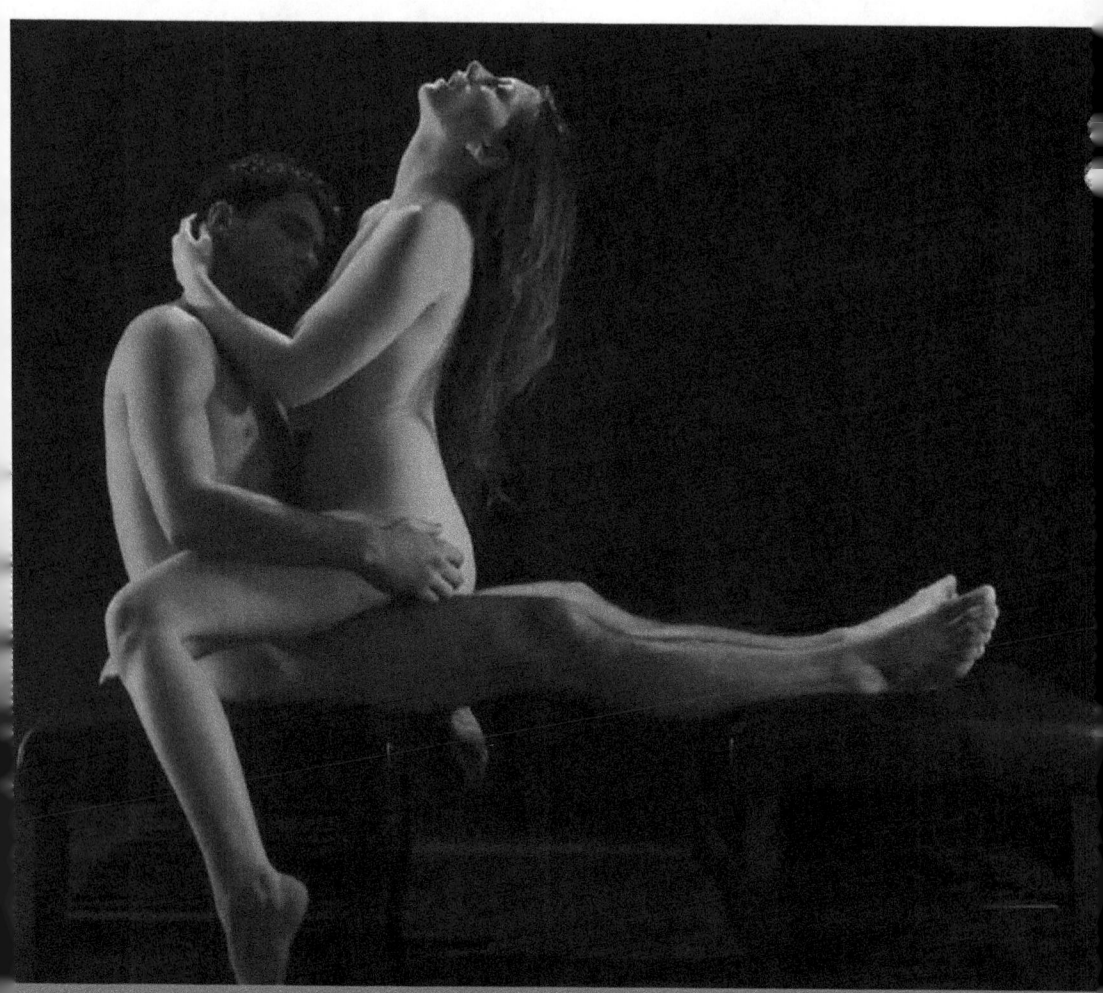

DAY 224

BRIDGING THE GAP

The man sits on one low piece of furniture while extending his legs across to another. The woman straddles her partner and lets him enter her deeply. His hands can come around and grab her buttocks.

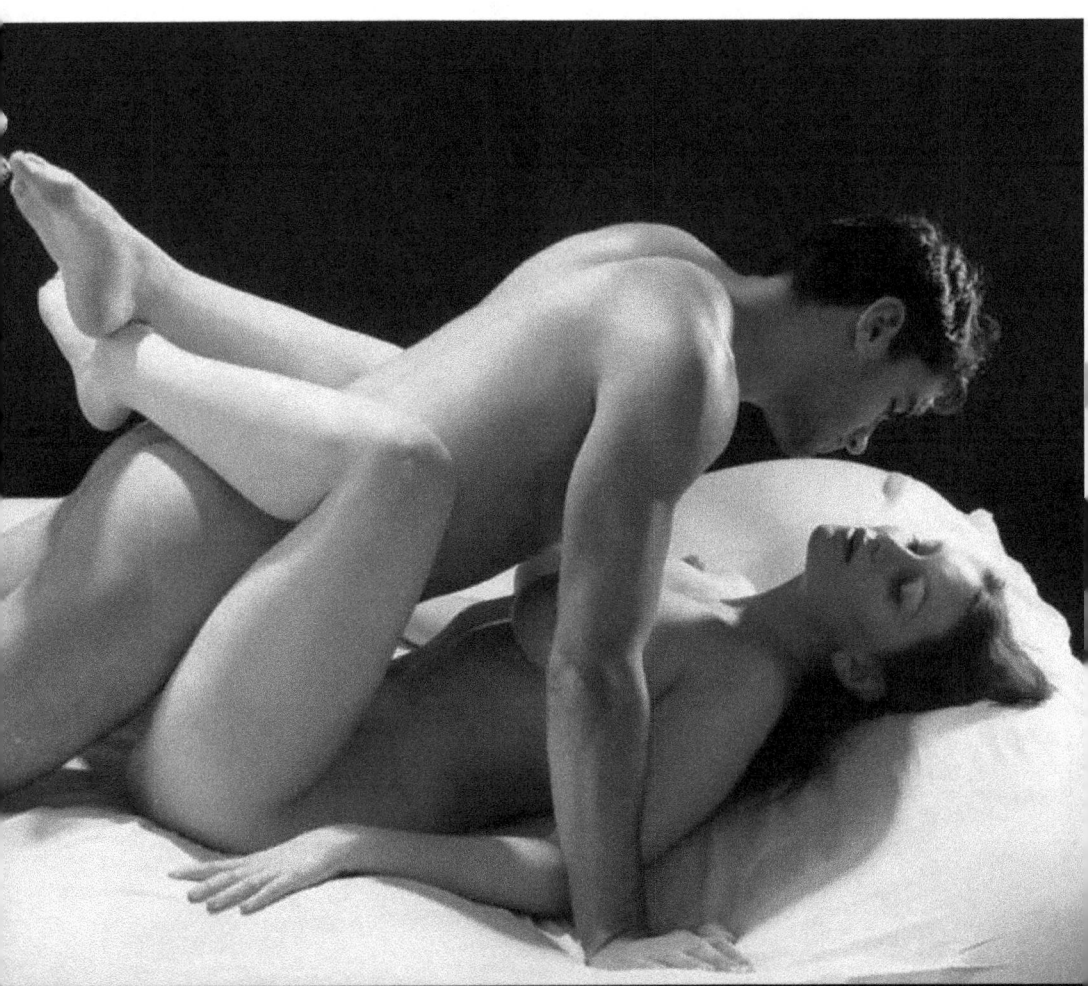

DAY 225

THAT'S A WRAP

He holds on to a chin-up or support bar standing straight with his legs shoulder length apart. She spreads her legs wide, wrapping her arms around his neck as she mounts his erect penis.

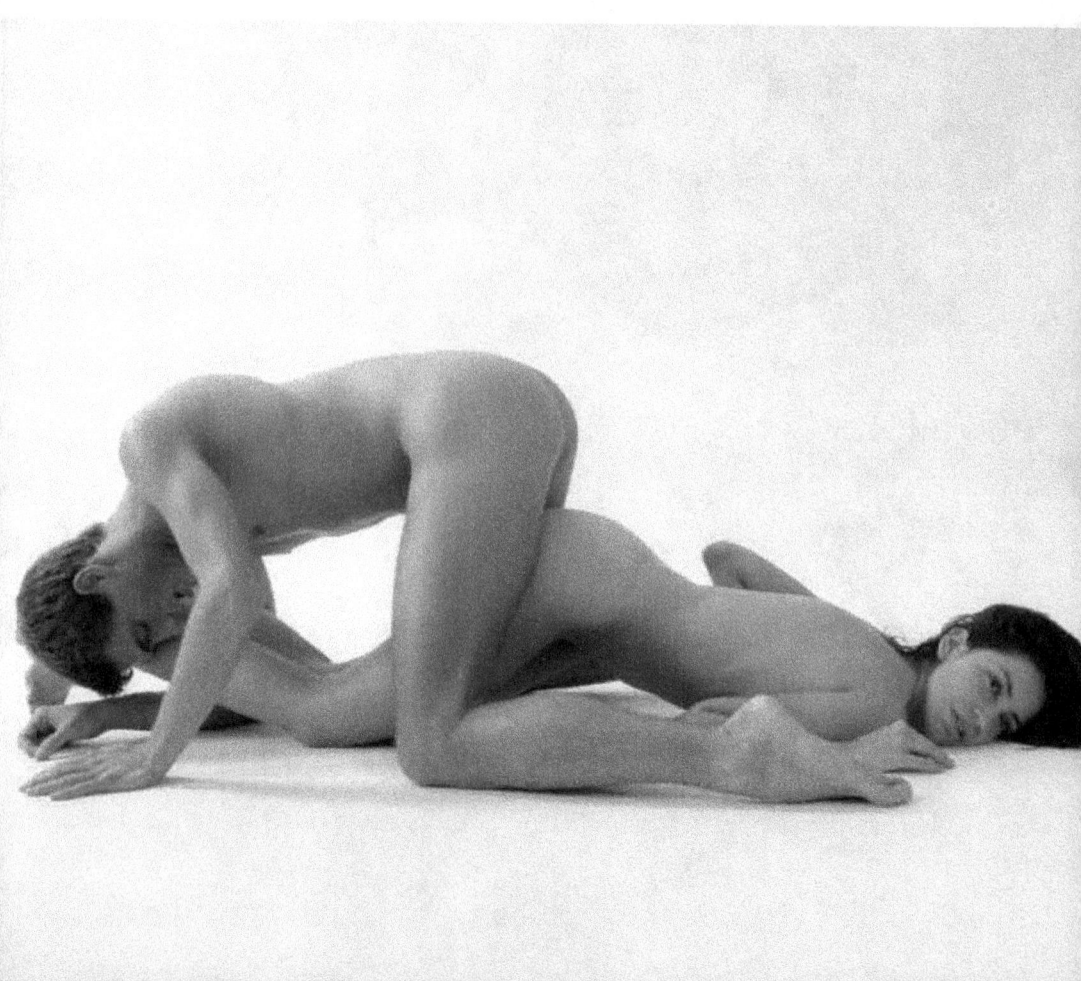

DAY 226

PEAKS AND VALLEYS

The woman positions herself on the floor with her buttocks raised. Her partner strikes a similar pose in the opposite direction as her enters her from above. The angles they create with their bodies are a work of art.

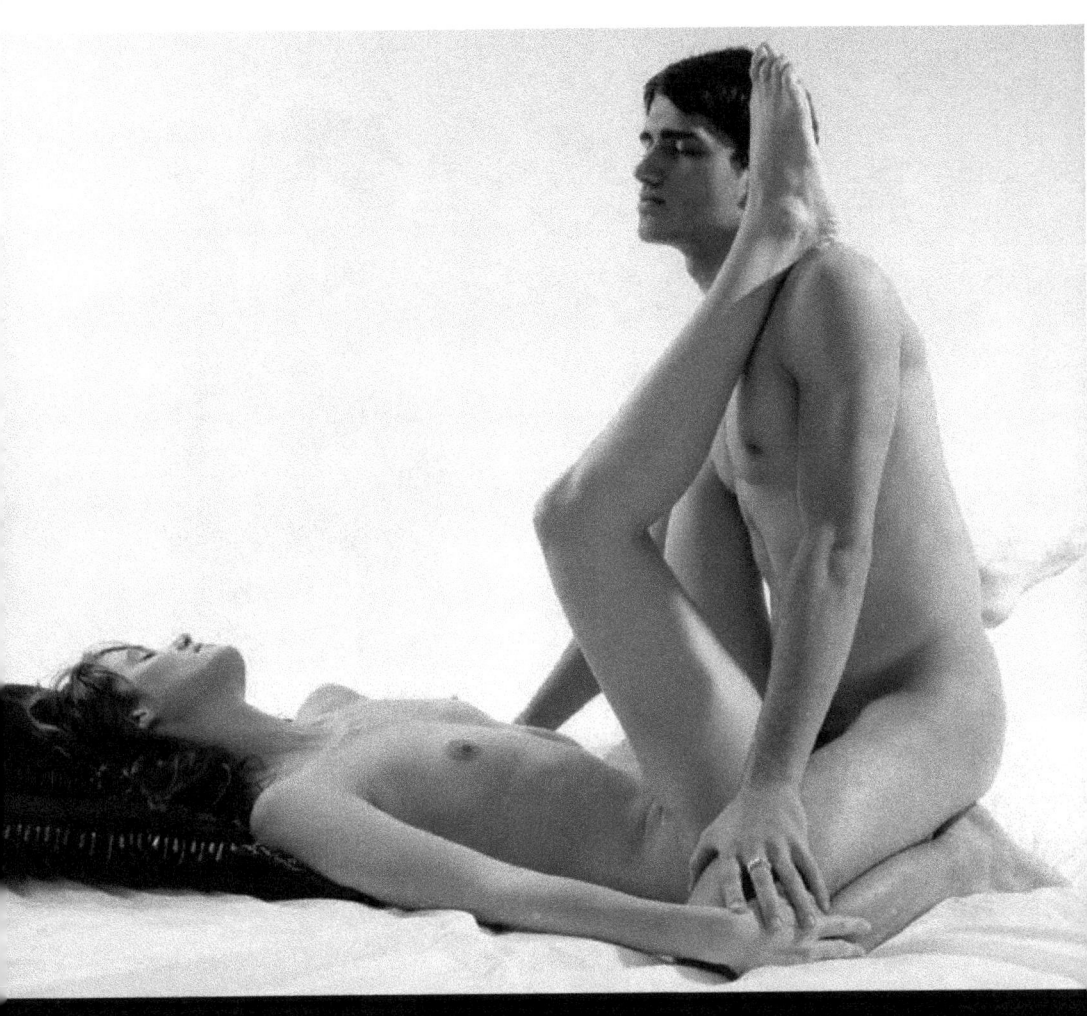

DAY 227

GET YOUR KICKS

An aerobic and erotic workout in one, this position allows the woman to alternately raise and lower her legs onto and off of her lover's shoulders in a pistonlike movement while his penis is inside of her. The sensation sends both hearts racing.

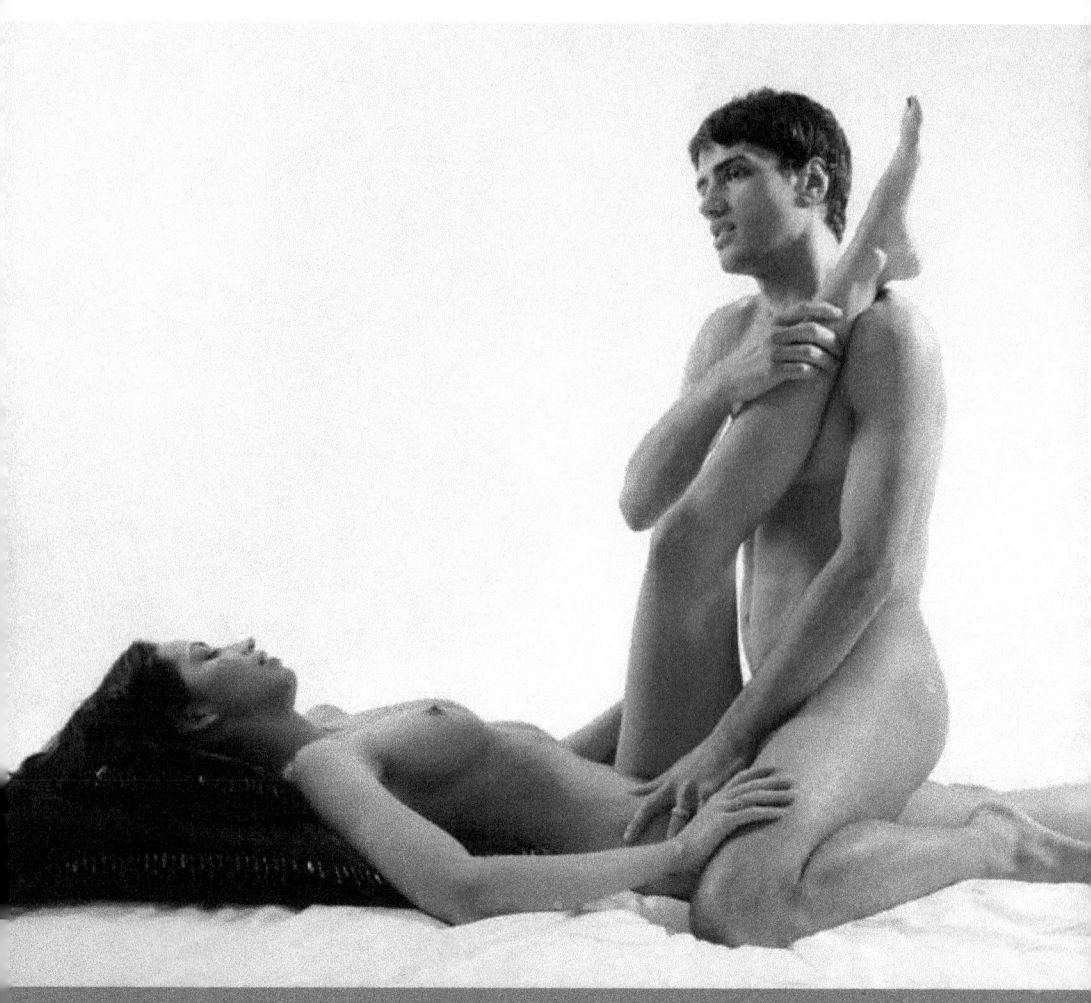

DAY 228

SPLIT DECISION

On her back, the woman positions her legs so that one is crossed over her partner's chest and the other is stretched out straight between his knees. As he gently holds her leg, his rhythmic thrusts register with both of them.

DAY 229

CRUISE CONTROL

His torso is flat against the bed with his shoulders back and arms out to the side. She squats on top of him, pulling one of his legs up like a gear shift. Moving from neutral to fourth never felt so satisfying.

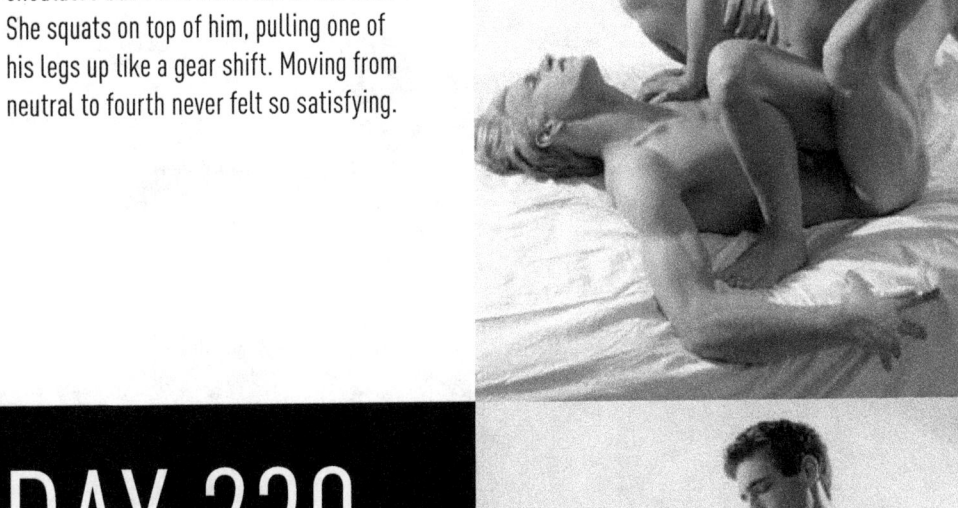

DAY 230

ARC OF TRIUMPH

Using her arms and shoulders, the woman brings herself into an almost plank pose with her hips lifted. The man positions himself between her thighs and enters her from a kneeling postion.

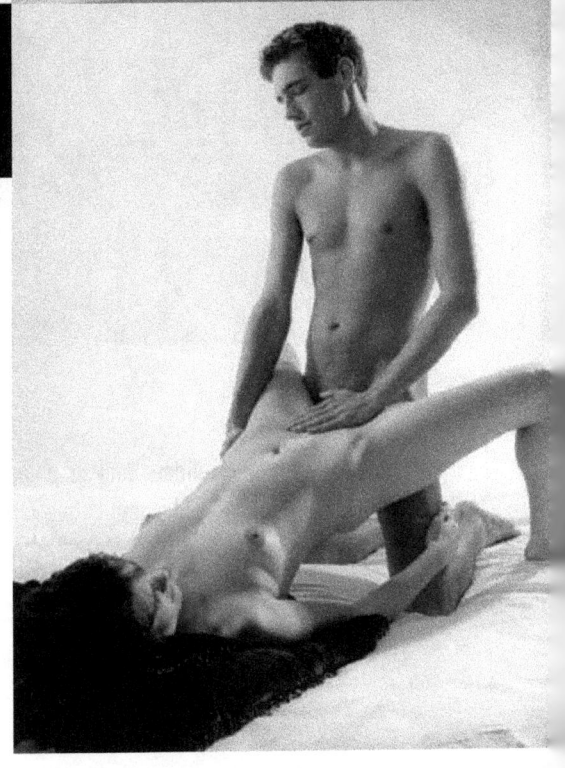

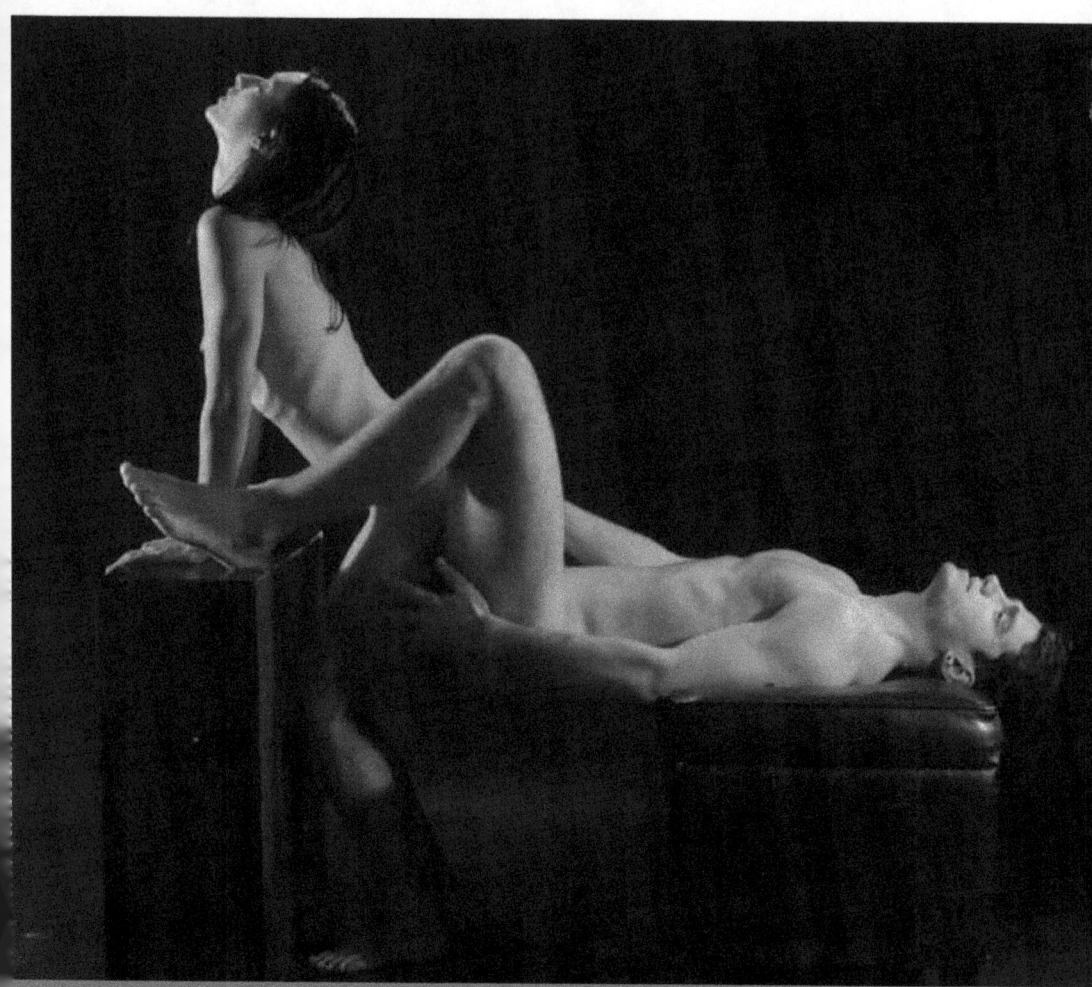

DAY 231

THE ALLEY CAT

He's got his head and shoulders back on a bench while his legs are open and feet planted on a higher piece of furniture. She gets between his legs and lowers her lubed anus onto his penis. It's purrfectly steamy.

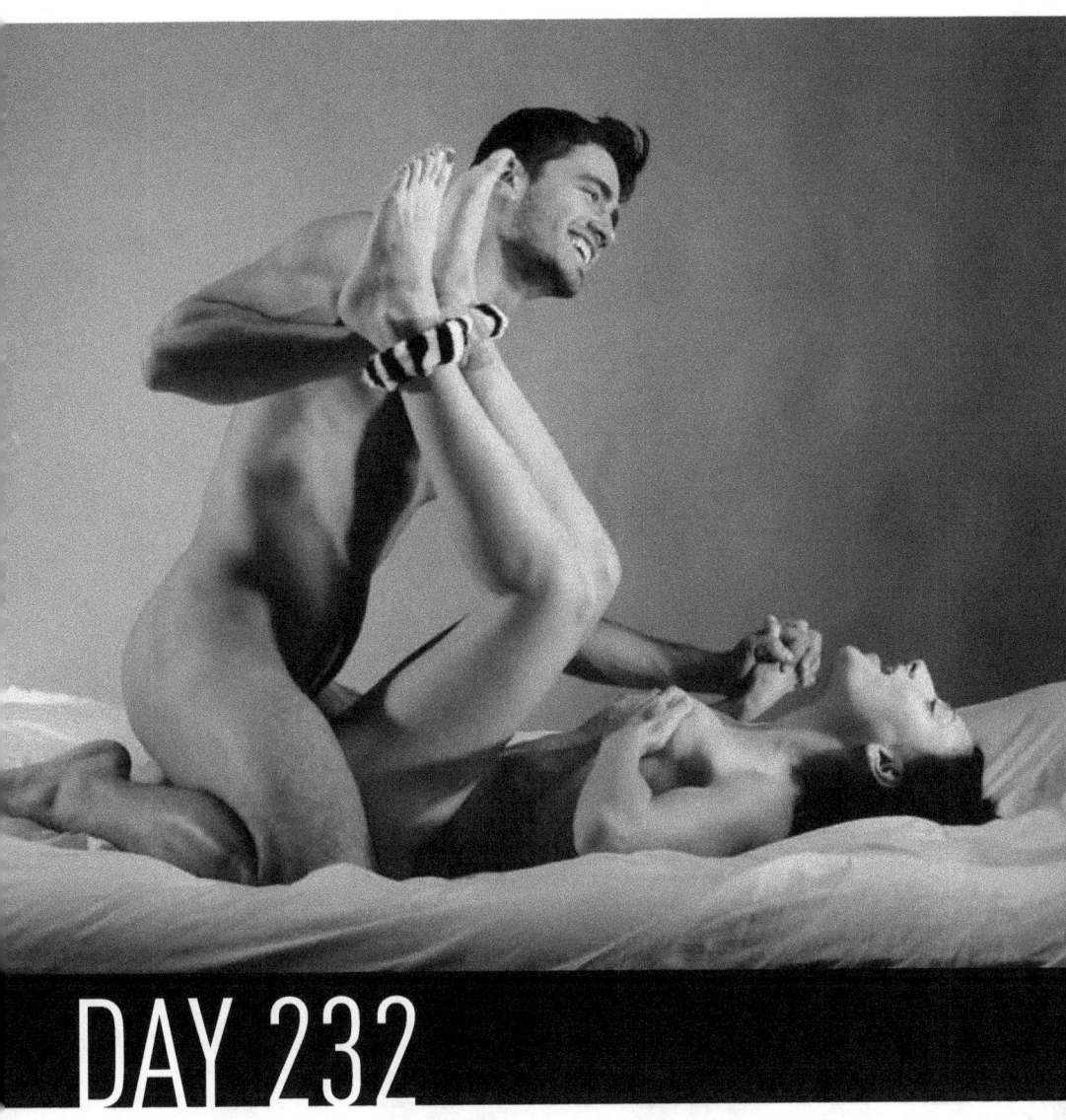

DAY 232

THE CAPTAIN AND THE SQUEAL

She's back on the bed with her feet cuffed together. As he penetrates his partner he grabs the chain between the cuffs and uses it to steer her legs and hips in all sorts of directions that will make them both squeal with pleasure.

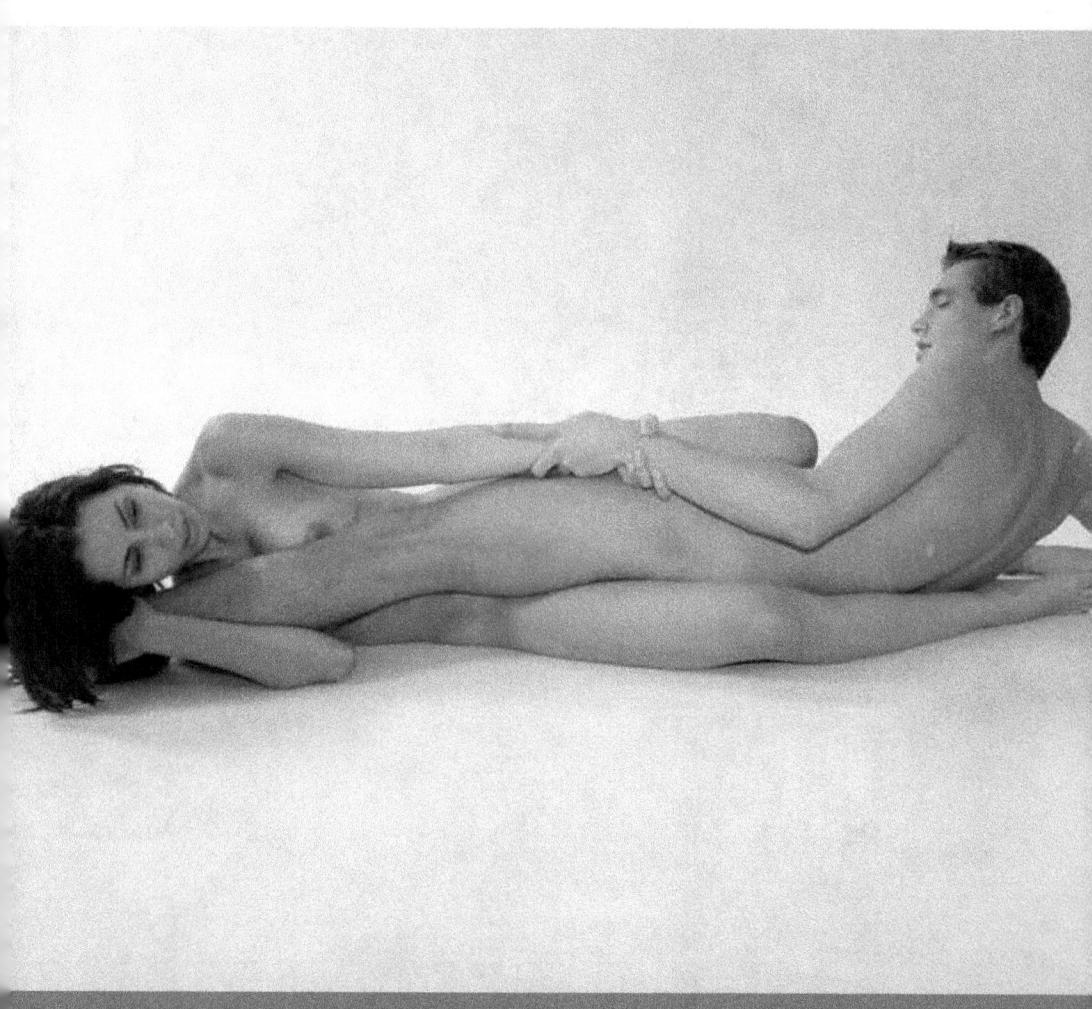

DAY 233

THE CHINESE RINGS

This move is not as puzzling as it appears. The lovers position themselves on their sides with the woman wrapping both of her legs around one of his. As their genitals meet in the middle they can link hands and pull each other back and forth.

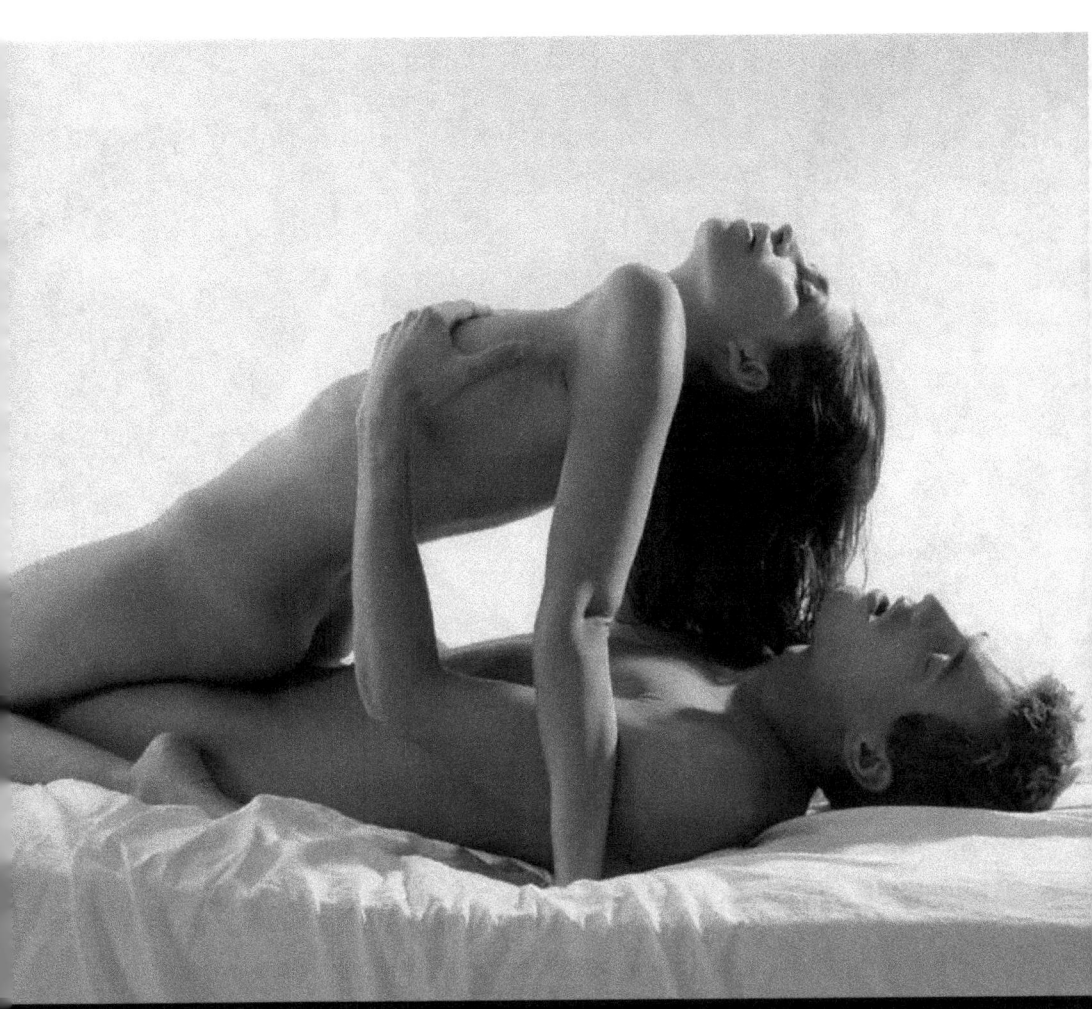

DAY 234

THE BACKDOWN

The man lies back on the bed as his partner mounts his penis from the top, lowering herself backward toward his chest. His hands are free to explore her breasts and clitoris.

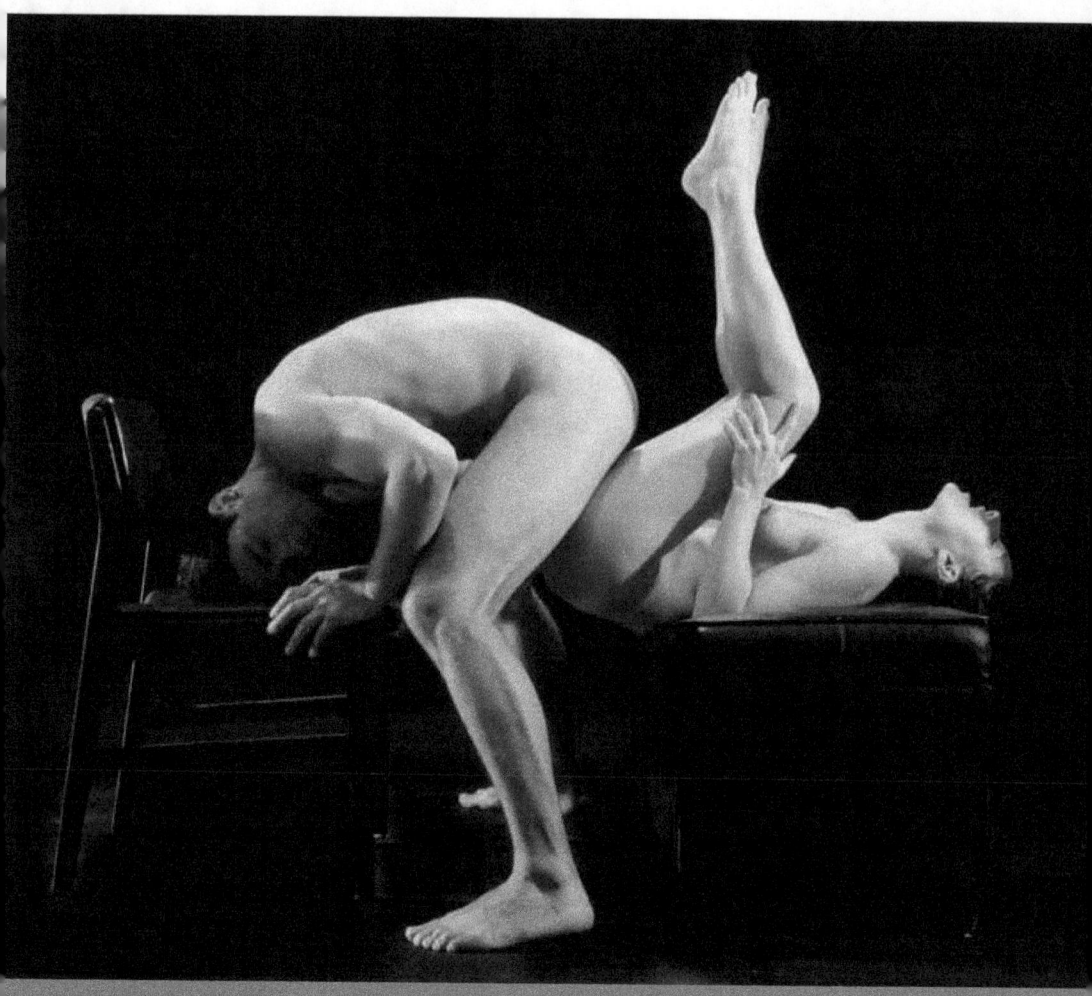

DAY 235

THE SPEAKEASY

The woman lies on an ottoman or low bench with her his lifted and her legs open and raised. Her partner bends over a chair and enters her from above. It's an unusual position, but fun once you get the hang of it.

DAY 236

STAND AND DELIVER

The man positions himself in a chair with one knee bent upward. The woman takes advantage of his pelvic tilt to straddle his thigh, mounting his upthrust penis from a standing posture. They both are free to move themselves toward climax.

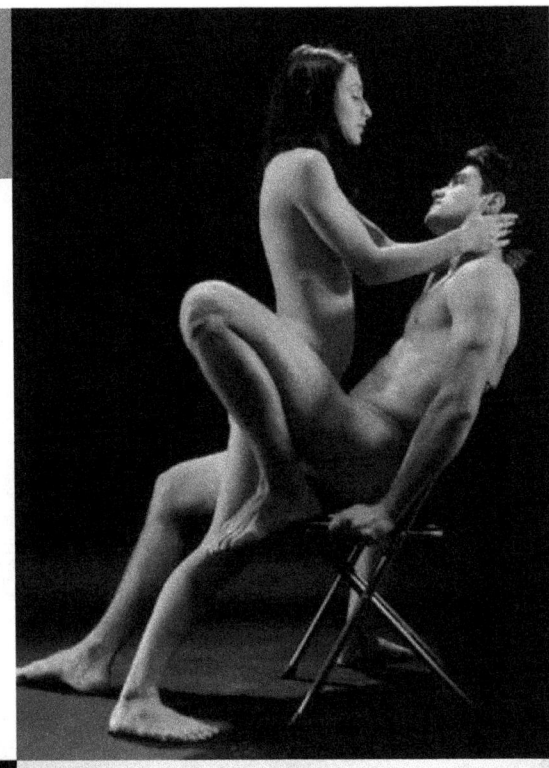

DAY 237

THE TRIPOD

Using her arms and shoulders, the woman brings herself into an almost reverse plank pose with her buttocks lifted. The man positions himself between her legs and enters her from a kneeling position.

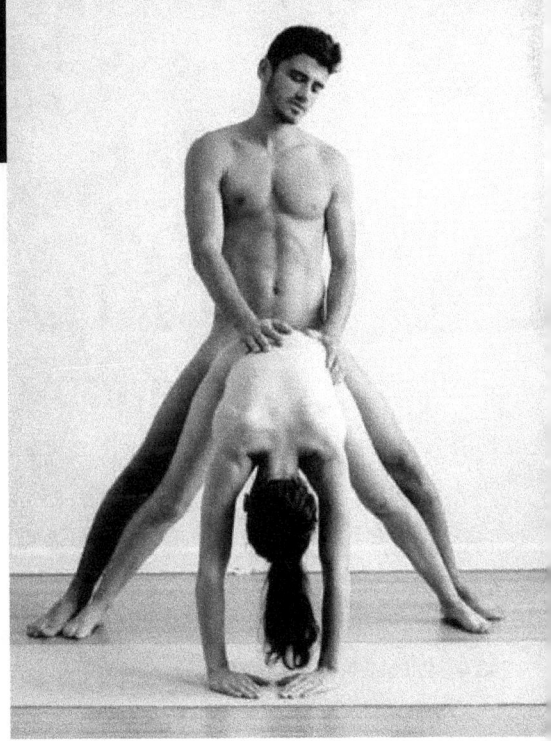

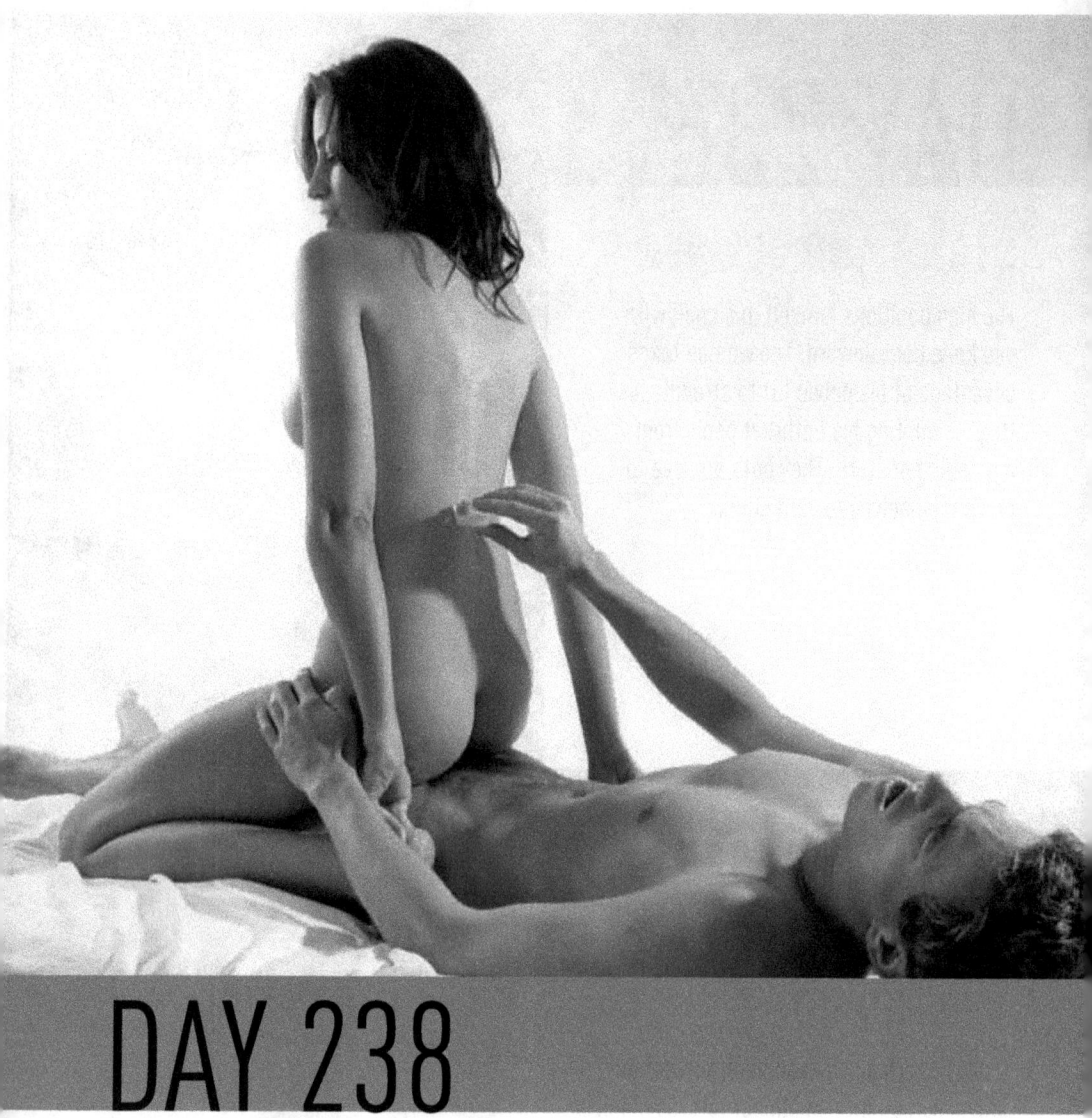

DAY 238

THE COLD SHOULDER

In this position the man lies on a bed as his partner straddles him facing away. As he penetrates her deeply he rubs an ice cube from her shoulder blades all the way down to the small of her back. The heat they create will make short work of that ice.

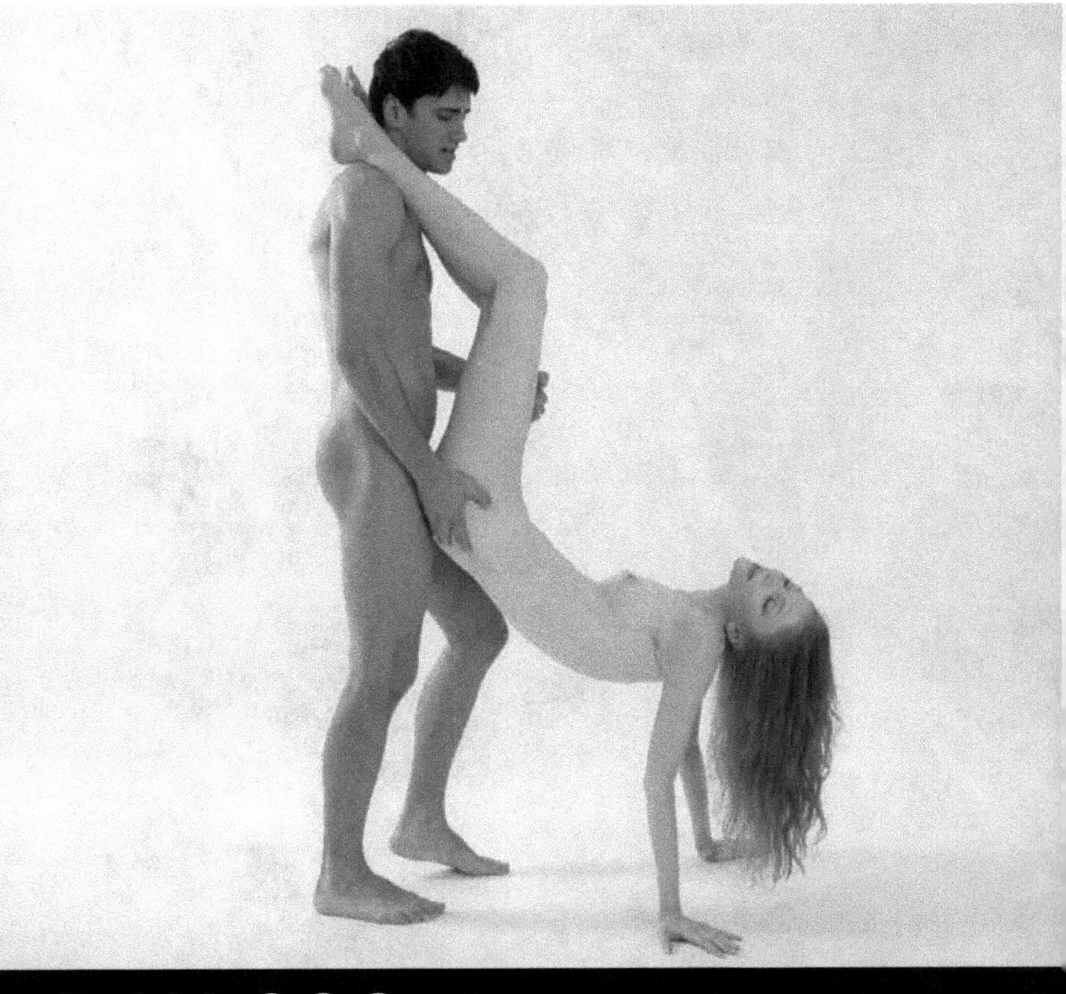

DAY 239

THE OBJECT OF DESIRE

From a standing position with her legs wrapped around his waist, she allows herself to fall backward as he supports her hips. With her palms flat on the floor she hooks her feet around his neck as he penetrates her. They're locked together in mutual desire.

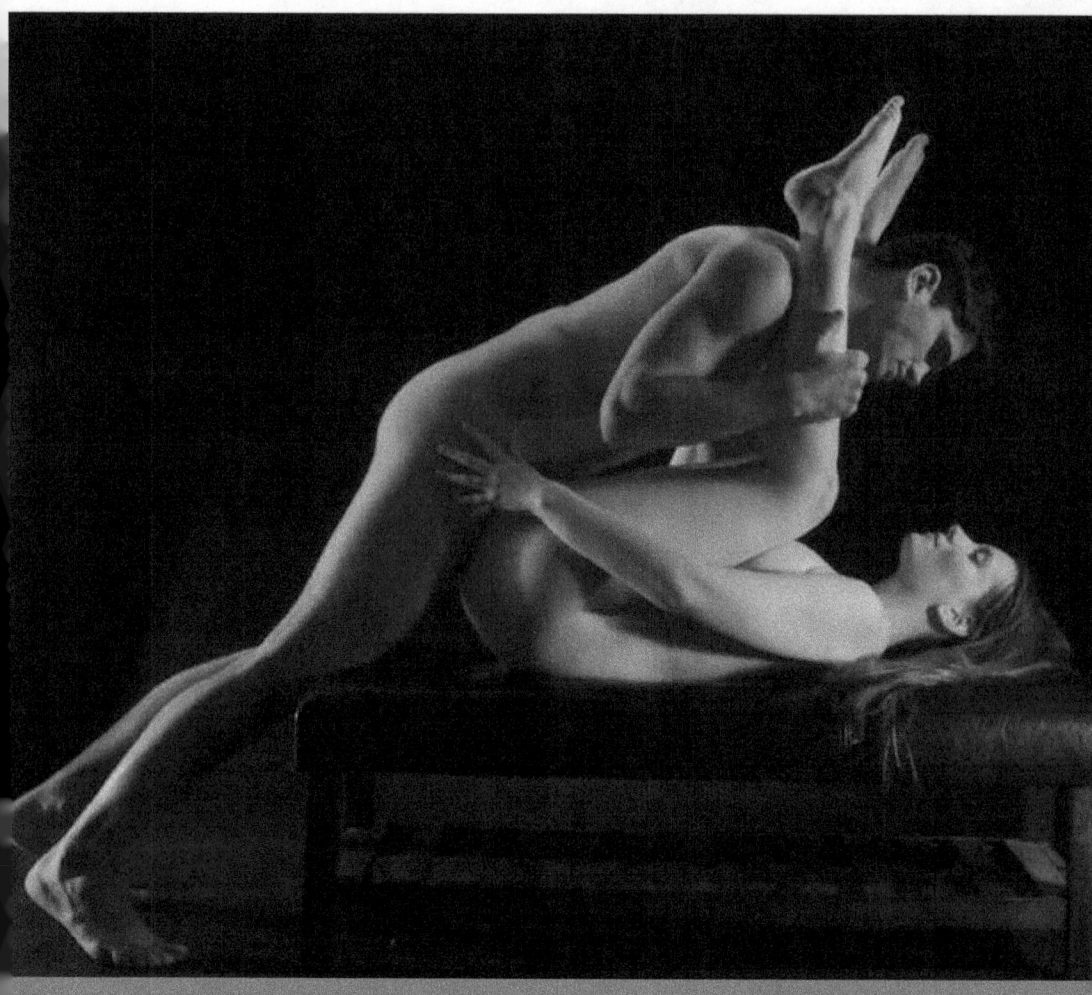

DAY 240

TOUCH YOU ALL OVER

The woman lies back on an ottoman or bench bringing her knees toward her chest and legs open. Her lover mounts her from a diagonal position. He runs his hands up and down her legs as she reaches for him too.

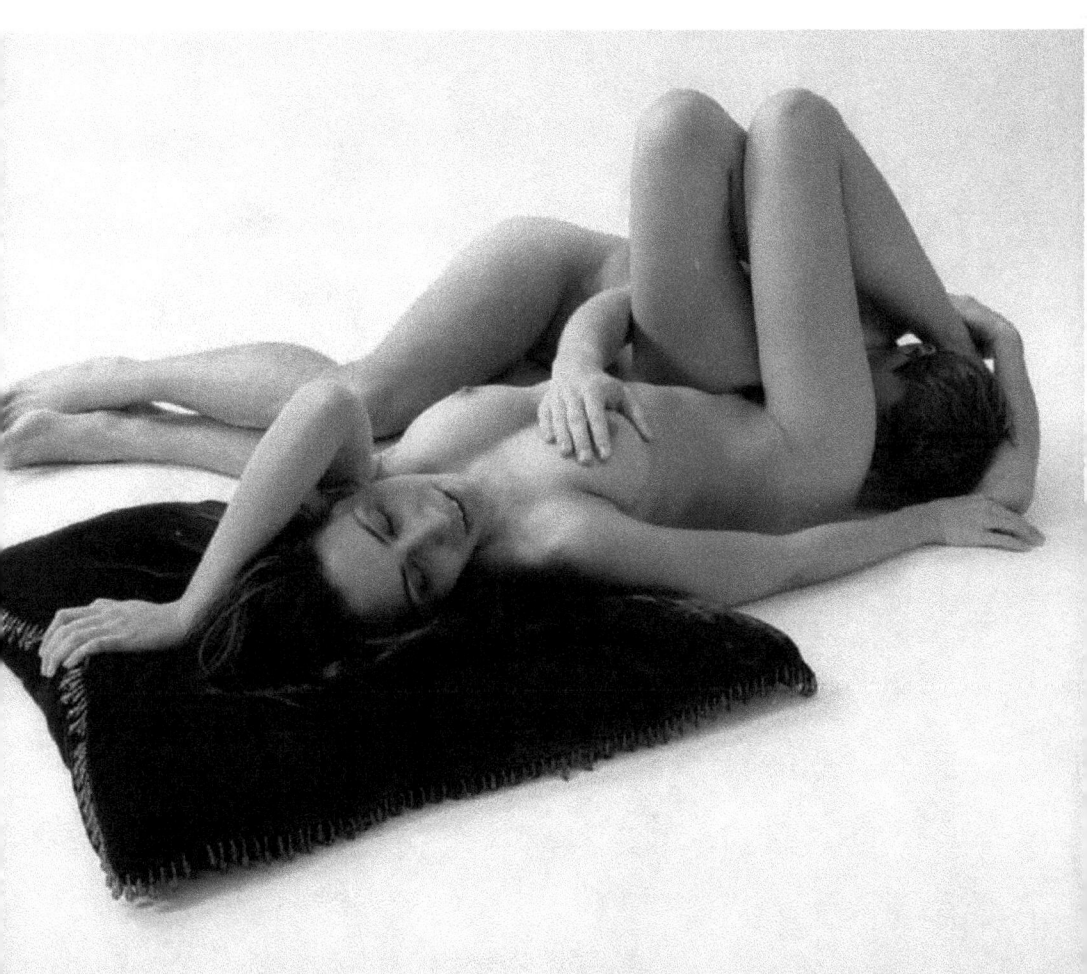

DAY 241

THE FEELING IS MUTUAL

The lovers lie next to each other head to foot. He gently moves her legs out of the way until his mouth has full access to her vagina. She returns the favor by stroking his penis with her hand.

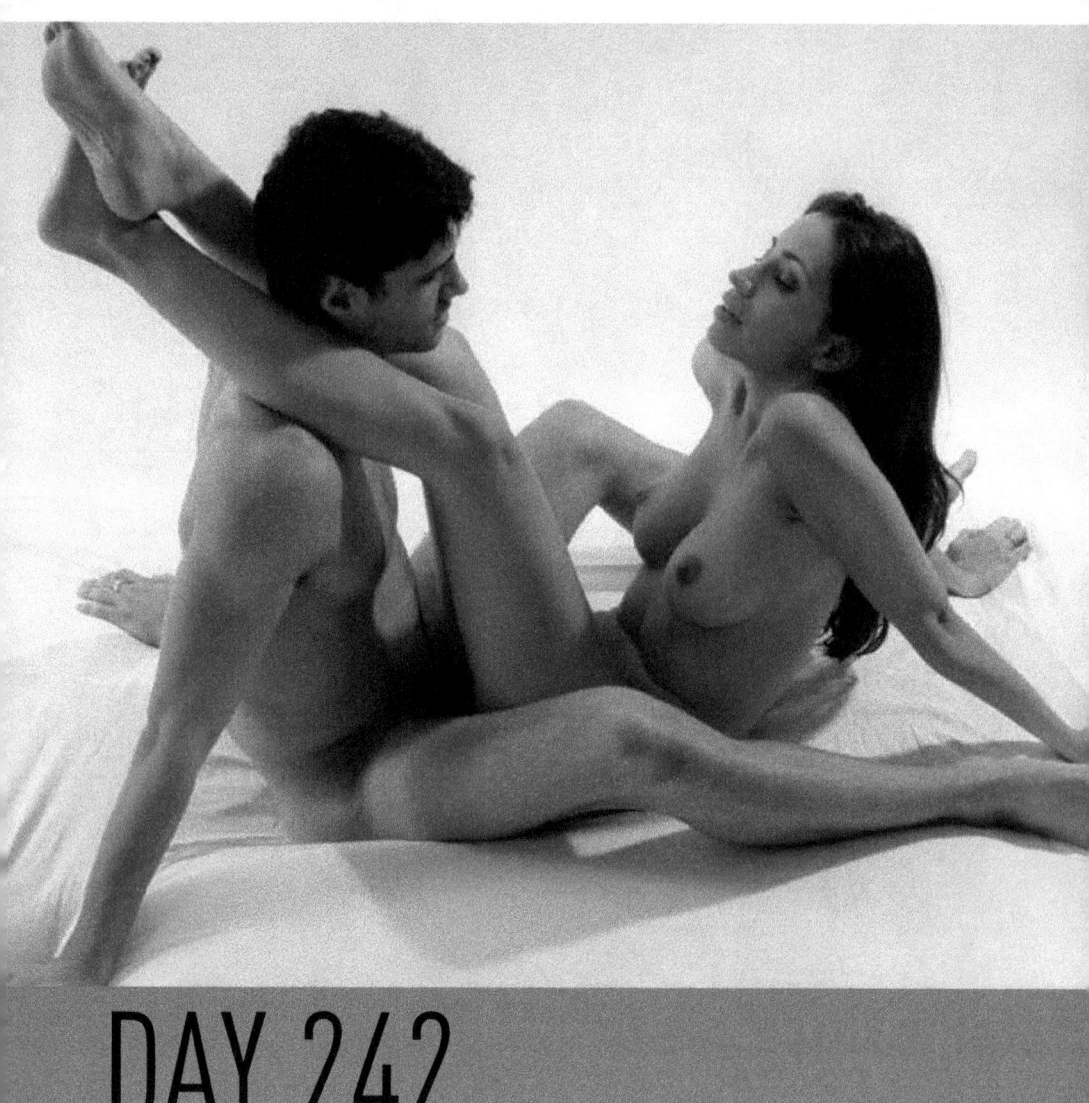

DAY 242

THE SCREW TOP

The man is seated with his legs apart and knees bent. As he enters his partner she rests her legs on his shoulders and hooks her feet behind his head.

DAY 243

BREATHLESS

As with some other pelvis-to-pelvis positions, this one starts with the woman in her partner's lap facing him. They both lean back slowly so as to maintain penetration. Rather than lots of physical movement, this one's about sharing each other's energy and being in the moment.

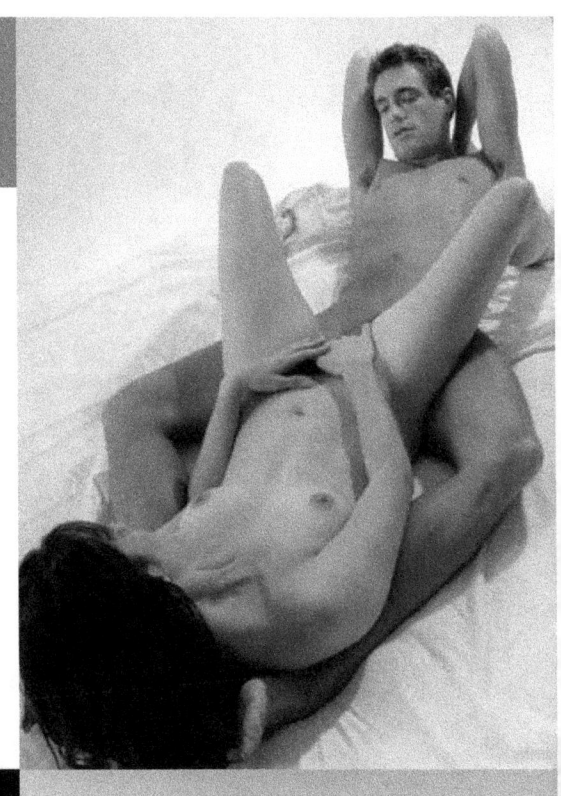

DAY 244

THE POW WOW

He's relaxed and on his back. She places herself on top, facing away from him, and crosses her legs yoga style. Hitting the G-spot from this position is always a distinct possibility.

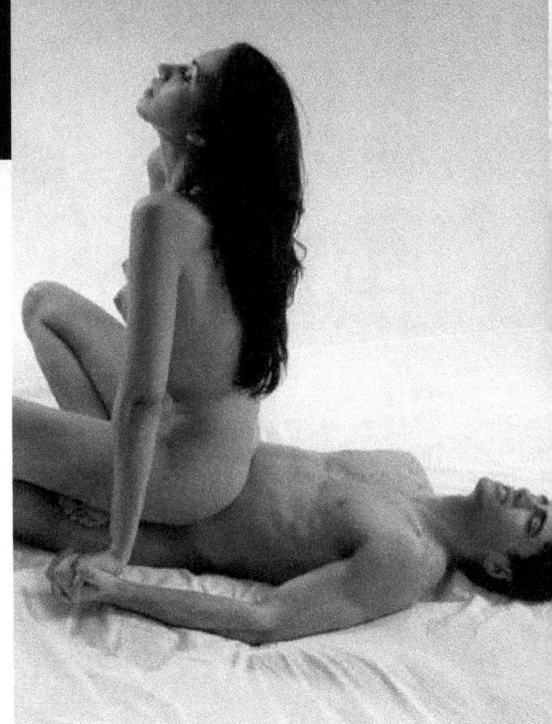

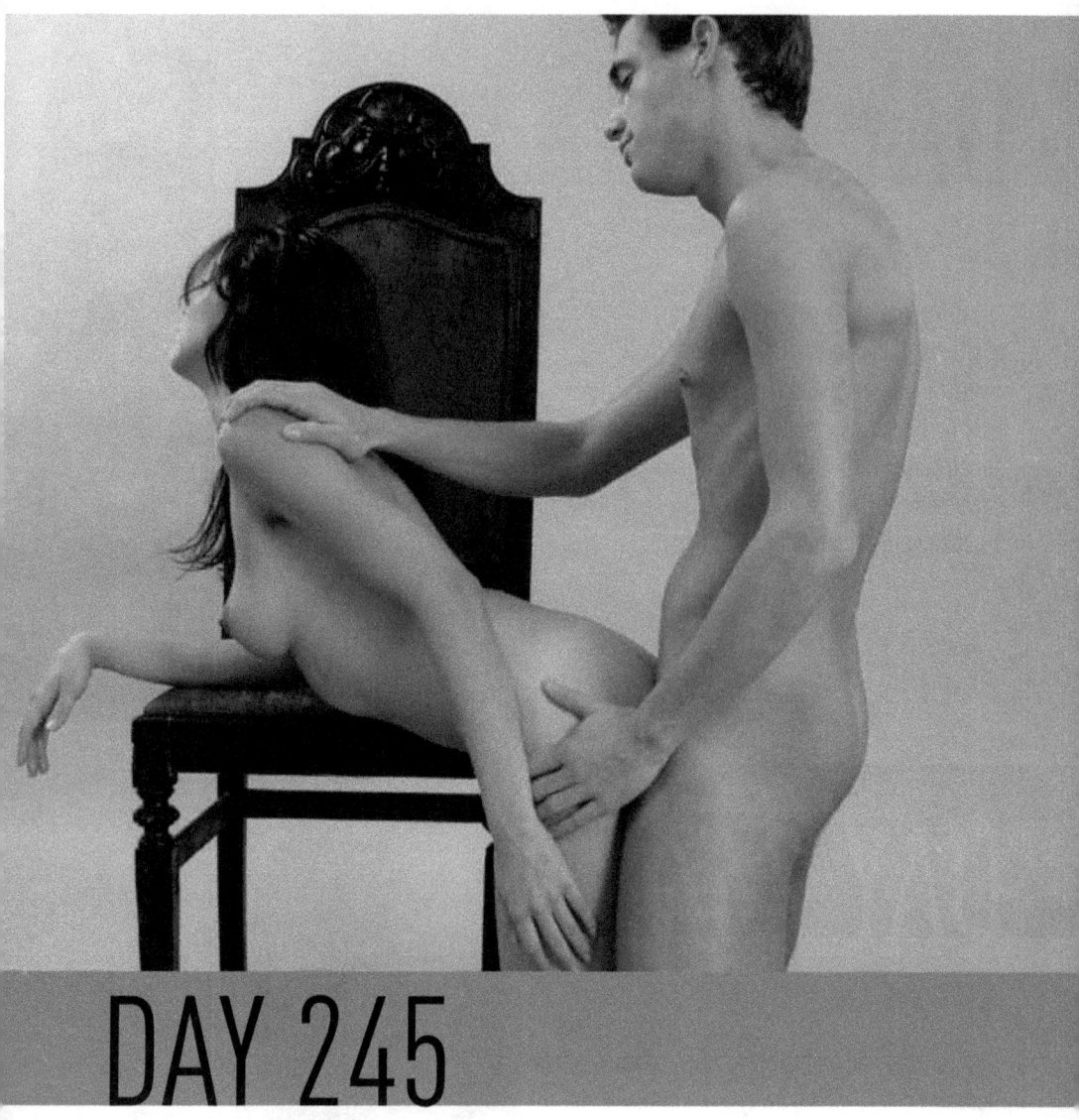

DAY 245

THE WELCOME GUEST

The woman gets on her knees and leans over a chair or the edge of a bed. Her partner penetrates her from behind keeping his legs outside of hers. His hands are free to guide her hips backward and forward on his penis.

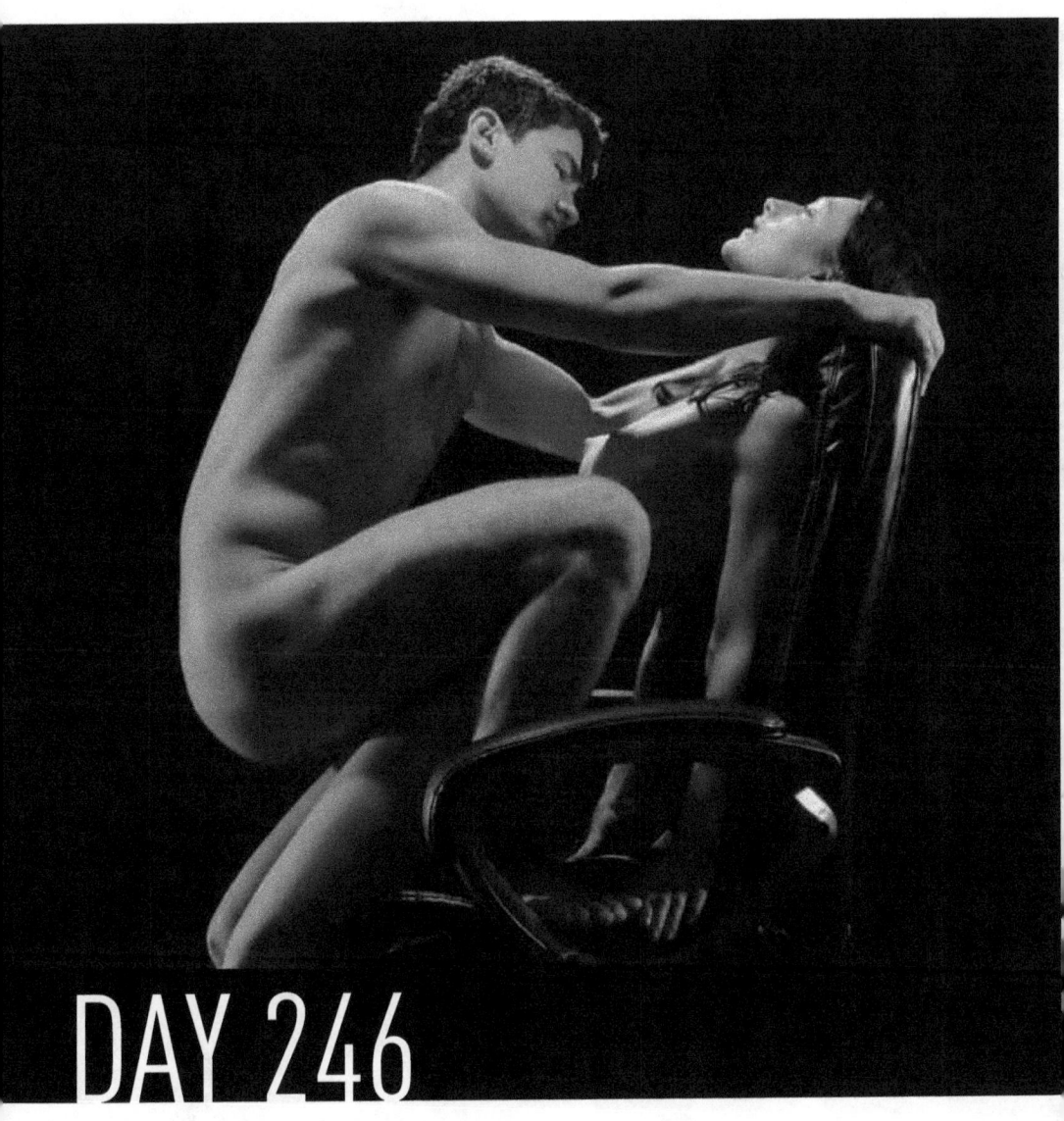

DAY 246

DOWN BOY

She sits on the edge of the chair with her legs apart and feet on the floor. He hops up on her like the horndog he is and penetrates her. The angle of entry allows for extra clitoral stimulation.

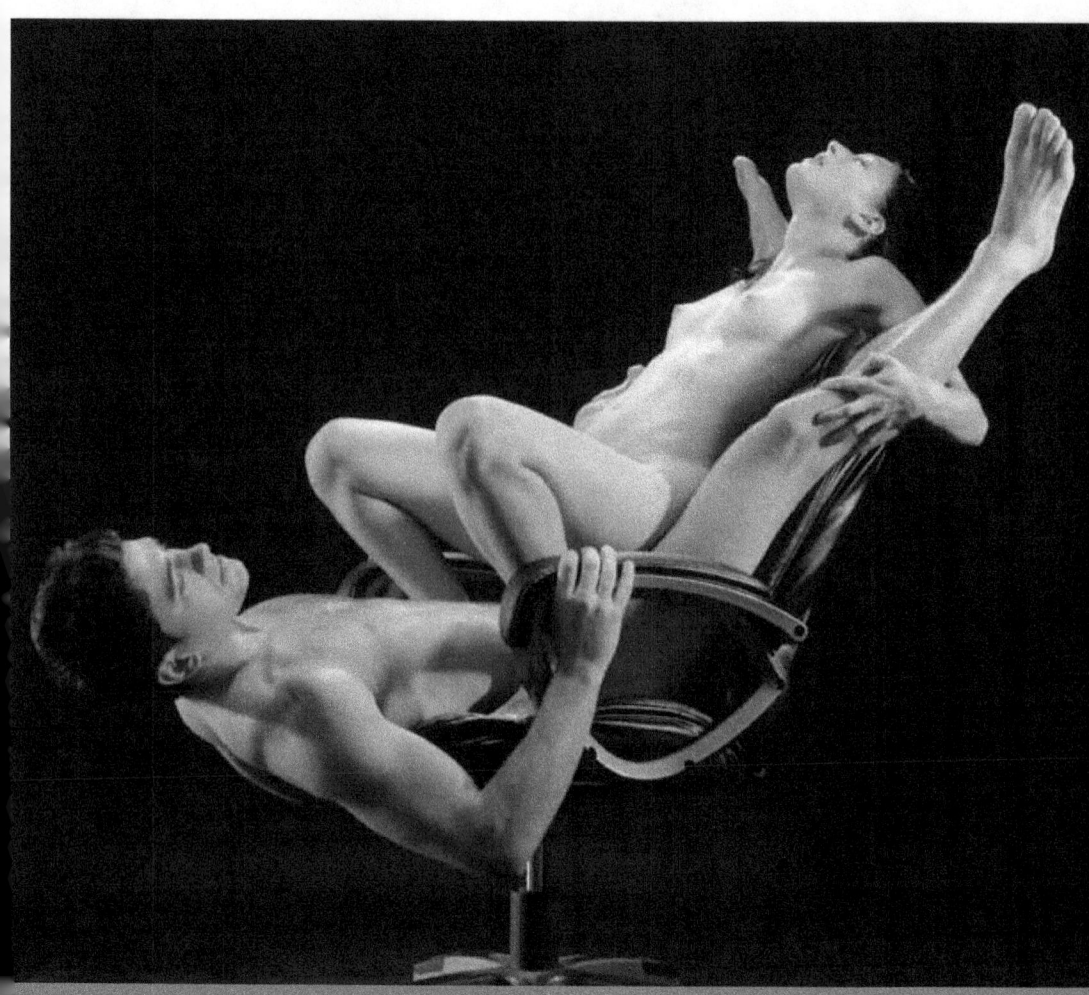

DAY 247

THE DAREDEVILS

Here's one that will send you head over heels, literally. The man positions himself upside down in a chair with his head hanging off the edge. His partner climbs up and mounts him, steadying herself by holding on to the chair's back.

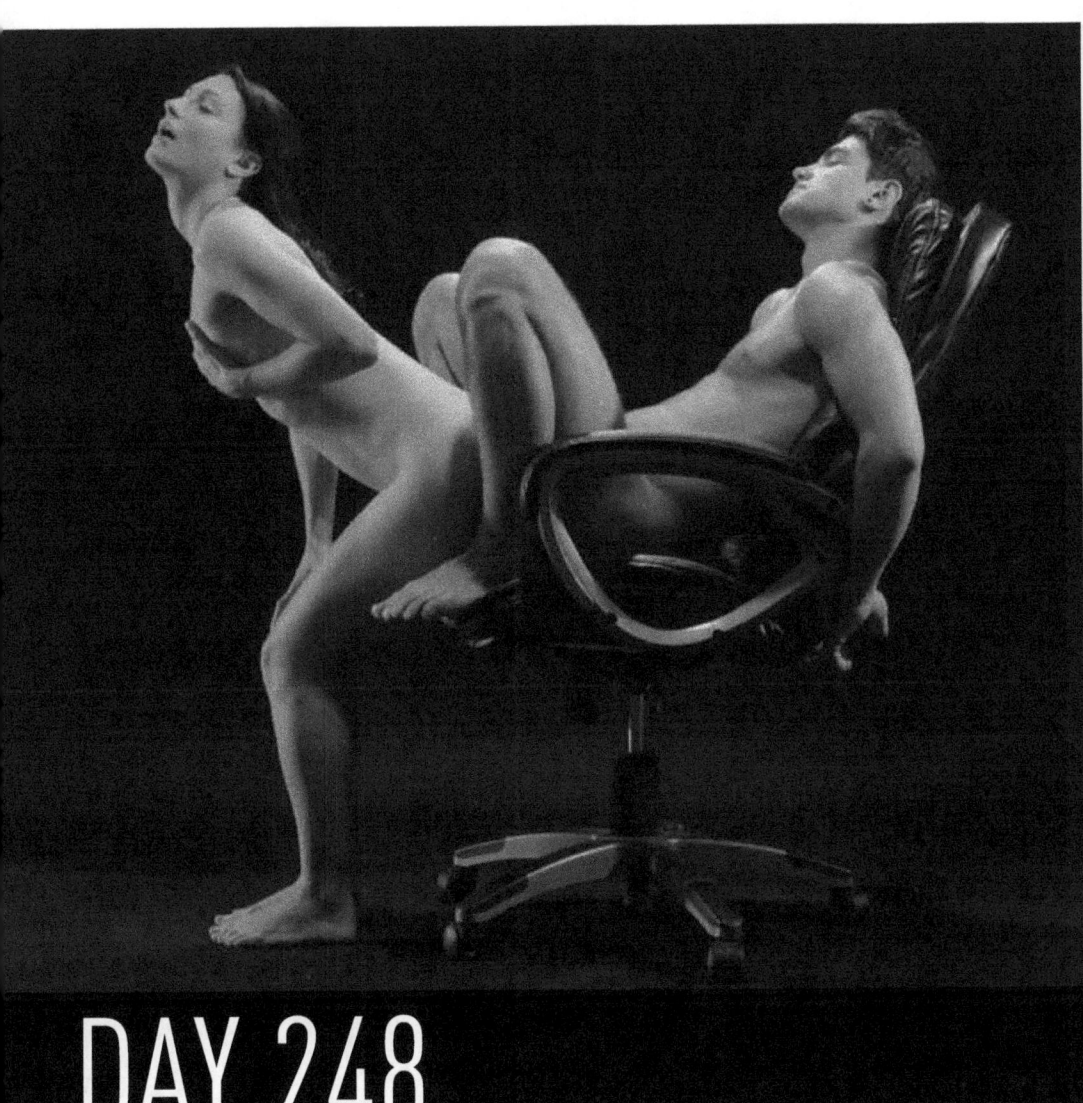

DAY 248

NO IFS, ANDS, OR BUTTS

The man places himself in a chair so that his feet are at the edge of the seat and his arms are holding on to its back. He lifts his pelvis so that his partner can mount his erect penis. She can back down into him as much as she pleases.

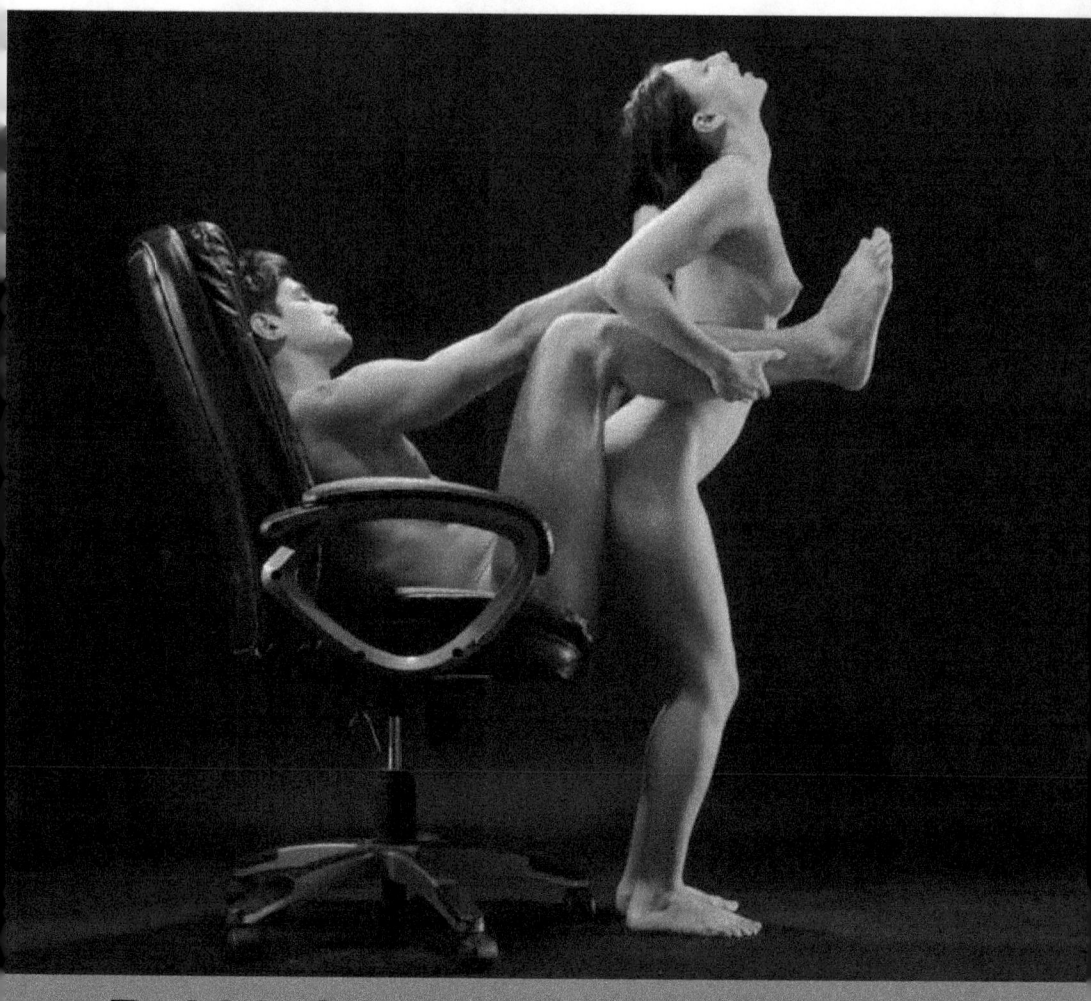

DAY 249

THE STABILIZER

He places himself low in a chair with his knees bent and legs open. His partner lubes up her anus and lowers herself onto his penis. She holds his legs for stability and for greater control over depth of penetration.

DAY 250

ALL YOU CAN EAT

The man lies back on the bed with his head right up against the edge. She straddles her partner's face and lowers her vagina onto his waiting mouth. He brings her to orgasm.

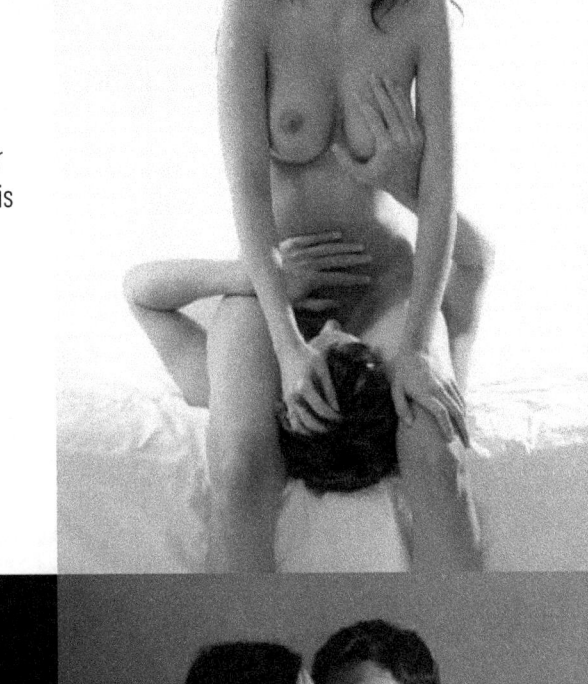

DAY 251

OH WHAT A KNIGHT

He leans back against the wall as his partner jumps into her lover's arms and mounts him. He's carrying her entire weight as she moves up and down on his penis. He can stay against the wall or carry her to the bedroom.

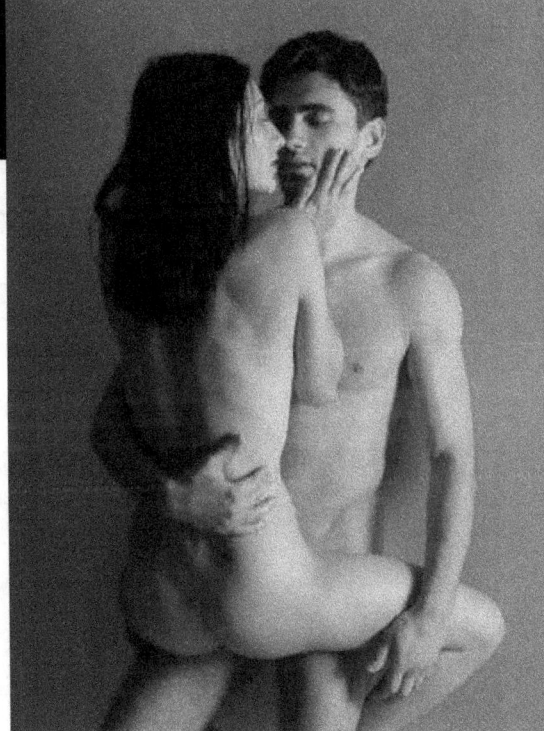

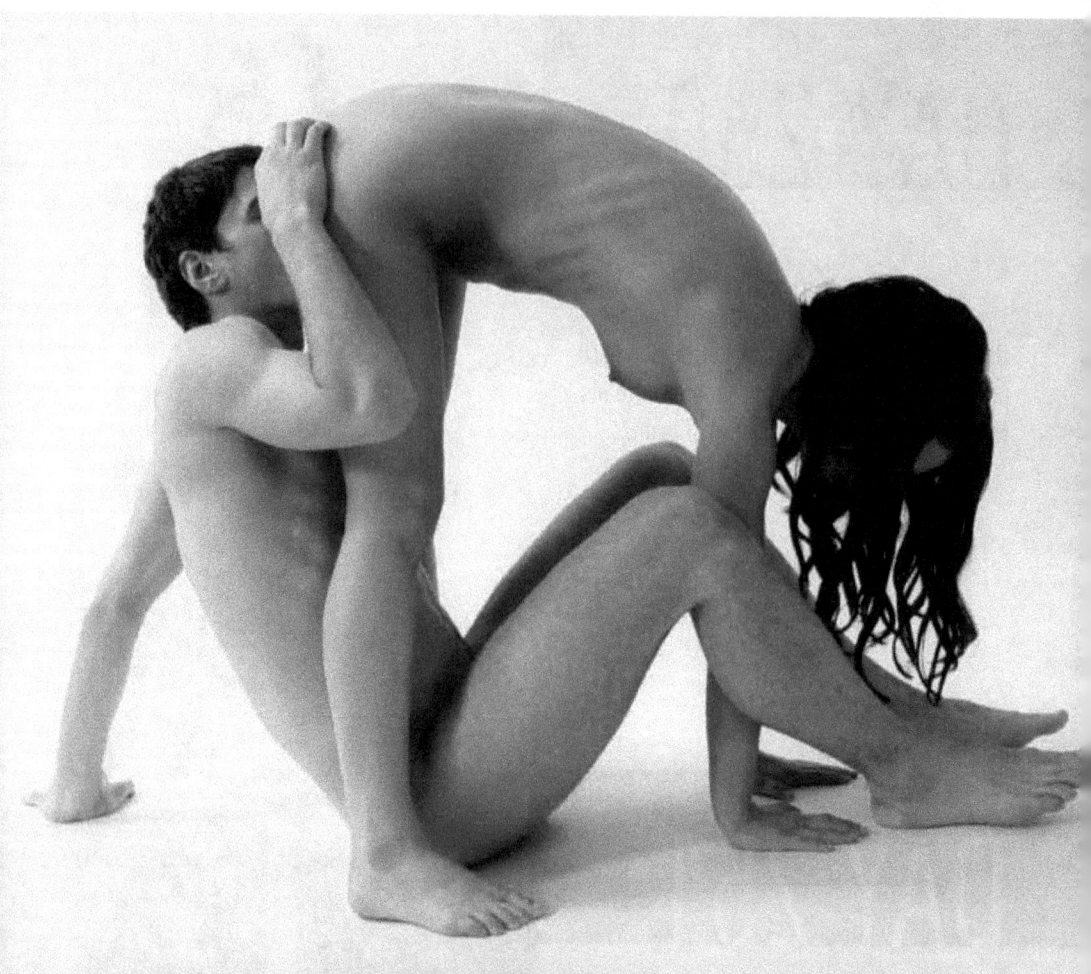

DAY 252

JACK AND JILL

She leans forward from a standing position and places her hands on the floor as though she's about to tumble. Her partner moves in between her legs from behind and uses his mouth and fingers to stimulate her vagina and anus.

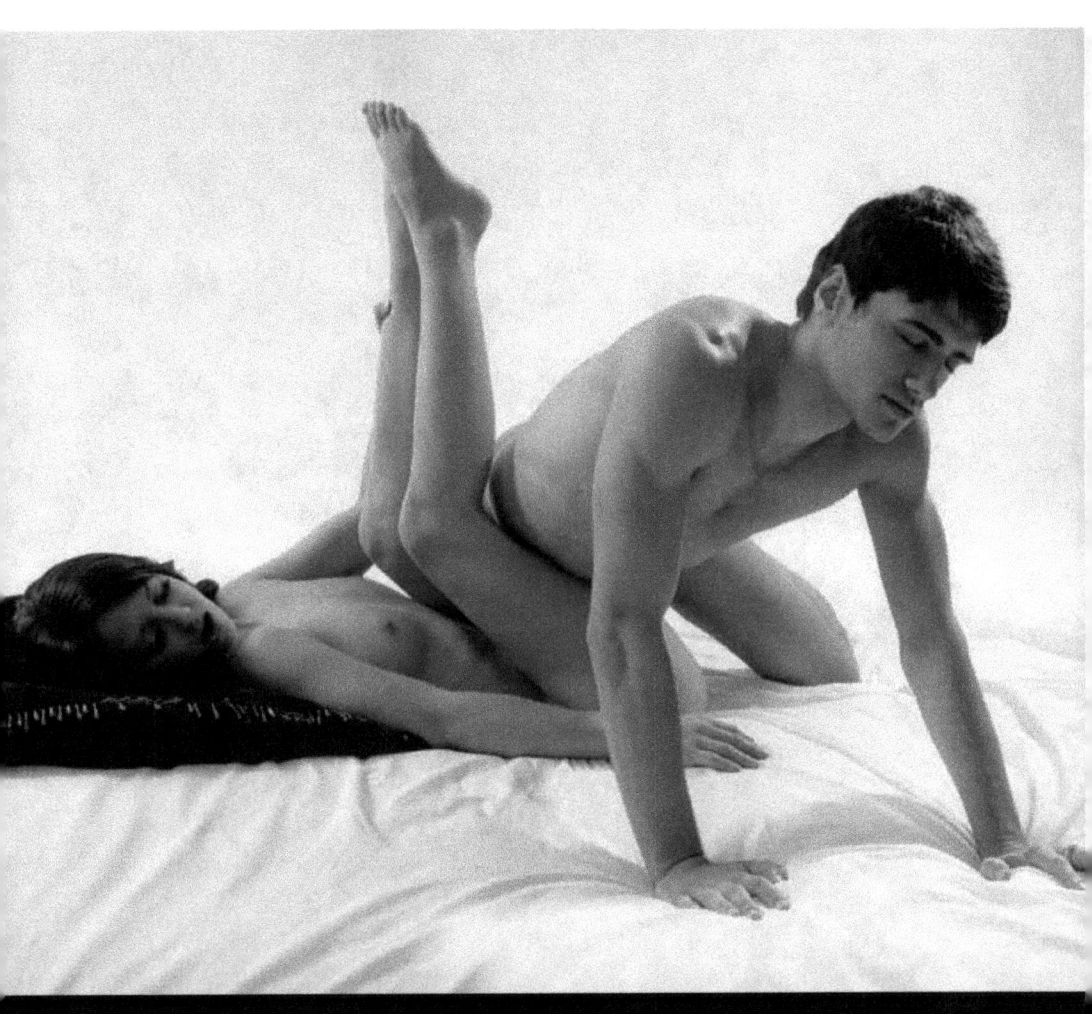

DAY 253

BODY SURFING

She's on her back with her knees bent in toward her chest and legs pointing up. He spreads himself across his partner. Together the lovers surrender to a current of passion.

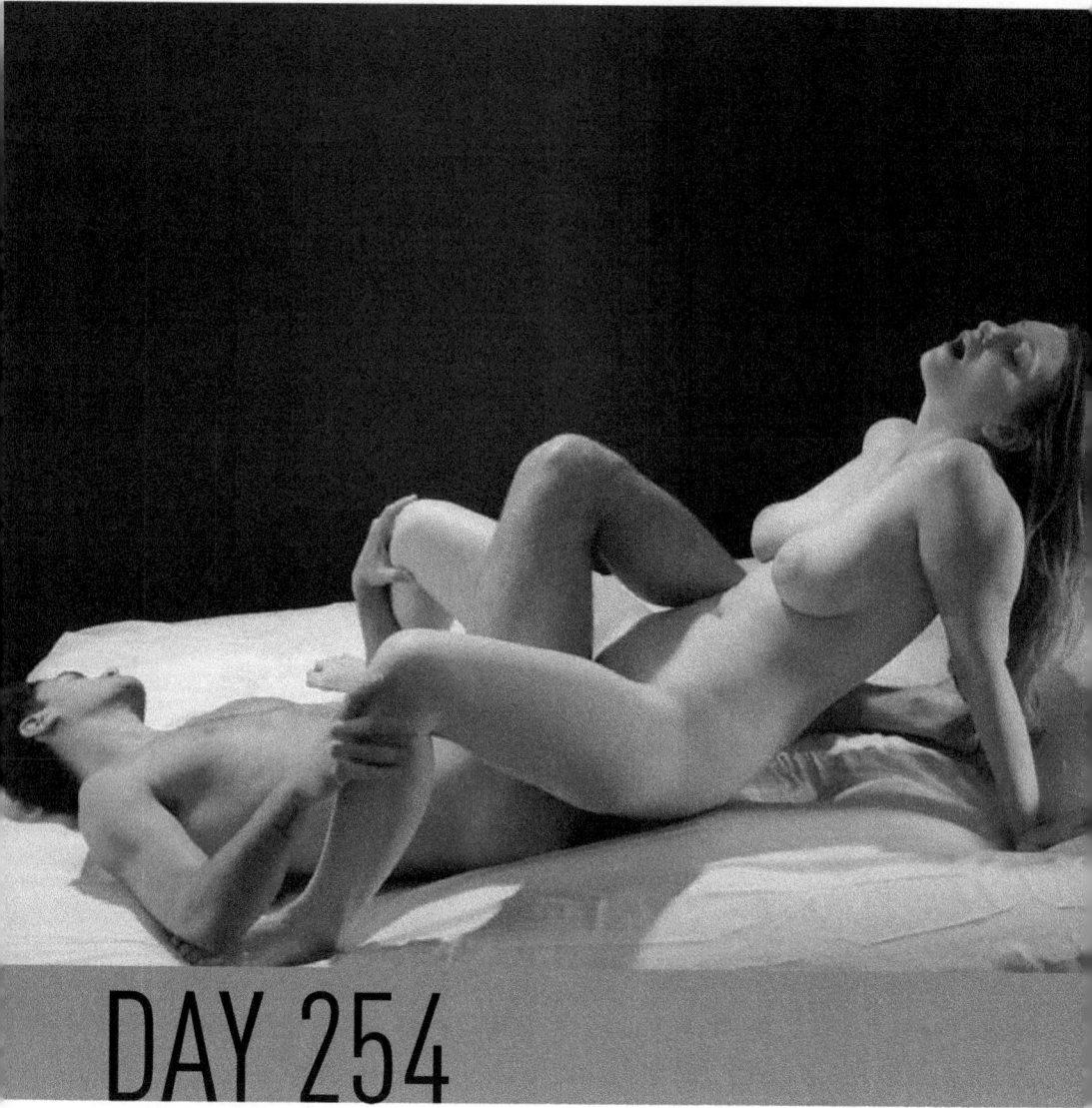

DAY 254

THE GRIND

He lies back on the bed with his knees bent and legs open. His lover slides in between as he penetrates her vagina. As both move their hips and legs, they create a fantastic friction.

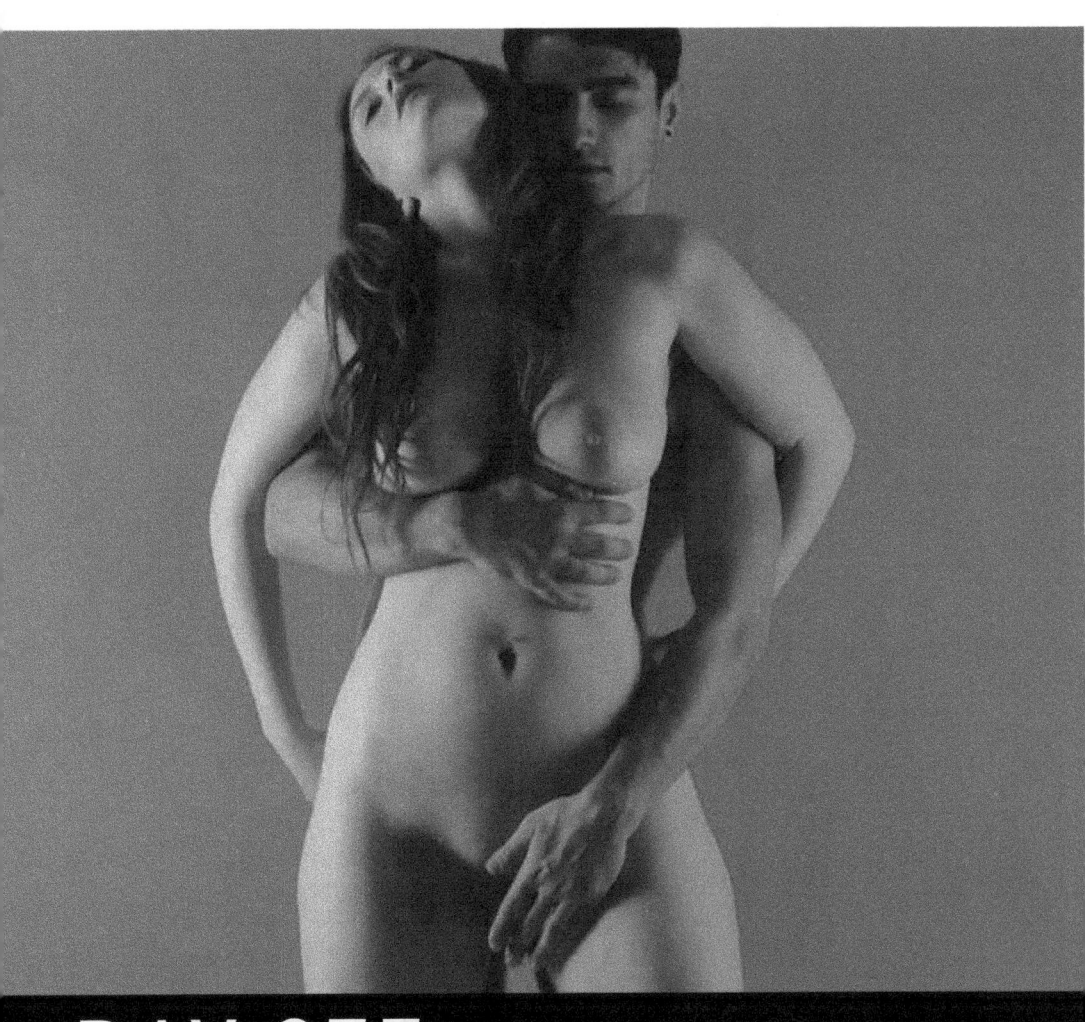

DAY 255

LEAN ON ME

He leans back against the wall with his legs slightly apart. His partner turns her back to him and takes a wider stance so that she's almost straddling his legs. As he enters her she leans back offering her neck for his kisses and brings her hands around to his buttocks.

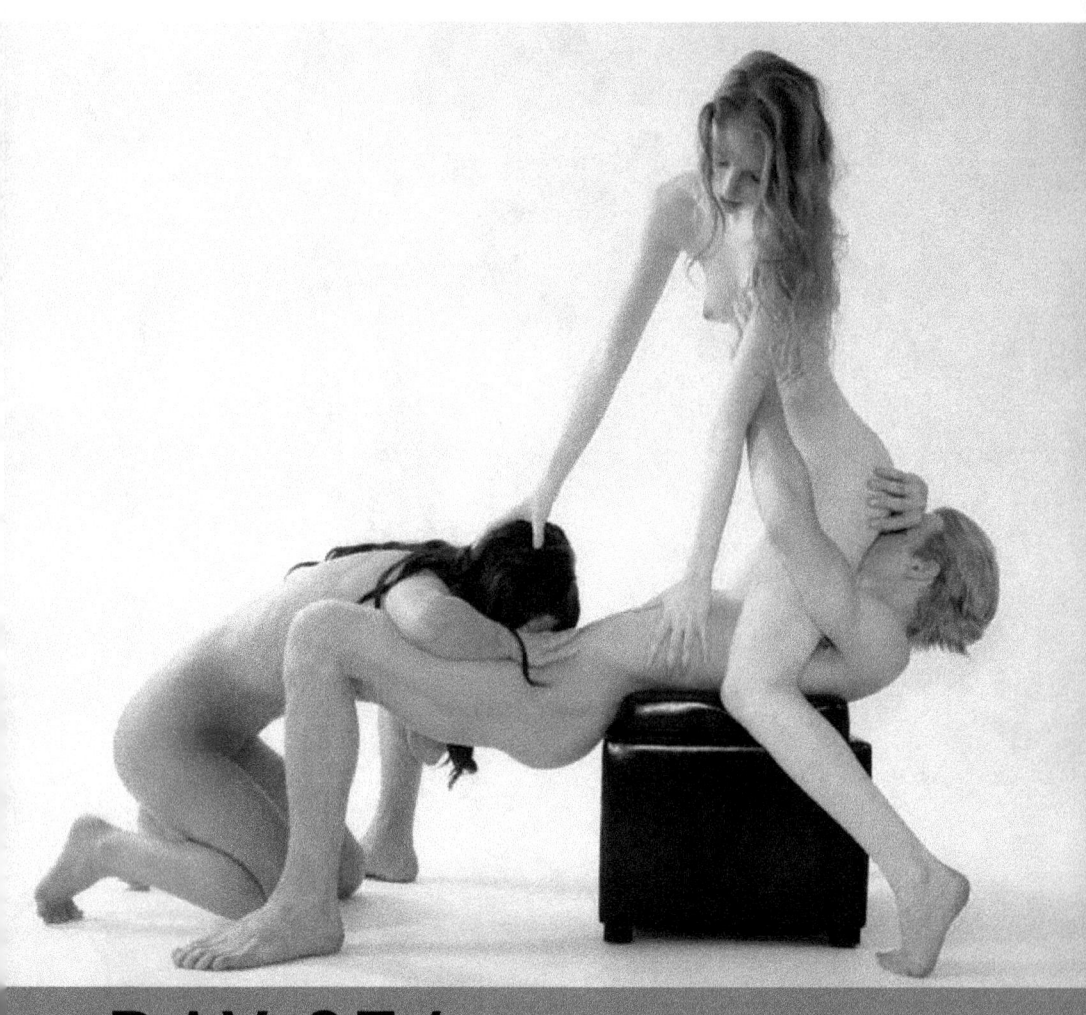

DAY 256

TABLE FOR THREE

The man lies back across an ottoman or low-lying table with his knees bent and feet on the floor. One woman lowers herself onto his face for some cunnilingus action while the other gets on her knees and gives him a blow job to remember.

DAY 257

BOUND FOR GLORY

She's on her knees with her eyes blindfolded and hands bound behind her back. Her oral senses are heightened as she takes his penis in her mouth.

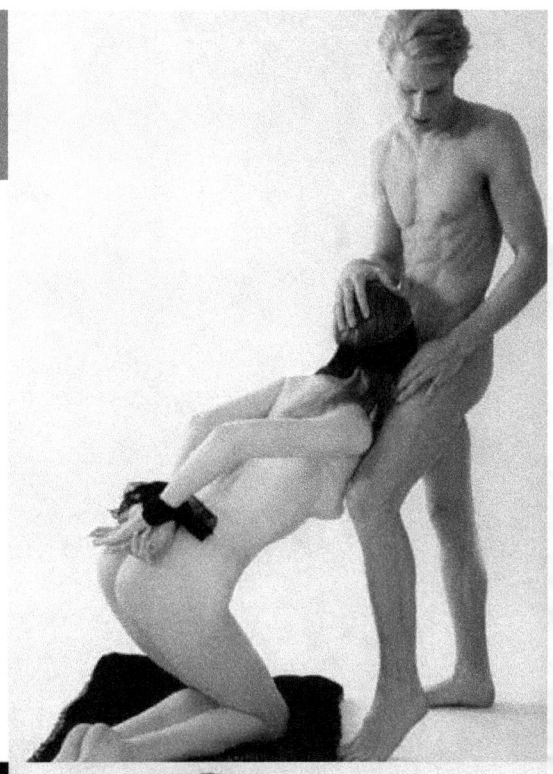

DAY 258

KNEEL APPEAL

The lovers kneel and face each other. She's in his lap with her legs spread apart and he's able to use his arms and legs to bounce her up and down.

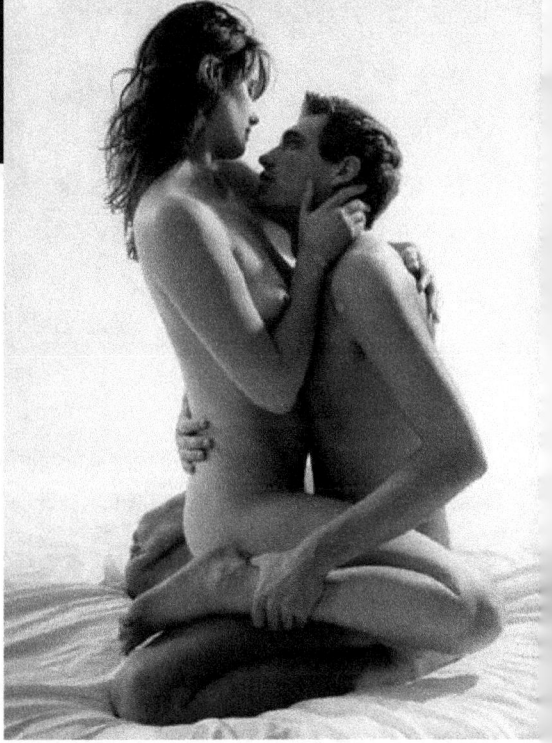

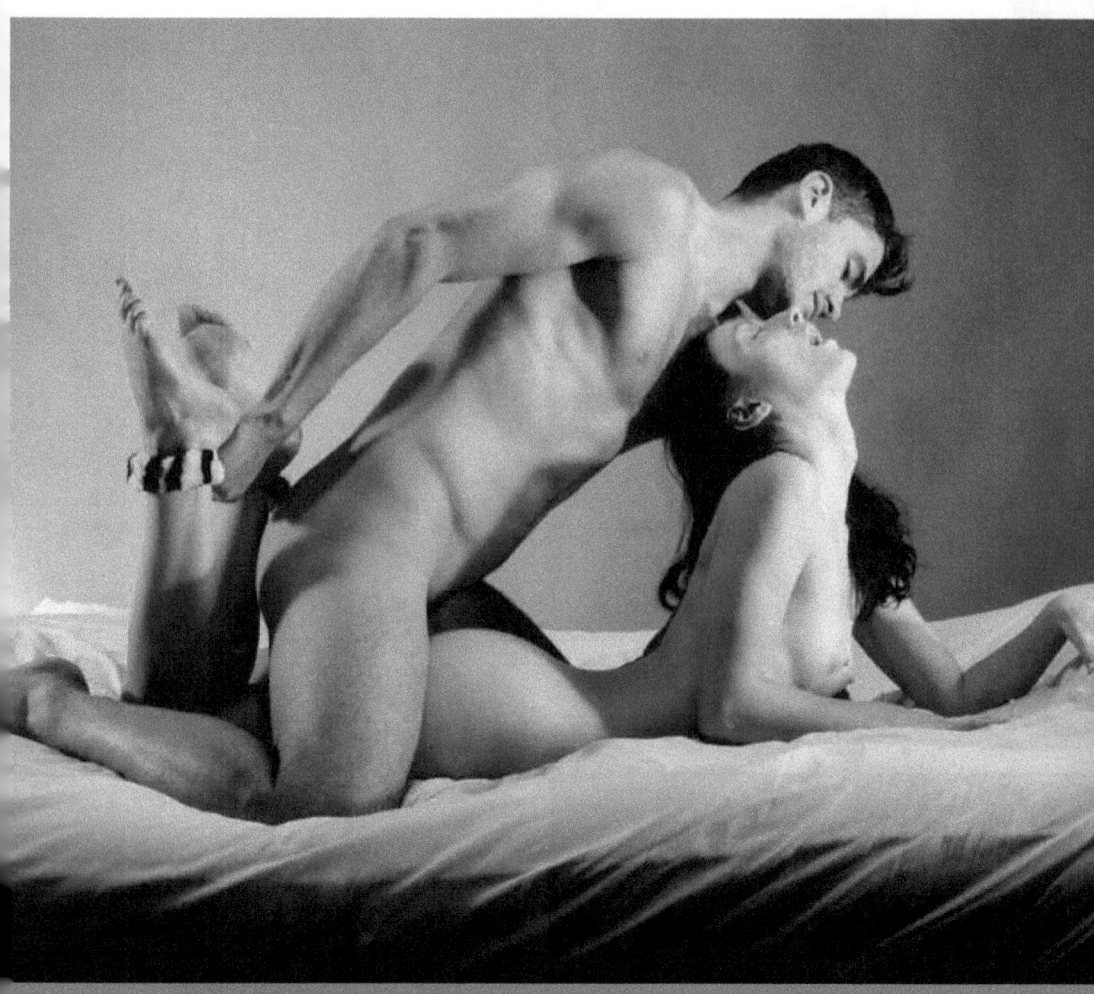

DAY 259

CALF ROPING

She lies on her stomach with her ankles cuffed together. As her partner enters her from behind, he gently pulls up on the cuffs. She lifts her torso in anticipation of his touch and kiss

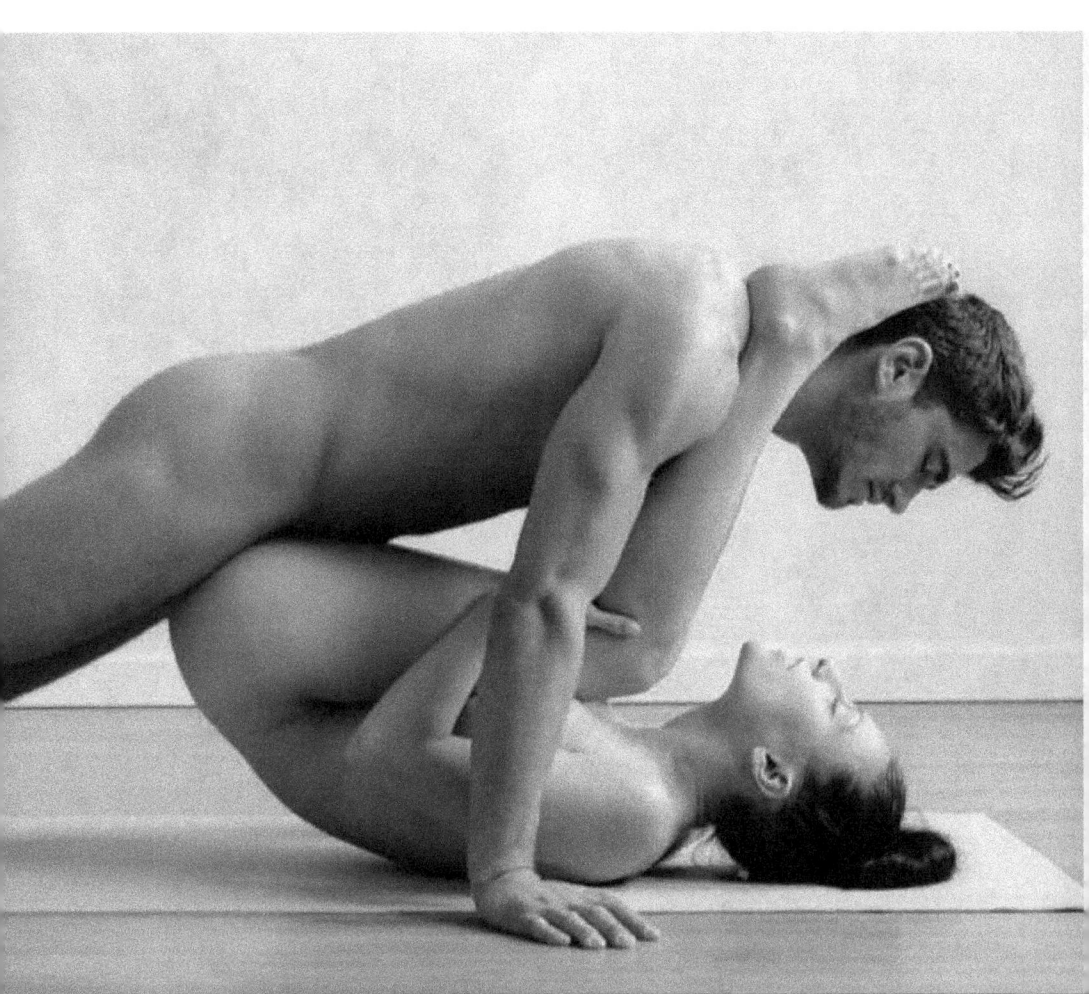

DAY 260

THE ROLLING BONE

She lies back on a yoga mat and tucks her knees in towards her chest. Her partner enters her deeply from a push-up position. As he thrusts away, she grabs her legs behind the knees and they are able to maintain a rolling rhythm.

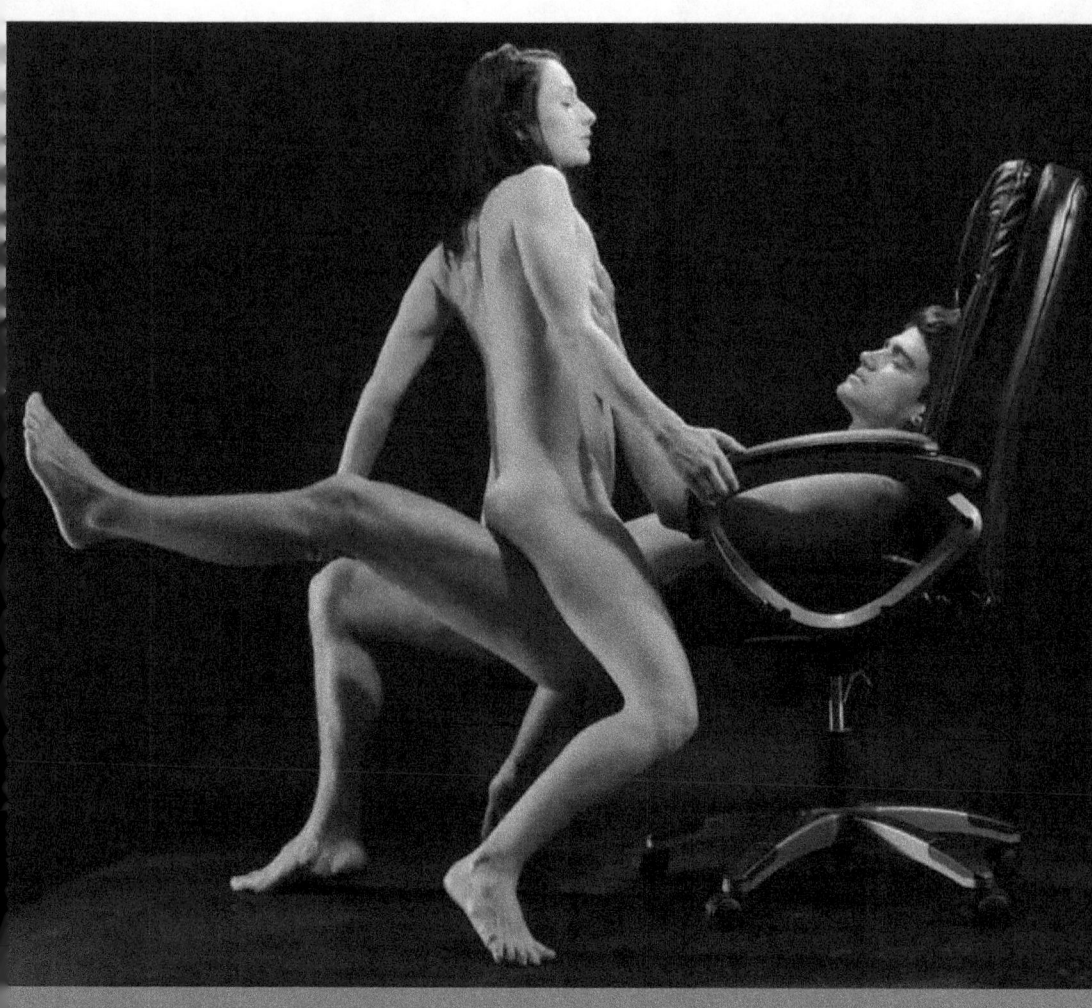

DAY 261

FLOATING ON AIR

He slouches down in a chair bringing one leg to the floor and the other one straight out. His partner straddles his leg as his penis penetrates her vagina. His hands are free to explore her breasts and clitoris.

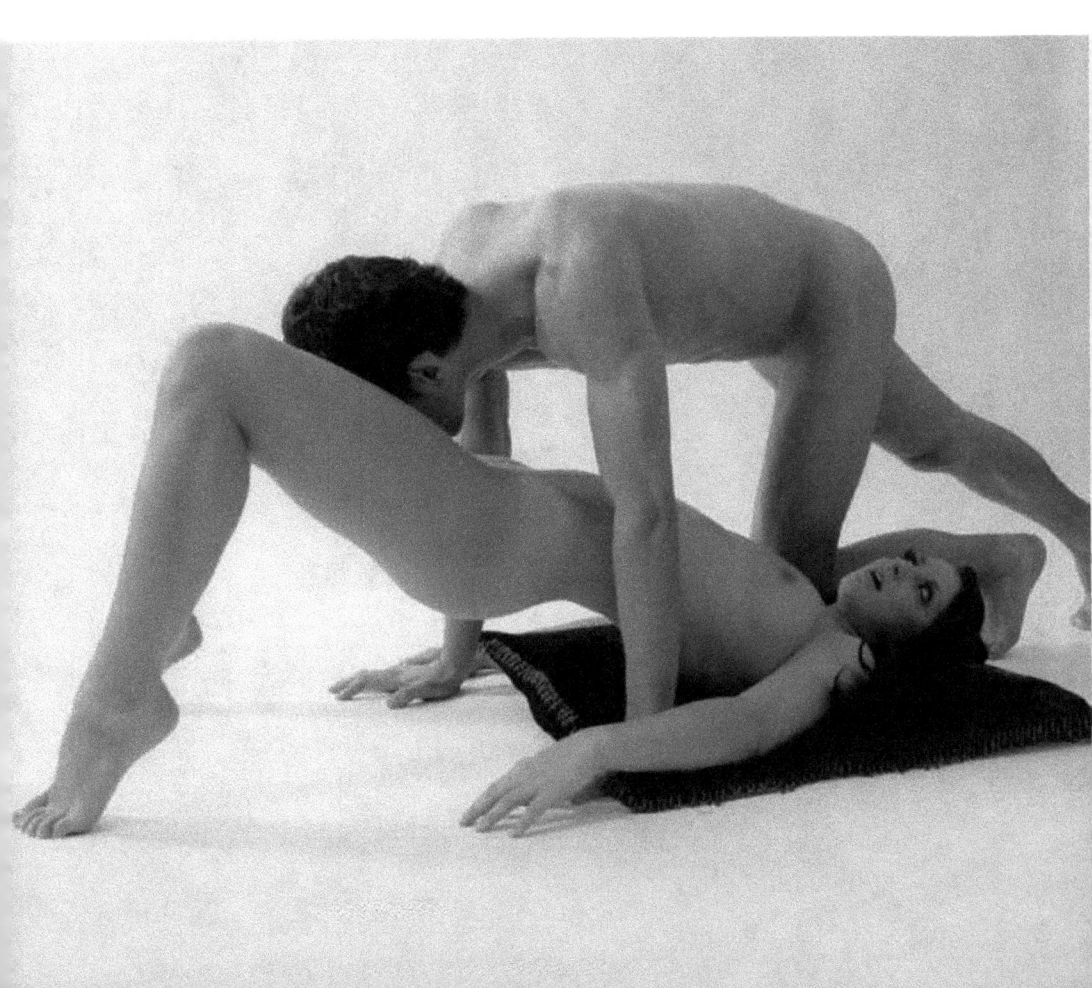

DAY 262

SENSATIONAL SUNRISE

From her back the woman presses her feet and hands into the floor so that her hips and back come up into a reverse plank position. Her lover comes in from the opposite direction and meets her elevated vagina with his mouth.

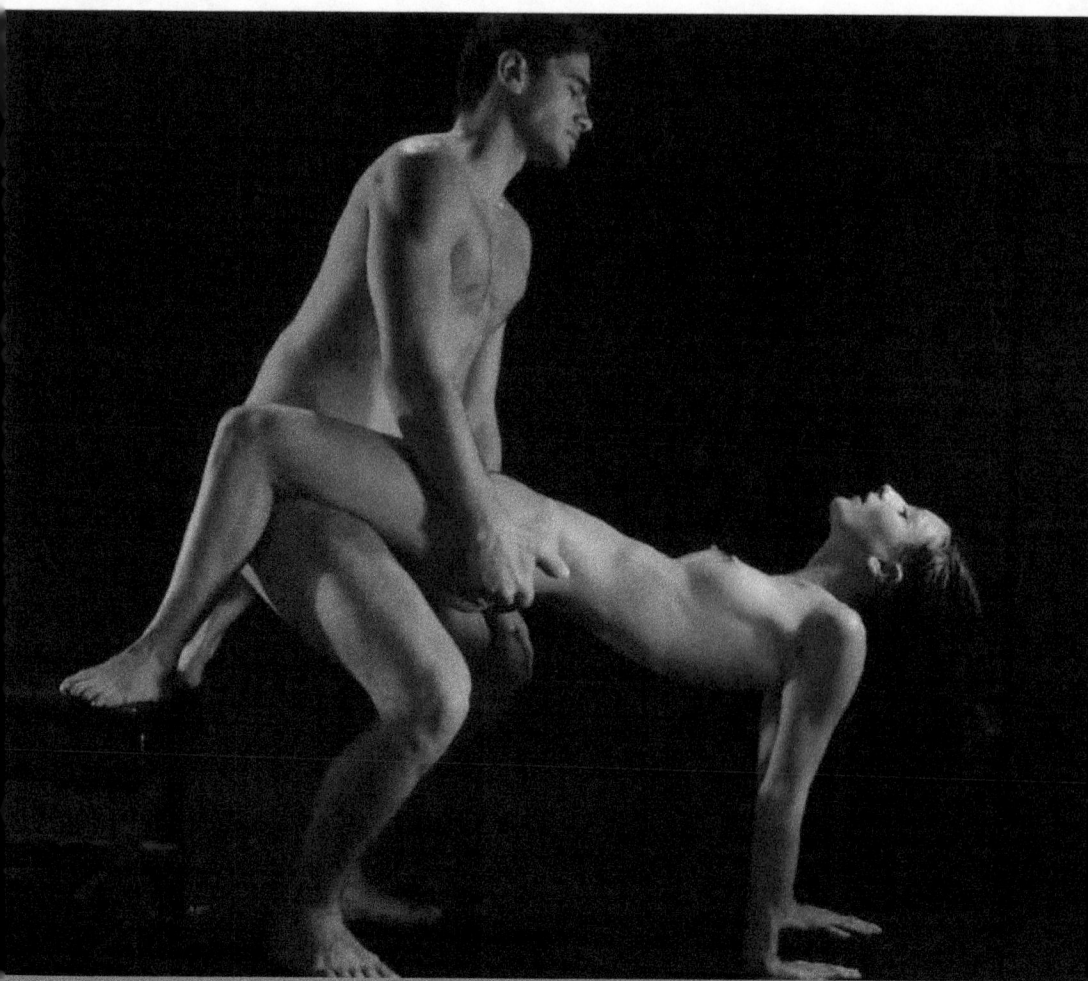

DAY 263

THE HOLLYWOOD ENDING

Like the old saying goes, it takes two to tango. The Man gently lowers his lover toward the floor from a standing position as though he's dipping her. Her hands are back while her feet rest on a table or bench. As he penetrates he may want to get closer and plant a passionate kiss on her.

DAY 264

OVERTIME ACTION

Nothing like a late day at the office to get you thinking about more pleasurable pursuits. She sits back against a file cabinet, bringing one foot up against its side. He leans in and penetrates her vagina, supporting her lower back with his hand.

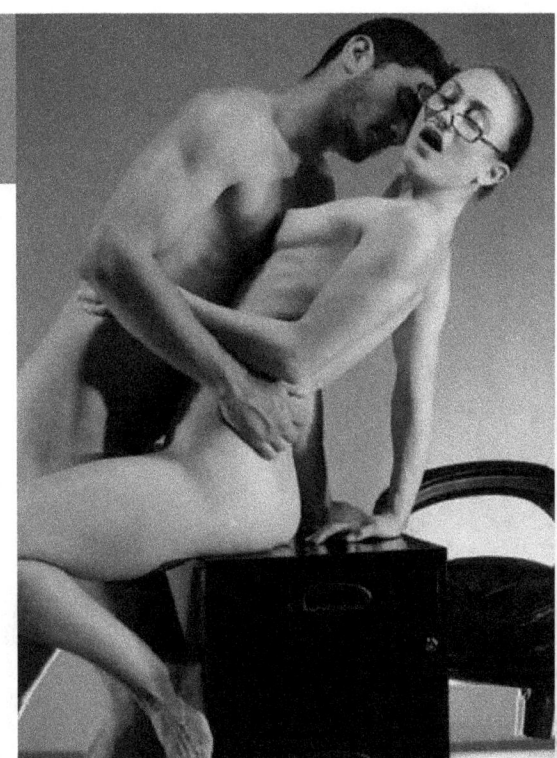

DAY 265

DOWNWARD DONG

She's seated on the edge of a chair with her toes touching the floor. He positions himself across her body so that his elbows are resting on the floor and his feet her up by her head. Her hands are free to roam across his butt and fondle his testicles.

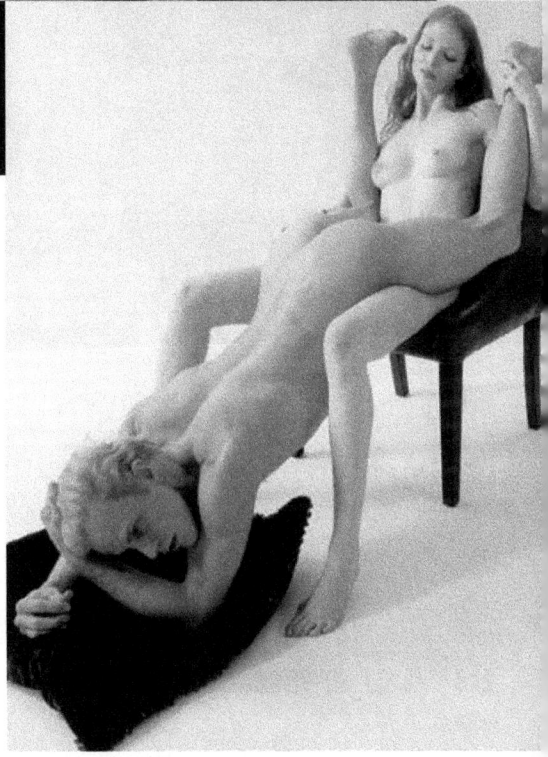

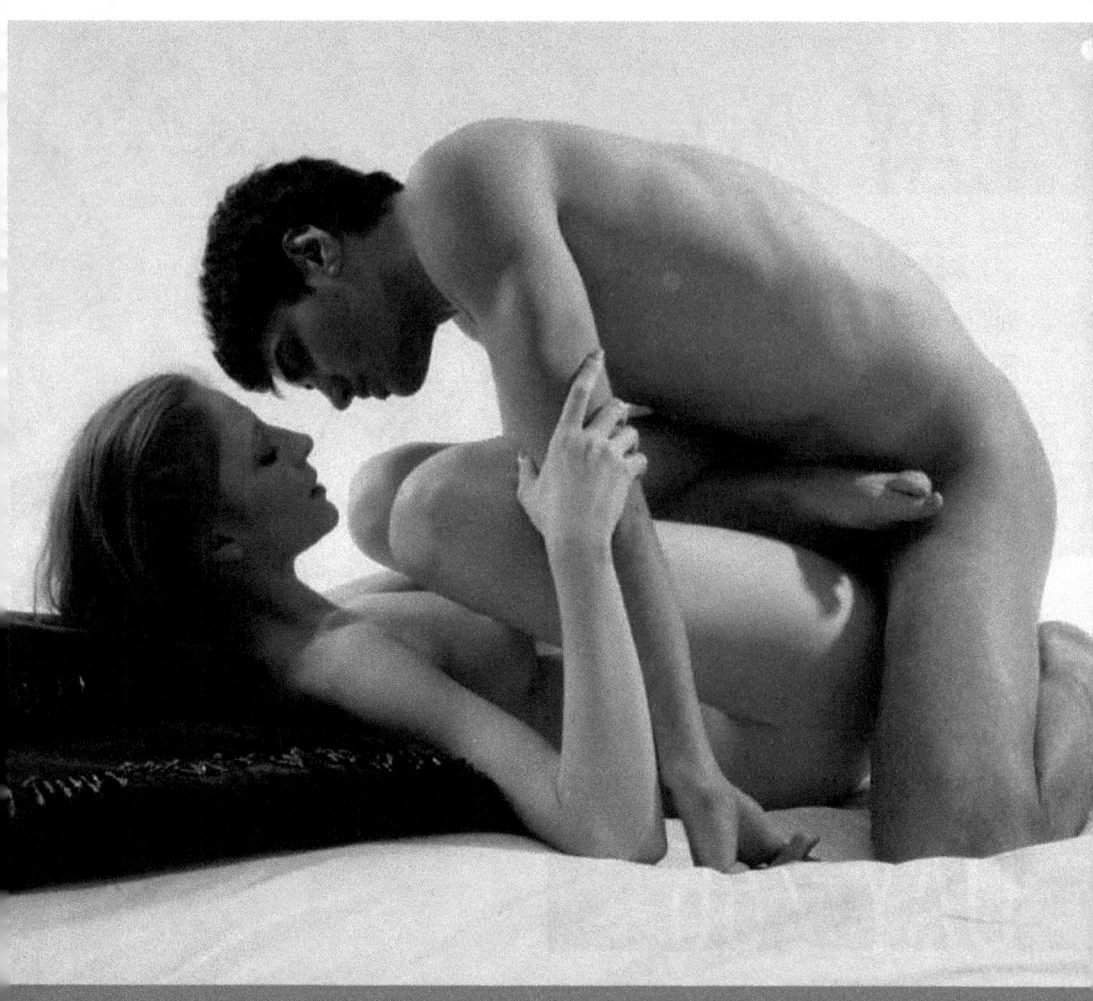

DAY 266

THE HAPPY LANDING

The woman lies back on the bed supporting her back and head with extra pillows. She brings her knees toward her chest and crosses her legs as her lover enters her from a kneeling position. Ample comfort surrounds this sometimes intense maneuver.

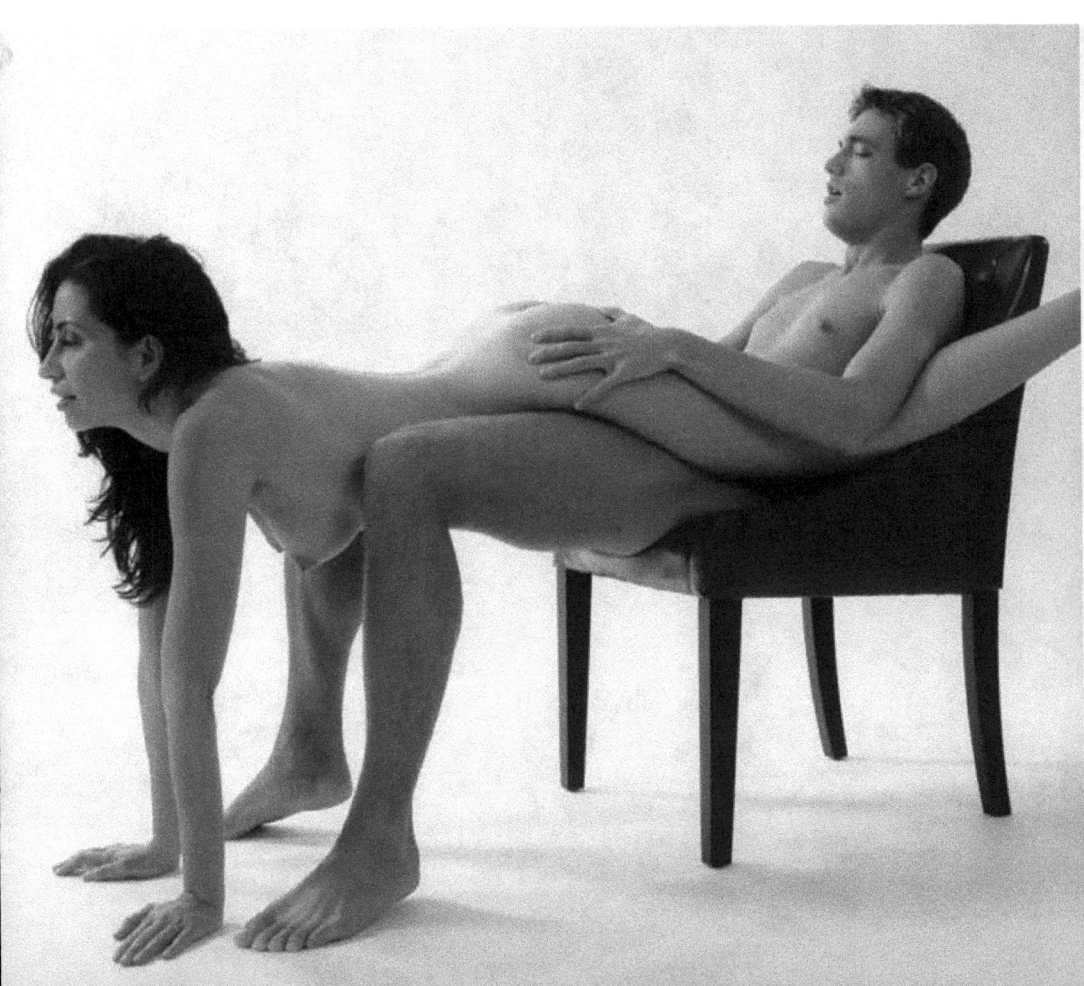

DAY 267

THE CHAMPIONSHIP BELT

He reclines back in a chair with his legs stretched out. She mounts him, facing outward, and lowers her hands to the floor as her thighs wrap around his waist.

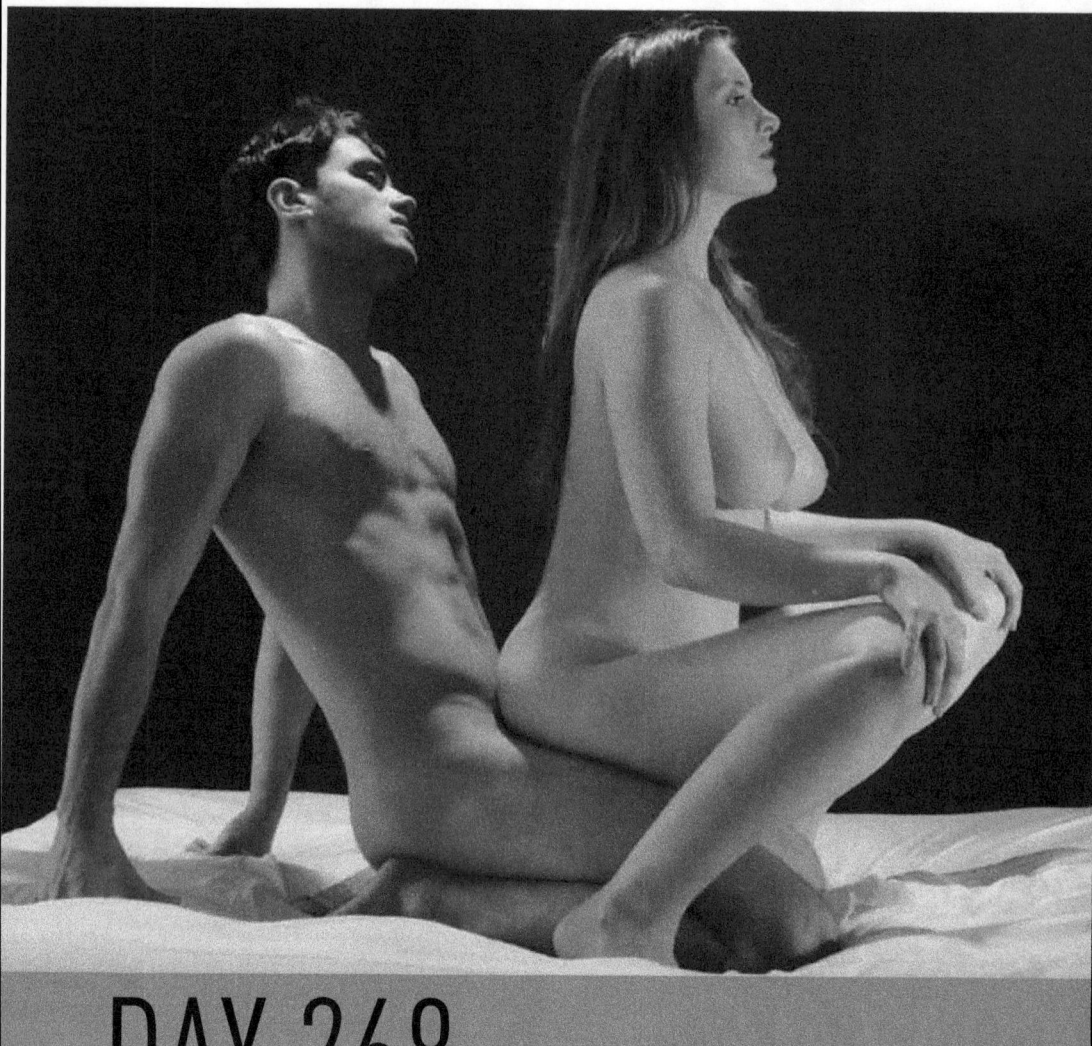

DAY 268

THE RUBBERNECKERS

The man gets up on his knees and leans back on his hands. His partner squats down onto his erect penis with her back facing him. She may be blocking his line of vision, but he likes the view just fine.

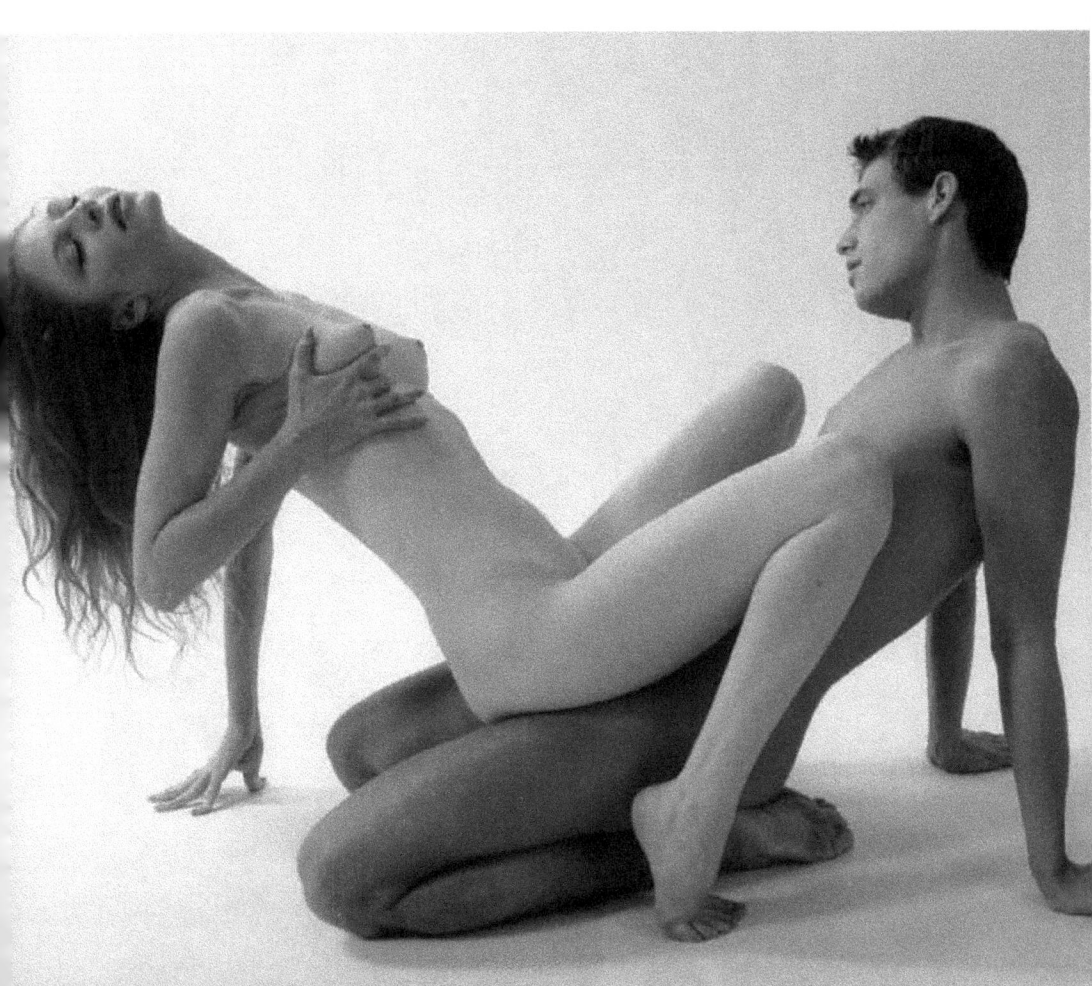

DAY 269

THE FLOOR EXERCISE

The man is on his knees leaning back on his legs with his hands back and to the floor. The woman faces him and mounts him, striking a similar pose to his own. Together, the lovers have plenty of flexibility for thrusting and bouncing.

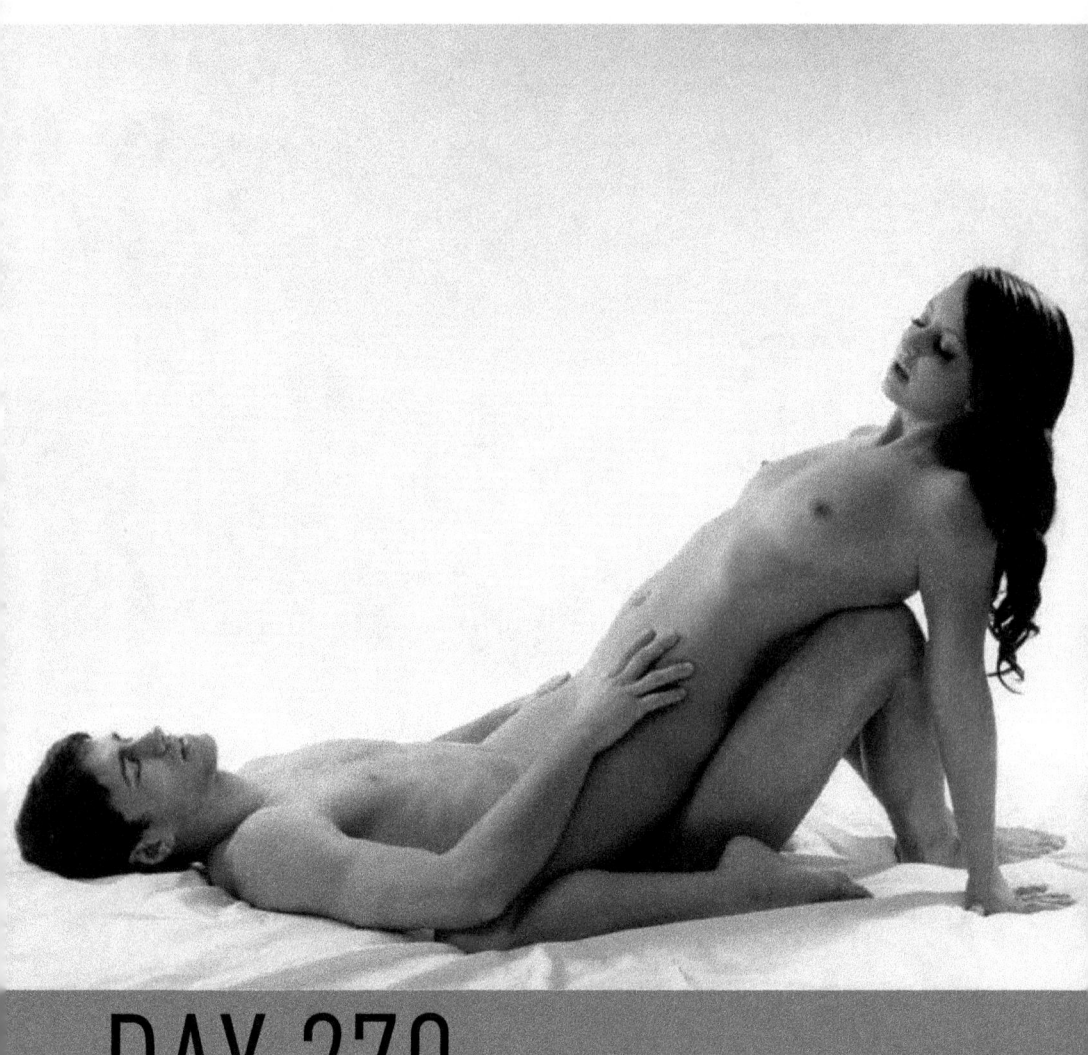

DAY 270

THE SCORCHING SLIDE

The man is on his back with his knees bent. The woman is on top facing her partner. She can then lean back against his thighs and slide up and down to her heart's content.

DAY 271

SCARY GOOD SEX

This advanced position starts simply enough with the man seated and the woman mounting him with her back to him. He then stands up, holding her forearms to support her. She leans outward and tucks her legs up against his thighs. This one requires a lot of strength, trust, and skill.

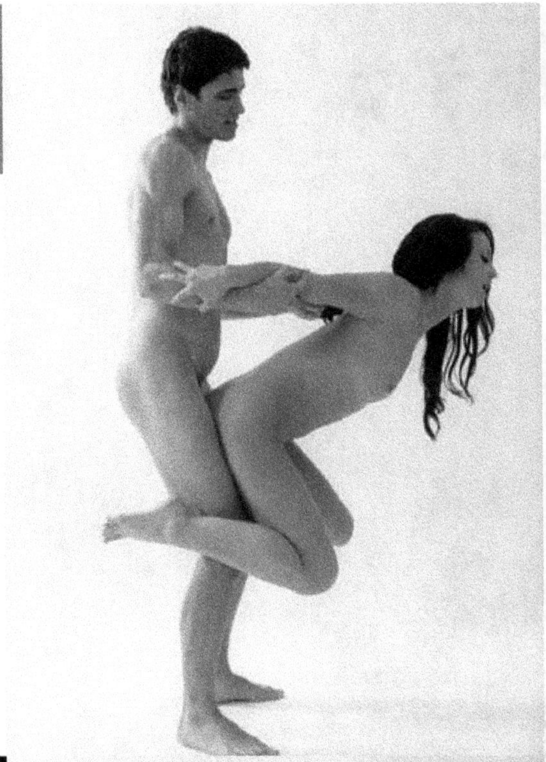

DAY 272

THE BUCKET LUST

The man positions himself on the edge of the bed or in a chair. She climbs into her partner's lap and reclines as though she's in a bucket seat. By hanging her legs over his arms she exposes her vulva and clitoris for his gentle touch.

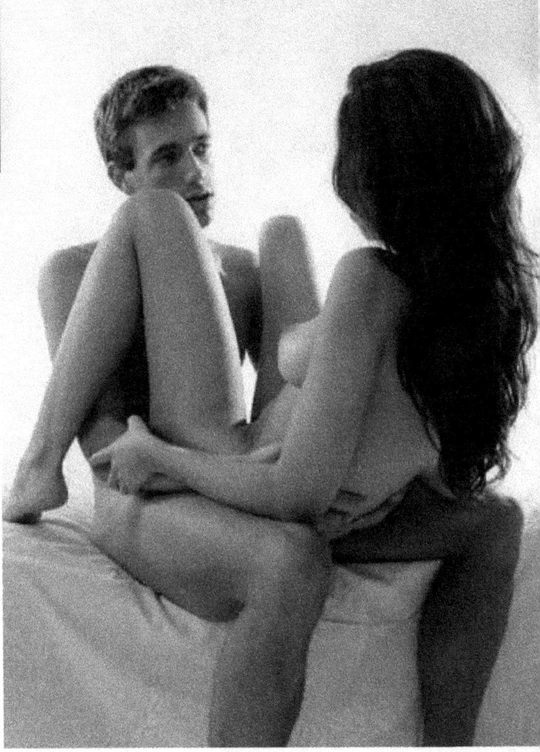

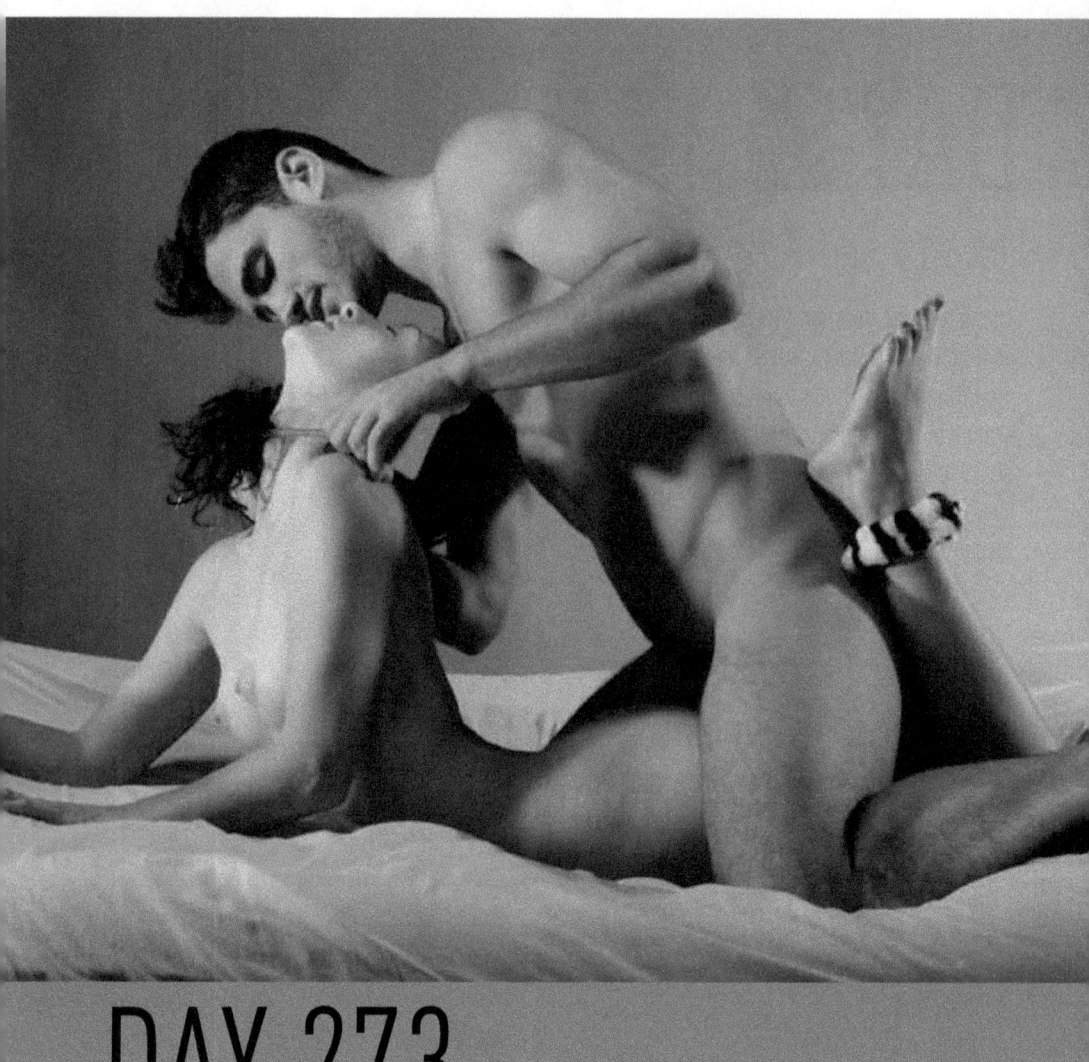

DAY 273

DRACULA'S KISS

The woman is stretched out on the bed on her stomach with her feet cuffed. Her lover straddles upper thighs and penetrates her from behind. He then uses his feathered riding crop to coax her throat upward so that he can kiss it and nibble on it like a vampire.

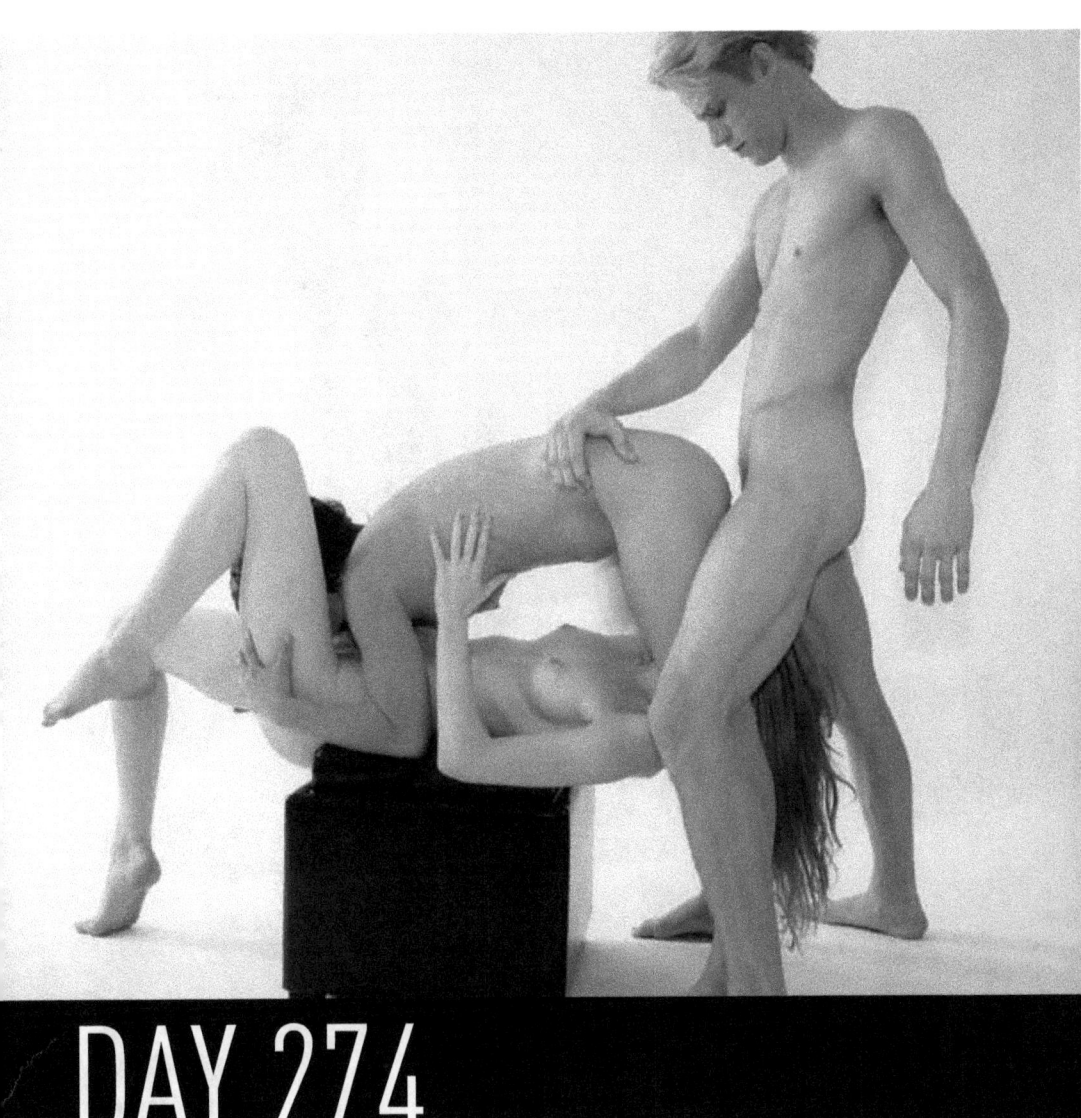

DAY 274

SCULPTED BEAUTY

One woman lies back across an ottoman or bench with one of her legs raised. The other leans over for a taste of her friend as the man penetrates her from behind. The woman on the bottom is free to return her girlfriend's oral pleasure and do likewise with the man's testicles.

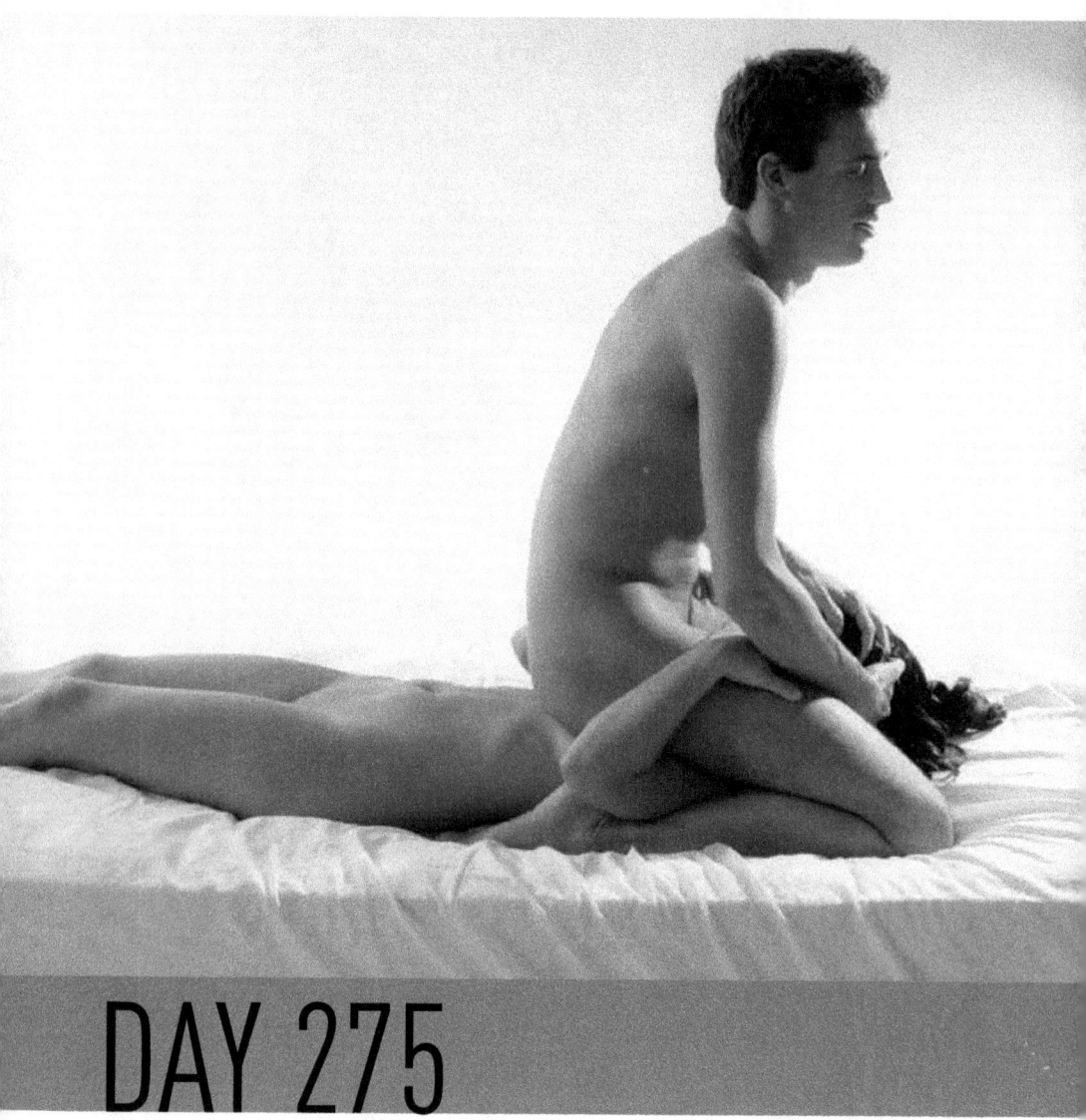

DAY 275

PLAY BALL!

The woman lies back on the bed while her lover straddles her shoulders. She licks and sucks his testicles while giving his penis a good old-fashioned hand job.

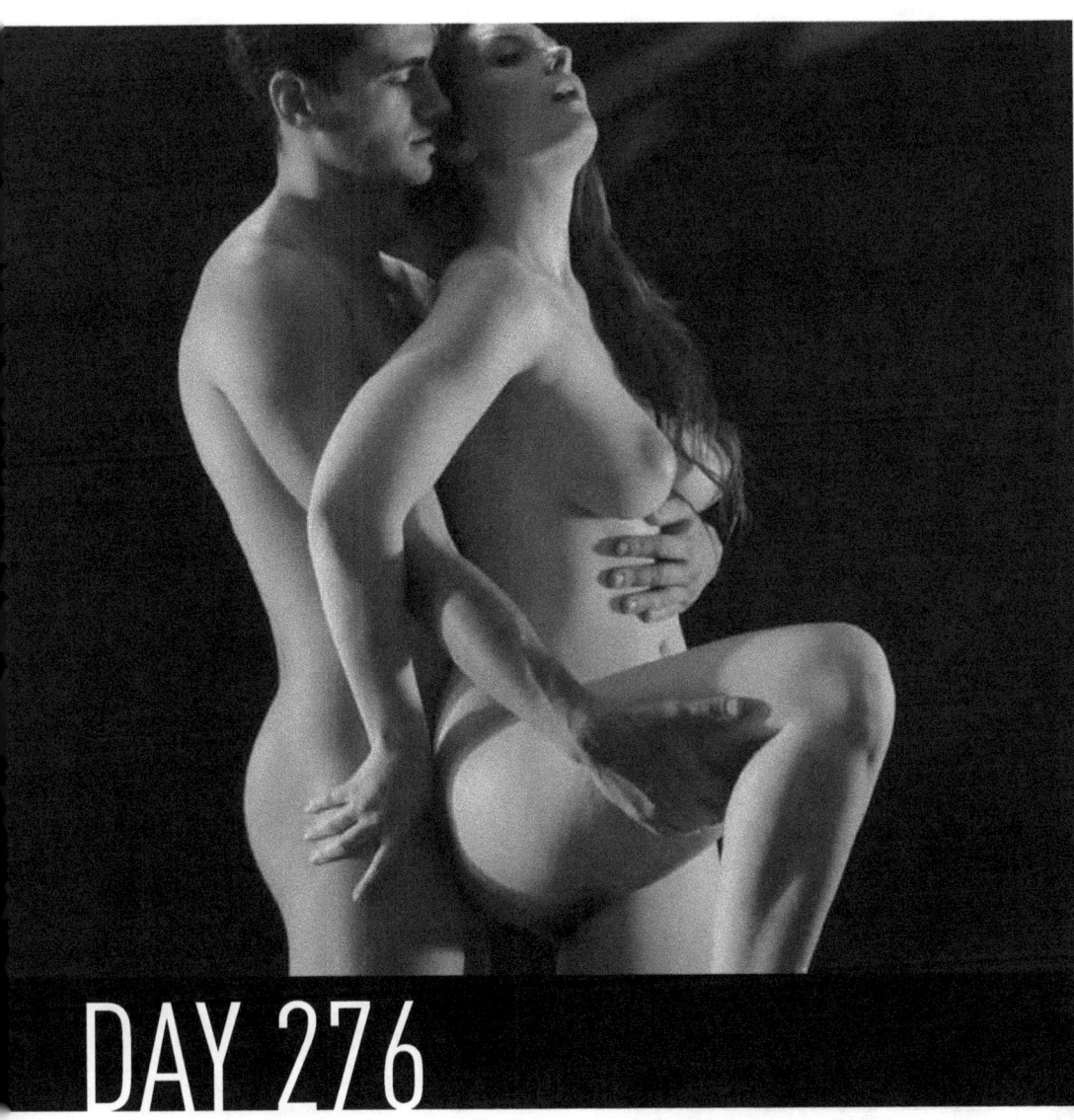

DAY 276

STRING DUET

She stands in front of her lover and brings one leg off the floor toward her chest. He supports her leg with one hand under her hamstrings as he enters her from behind. She can bring her hand back to fondle his testicles or touch his buttocks.

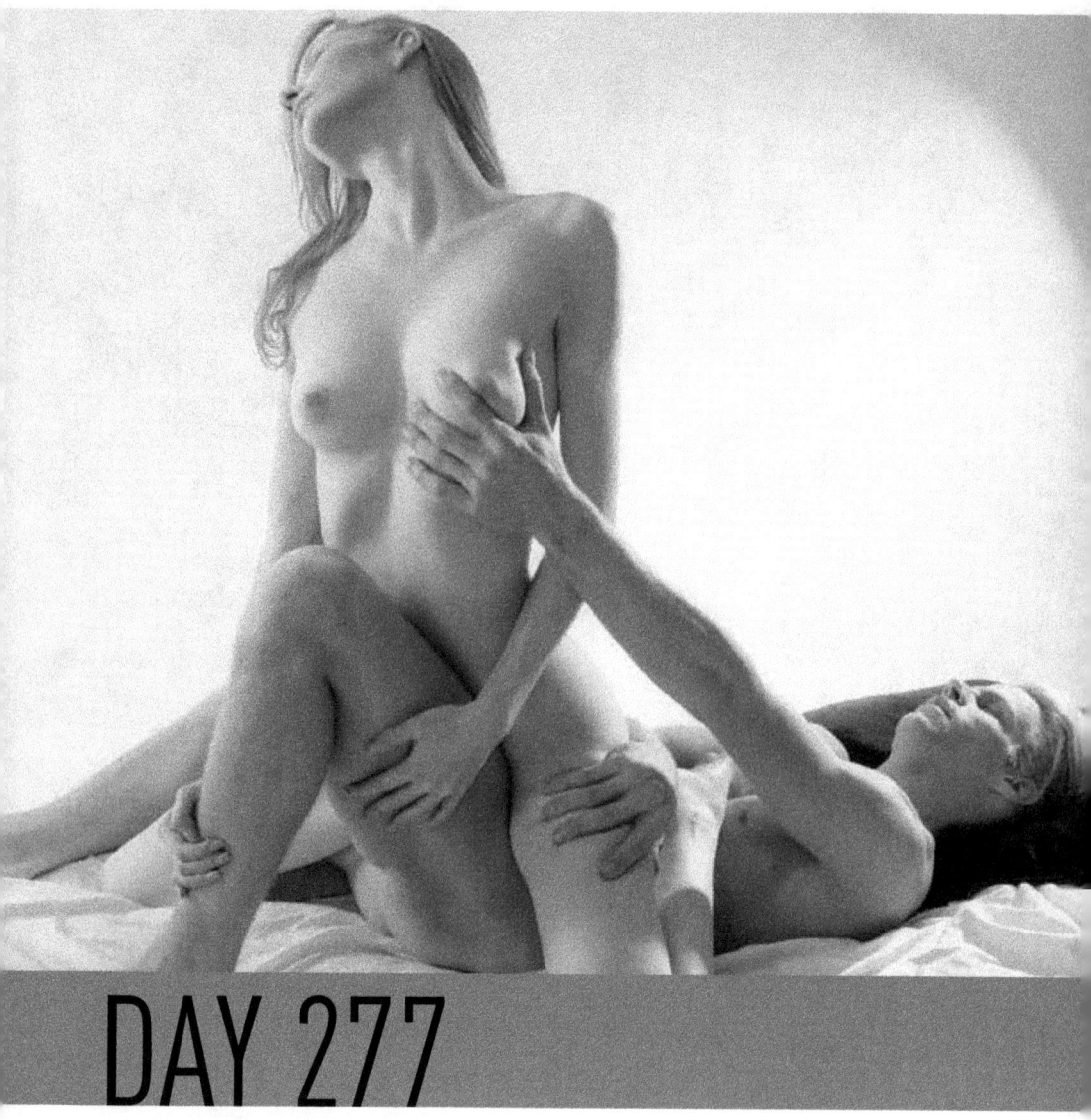

DAY 277

THE SCRATCHING POST

The man lies back on the bed with one leg stretched out and the other bent at the knee. His lover straddles his leg sideways and lowers herself onto his penis. From this position any movement will also stimulate her clitoris.

DAY 278

CORE-PULATION

Anyone up for a workout? She places her legs on a chair and lengthens her core by reaching down to rest her hands on the floor. Her partner squats over her and penetrates her from behind.

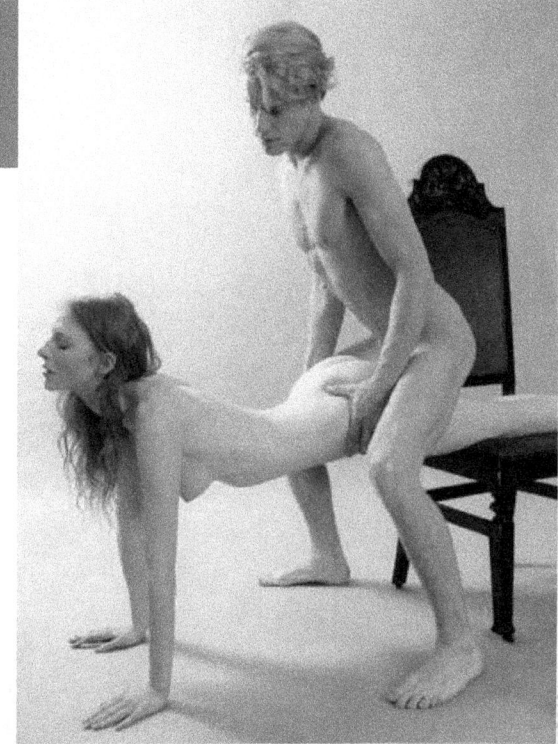

DAY 279

SPANKS A LOT

The woman sits in a chair as her obedient partner stretches himself across her lap and offers up his buttocks. She dishes out a firm spanking as a prelude to other pleasurable penalties to come.

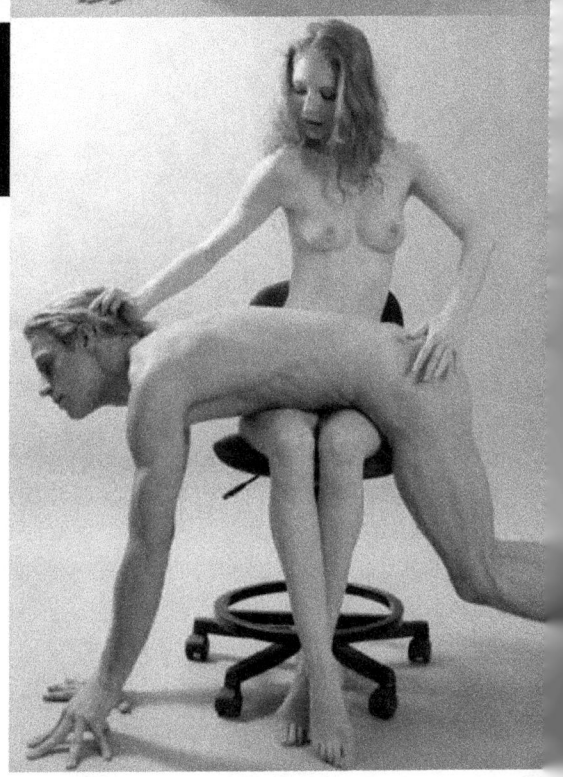

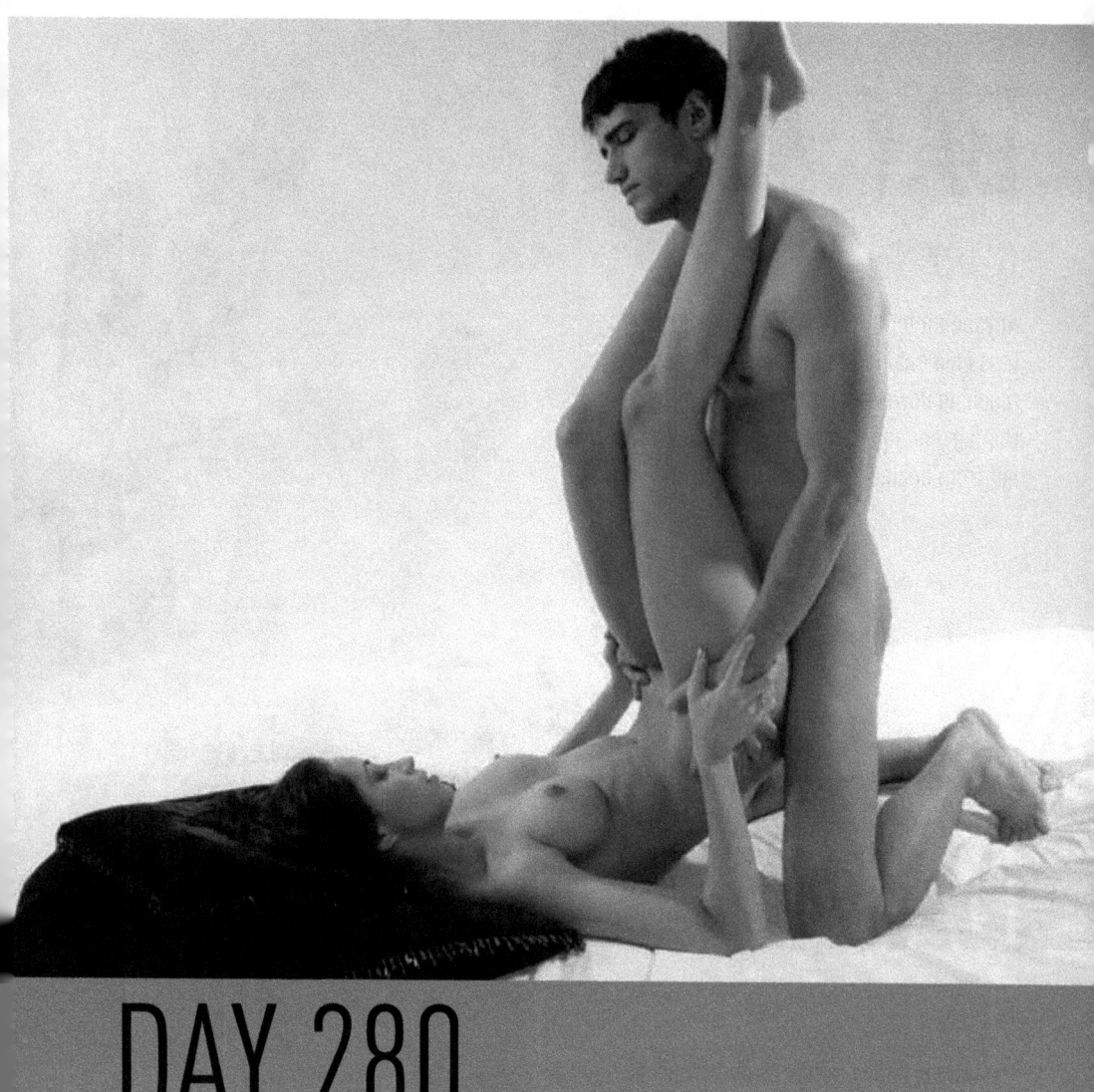

DAY 280

THE SHOULDER STAND

The woman supports her weight on her shoulders as she lifts her legs up and around his neck. He enters her from a kneeling position while offering additional stability by holding onto her legs. This one sends pleasure pulses rushing from head to toe.

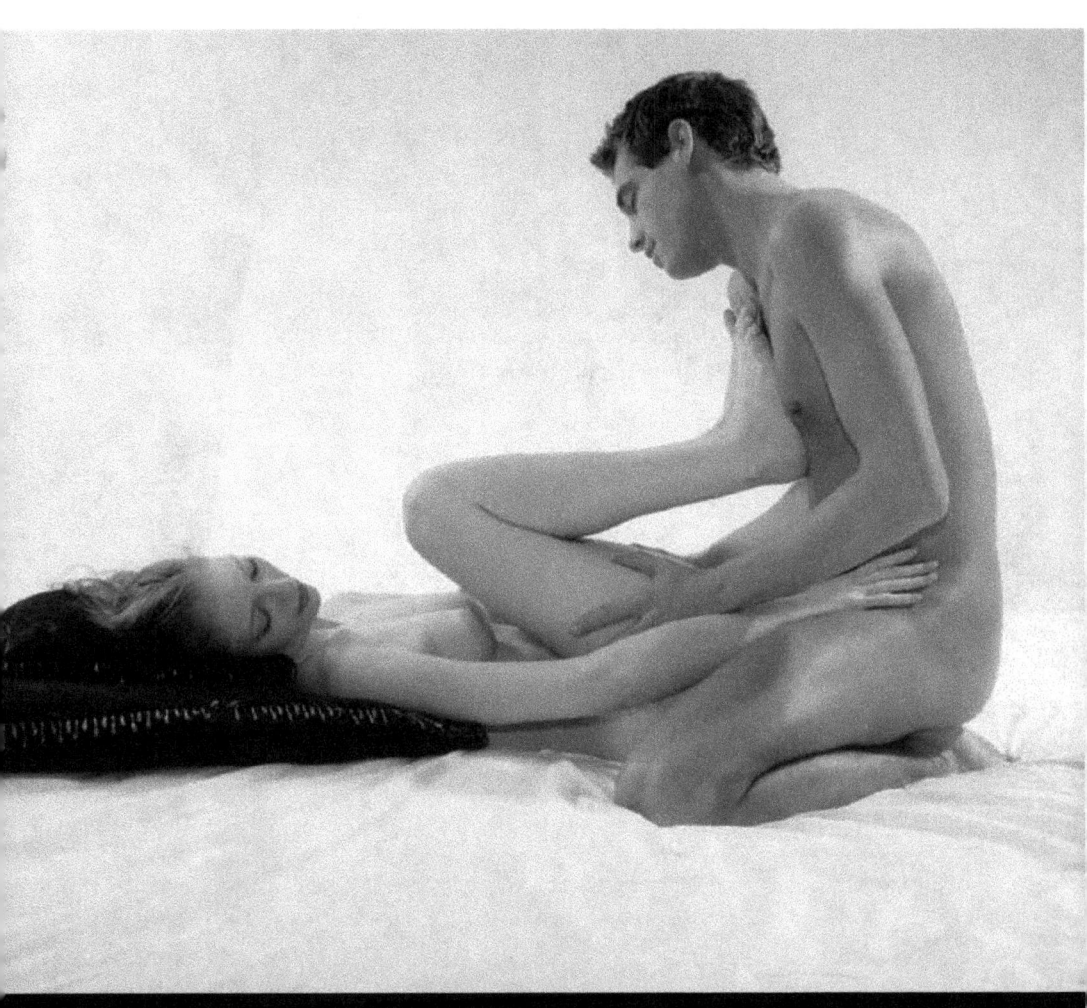

DAY 281

THE PUSHING MATCH

The woman is relaxed and on her back while he sits back on his legs. She lifts her feet and gently presses them against his chest. Together they create a rhythm between his penetration and the light push-back from her feet.

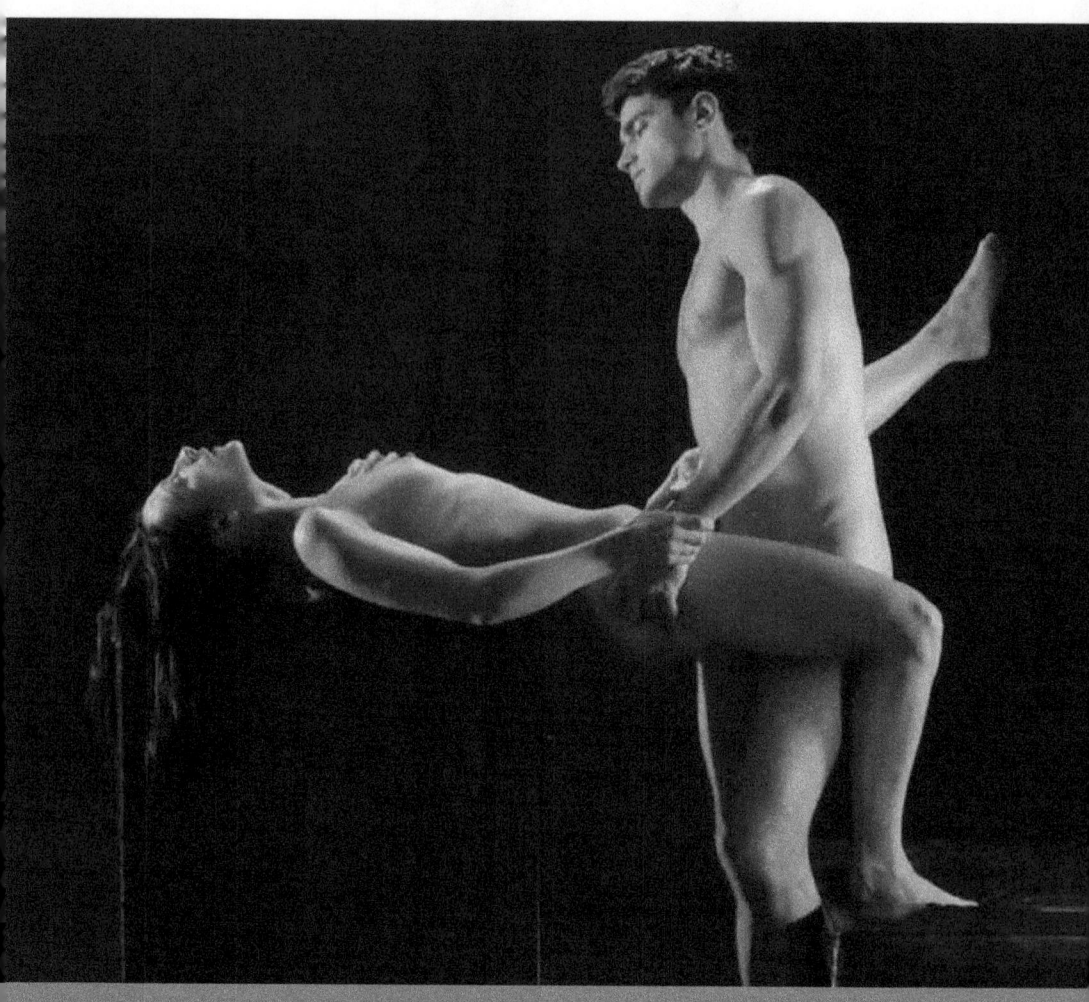

DAY 282

DOCKING BAY

She lies her head and torso back against a table or dresser and dangles one of her feet down to a bench or ottoman. As her partner enters her from a standing position she flares her other leg out to the side, giving him ample room for deep penetration and clitoral stimulation.

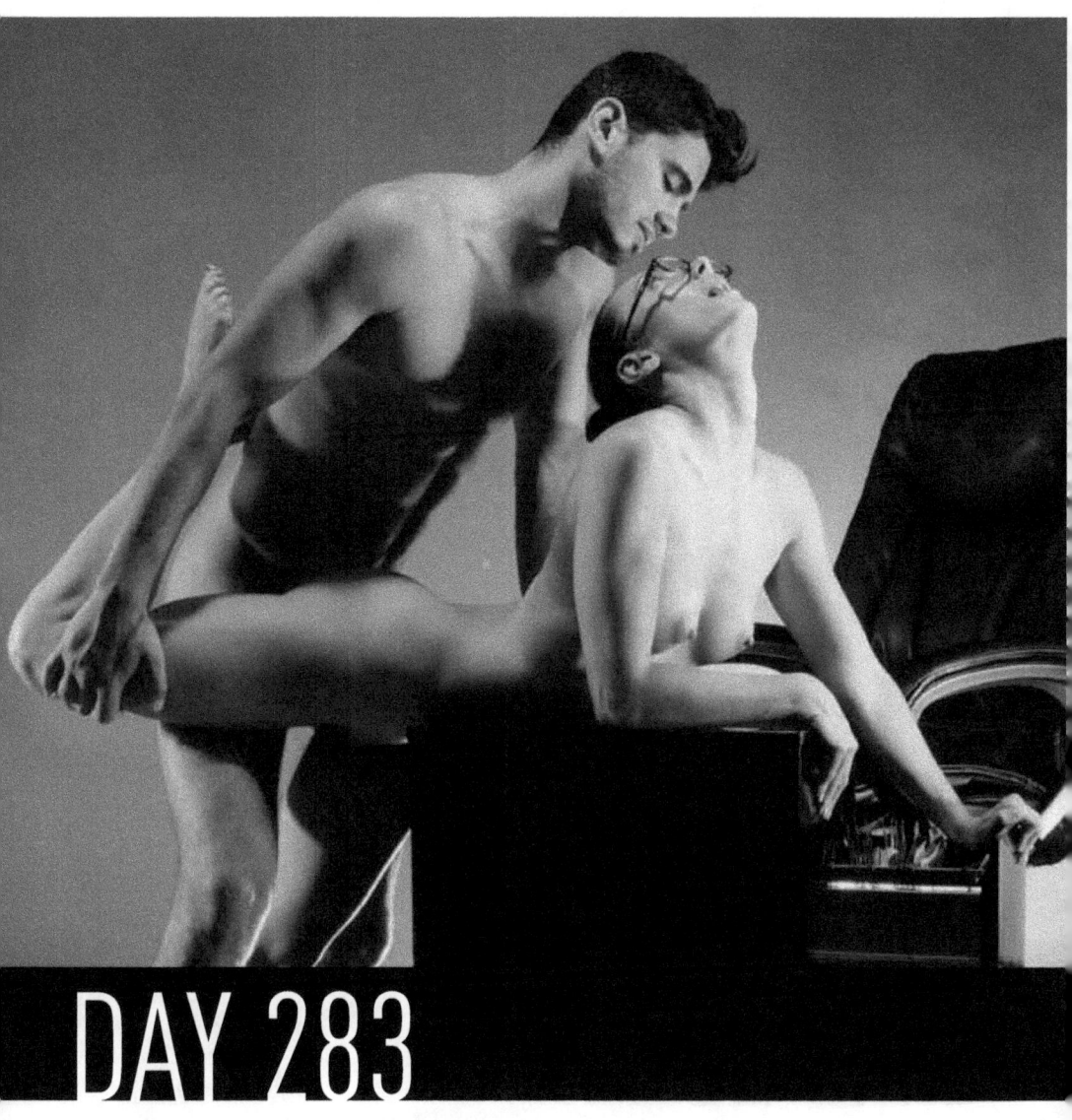

DAY 283

THE FILING EXTENSION

She nakedly sprawls across the top of a file cabinet, letting her hand pull the drawer out to extend even farther. He comes in from behind, gracefully lifts her leg up, and enters her.

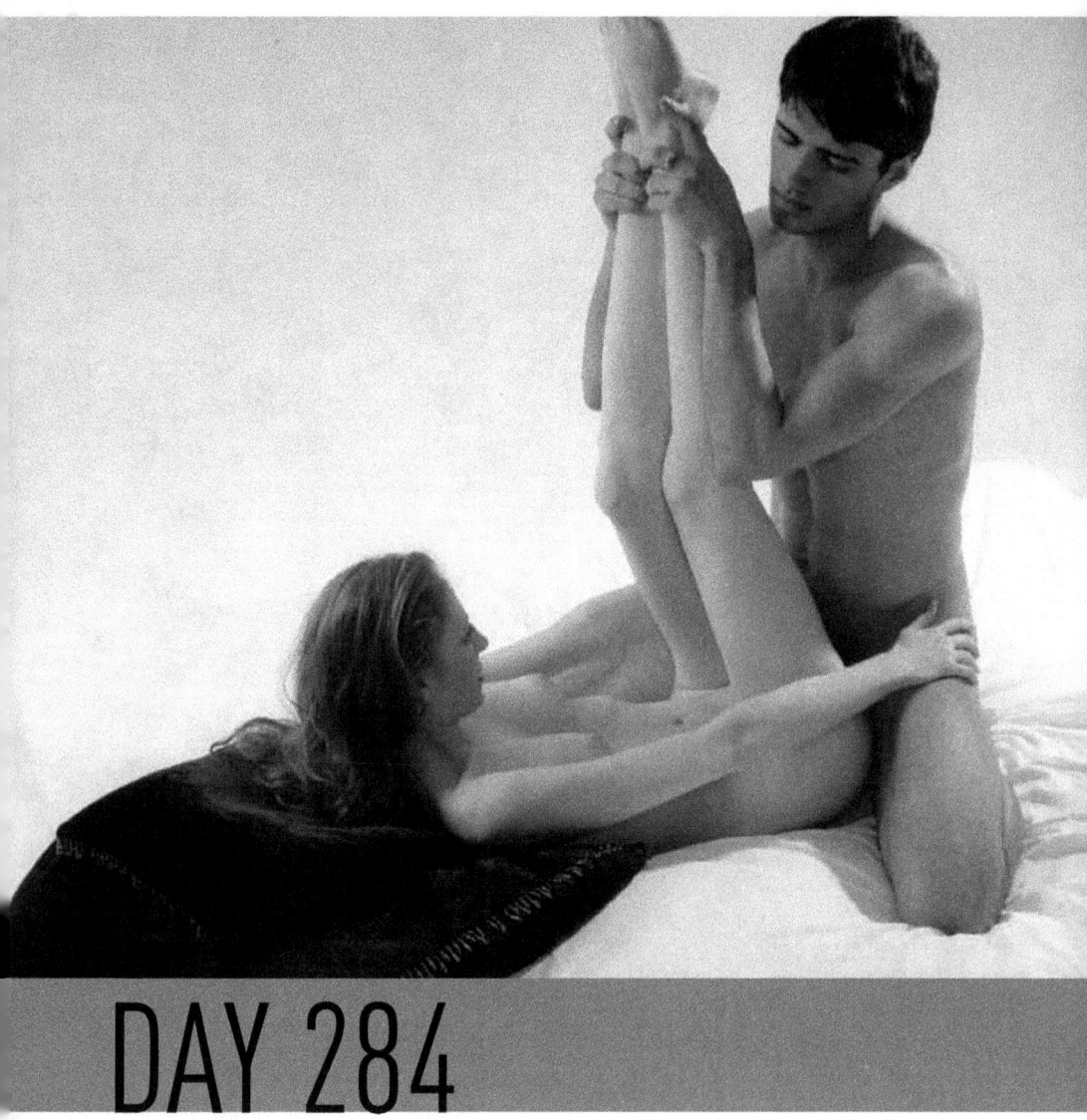

DAY 284

PUSHING PLEASURE

The woman lies on her back and brings her legs up. He lover grabs her ankles and penetrates her from a kneeling position. He can push her legs back toward her to change the entry angles and sensations.

DAY 285

THE PLAYFUL KITTEN

The man starts on his knees and leans back so that his buttocks are touching his feet and his hands are behind him. She climbs on top, distributing her weight to the balls of her feet. Together, they can bounce, rock, and sway.

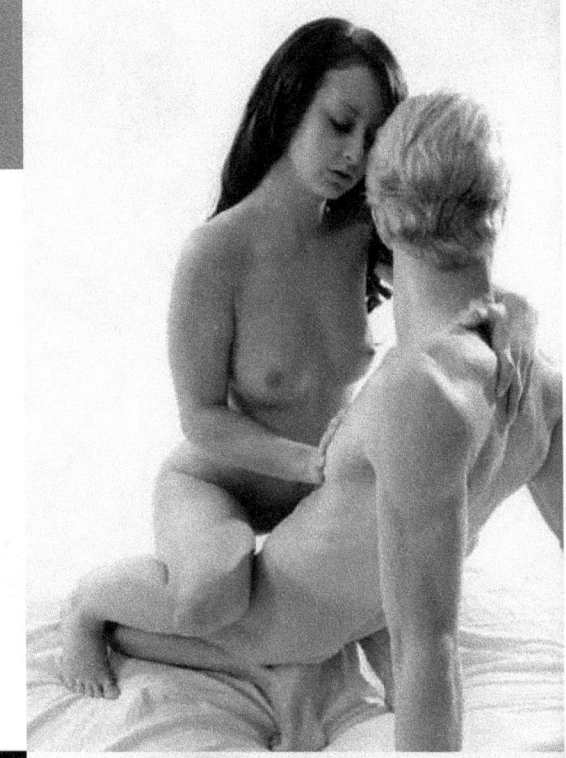

DAY 286

COME TO PAPA

He's in a kneeling position in between her legs, while she sits in his lap facing him. There's plenty of room for hugging, kissing, and hair tousling with this one.

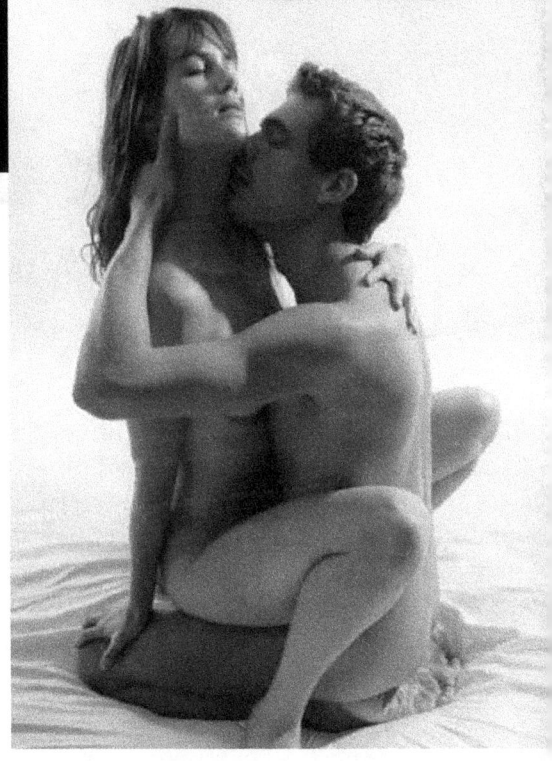

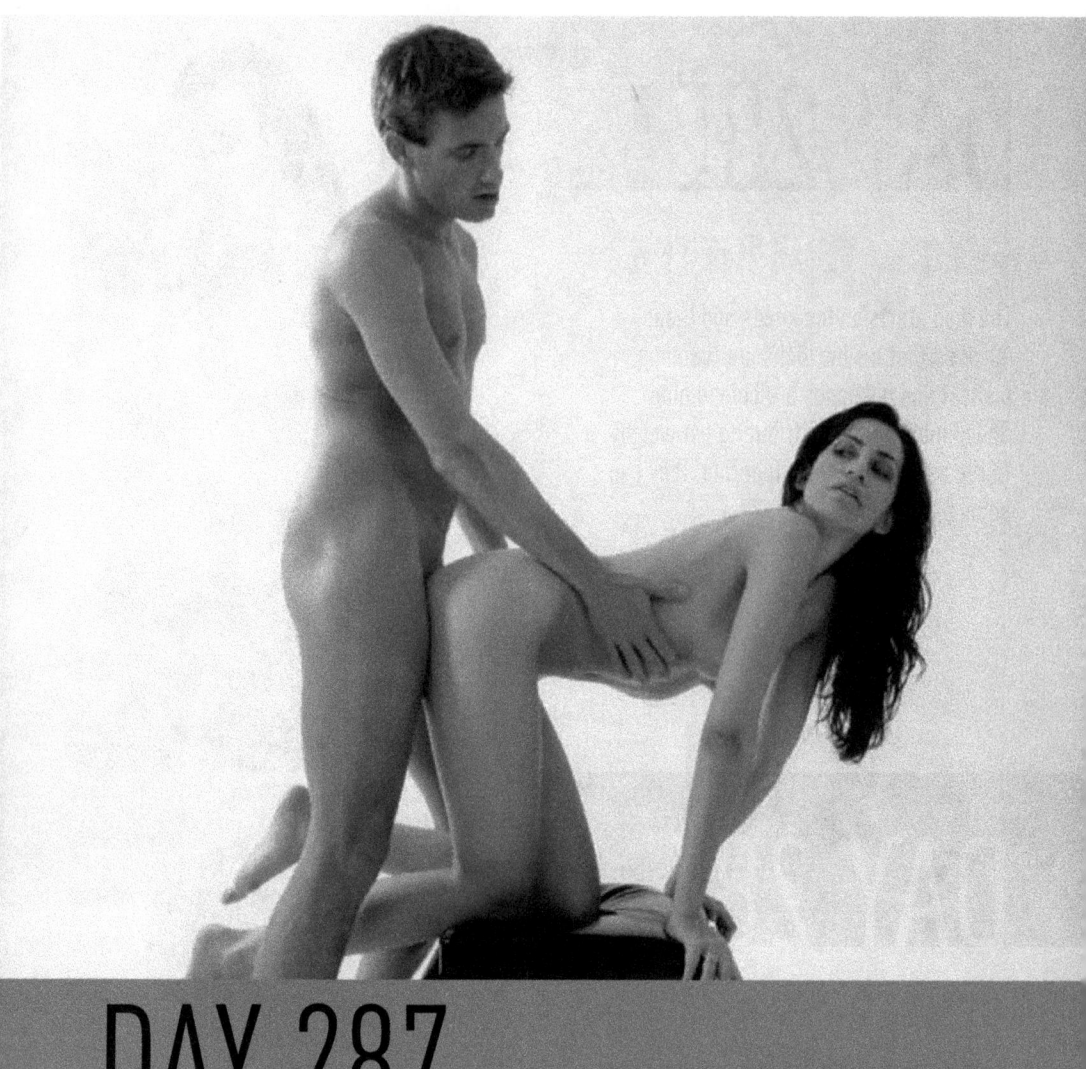

DAY 287

DOGGY DELIVERY

She's assumes a rump-up doggy position up in a chair as he mounts her from behind. His hands may wander to her clitoris or elsewhere.

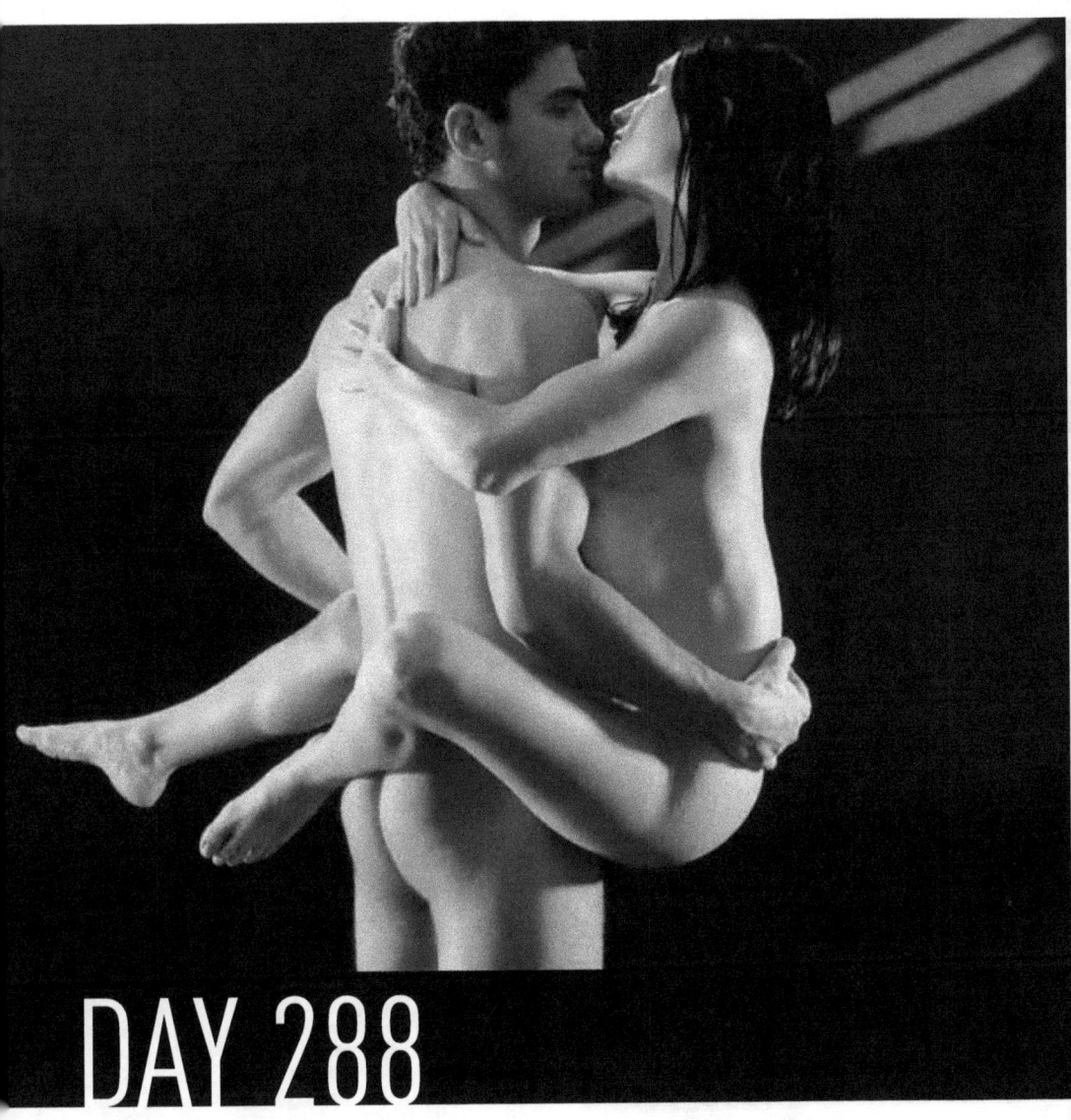

DAY 288

THE HAPPY HOOKER

The lovers start on their feet facing each other. She wraps her arms around him as he lifts her up and enters her. She slyly hooks one leg around his butt, pulling him closer.

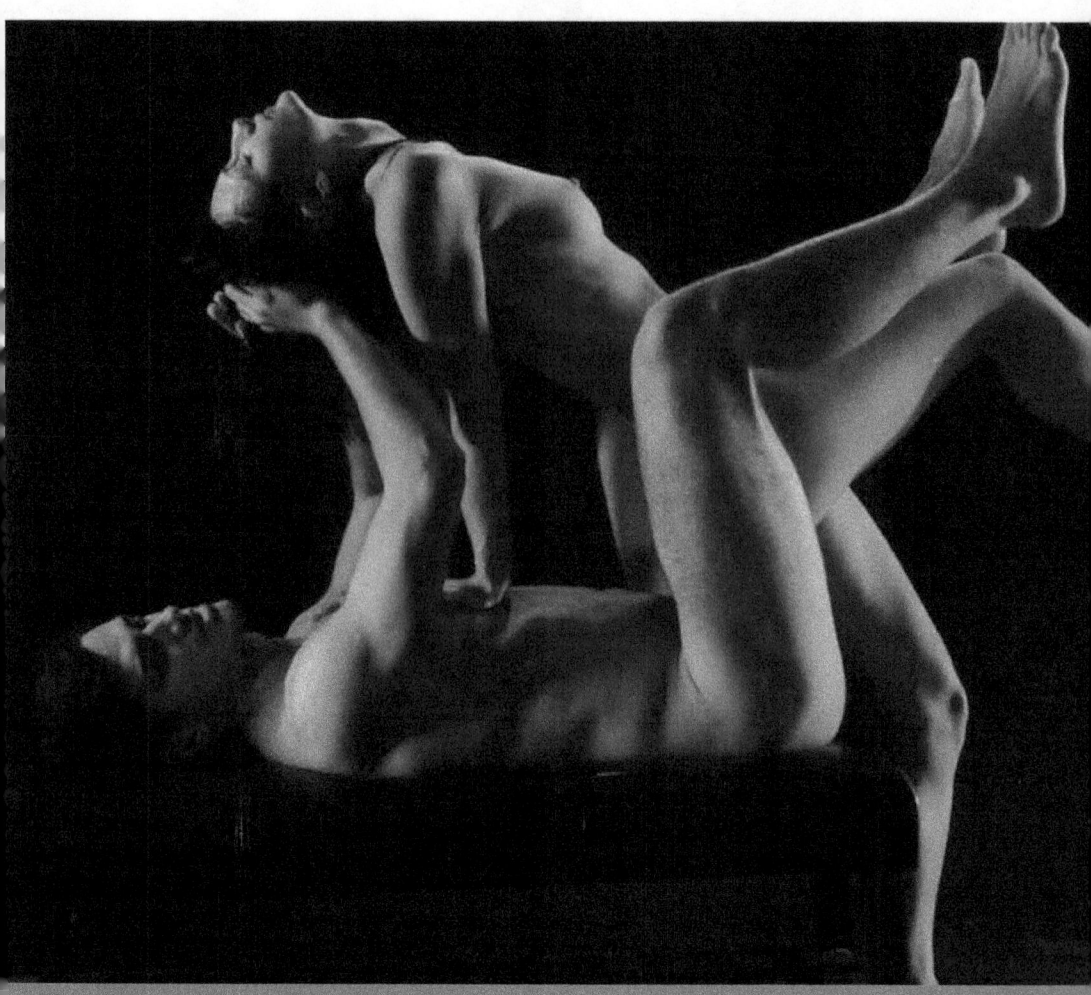

DAY 289

CLIMBING CLIMAX

He lies back against a bench or ottoman, opening his legs and raising them up. She takes her cue and climbs on top of him. As he enters her, they can both move their legs to increase the pleasure of the moment.

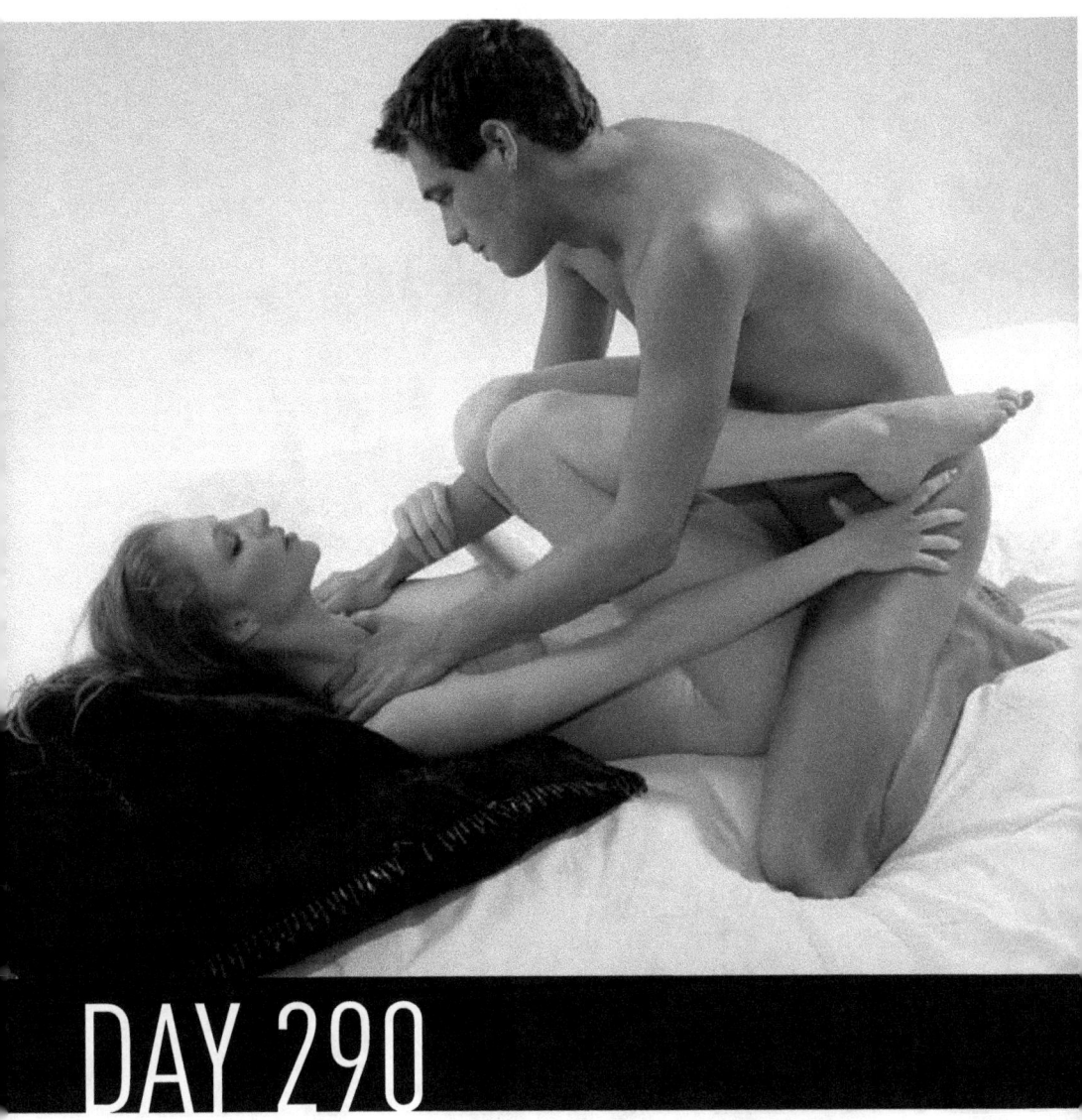

DAY 290

INNER BEAUTY

Opening her legs and resting her feet outside her lover's thighs, the woman invites him to experience a deep passion that will send both their minds and bodies spinning.

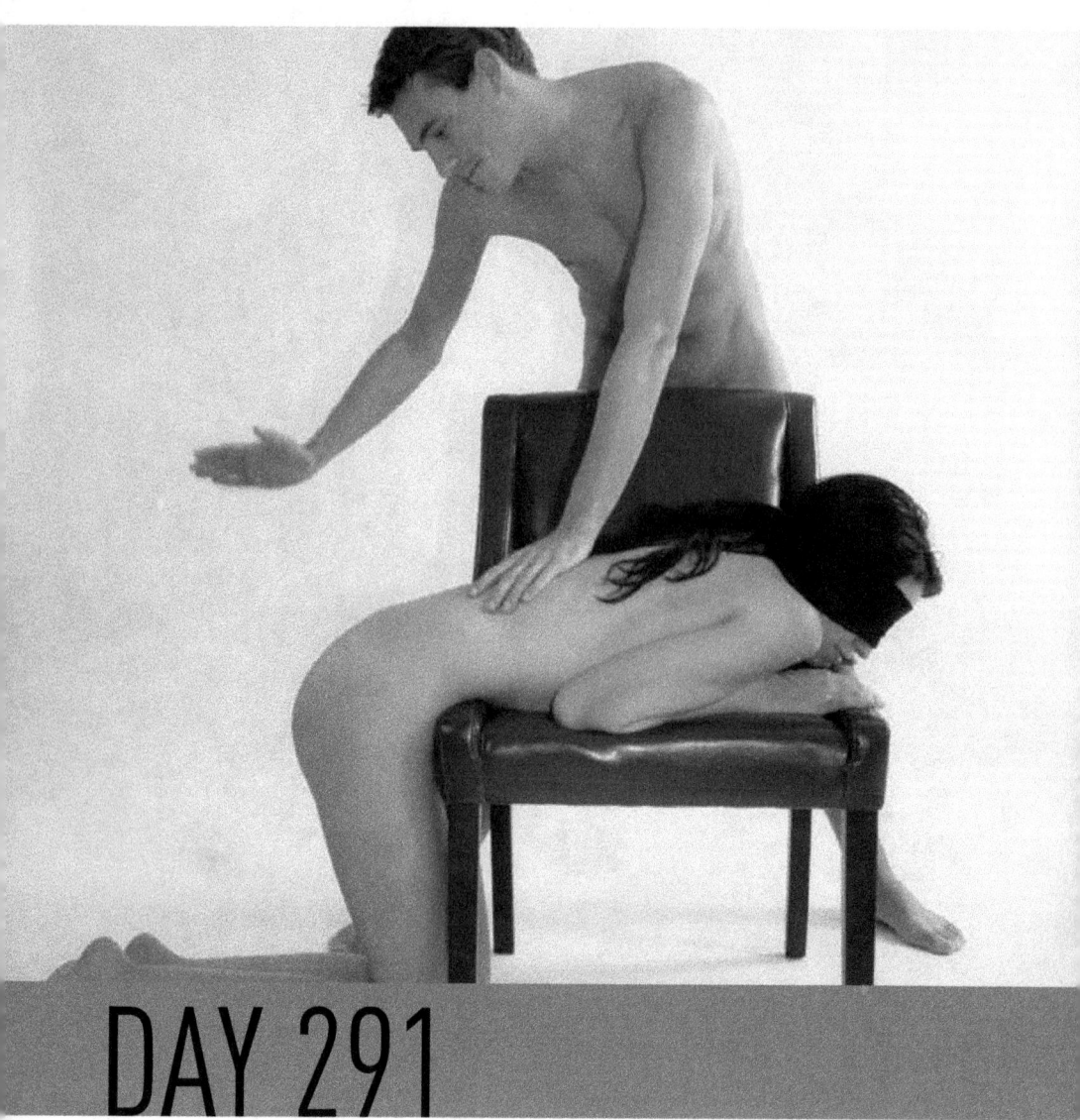

DAY 291

SLAP HAPPY

The woman is blindfolded and kneeling over the seat of a chair. Her lover braces one hand on her back as he asks her for the magic word. Once she utters it, he delivers a firm slap to her buttocks. He then soothes the sting by paying attention to her pleasure points.

DAY 292

LIKE A PRAYER

The man and woman both get down on their knees as he moves in between her legs and enters her from behind. He can kiss her neck as he runs his hands from her breasts down to her clitoris.

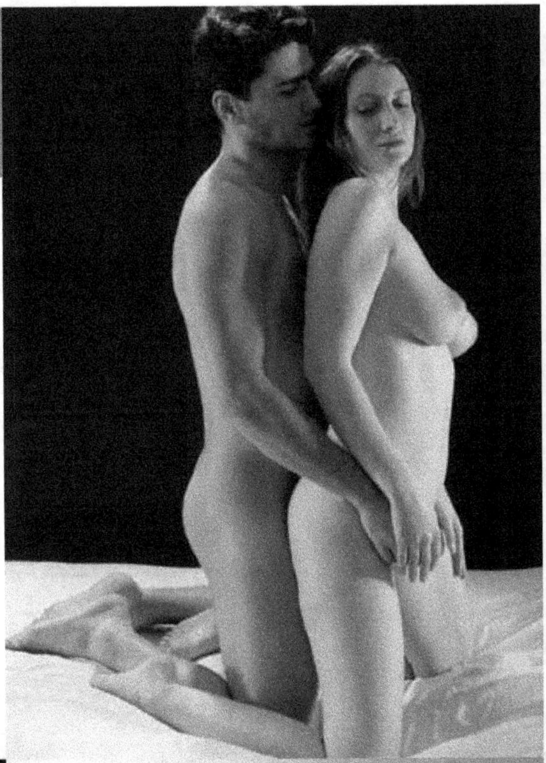

DAY 293

TAKE A PLOW

The woman rests her forearms on a chair or the edge of a bed. Her partner lifts her at the waist and enters her from behind as she wraps her legs around his back.

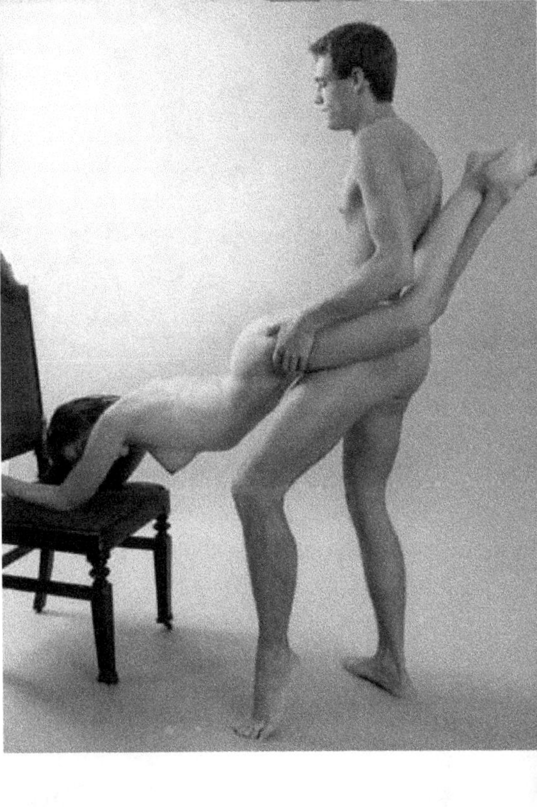

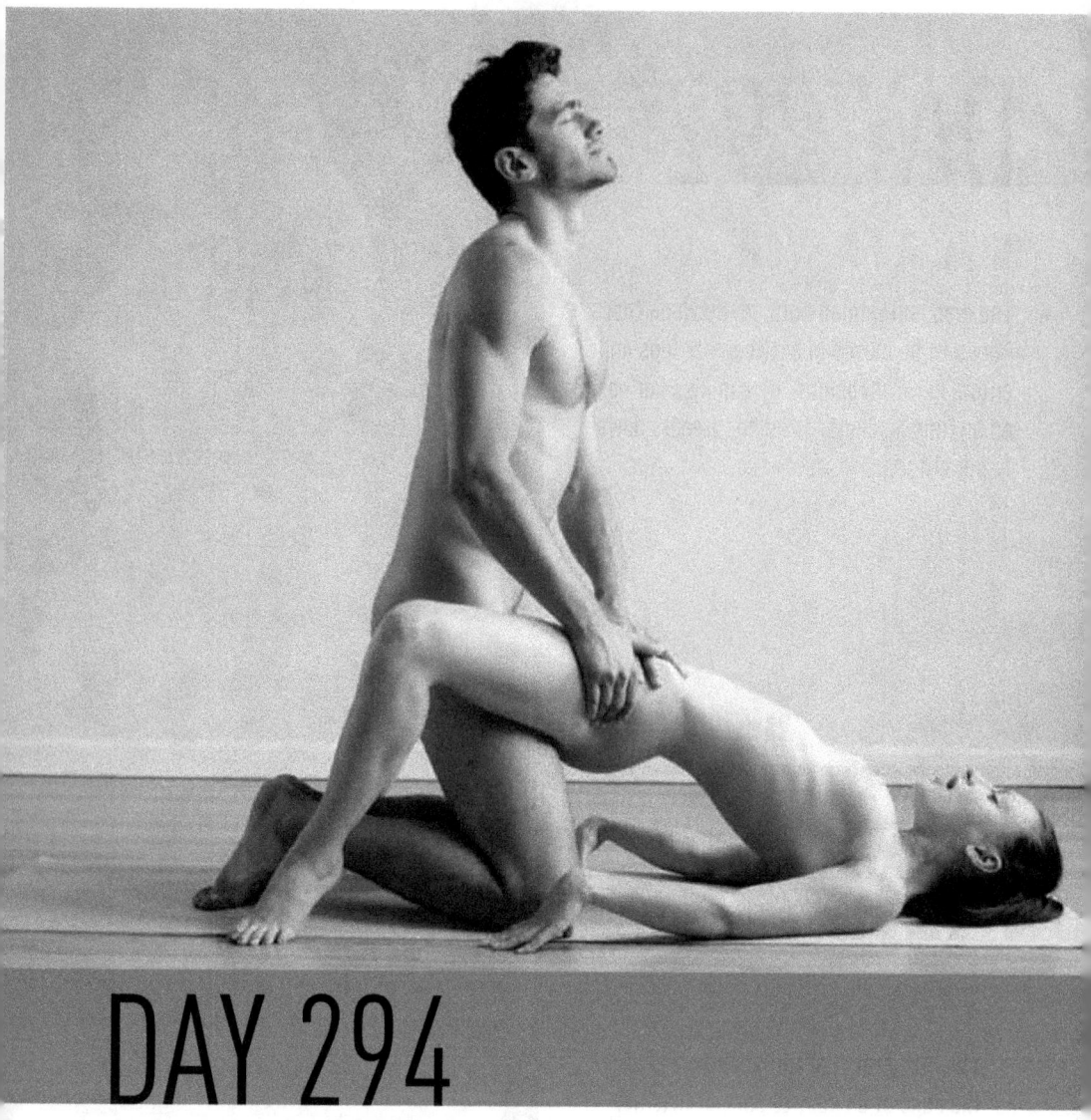

DAY 294

UP, UP, AND AWAY

She lies flat on a yoga mat and places herself in a bridge position with her pelvis lifted up high. Her lover penetrates her from his knees and lifts her hips with his hands, bringing her even higher and manipulating the angle of entry.

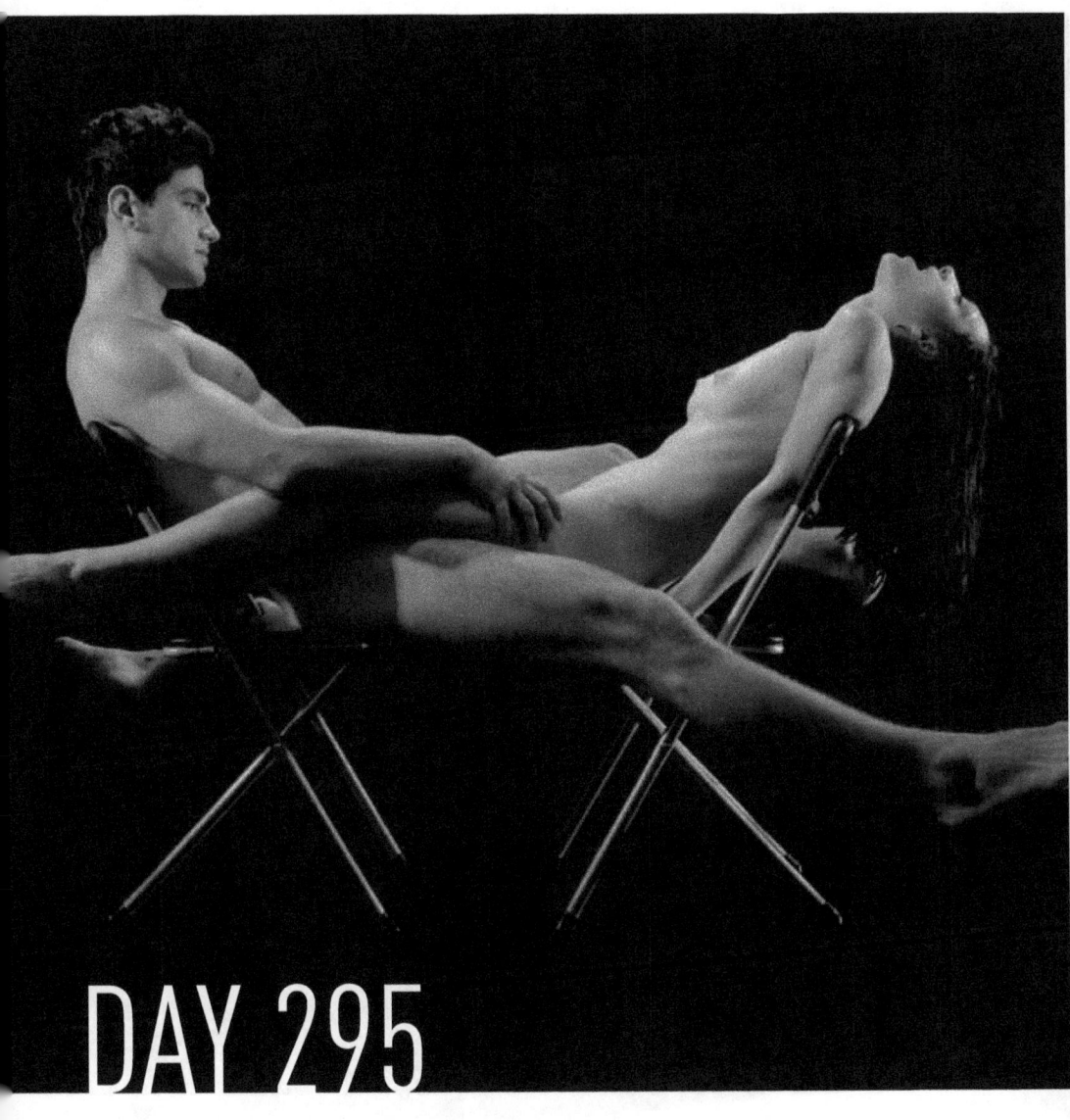

DAY 295

THE CHAIR-RAISING ADVENTURE

The man and woman each pull up a chair and face each other. He opens his legs and extends them as she brings her legs over his thighs, allowing him to enter her anus. They can pull each other as close as they like.

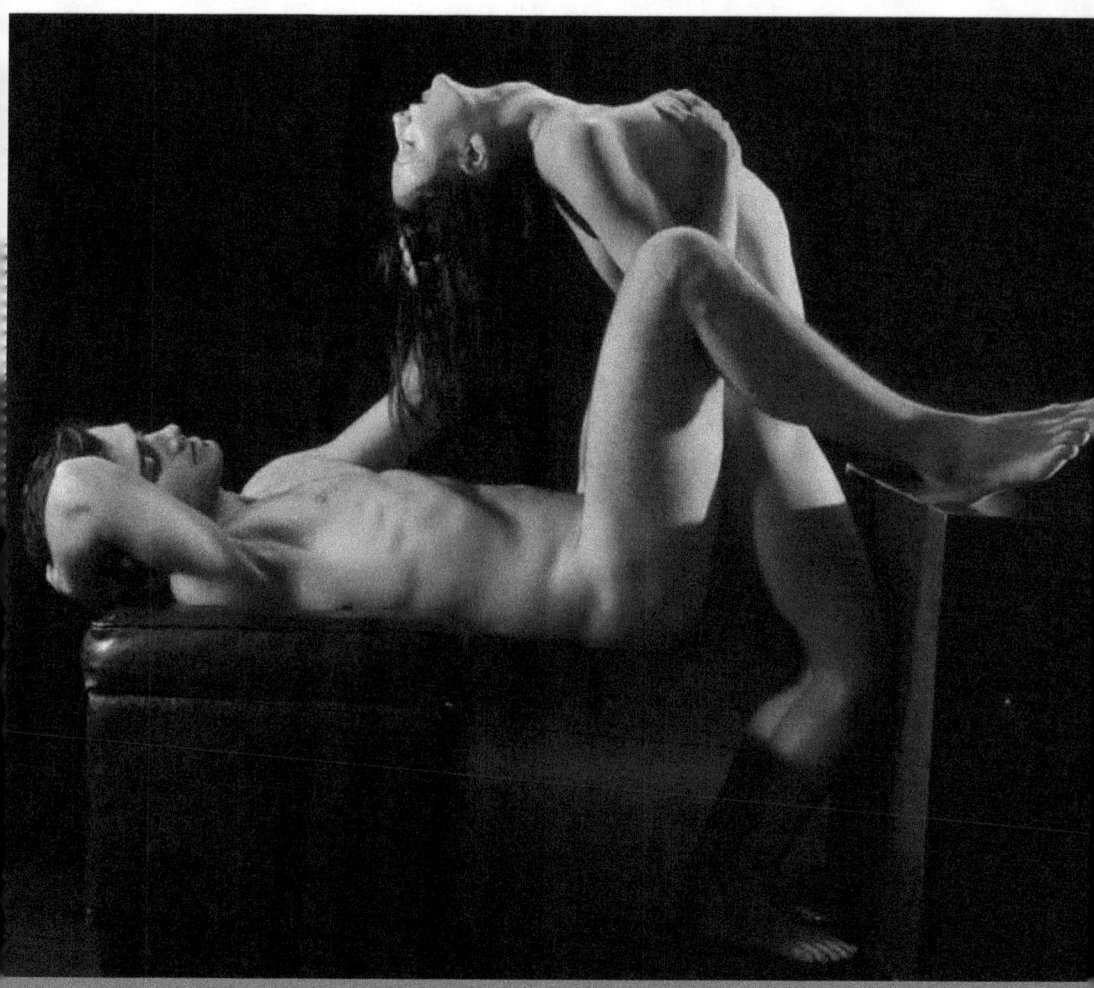

DAY 296

THE HAIR SALON

If you don't have the hair length for this one, you can always use a wig. The man places his head and shoulders on an ottoman with his feet raised up against something higher. His partner gets between his legs, lowering herself onto his penis. As he enters her, she leans back so that he can stroke her locks.

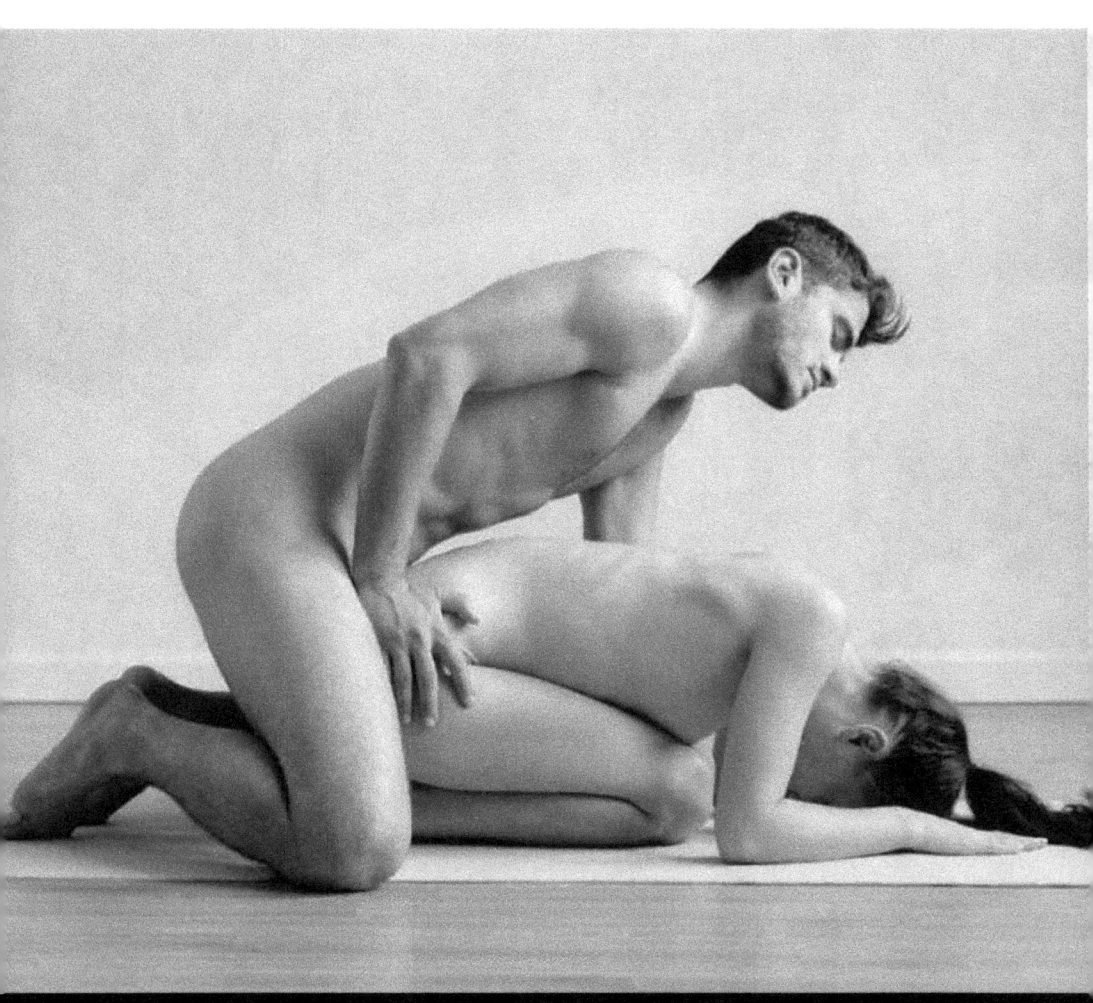

DAY 297

BABY GOT BACK

The woman assumes a common yoga pose. sitting back on her heels with her head down and back extended. She relaxes her breath as her lover lubes them both up and enters her anally.

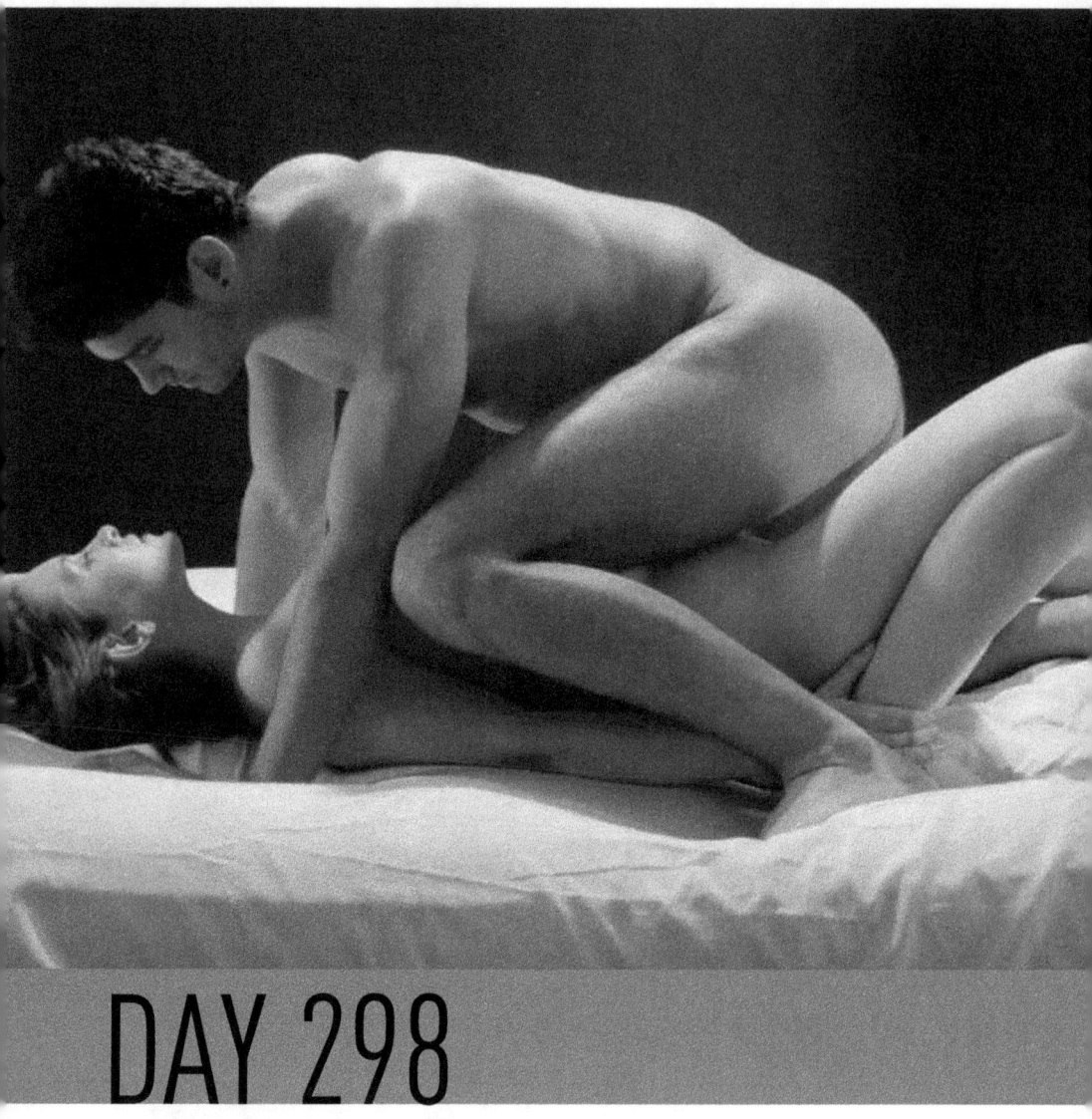

DAY 298

OVER, UNDER, SIDEWAYS, DOWN

She lies back on the bed and bends one leg at the knee while grabbing her ankle. She subtly twists her body to the side extending her other leg outward as her lover moves in from the top and enters her. Arms and legs are everywhere as they lose themselves in the moment.

DAY 299

THE JACKHAMMER

He sits on the edge of the bed as his partner brings her legs up to his chest and gets into a semi-headstand. As he penetrates her from above he supports her legs to take any potential stress off of her neck.

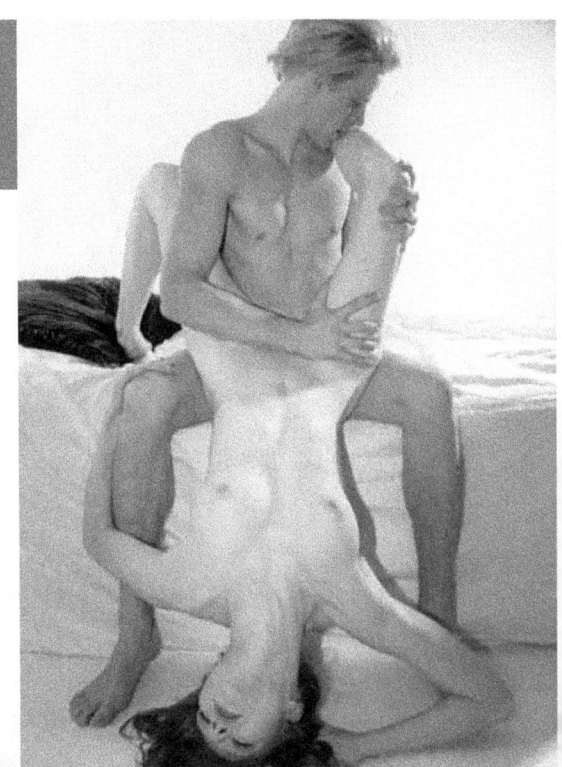

DAY 300

THE SEAT SAVER

As the man sits on a short stool or a chair his lover sits in his lap facing him and mounts him. The couple are as close as can be and she's able to dictate the action by pressing her feet into the seat.

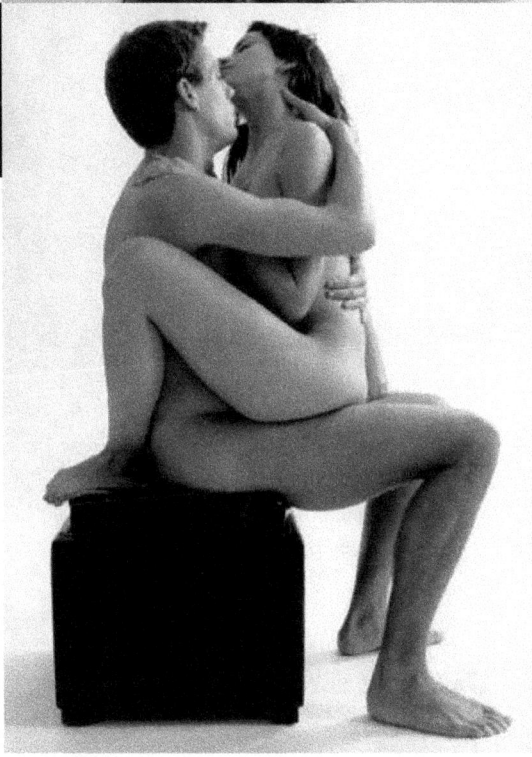

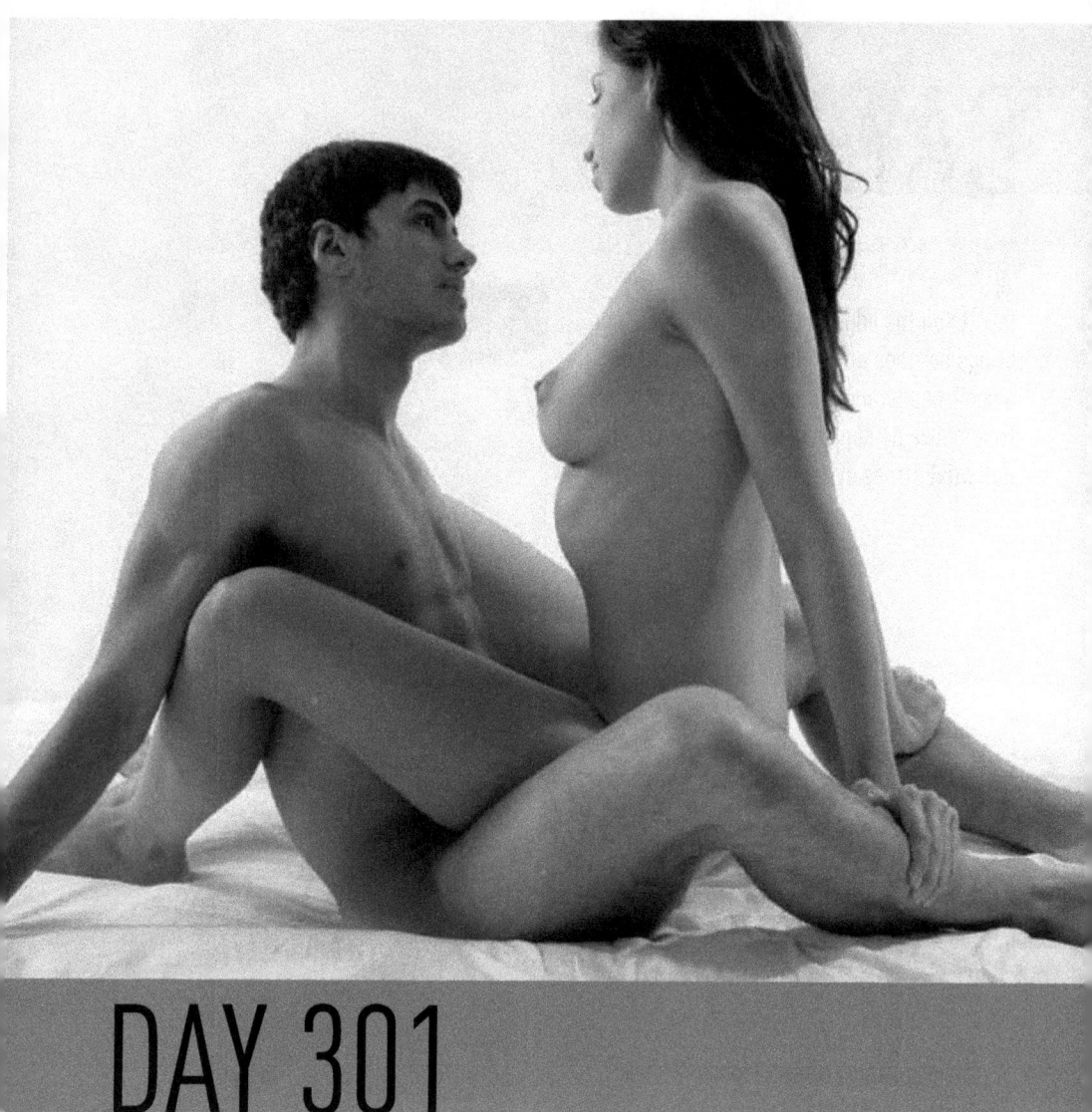

DAY 301

LOST IN YOU

He's seated with his knees bent and legs open. She drapes her legs over his and makes herself comfortable. They are now in a perfect position to stare into each other's eyes and kiss as they make love.

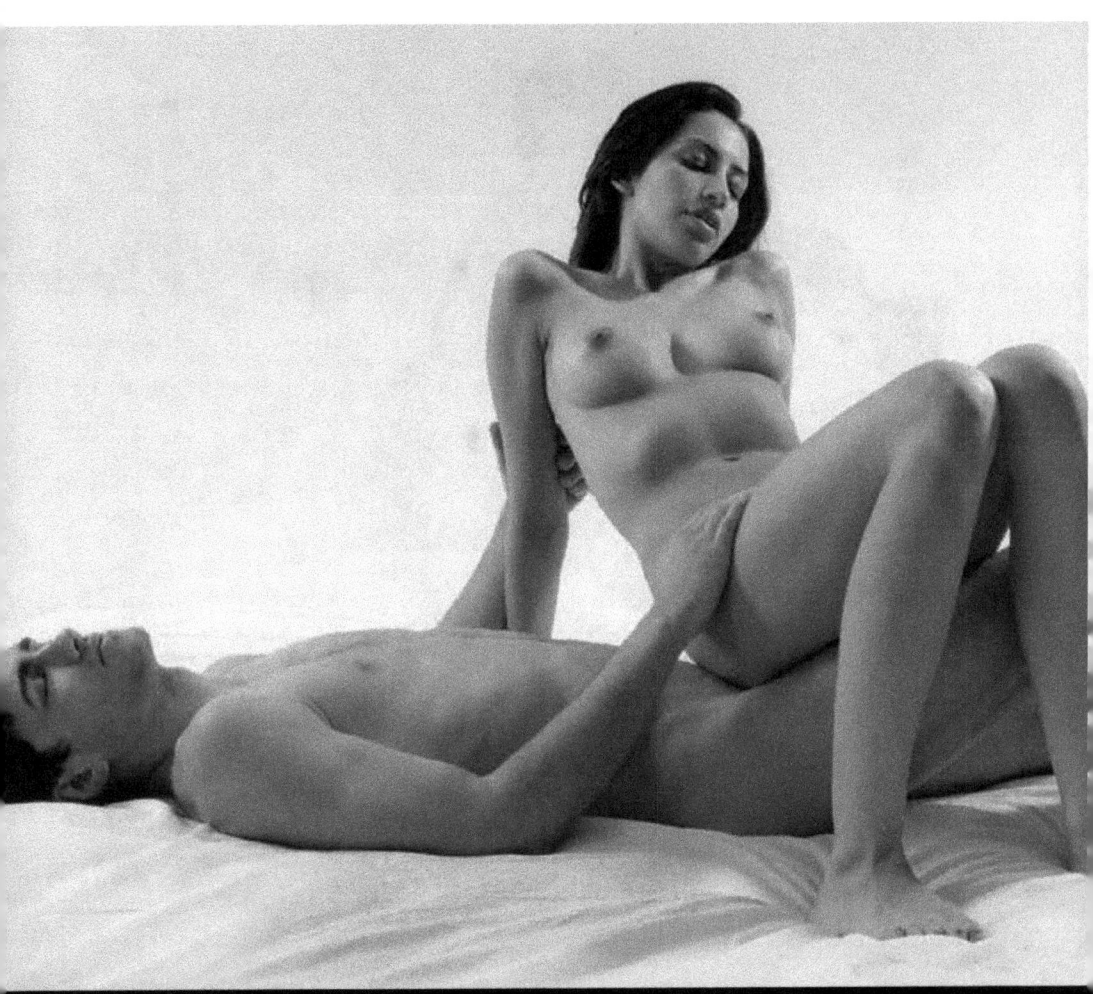

DAY 302

G-SPOT ROULETTE

The man lies on his back with his legs stretched out as his partner climbs on top. Once there she's free to experiment with penetration sensations by spinning herself a full 360 degrees. G-spot contact spells j-a-c-k-p-o-t.

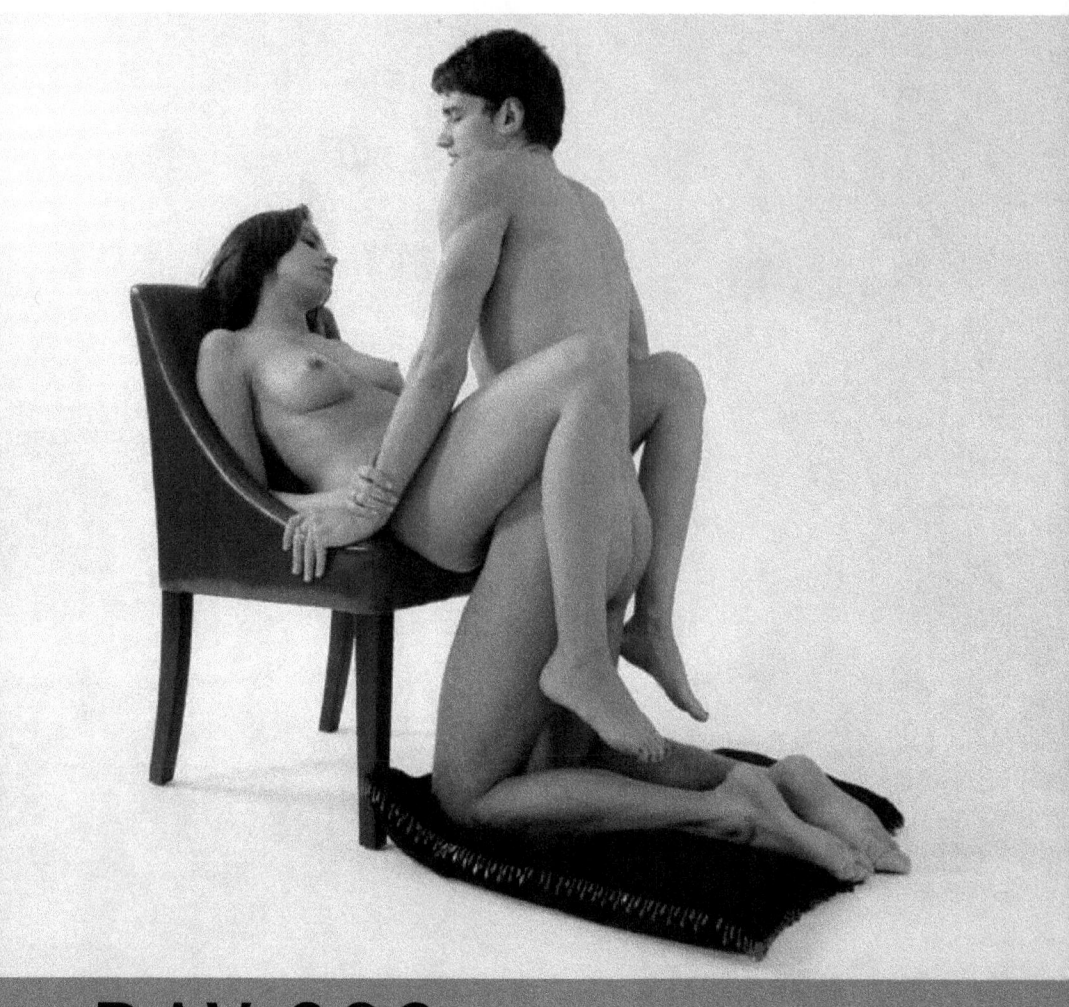

DAY 303

EASY DOES IT

There's just no substitute for a nice comfortable chair. In this position, the woman reclines in one, while her lover gets on his knees before and enters her. She can lock her legs around his waist if the mood strikes.

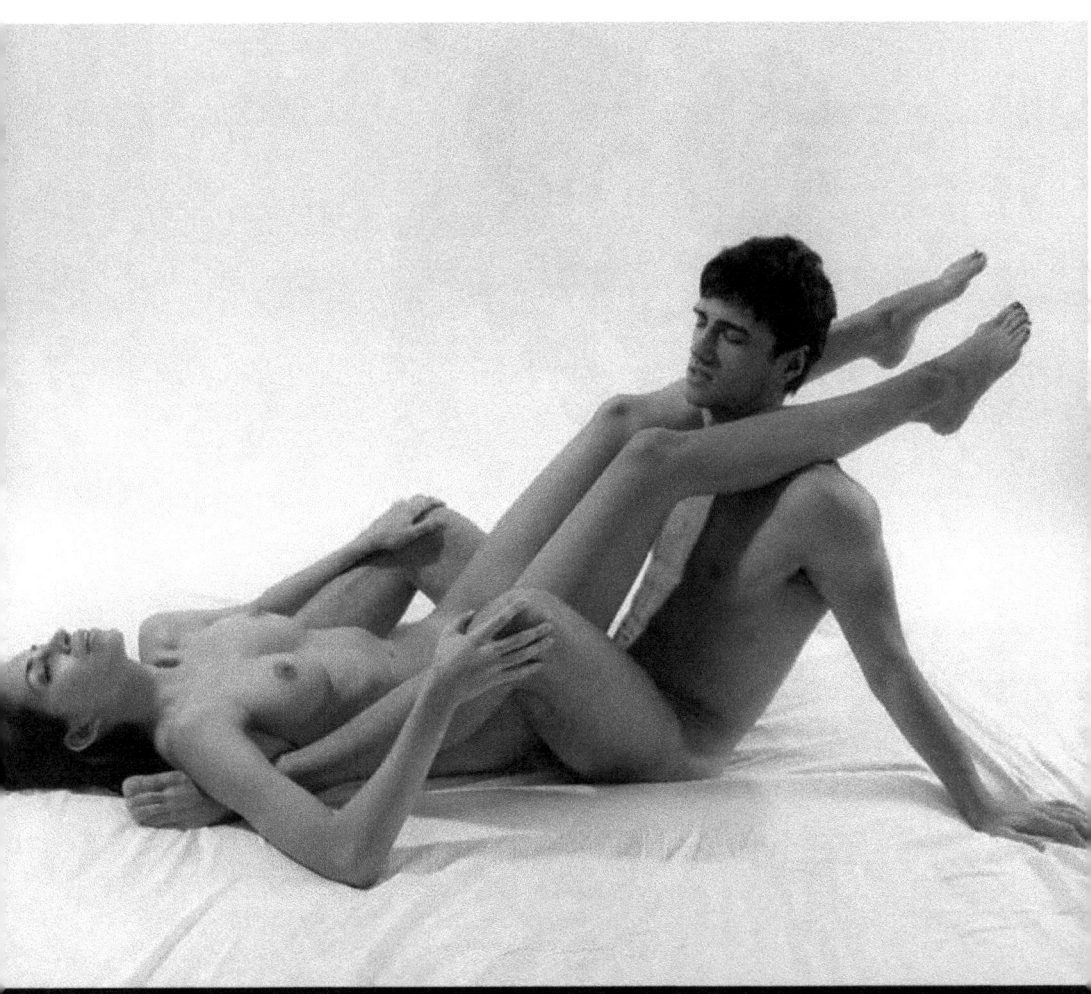

DAY 304

THE NECK BRACE

Starting in his lap, the woman reclines all the way back so that most of her weight is on her head and shoulders. She then snakes her legs up and clasps them behind her lover's neck.

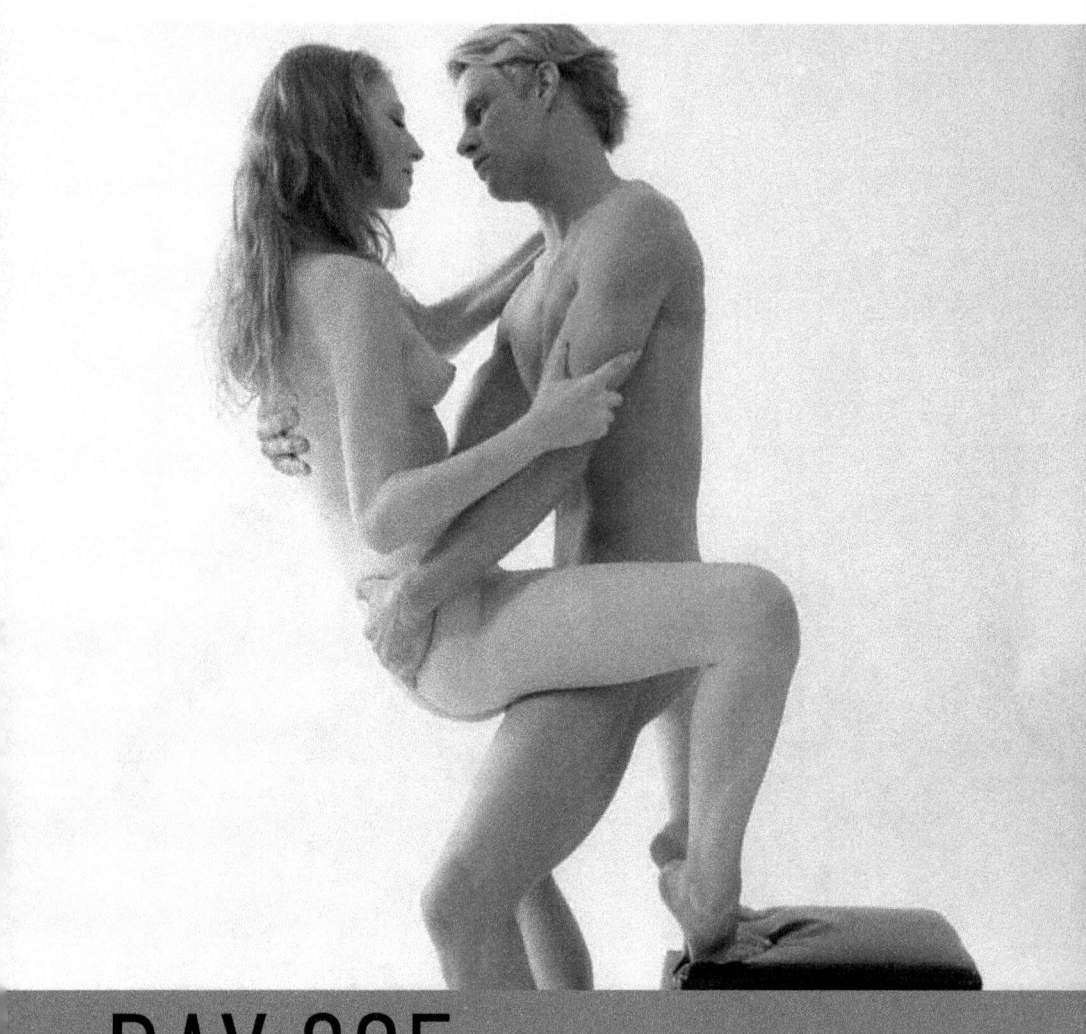

DAY 305

STEPPING IT UP

He's standing with his knees slightly bent as his lover climbs onto his erect penis. She places her feet on a nearby stool or step and grabs on to her partner's arms. Who needs a stair-climber machine when you've got this kind of workout?

DAY 306

ON YOUR TOES

The woman gets up on her tiptoes and places her hands against the wall. Her lover applies lube to her anus and his penis and enters her from behind.

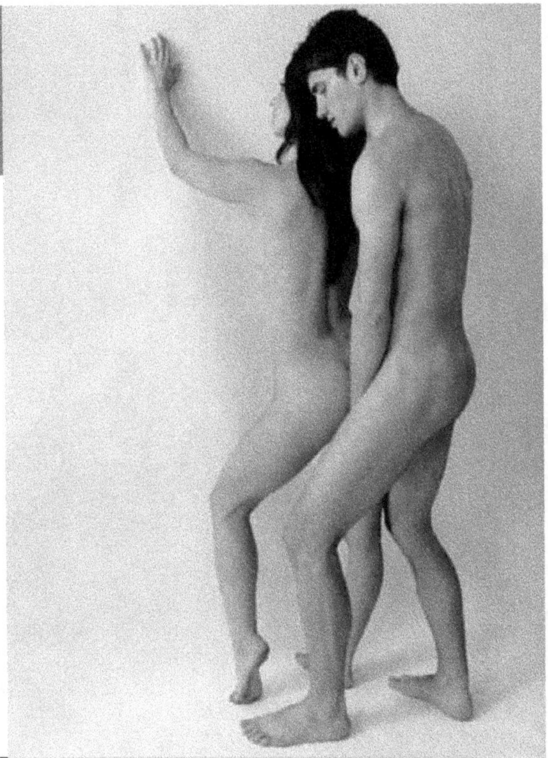

DAY 307

POINTS OF INTEREST

The man sits bedside with his legs wide apart. The woman bends before him, placing her hands on his ankles, giving her lover full access to perform all sorts of oral and manual stimulation.

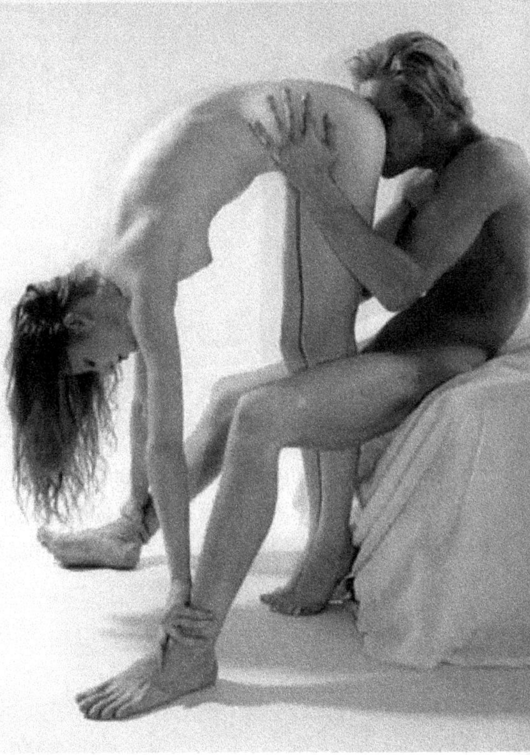

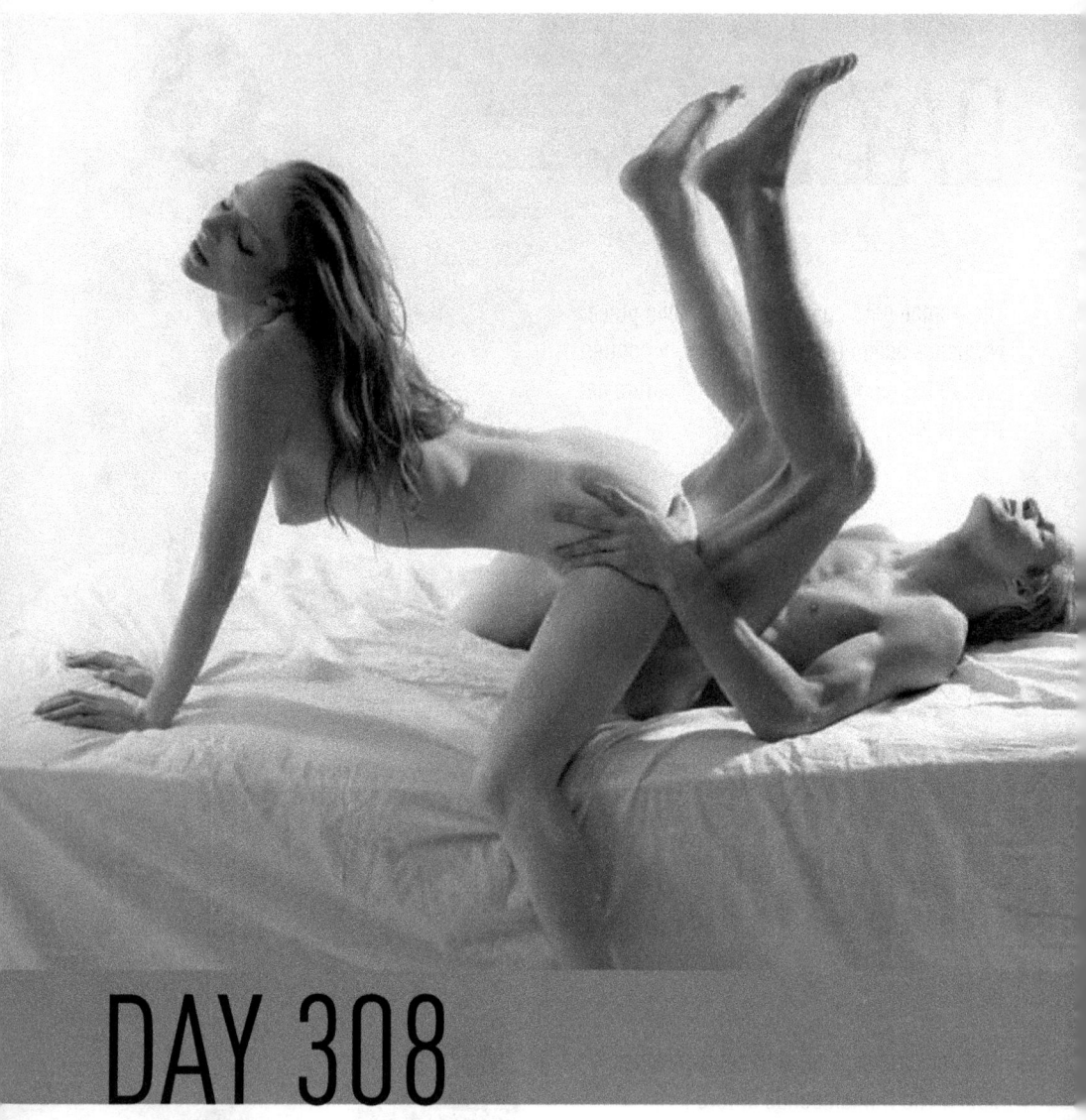

DAY 308

THE HEDGE TRIMMER

He lies back on the bed, and brings his knees to his chest with his legs spread wide open. She has one knee on the bed and one foot off as she backs herself onto his erect penis. Not a bad way to trigger some G-spot stimulation.

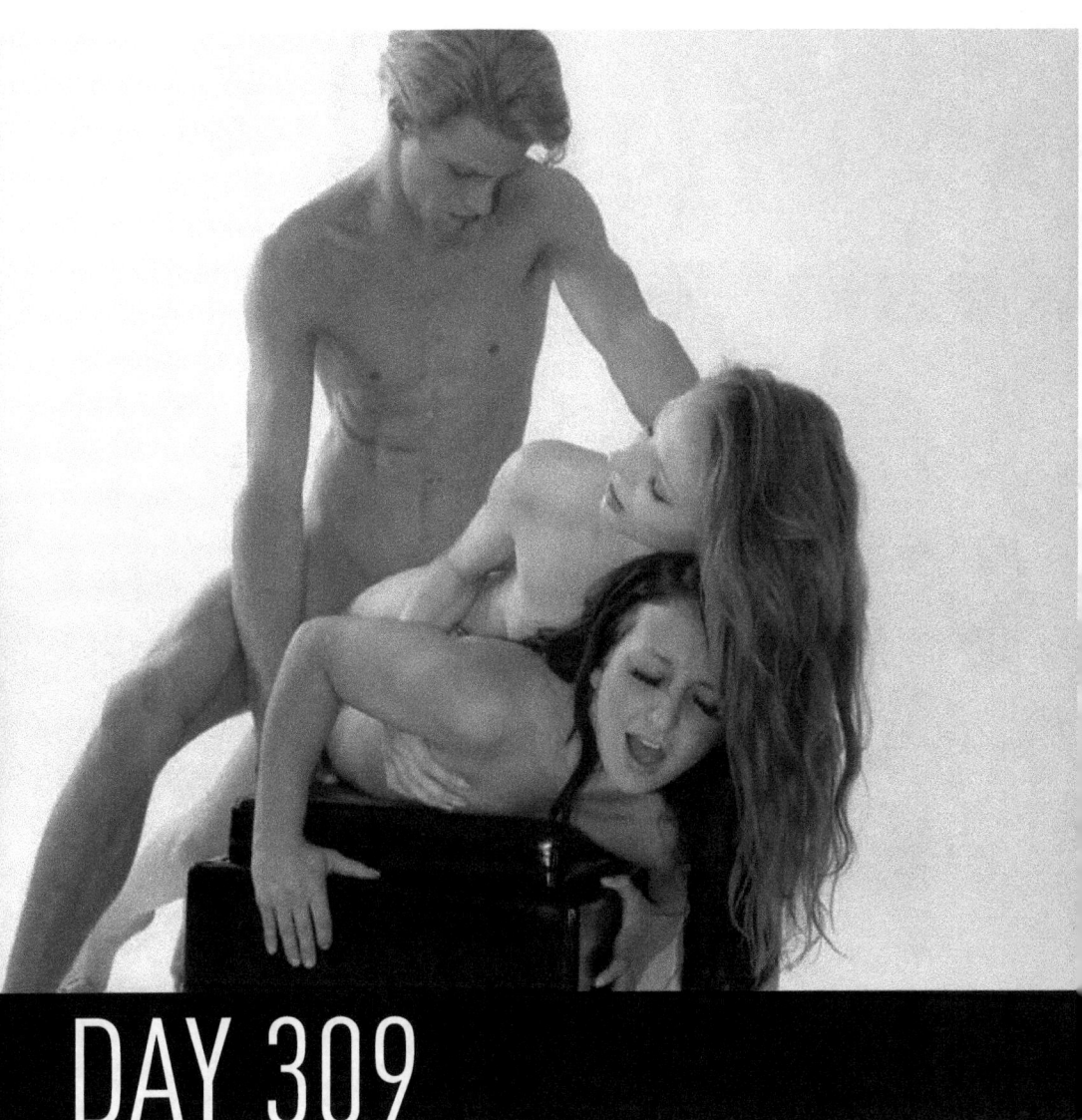

DAY 309

THE TRIPLE-DECKER SANDWICH

The first woman positions herself stomach-down on top of an ottoman, and her friend then lies facedown on top of her. The man takes turns penetrating each of them from behind.

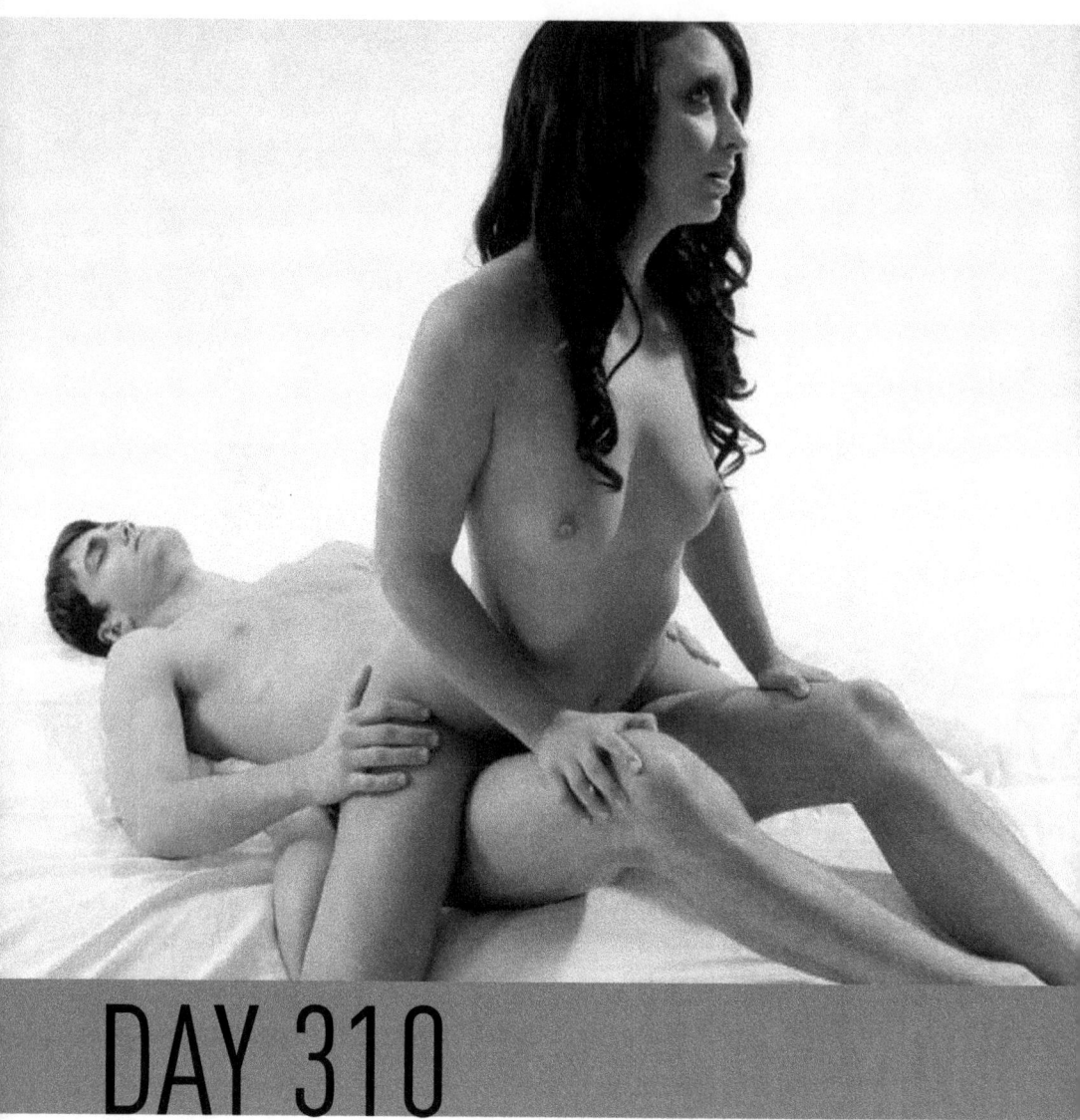

DAY 310

INSIDE AND OUT

He's on his back with his legs slightly bent. She faces out away from him as she lets him inside her. She can place her hands on his thighs to steady herself.

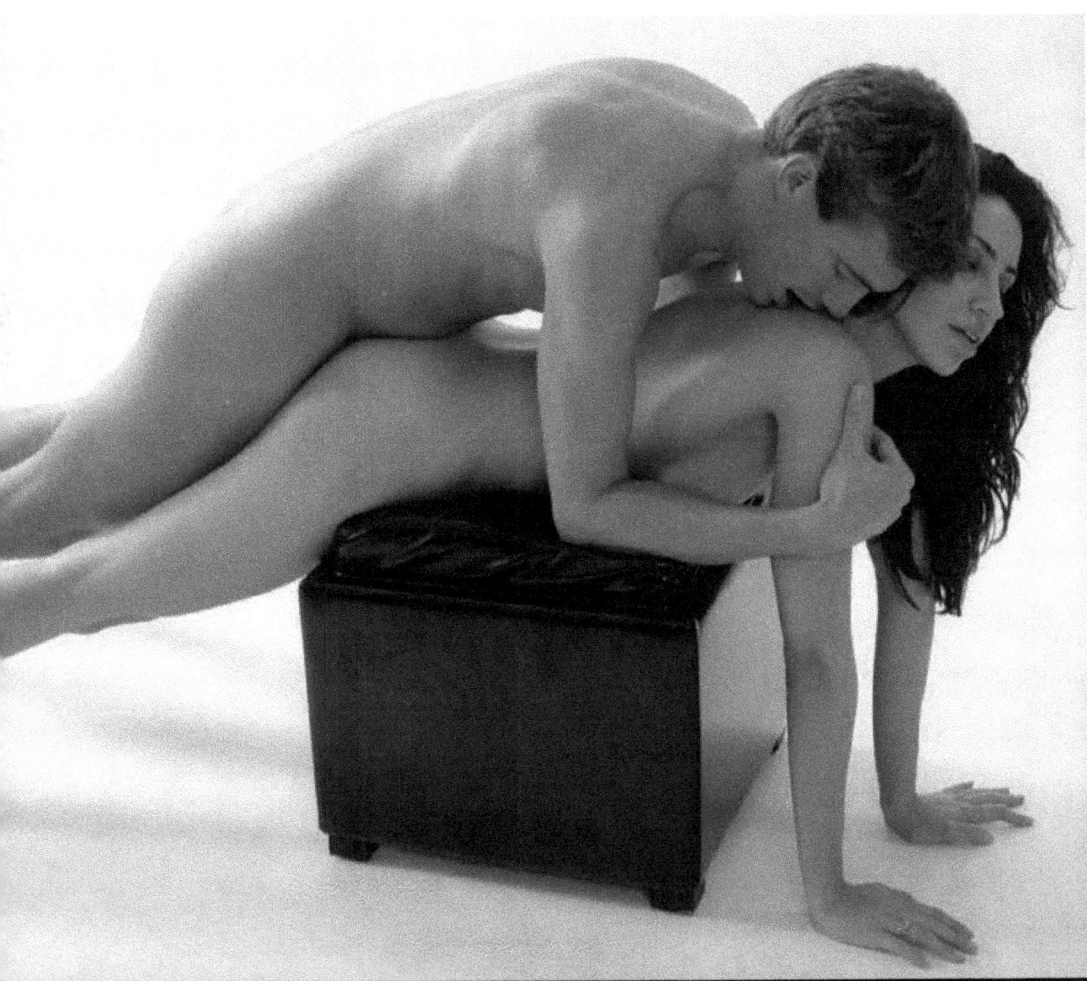

DAY 311

THE MERGER

She sprawls herself over an ottoman, placing her hands on the floor and extending her legs back. He lies his body atop hers, connecting with her completely as he enters from behind.

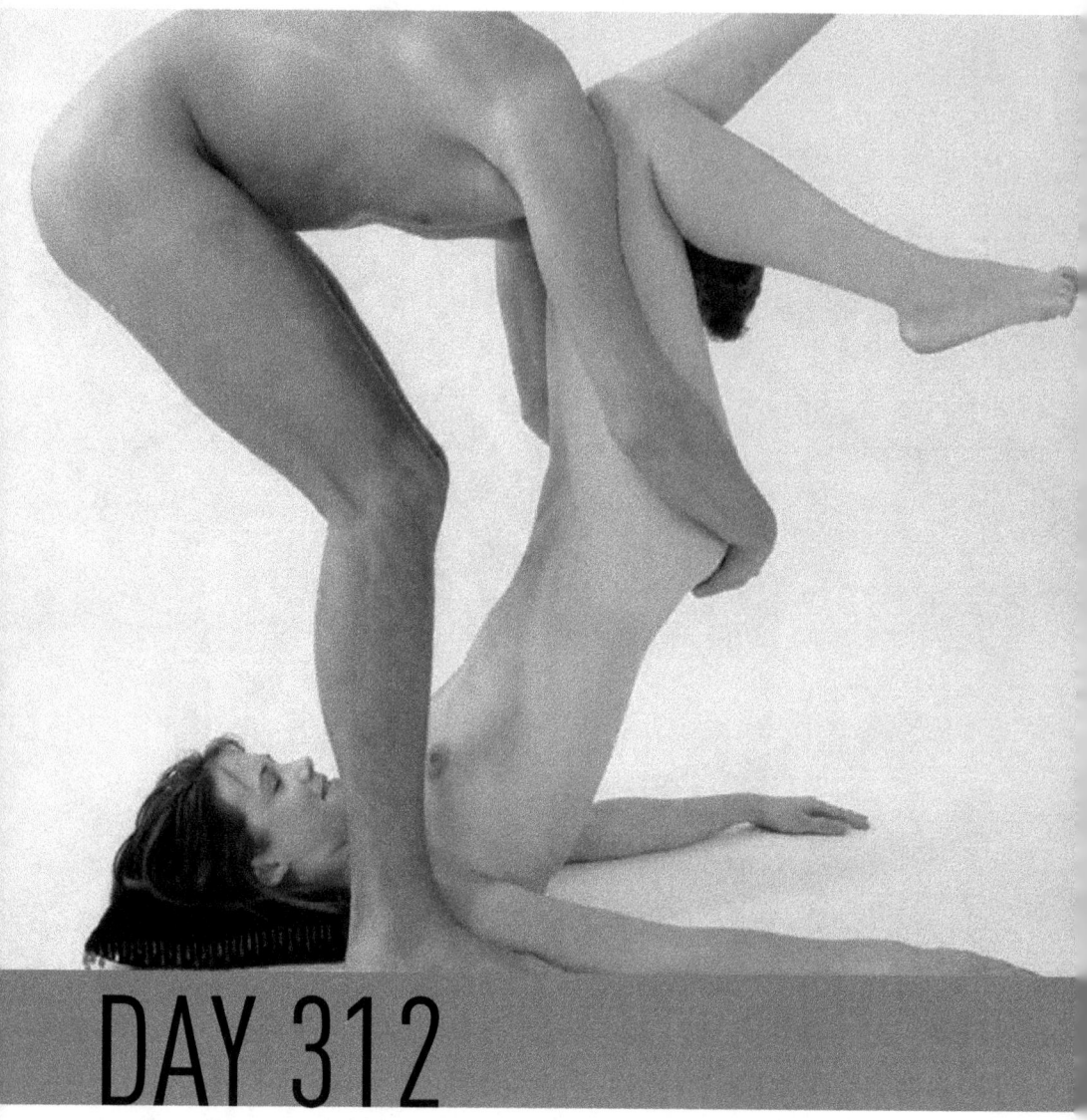

DAY 312

THE HONEY POT

The woman lies on her back with her partner straddling her in a standing position. He bends down lifting her from the waist and buttocks as her weight shifts to her shoulders. He lowers his mouth to sample her sweet treat.

DAY 313

KICK YOUR FEET UP

The man stands up straight with the backs of his legs against a chair. His partner stands in front of him as he lifts her up. As he penetrates her from behind, she can place one or both of her feet on the seat of the chair to gain some traction.

DAY 314

THE BELL RINGER

The man leans back against a wall, holding on to a support strap or belt, while bringing his feet out away from him. His lover straddles his legs, allowing him to enter her from behind. They swing and sway toward and ear-ringing climax.

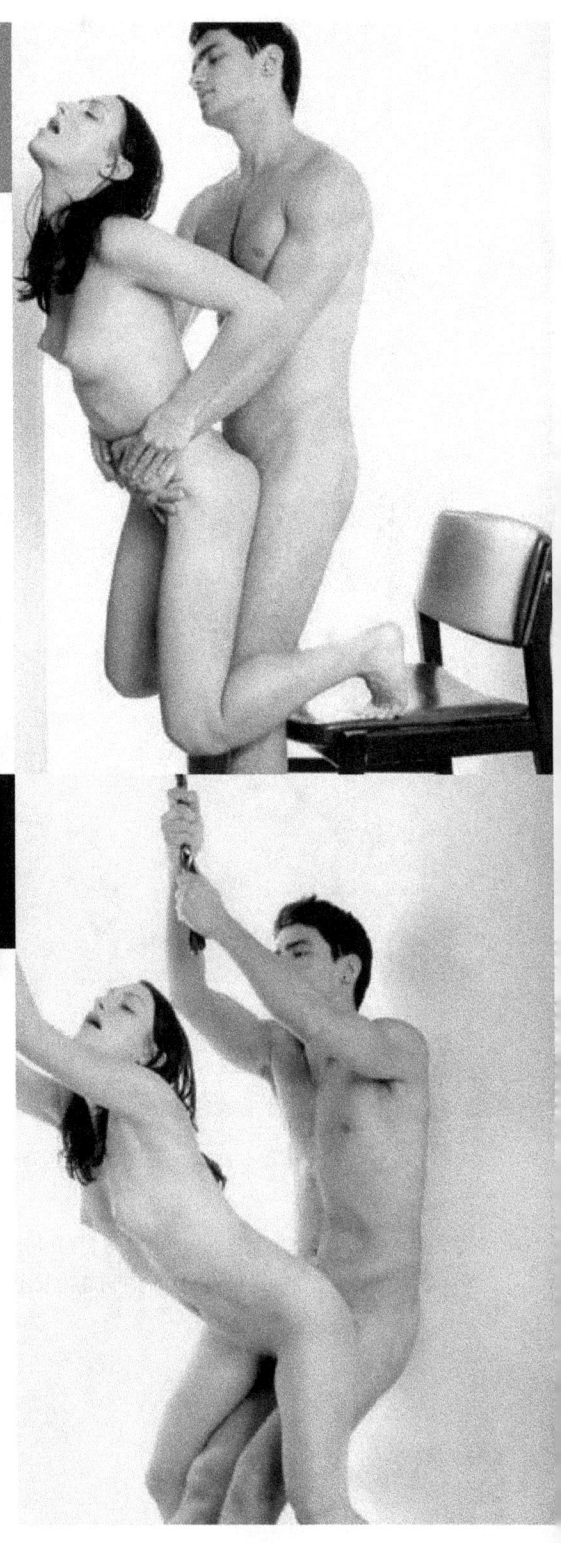

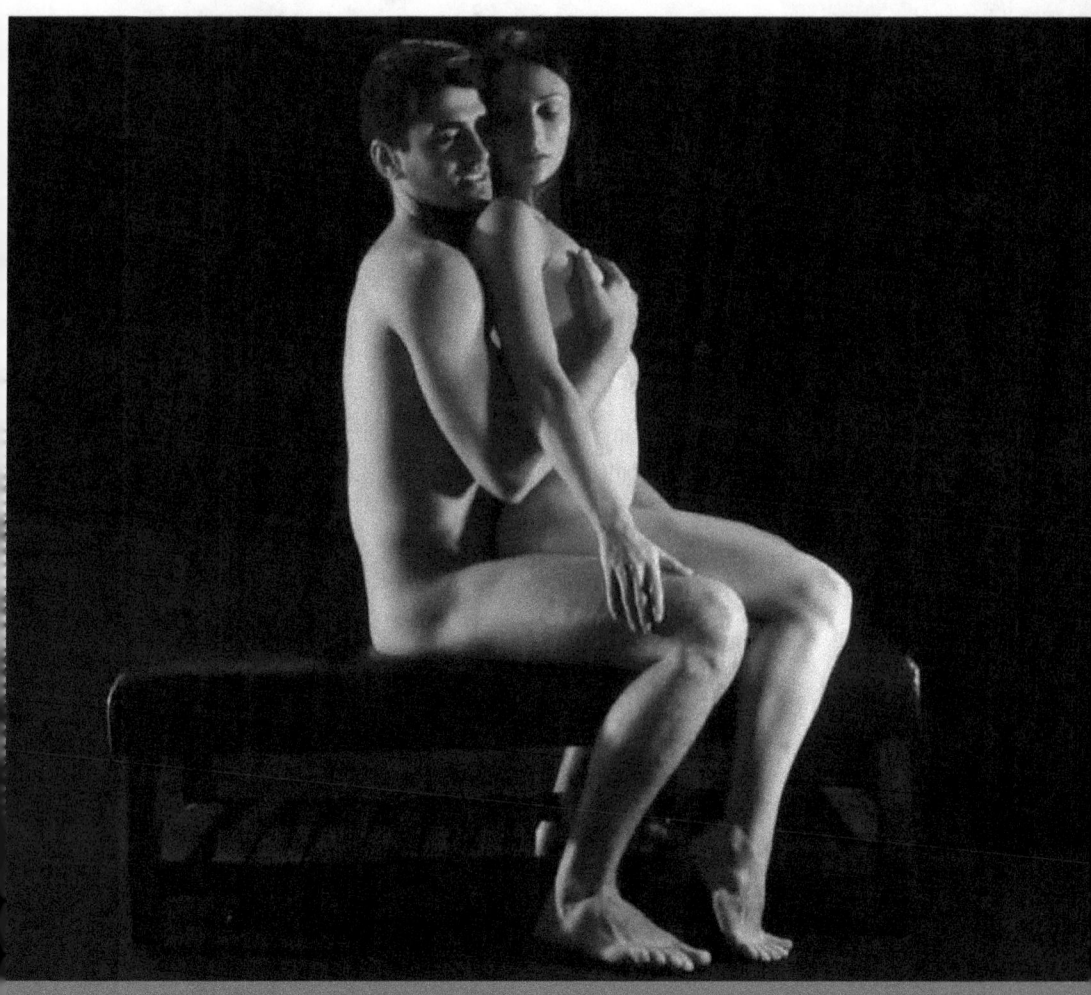

DAY 315

IS THIS SEAT TAKEN?

He sits on a bench, straddling it. His lover takes a seat in his lap as his penis penetrates her vagina. He brings his hands around to touch her breasts and stroke her clitoris.

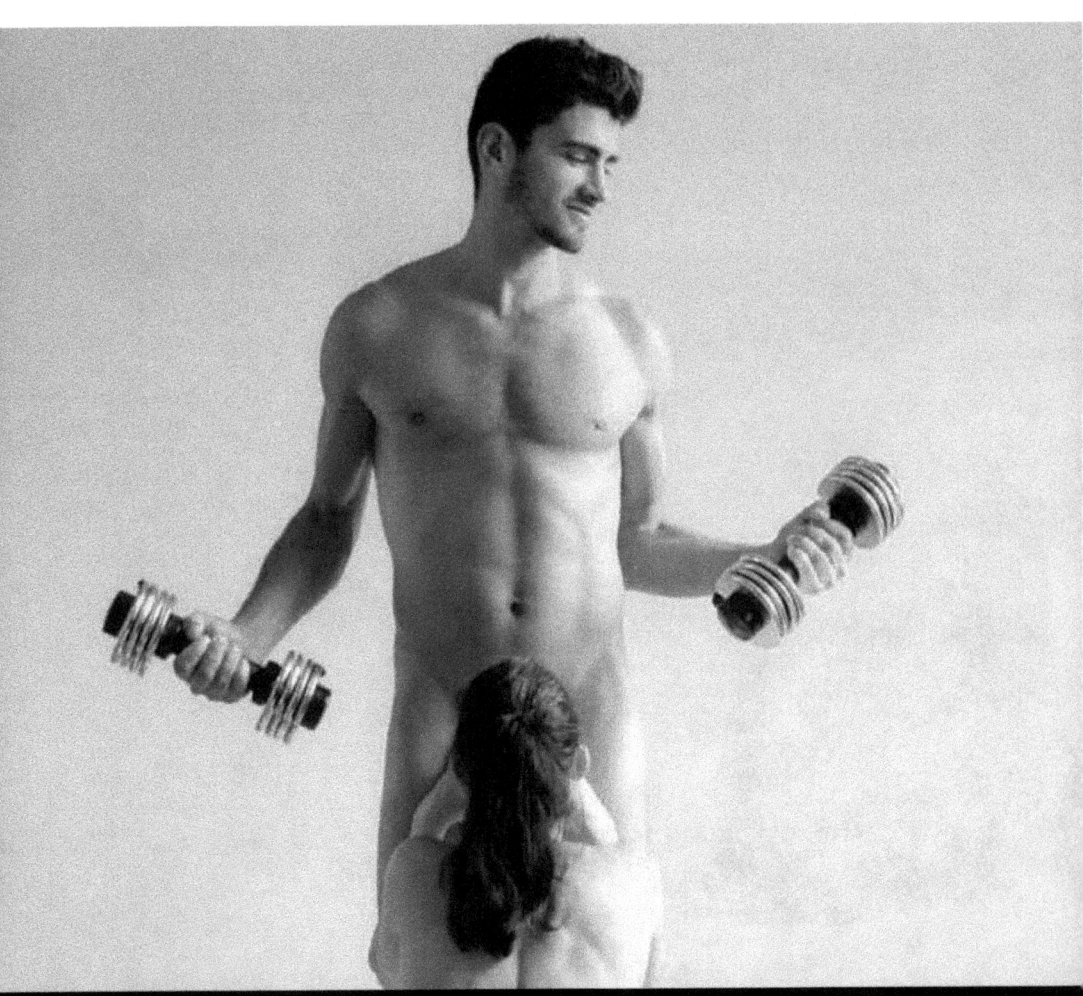

DAY 316

THE CURL FRIEND

He stands up straight and starts curling some dumbbells. His lover seizes the opportunity, drops to her knees, and gives his favorite lower body muscle an oral workout.

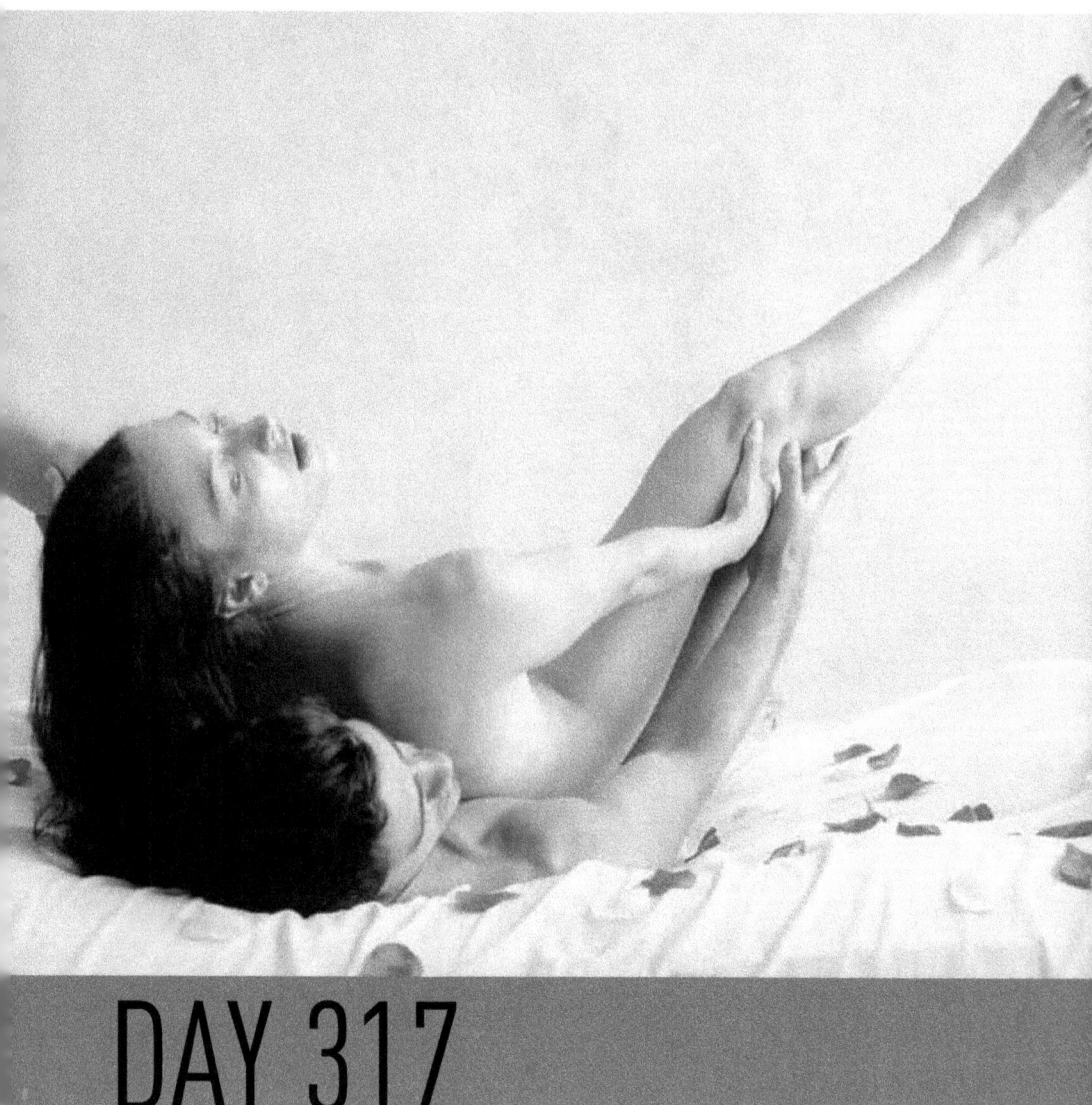

DAY 317

THE ROSE GARDEN

The couple scatter rose petals across the bed as the man lies back straight with legs extended. She lubes up and lowers herself onto him so that he's able to enter her anus. She fans her legs out to the side, opening herself up to his upward thrusts.

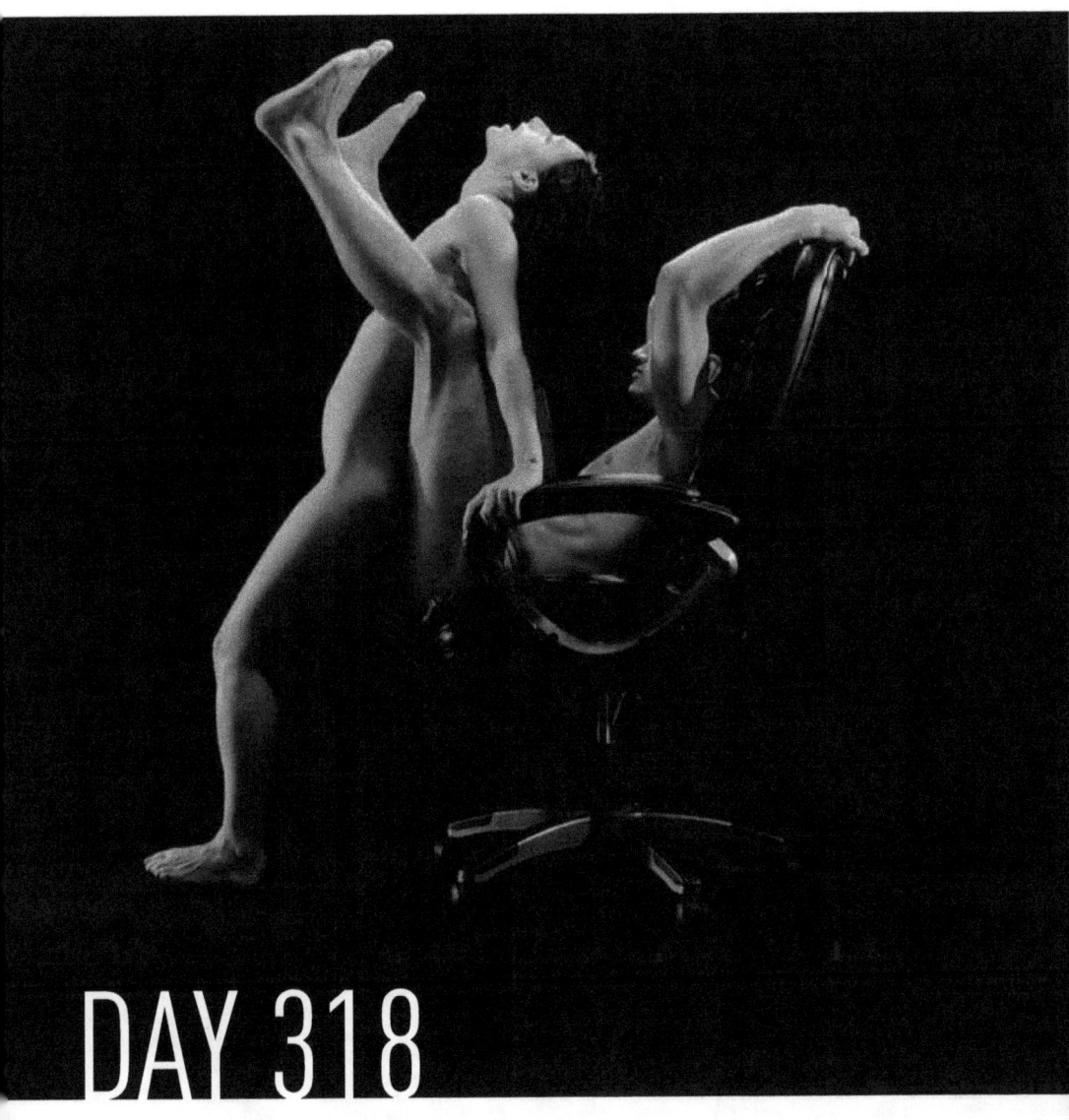

DAY 318

DANGEROUS CURVES

The man slides down in a chair curling himself into a "U" shape with his arms and legs in the air. His partner backs in toward him and lowers herself onto his penis. From here on, she controls the depth of the penetration and pace of their movements.

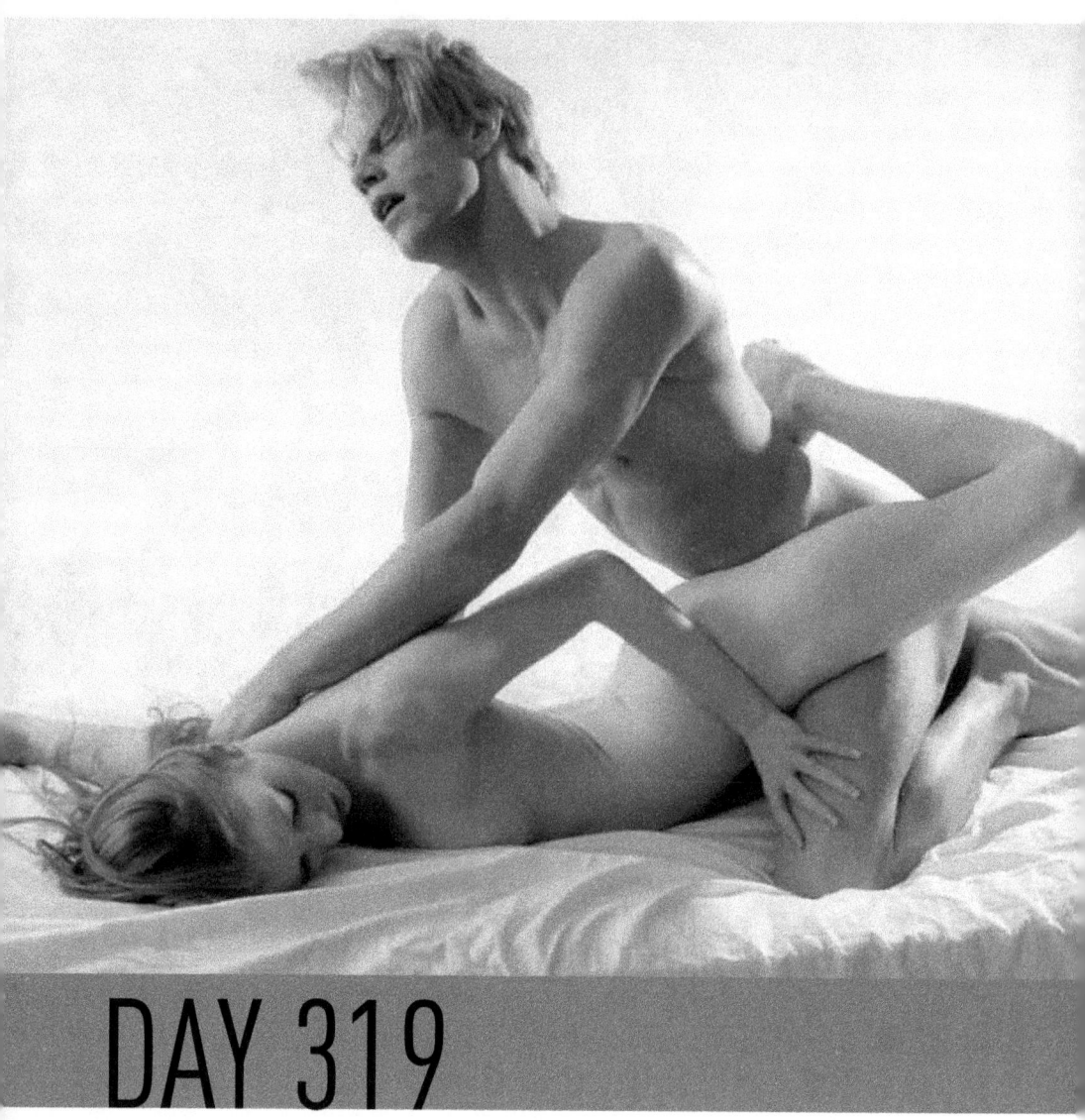

DAY 319

"A" FOR AROUSAL

The woman lies on her stomach with her legs fully extended. As her lover enters her from behind, she swings her leg around to touch the small of his back. The penetration is deep and the body contact sublime.

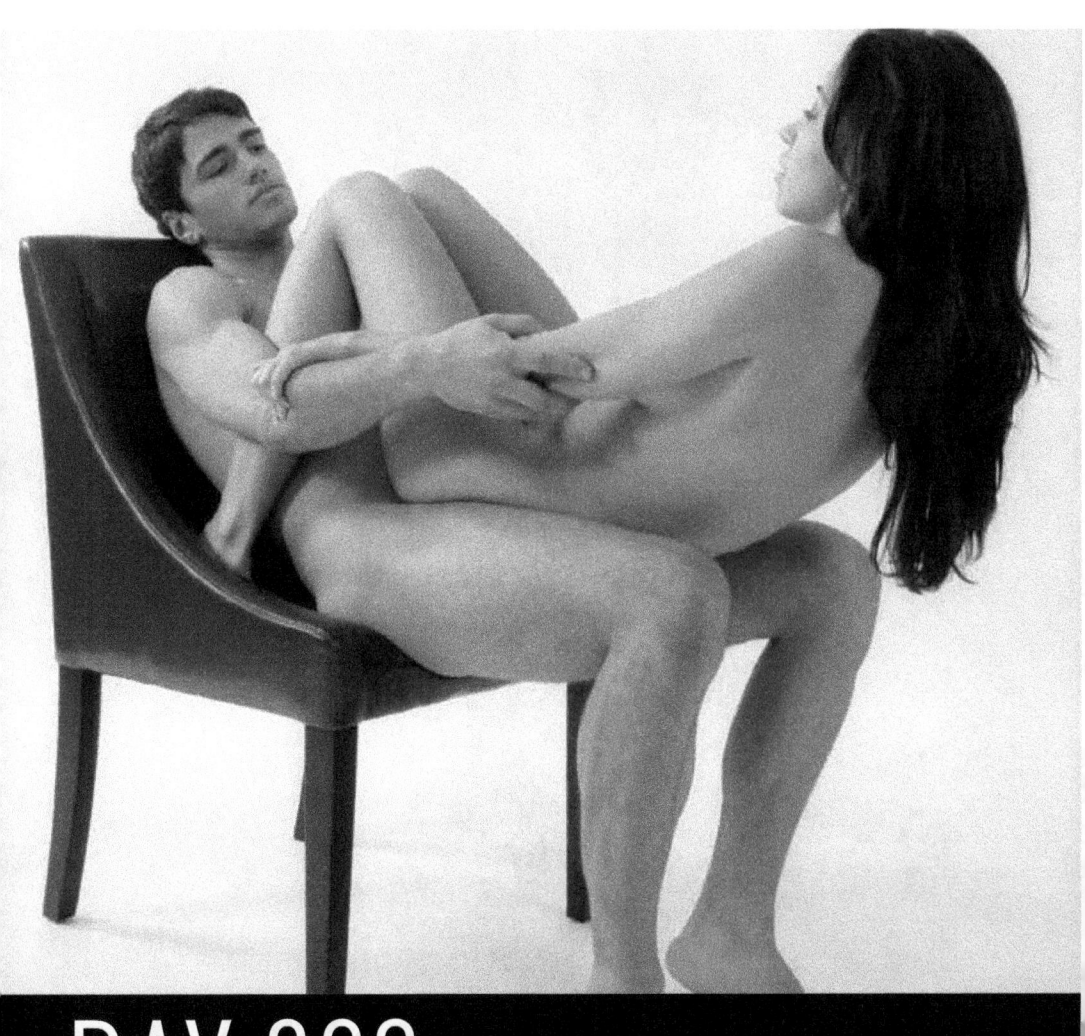

DAY 320

THE LOVE TUG

He positions himself low in a chair while his partner climbs on top facing him. As he penetrates her, they grab on to each other's forearms for both movement and support.

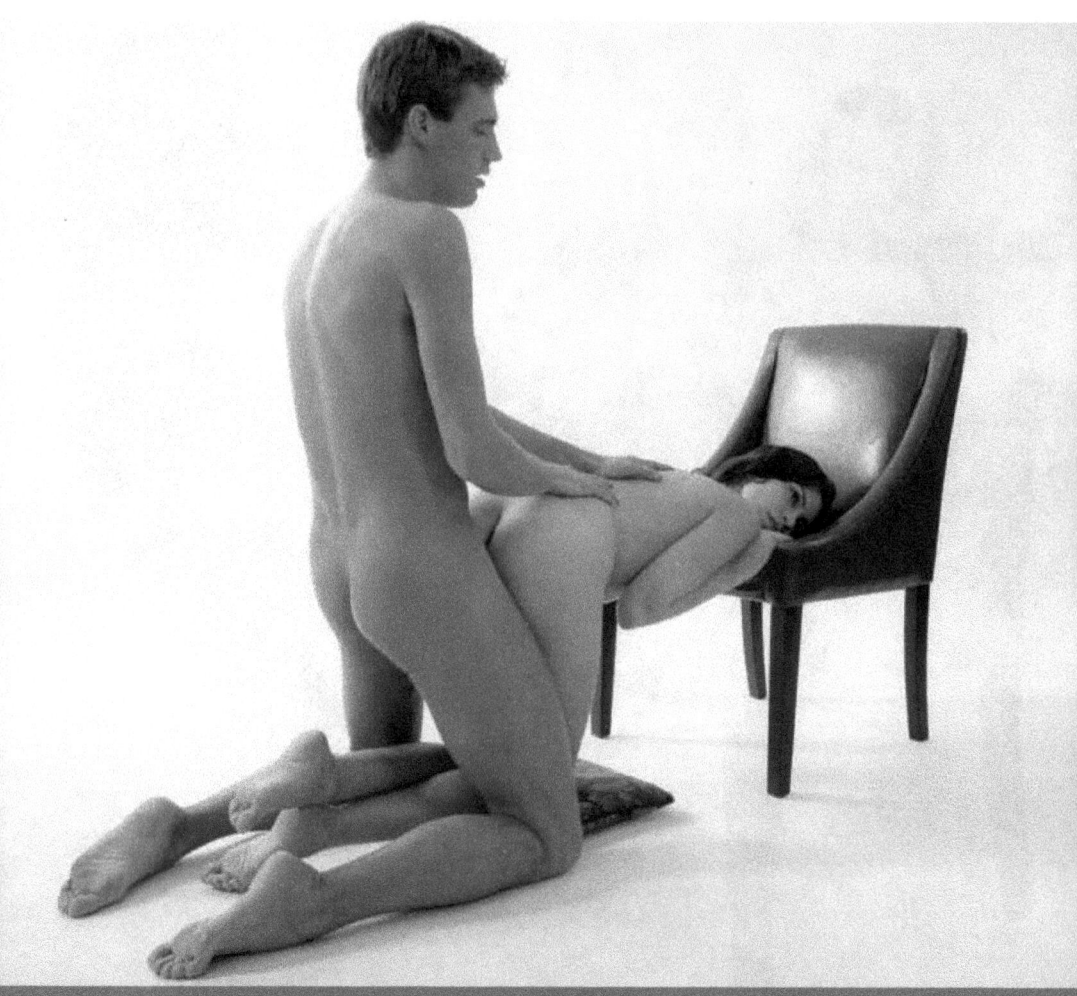

DAY 321

I GOT YOUR BACK

In this doggy-style variation, the lovers employ a chair. She's on her knees with her head and torso resting against the seat of the chair. Her partner enters her from behind from a kneeling posture with his legs outside hers. A pillow comes in very handy.

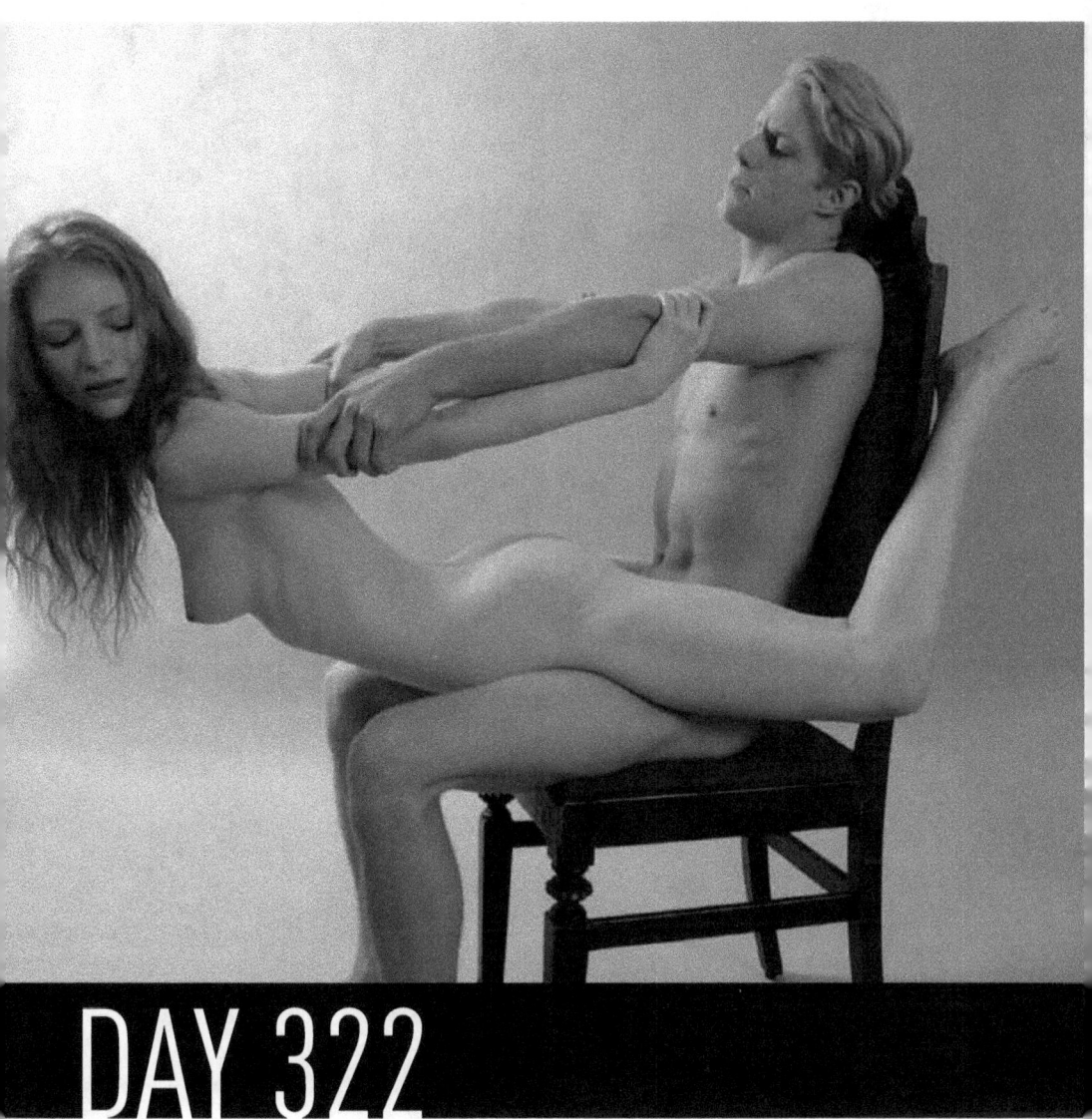

DAY 322

COME FLY WITH ME

The man sits in a chair as his lover mounts him facing away from him. He holds onto her wrists or hands as she drops forward.
He thrusts away as they prepare for
a tantalizing takeoff.

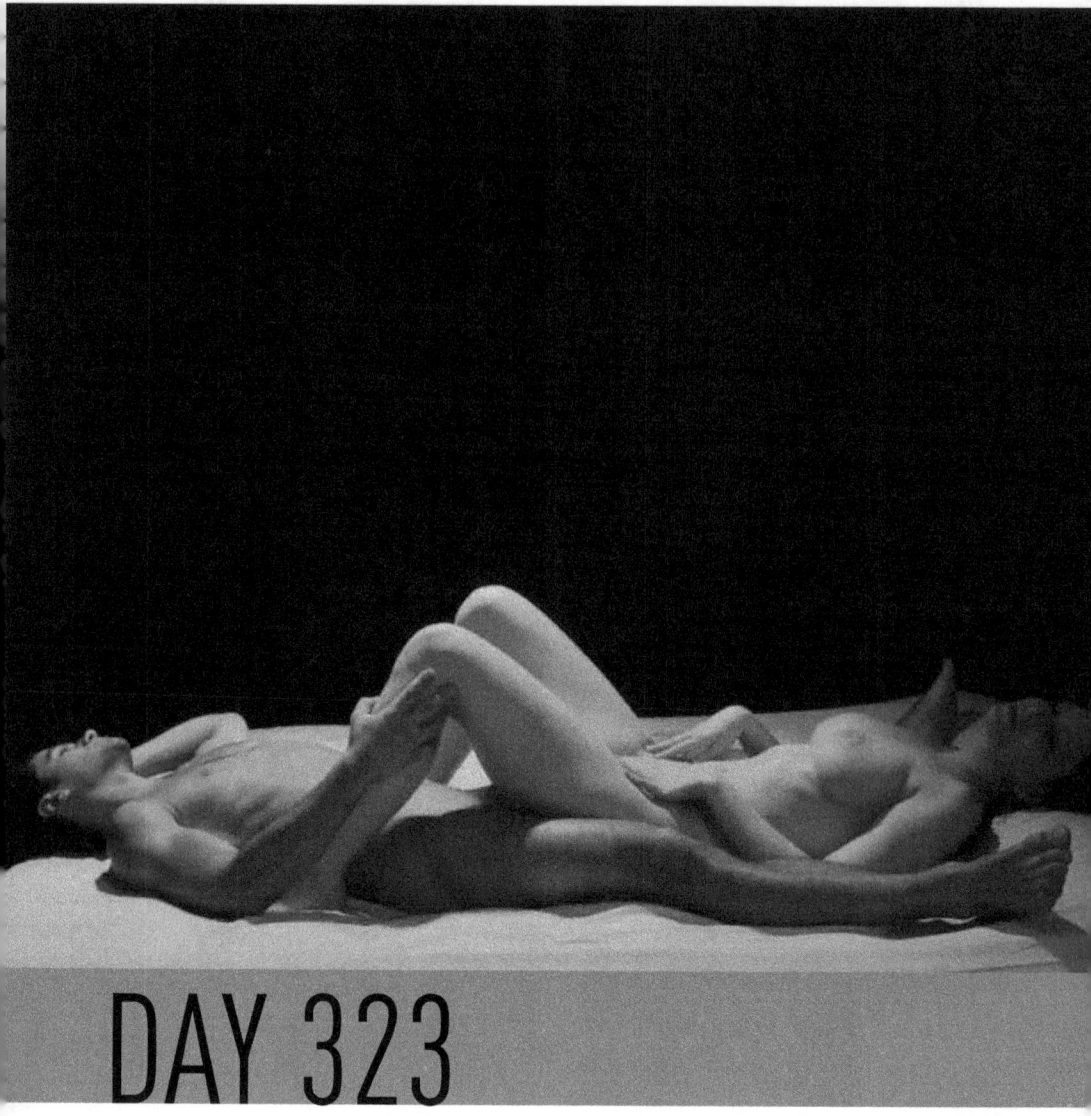

DAY 323

THE KNOCKOUT

They're down, but certainly not out. He stretches out on the bed with his legs open. His lover lies back on top of him in the opposite direction as he enters her. They can stroke each other's legs and feet.

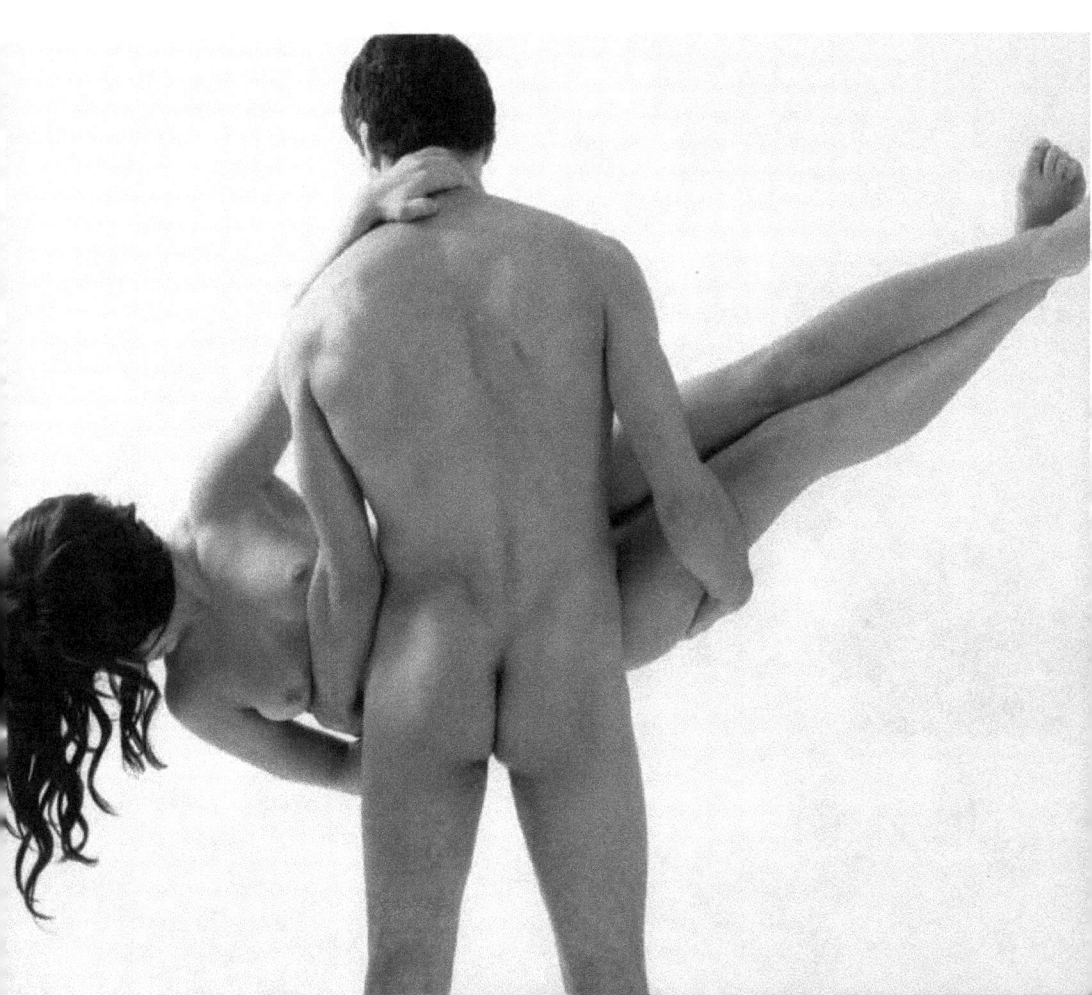

DAY 324

FRISKY BUSINESS

From a standing position, the man lifts his lover by the waist and legs and holds her body perpendicular to his. She gives him a lift of his own by stroking the underside of his penis.

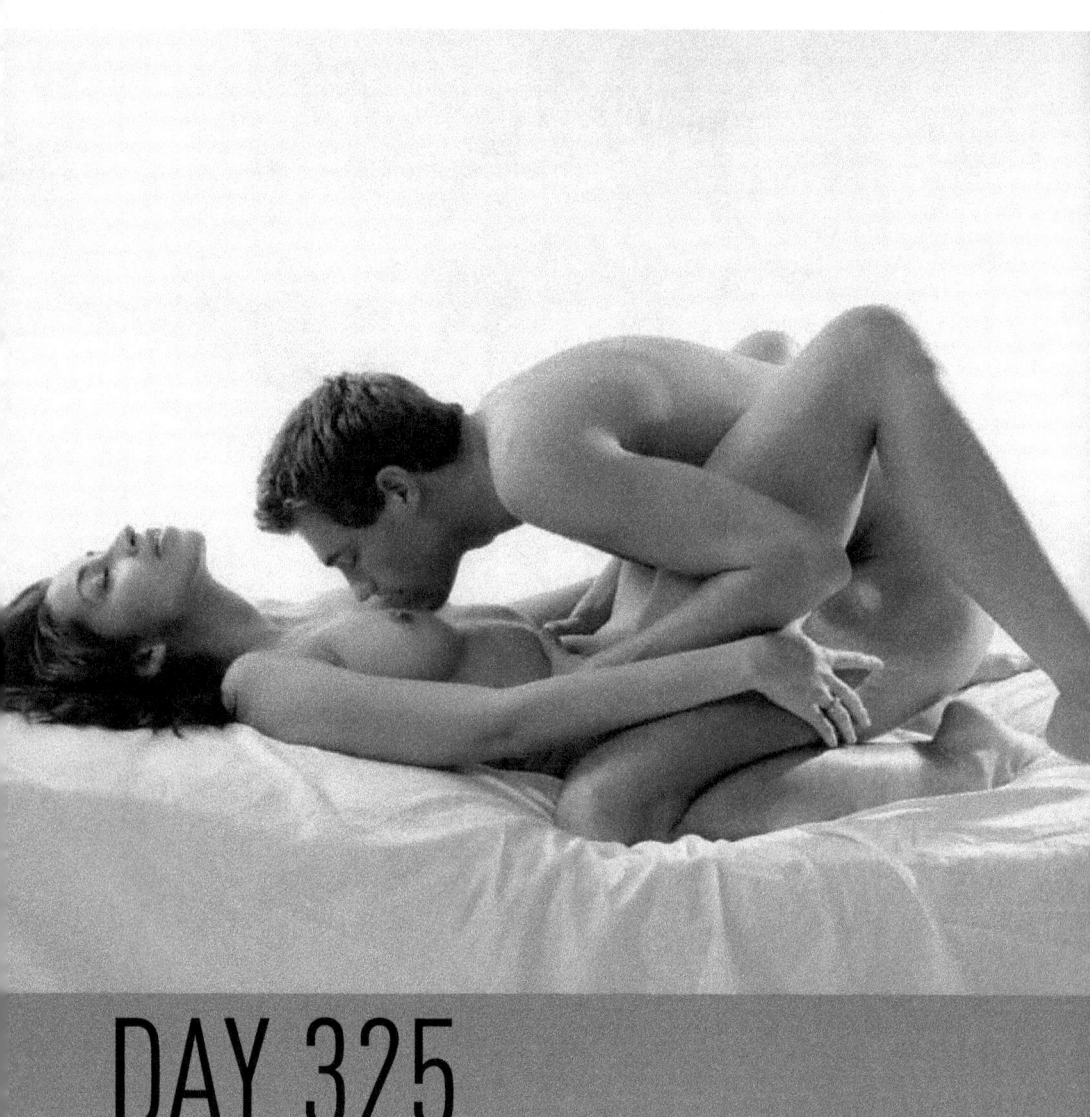

DAY 325

THE SLOW BURN

The woman lies on her back and parts her legs while her lover enters her from a kneeling position. He ups the ante by lavishing her body with slow, deep kisses.

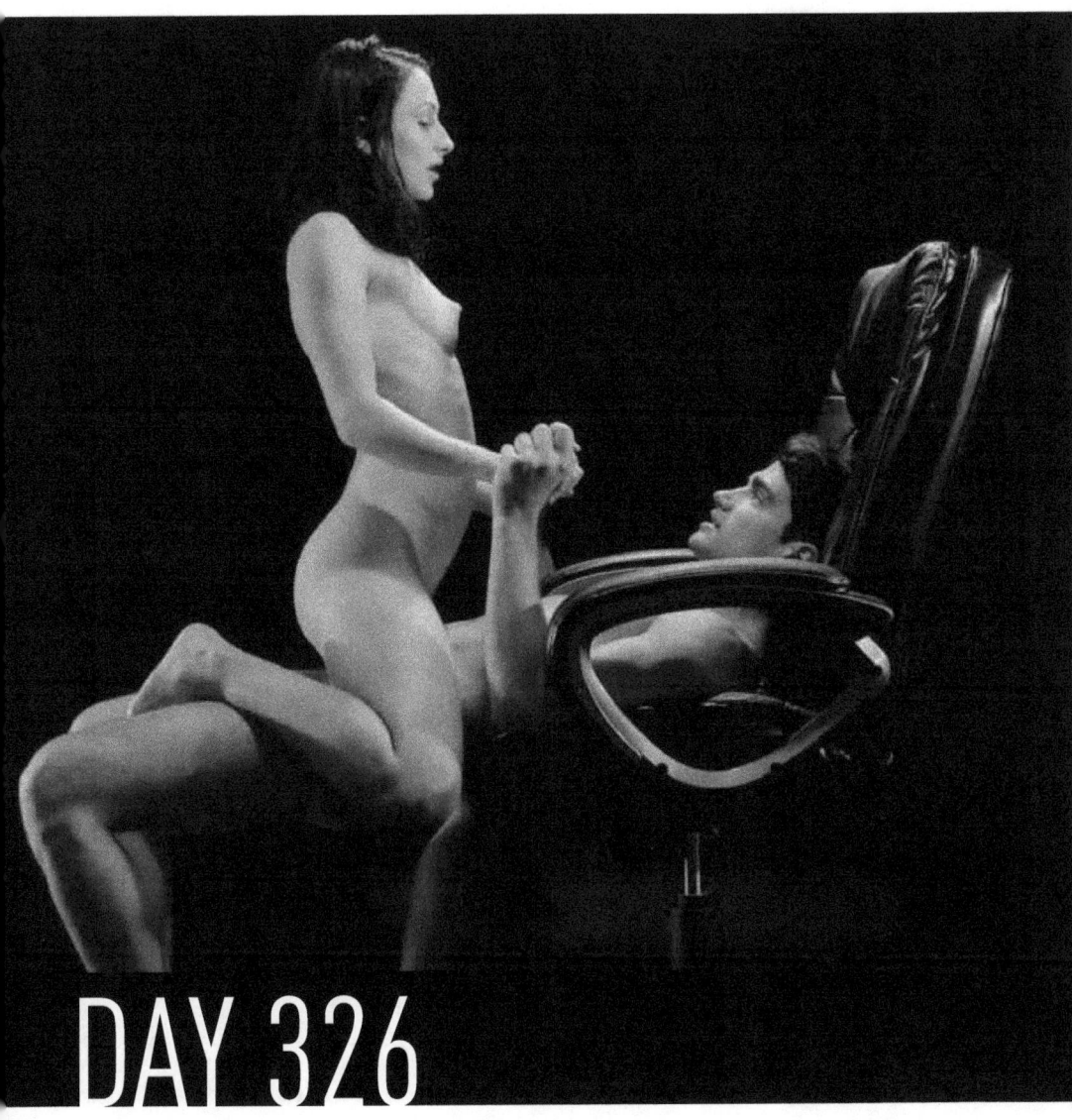

DAY 326

COMING ATTRACTIONS

He places his head and torso low in a chair with his legs out and feet on the floor. She likes what she sees and mounts his member, hooking her feet up over his thighs. They lock hands as they head toward a terrific climax.

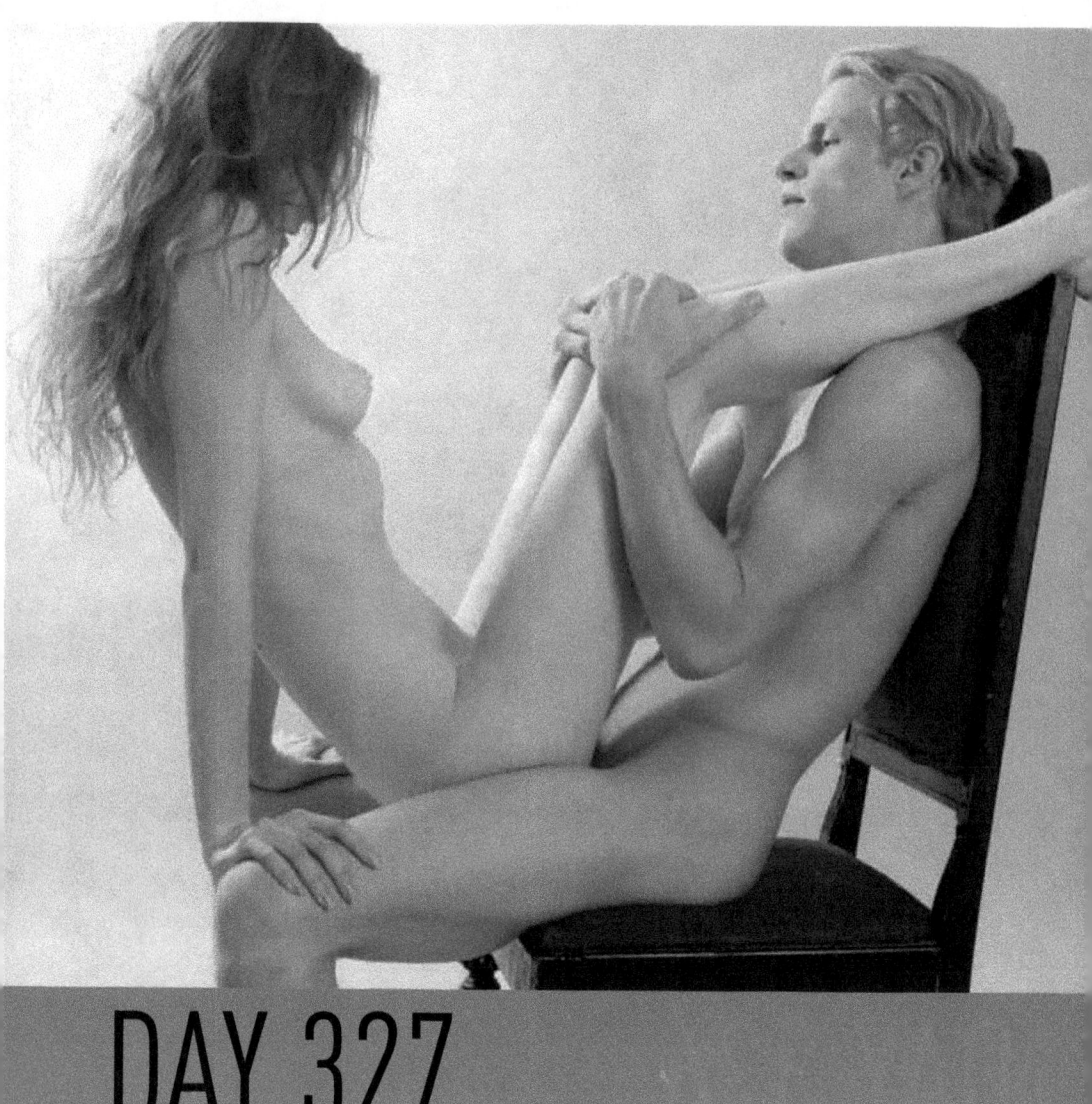

DAY 327

THE LUSTY LOUNGE

The man sits on the edge of a chair with his legs spread wide enough to provide an ample seat for his partner. She lubes her anus and brings her legs up over his shoulders. As he penetrates her he can squeeze her legs together to vary the sensations.

DAY 328

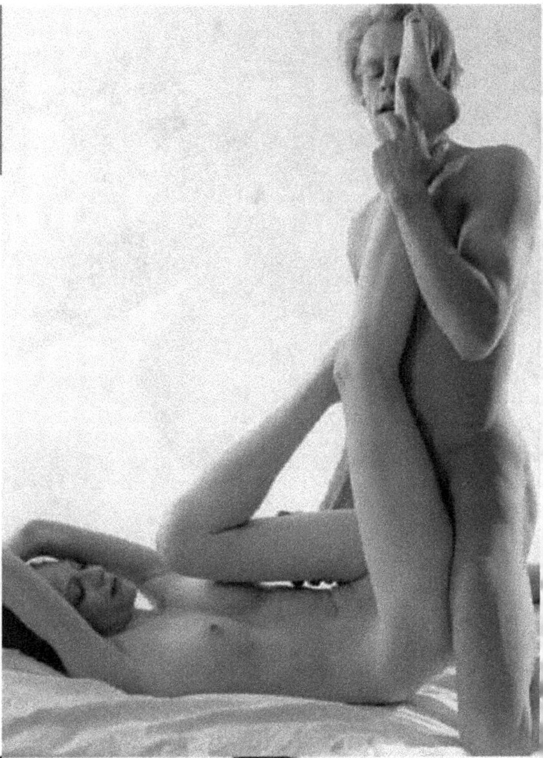

GROWING ATTRACTION

She's on her back as her lover lifts her hips and penetrates her from a kneeling position. As he thrusts inside her, she runs her legs up his chest like vines up a wall.

DAY 329

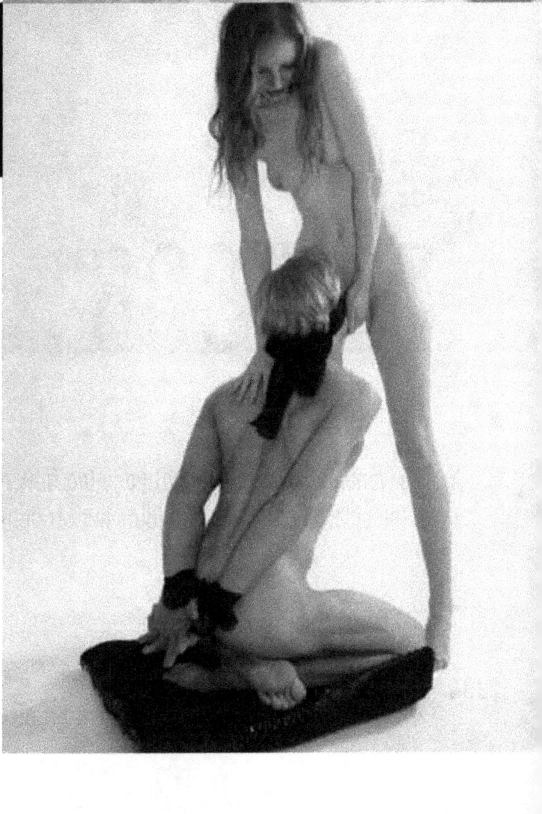

BLIND MAN'S MUFF

The man kneels before his partner, blindfolded with his hands bound behind his back. The woman guides his head between her legs. His heightened senses only increase the oral pleasure to follow.

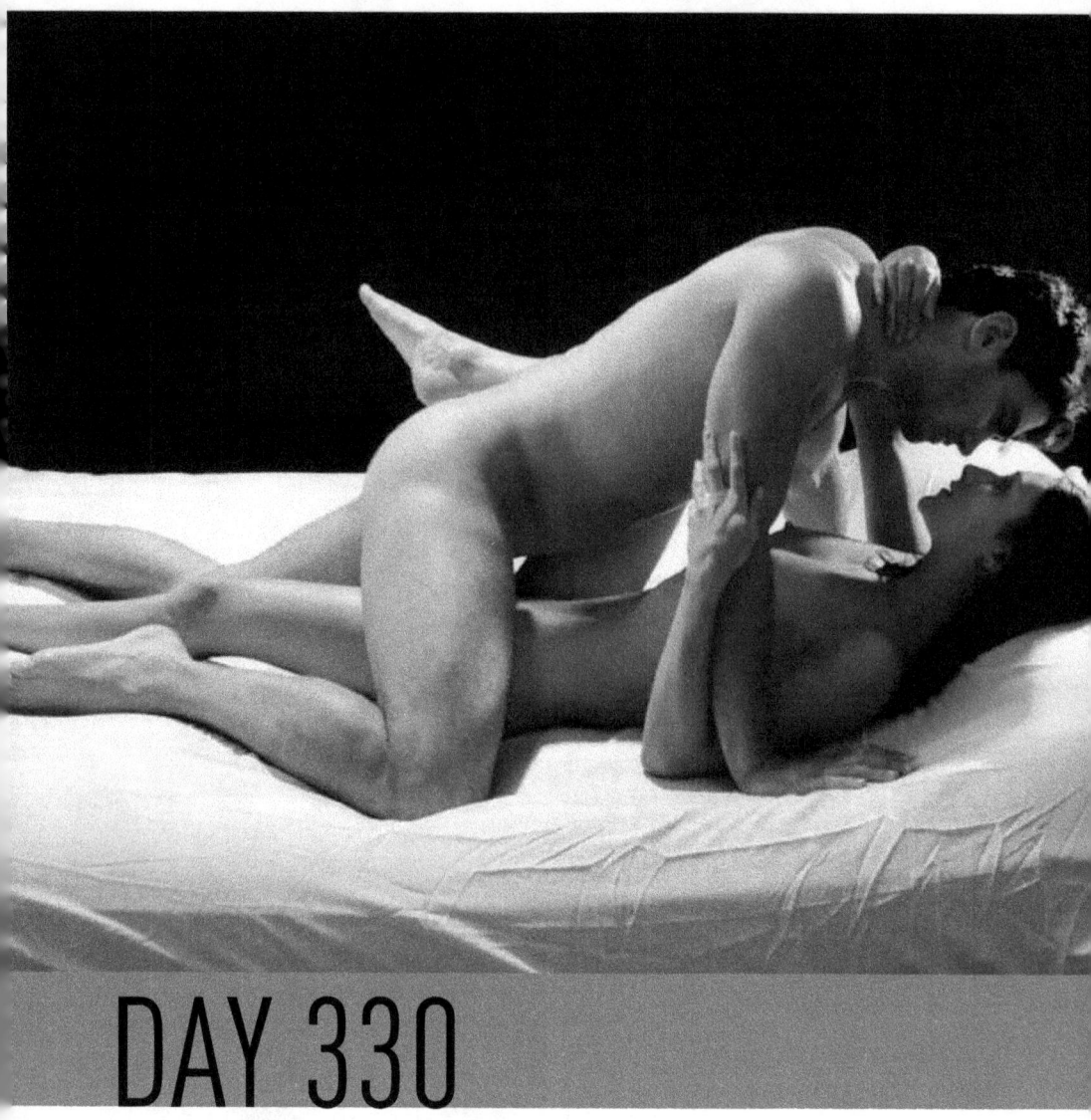

DAY 330

THE STRADDLE ROYALE

The woman is on her back with one leg fully extended and the other bent at the knee and out to the side. Her partner straddles her straightened leg and penetrates her vagina.

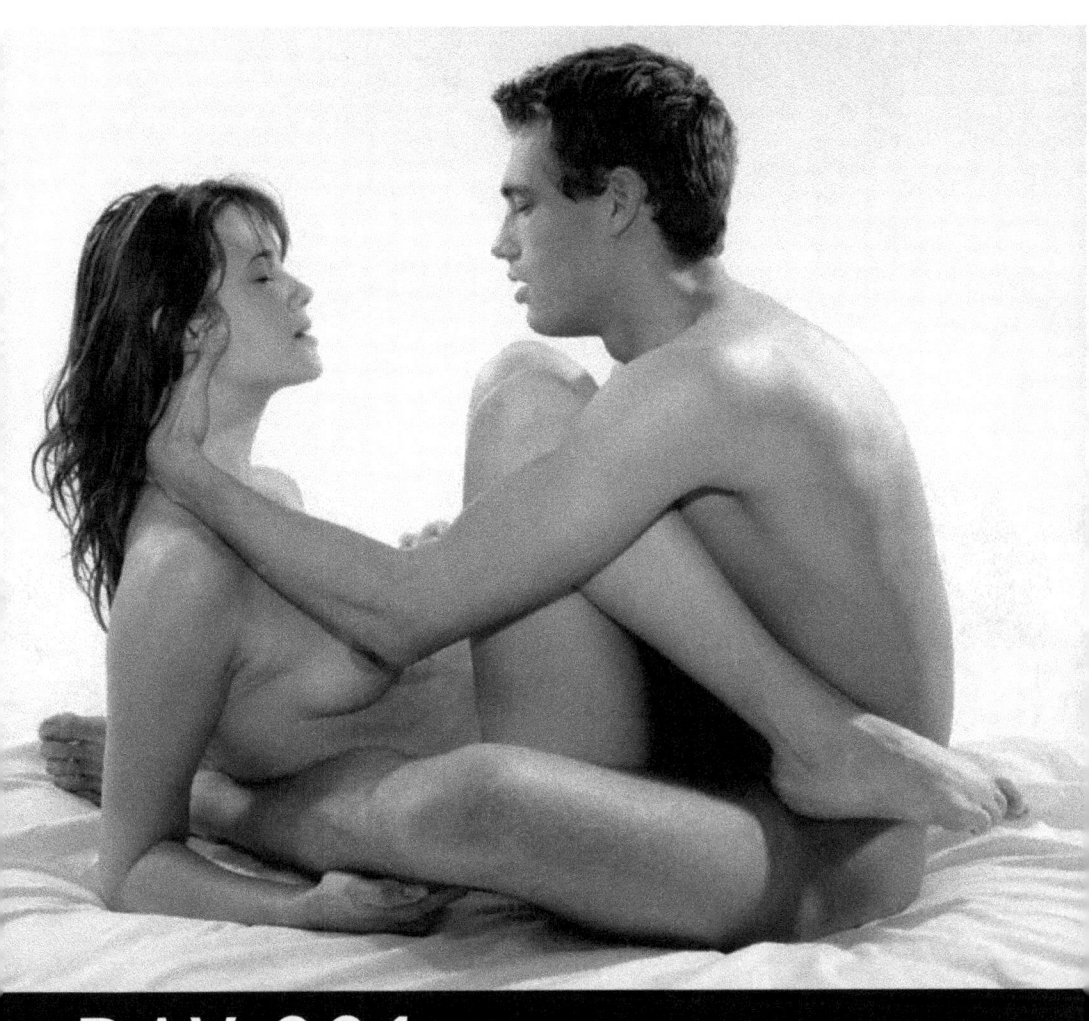

DAY 331

THE COCOON

He opens his legs wide and invites her in. She reclines slightly and brings her shins up to his chest. Once penetration is achieved he's able to add to the stimulation by rhythmically pressing her thighs inward.

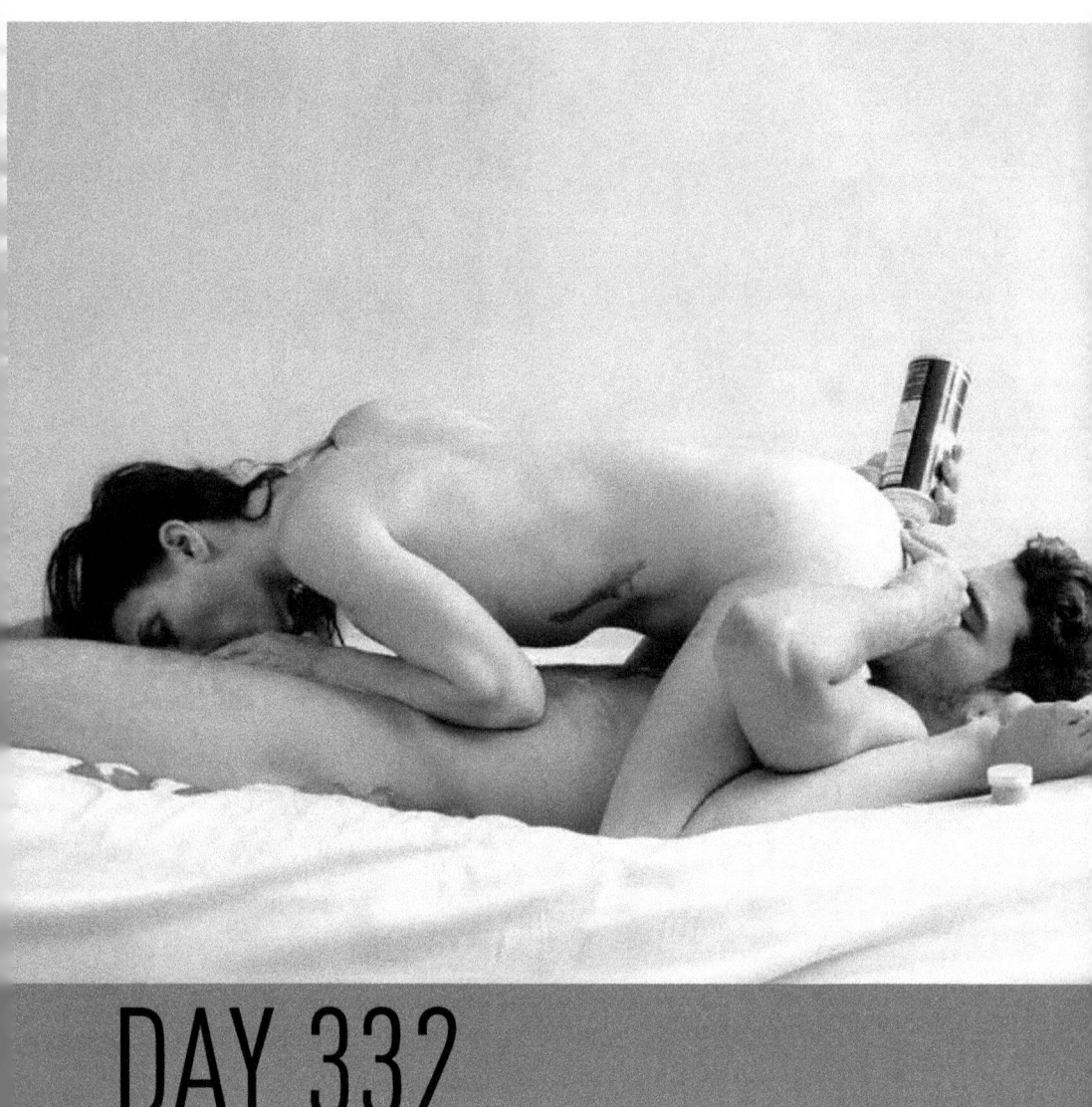

DAY 332

THE WHIPPED-Y NINE

The lovers arrange themselves in a classic 69 position with the woman on top. As she pleasures him with her mouth, he applies a little whipped cream to the areas on his menu.

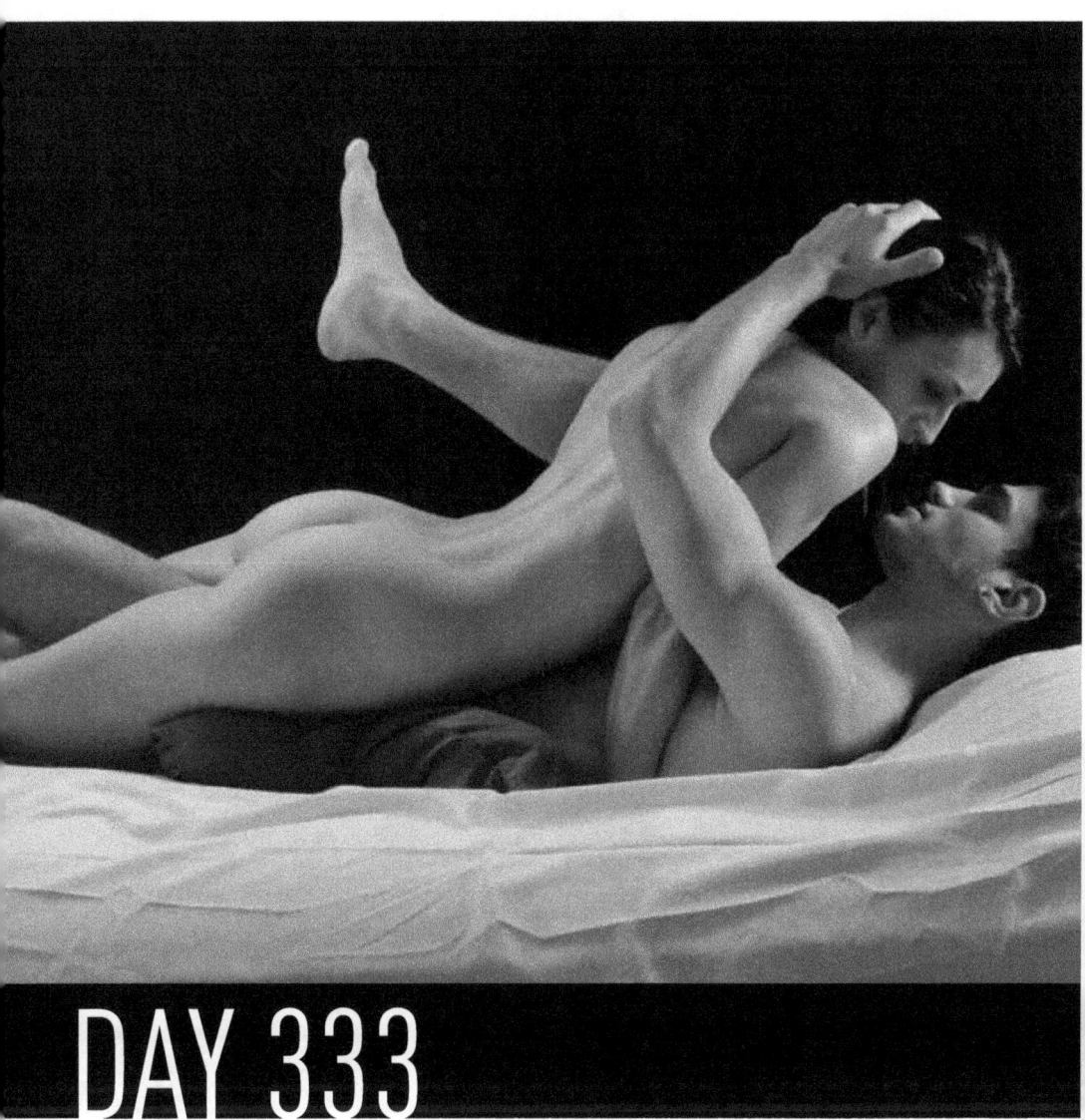

DAY 333

ROLE REVERSAL

The man lies back on the bed, keeping one leg straight and bringing the other out to the side. His partner takes the initiative, straddling his leg and mounting his penis. There's lots of clitoral stimulation for her in this position.

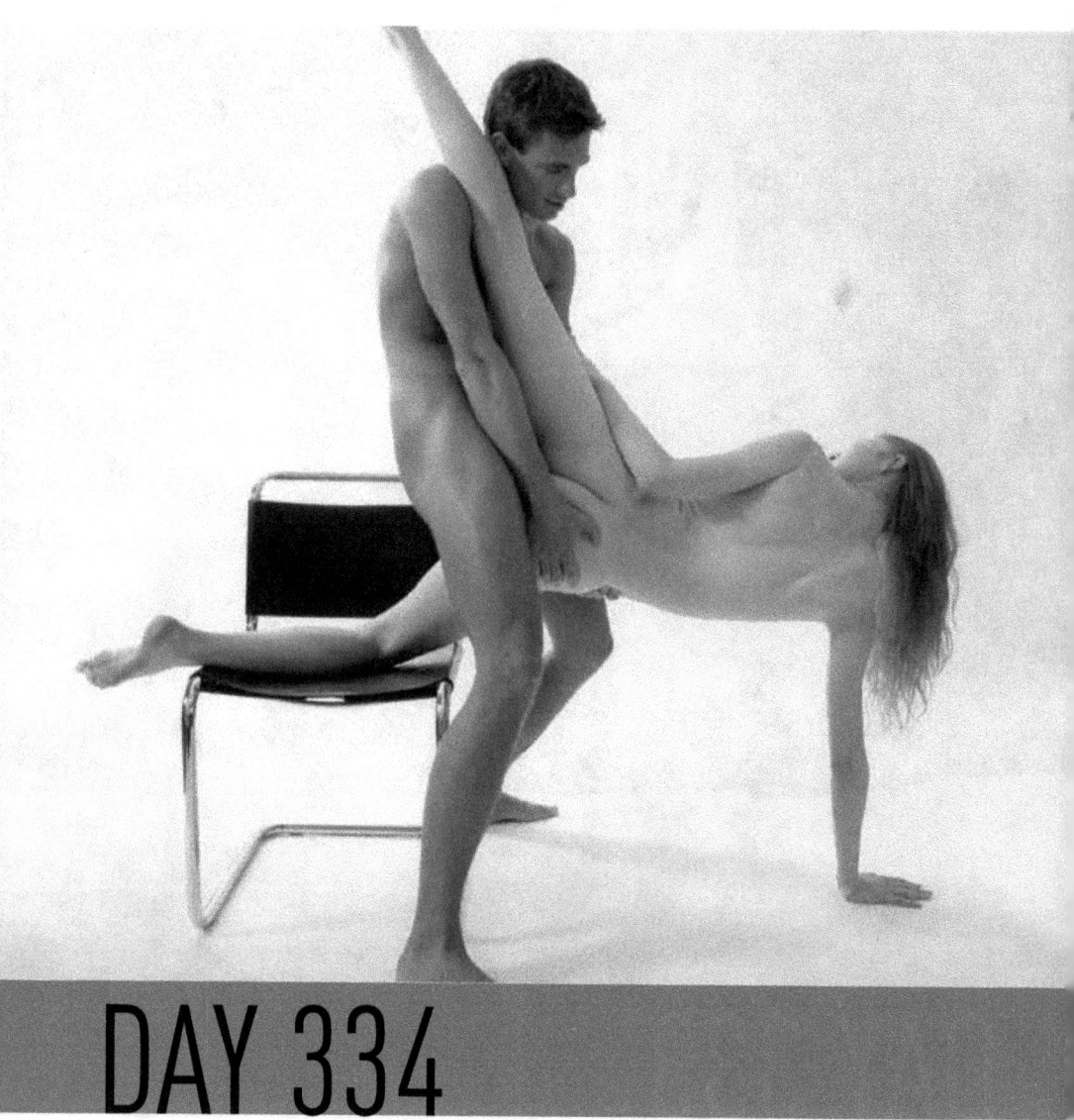

DAY 334

THE BUZZ SAW

Ready to test your athleticism? The woman places her leg on a chair while she extends one arm down to the floor, basically holding herself in a horizontal position. As her partner penetrates her, she lifts her other leg and rests it on her shoulder. He lends further support by wrapping his hands around her waist or buttocks.

DAY 335

PUMP YOU UP

The woman grabs a pair of dumbbells and stands up straight as her lover penetrates her from behind. As she presses the weights upwards he thrusts away and uses his free hands to massage her breasts and clitoris.

DAY 336

THE PULLEY PARTY

For this one you'll need an exercise resistance band, belts, or some other kind of support straps. He lies on the floor as his lover straddles him, allowing his penis to enter her. She grabs on to two support straps which complement her bouncing motion.

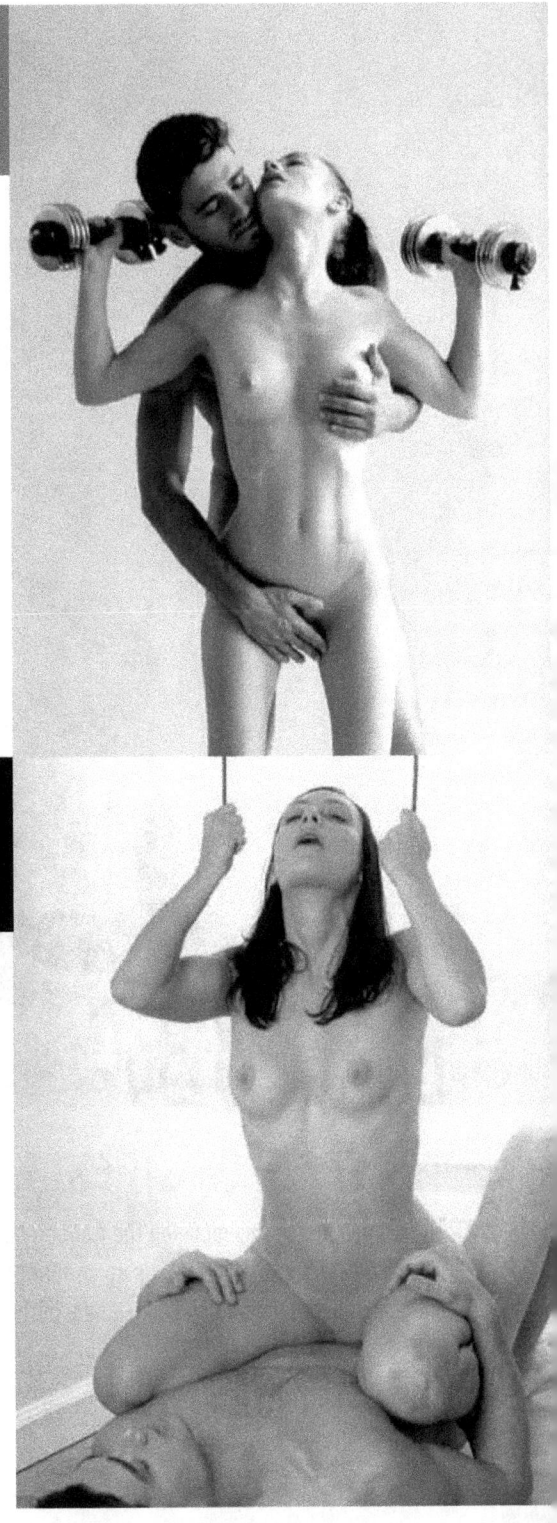

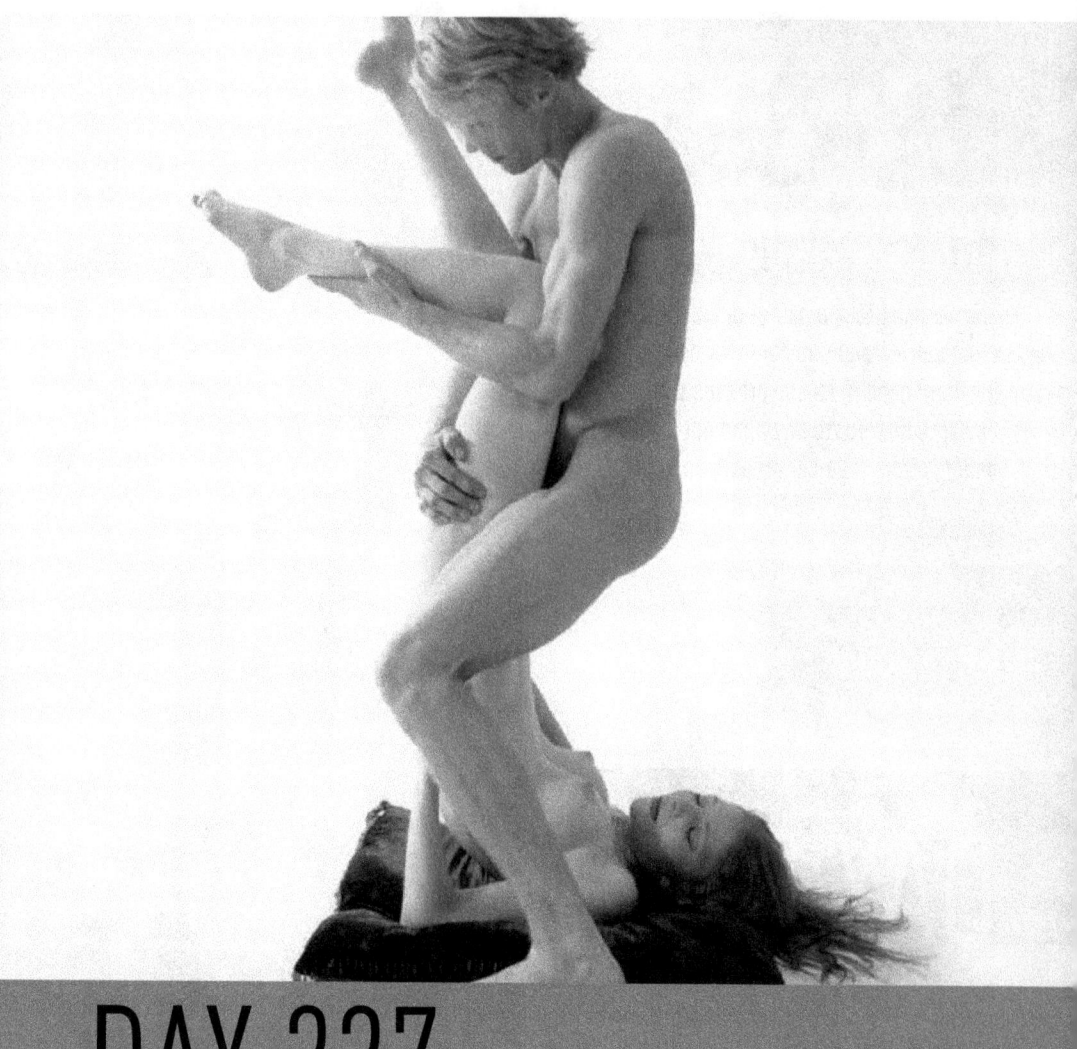

DAY 337

THE FEATS OF STRENGTH

The woman starts this move on the floor on her back. She shifts her weight to her shoulders allowing her lover to lift her legs up so that they can achieve penetration. Concentration and communication are key here—and a pillow doesn't hurt either.

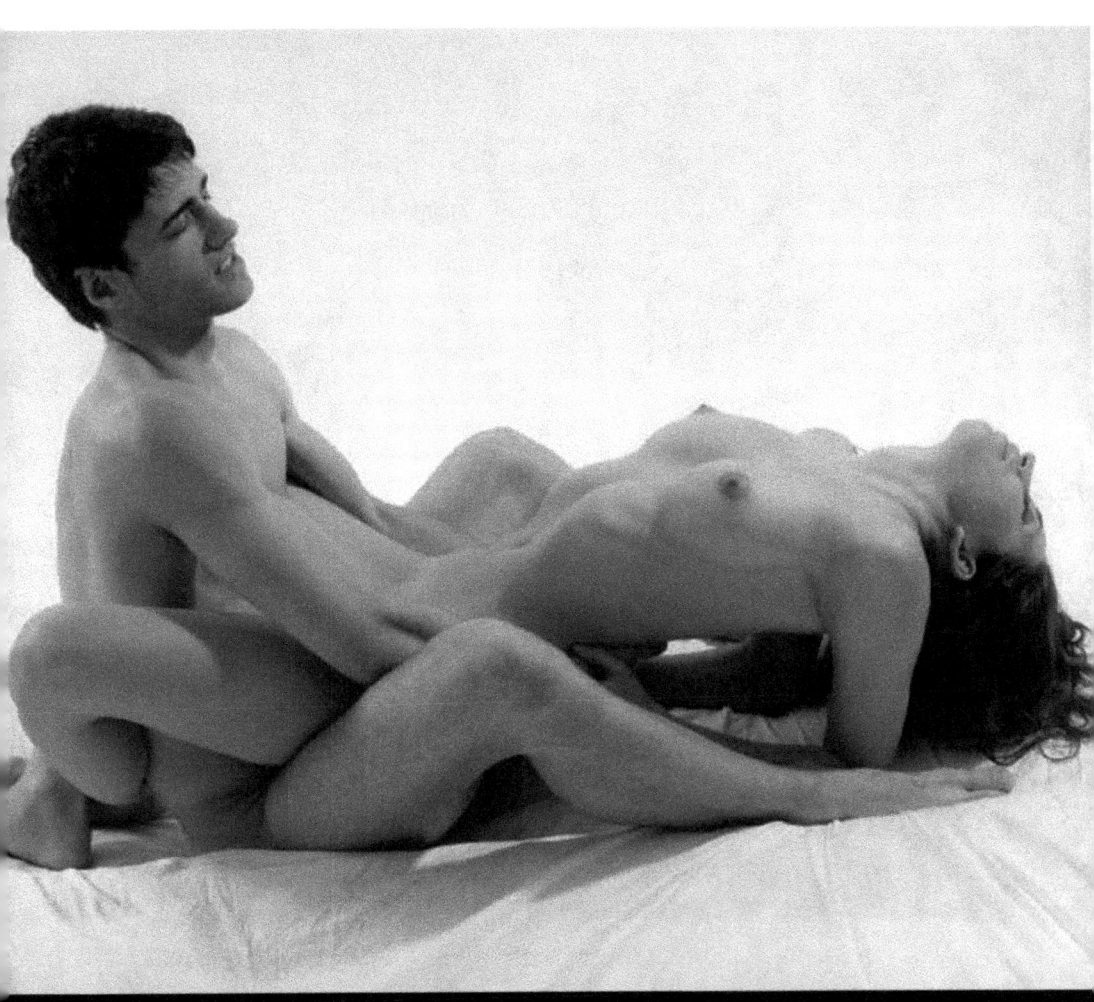

DAY 338

CAN'T LET YOU GO

The woman first climbs onto her lover's lap and then leans back on her elbows and locks her legs around his waist. He can either hook his hands under her lower back for support or use them on her breasts and clitoris.

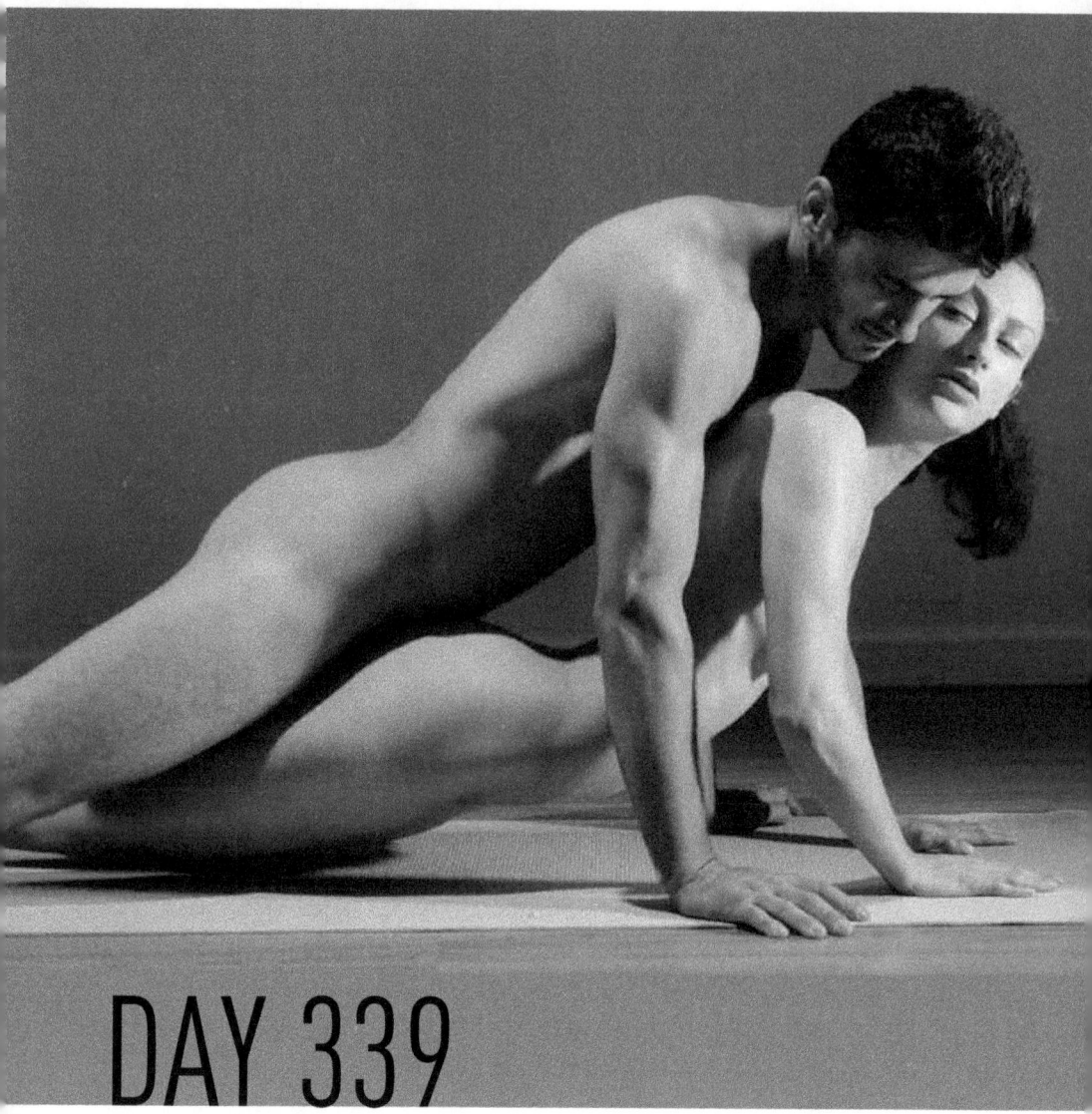

DAY 339

THE PASSIONATE PUSH-UP

The woman gets down on the floor into a push-up position. Her partner strikes a similar pose, with his arms outside hers, as he enters her from behind. In concert, they do as many push-ups as they can without breaking penetration.

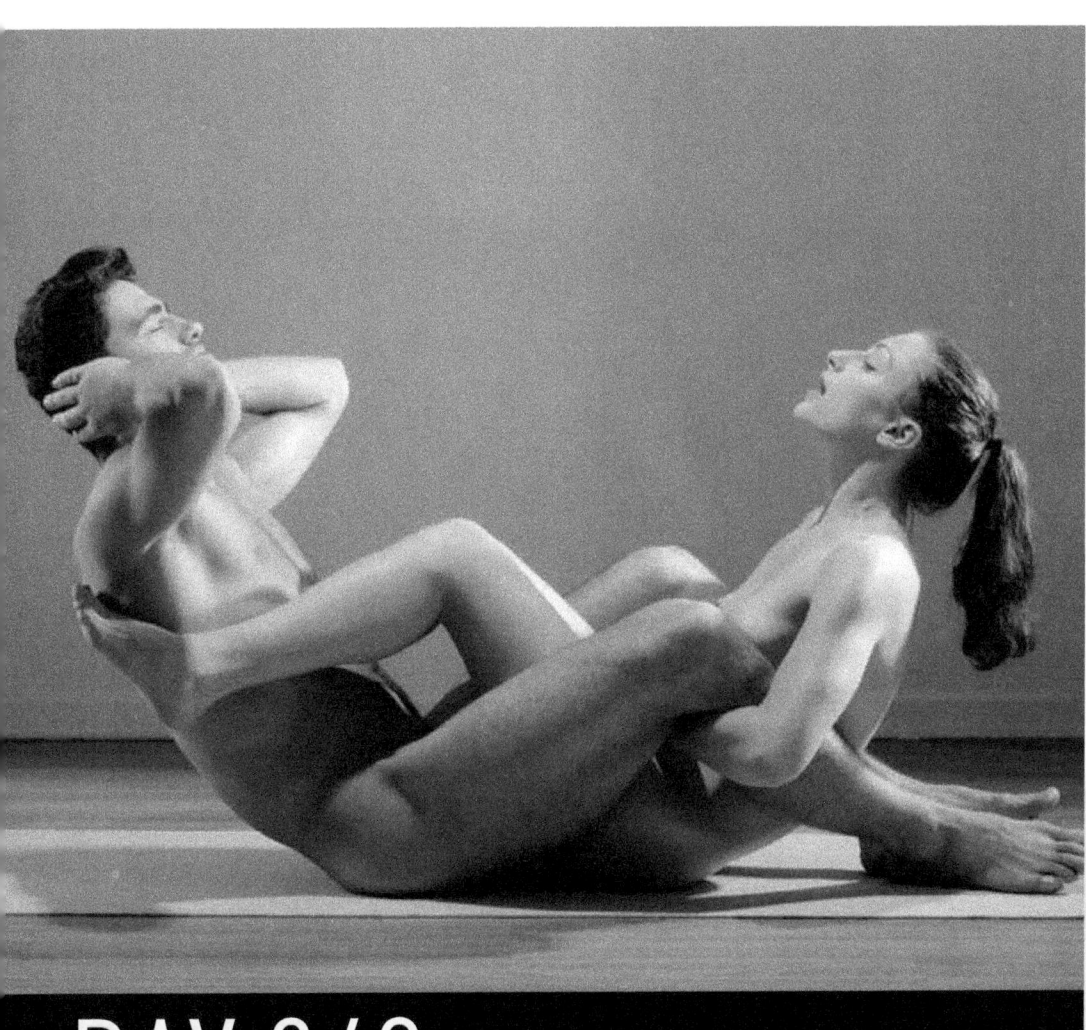

DAY 340

CAPTAIN CRUNCH

He sits on an exercise mat with his legs open while his partner, facing him, moves herself in as close as she can get. As he penetrates her vagina she anchors his legs, allowing him to work out his abdominals while they're having sex.

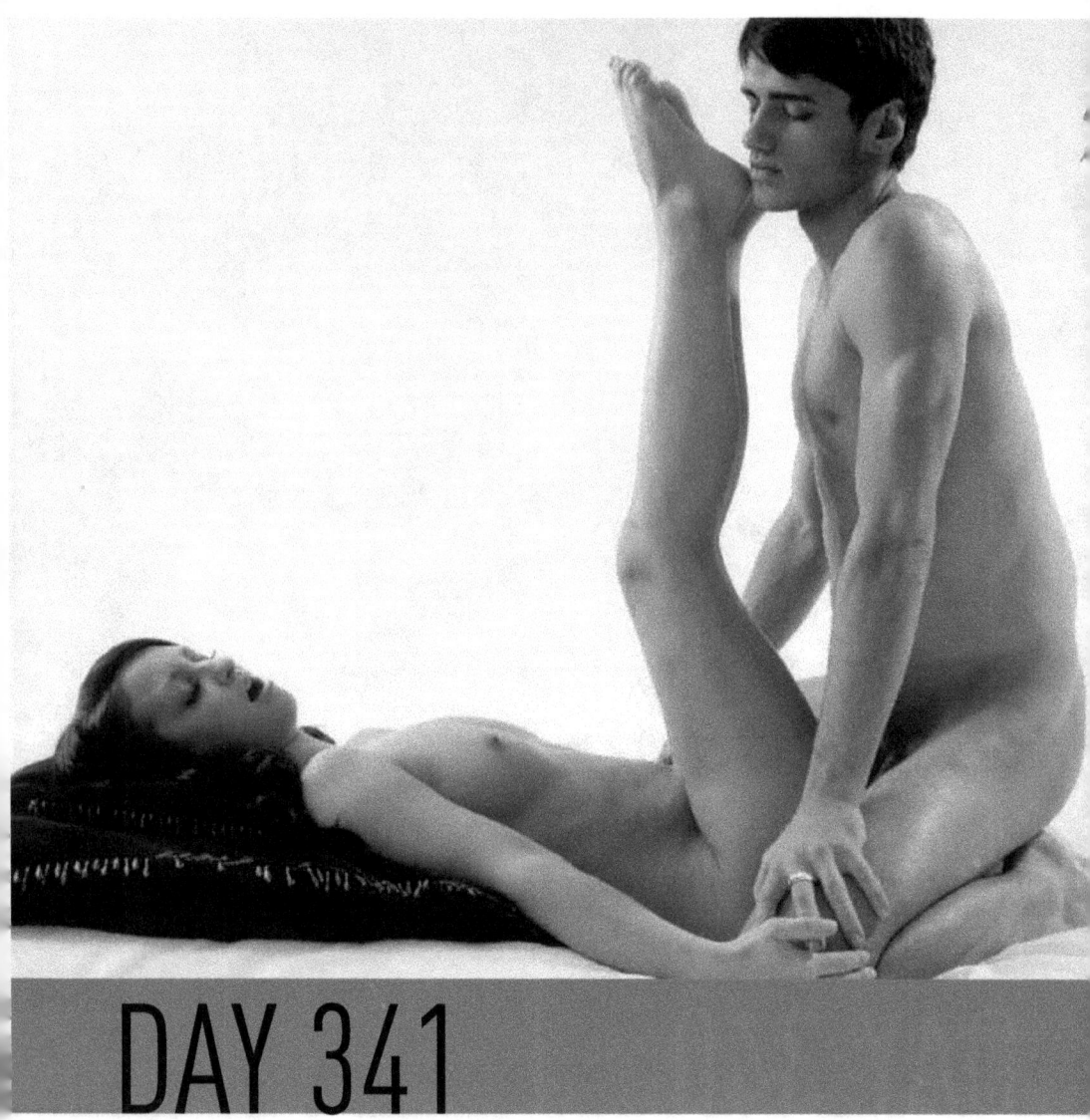

DAY 341

CHIN MUSIC

The woman lies back on the bed and lifts one leg up so that her heel is even with her partner's chin. He enters her from his knees and is in the perfect position to manipulate her clitoris with his fingers.

DAY 342

WINTER WARMTH

Nothing staves off the cold temperatures like a warm embrace. He gets into a squatting position while she lowers herself down and mounts him. She wraps her arms around him and the two lovers bounce and rock toward climax.

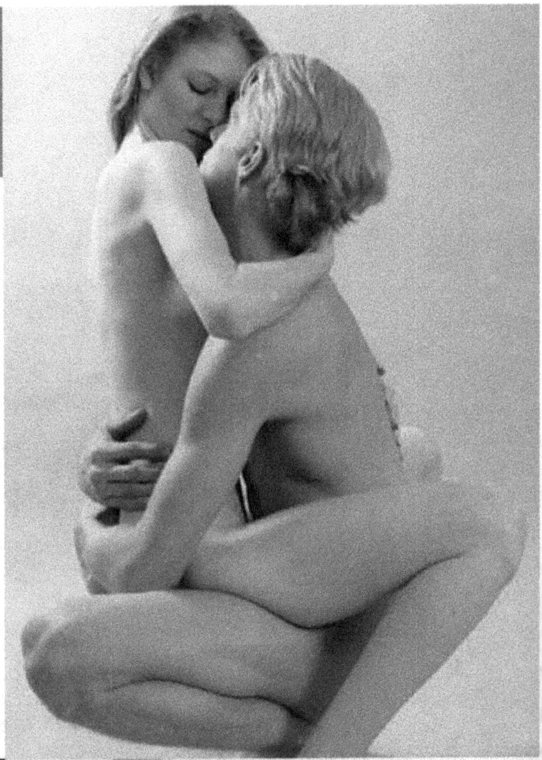

DAY 343

THE NECTAR DETECTOR

The woman positions herself in what amounts to a yoga shoulder stand, with her legs pointing straight up and her hands flat on the floor. Her partner gives her extra lower-back support as he dips his face between her legs—and makes this challenging move worthwhile.

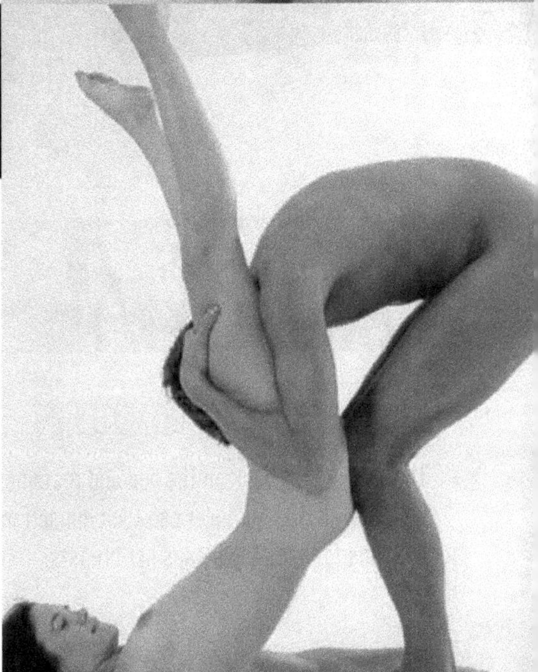

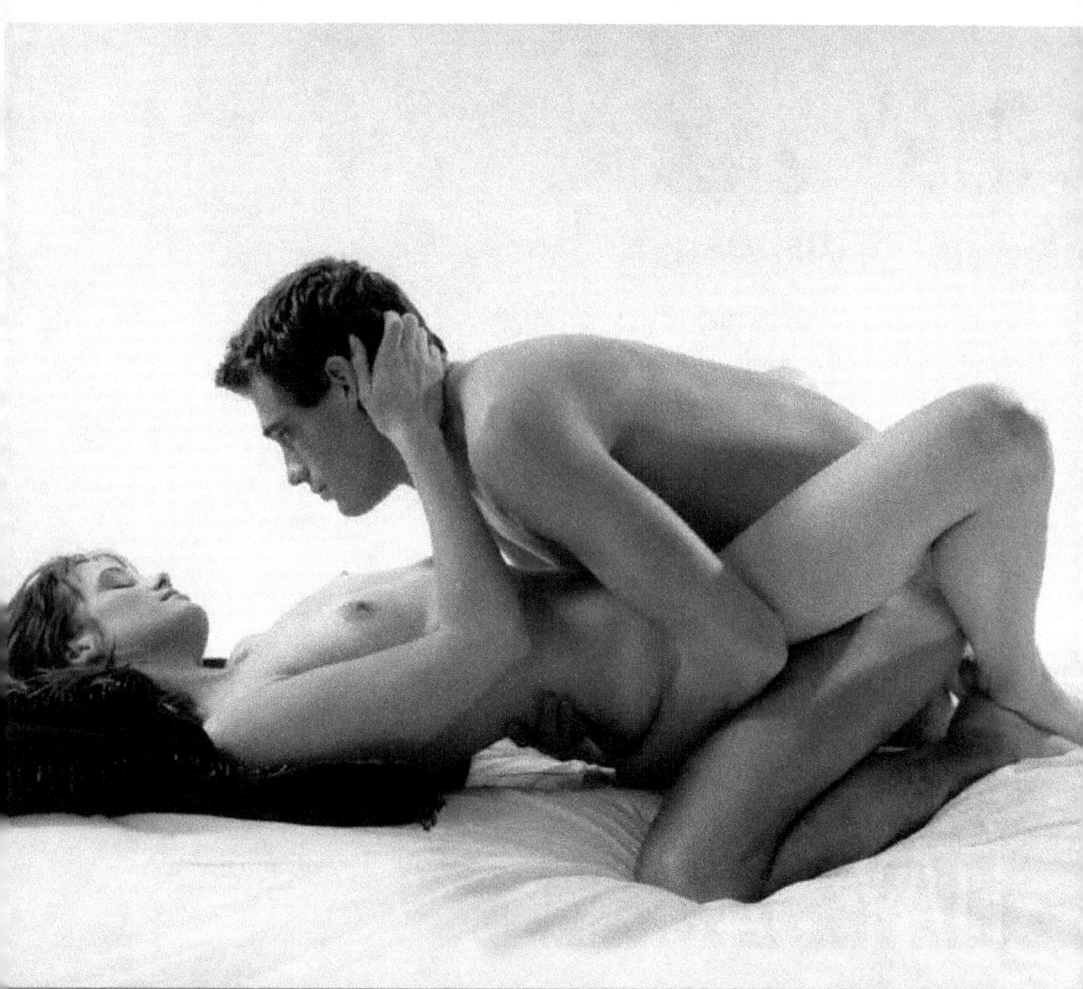

DAY 344

TUCK, TUCK, GOOSE

The woman lies back on the bed and rests her head and shoulders on a cushion and arches her back so that her lover can tuck himself in underneath her. As he penetrates her anally, he leans forward and kisses her breasts.

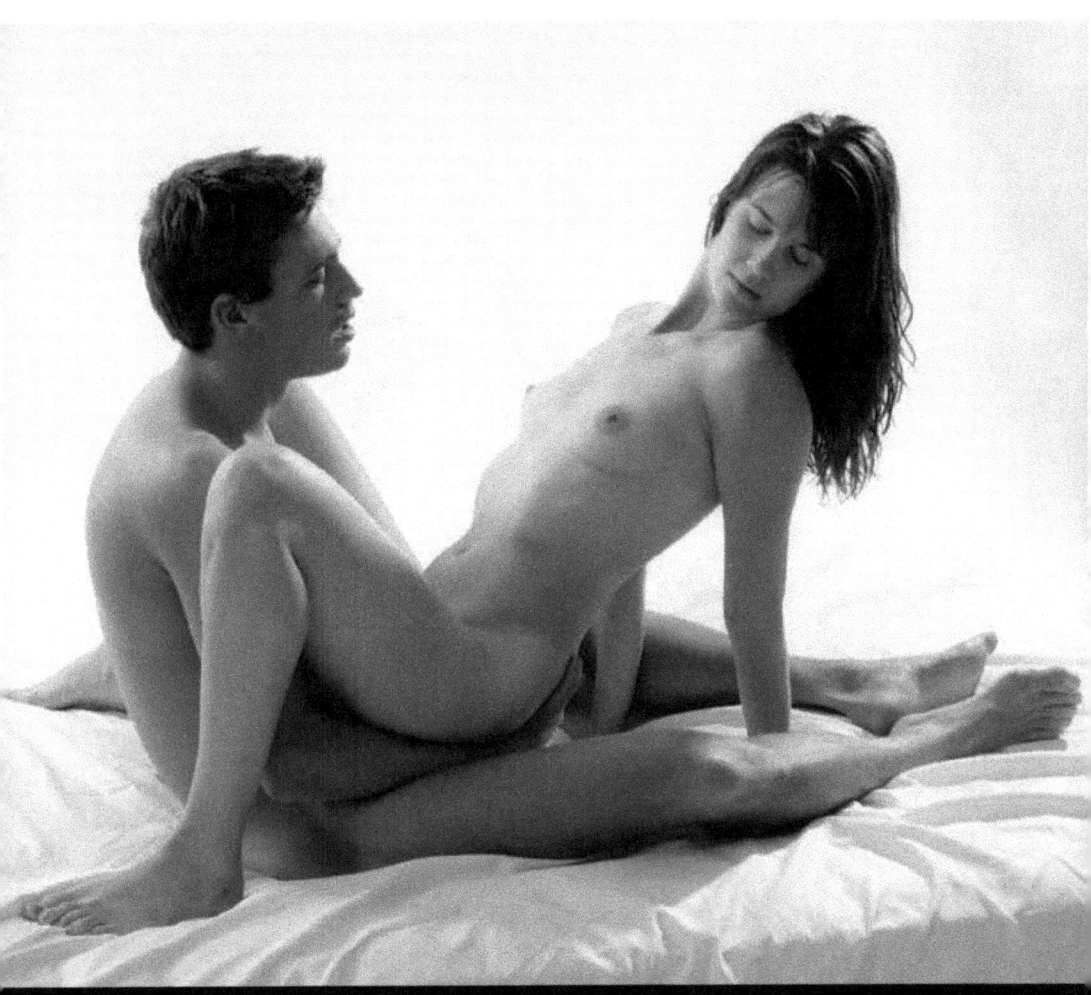

DAY 345

THE BUTTER CHURN

In this anal position the lovers lube up before moving to the bed. The man sits up with his legs extended. His partner moves herself high up in his lap and lowers herself onto his penis. He offers support as she makes slow circular movements with her hips.

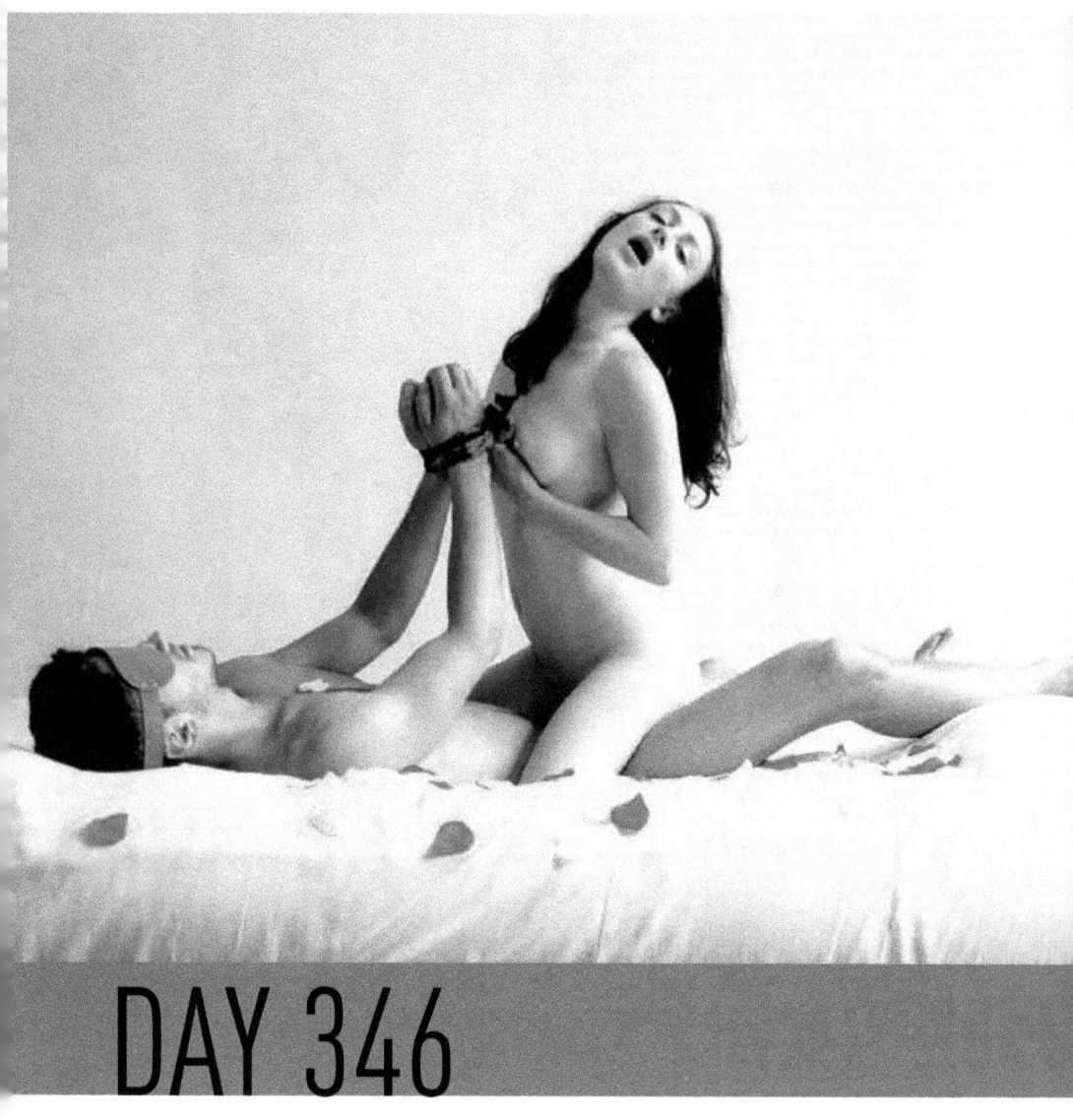

DAY 346

BIND MAN'S BUFF

He's on his back with his eyes blindfolded and his hands bound. His lover straddles him, allowing his penis to enter her. As she bounces up and down, she pulls his hands upwards, for an even deeper penetration.

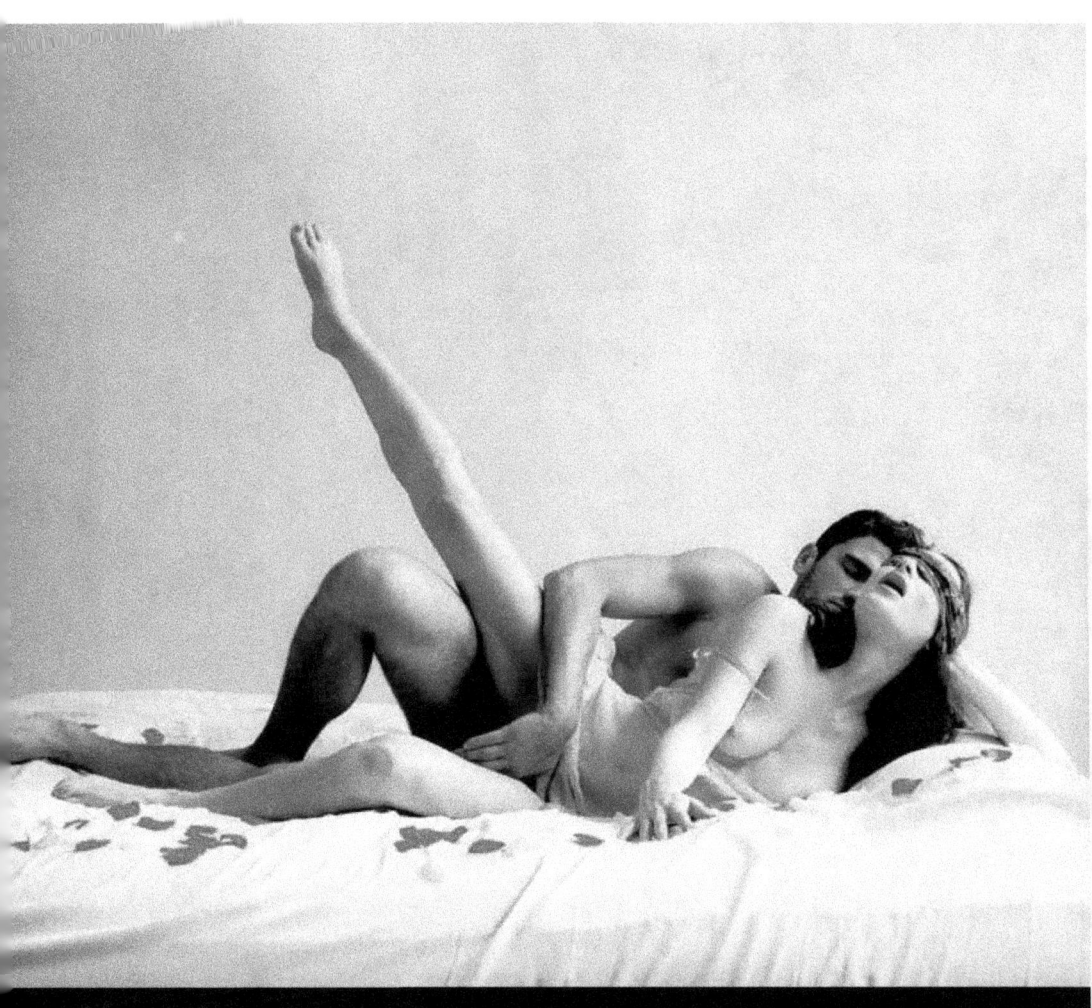

DAY 347

THE HOT BUTTON

The lovers lie on the bed side by side with the man behind his blindfolded partner. She lifts her top leg up high, allowing him to penetrate. The added bonus of this position is that he has ample access to her clitoris.

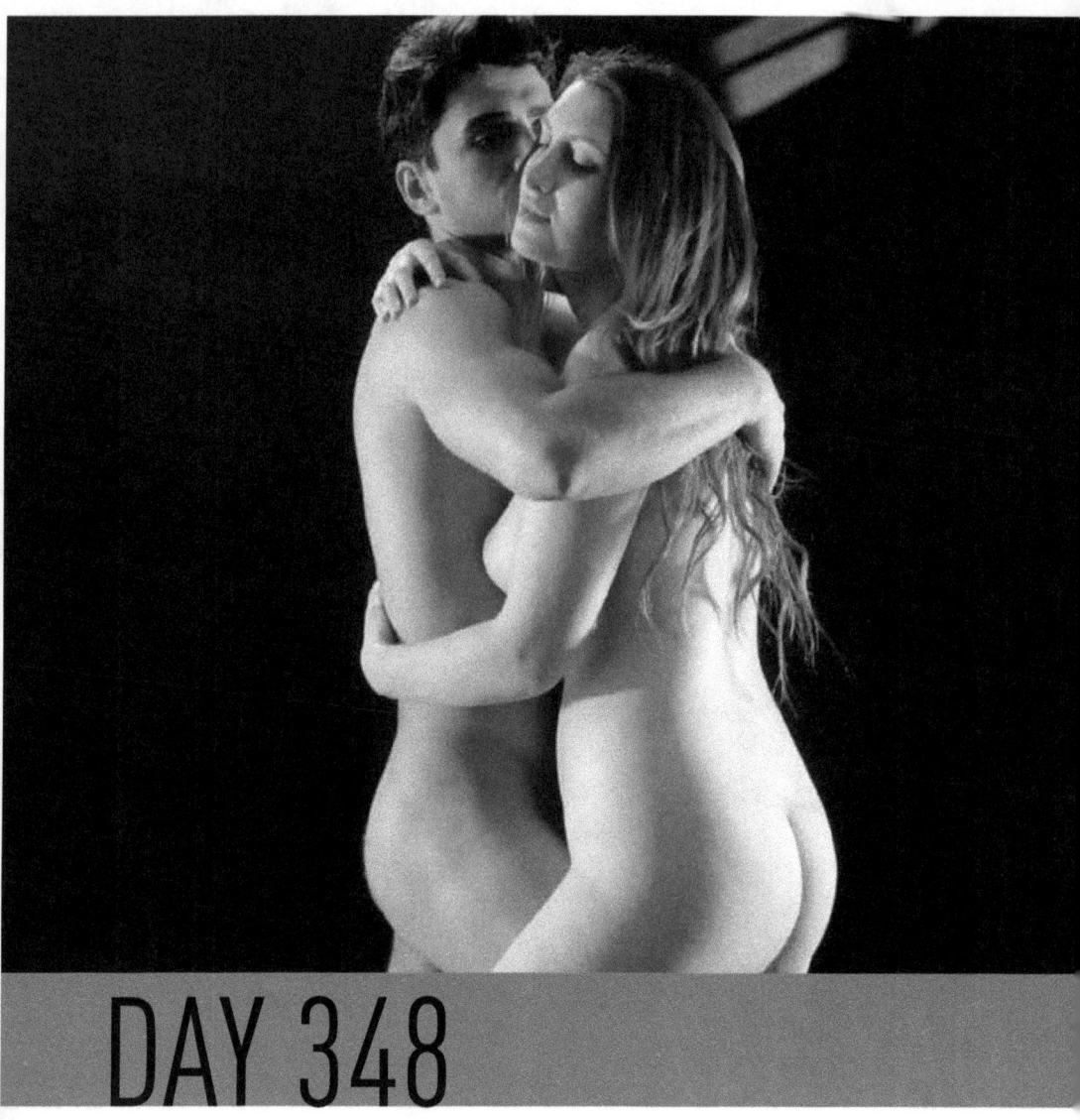

DAY 348

DIRTY DANCING

The lovers start in a standing posture, wrapping their arms around each other. The man penetrates the woman's vagina and they are free to move whichever way the mood takes them. It's up to them who will take the lead.

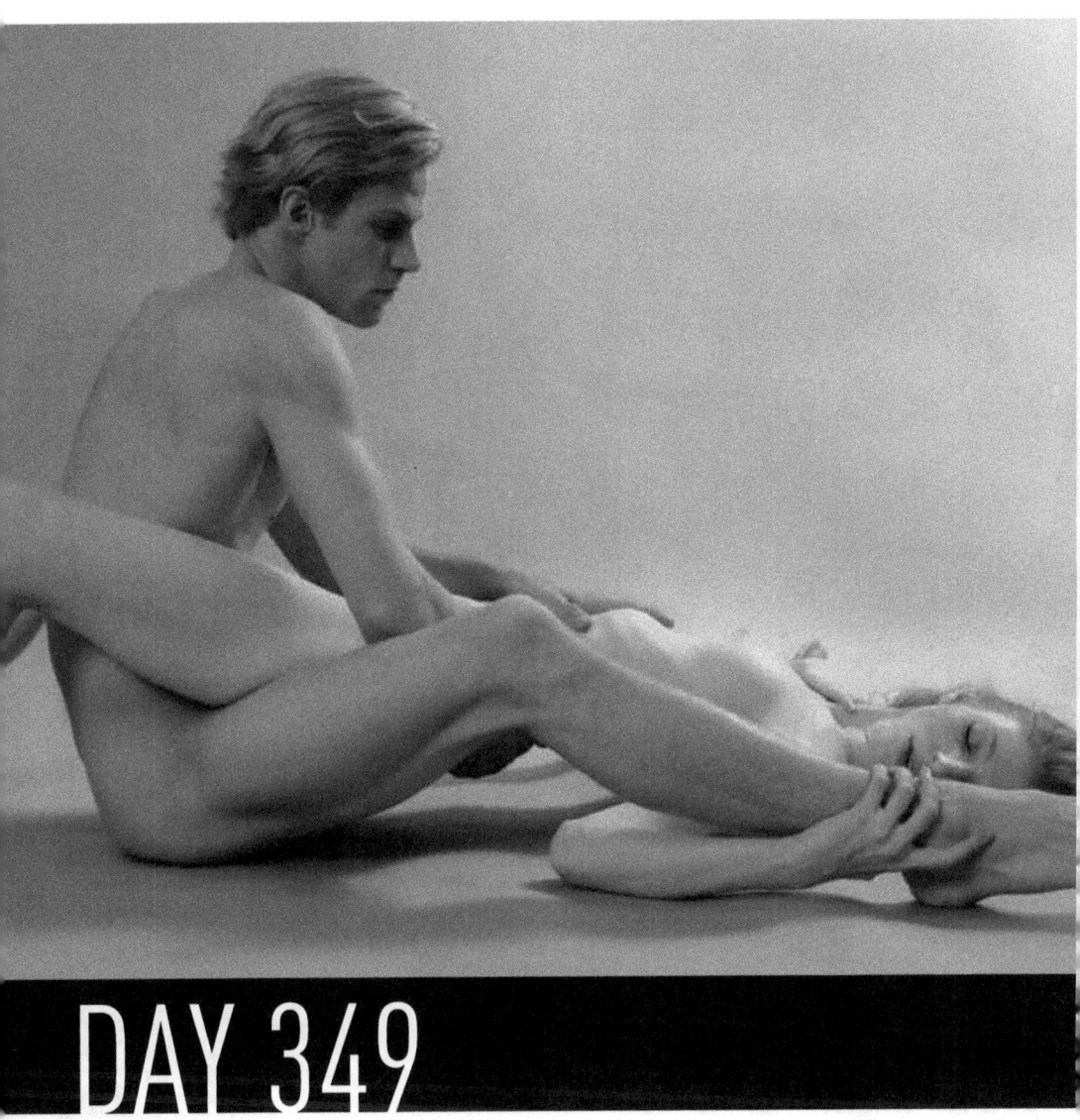

DAY 349

SPELLBOUND

He sits up with his legs wide apart. She lies back and drapes her legs over his upper thighs as he penetrates her. She falls under his influence as he takes hold of her hips and guides all their movements.

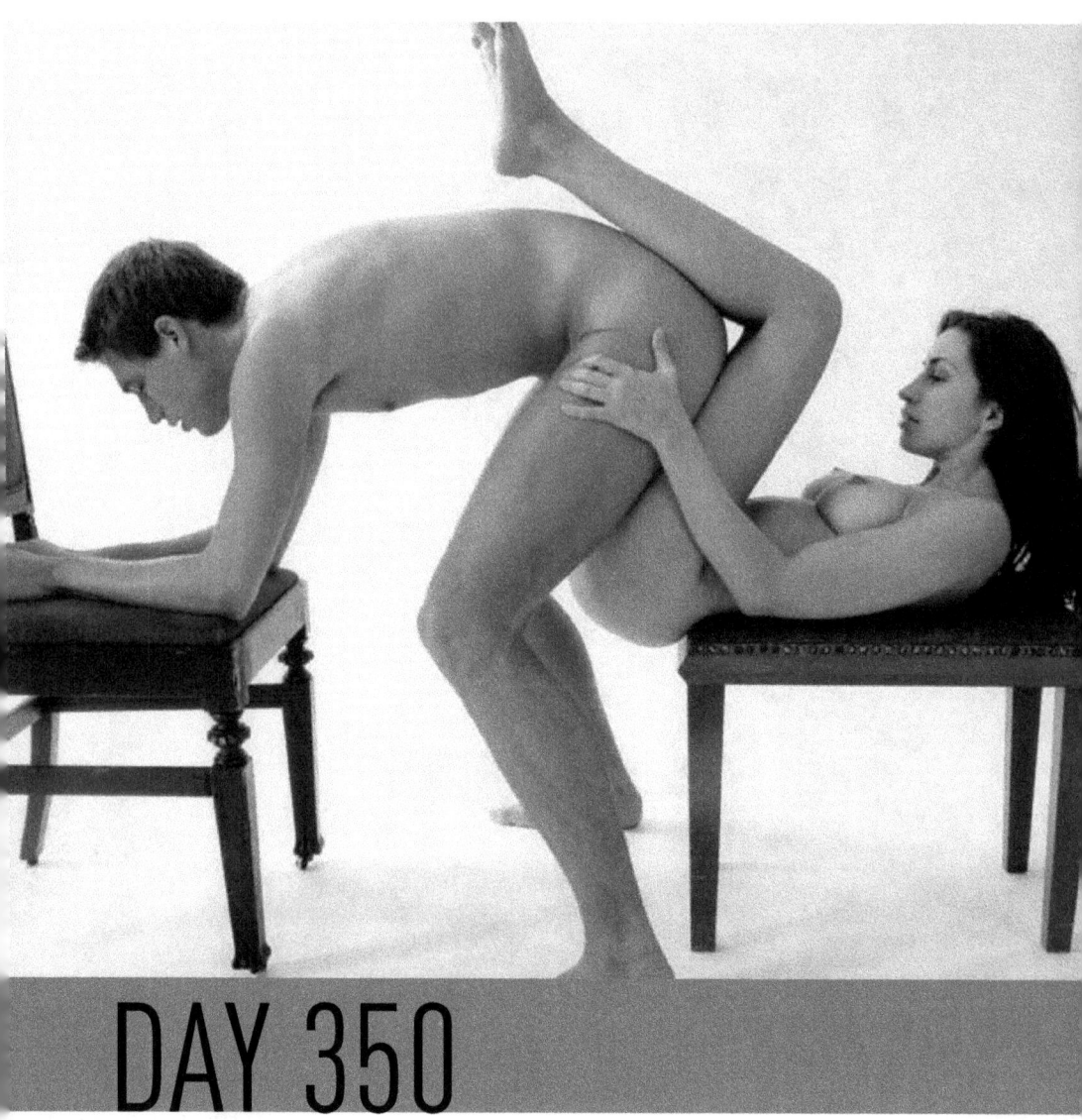

DAY 350

THE BERMUDA TRIANGLE

Sometimes getting lost during sex is a good thing. She lies back against an ottoman or padded stool while her lover rests his head forward on a chair and enters her from a bent position. They're delightfully disoriented.

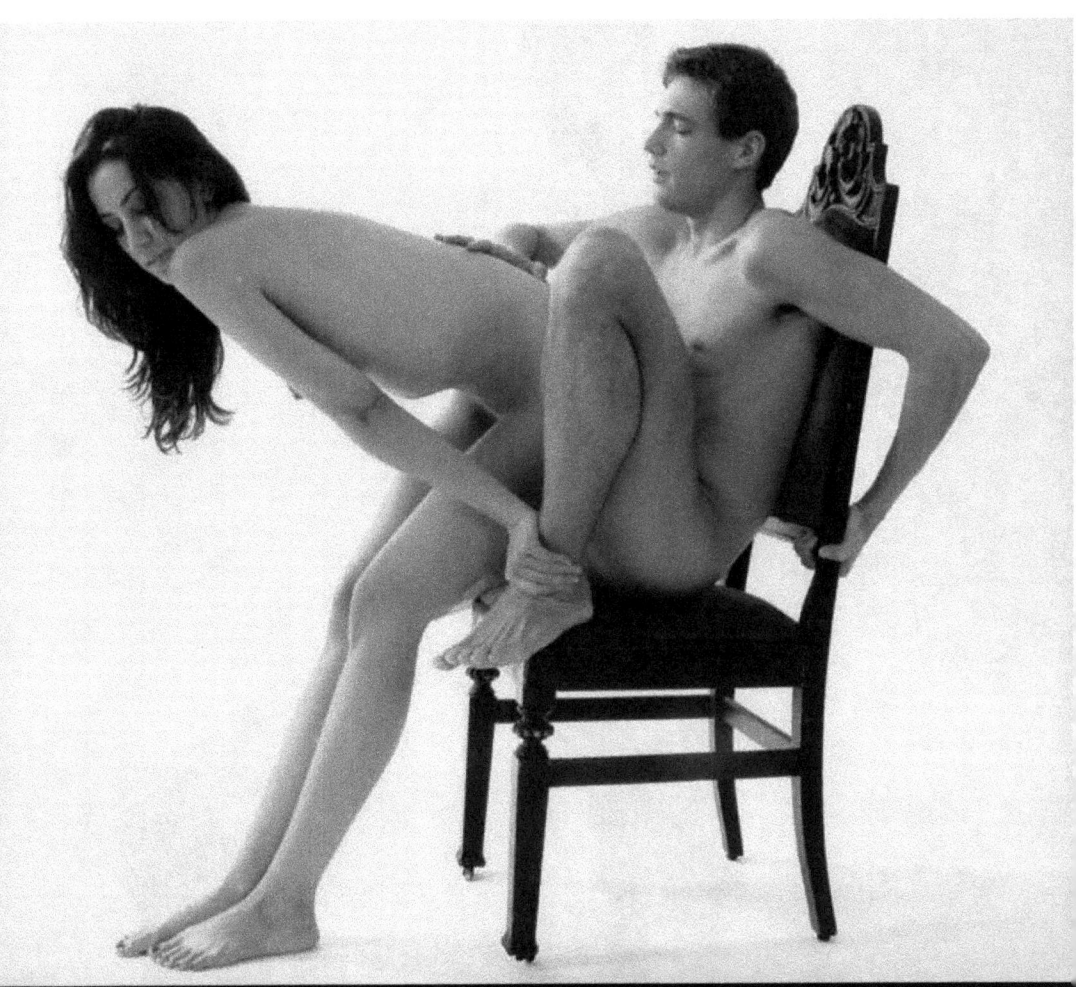

DAY 351

CAN YOU SQUEEZE ME IN?

The man squats in a chair with his heels pressed against the edge of the seat. From a standing position she lowers herself down onto her lover's penis. Her legs are closed keeping the penetration tight.

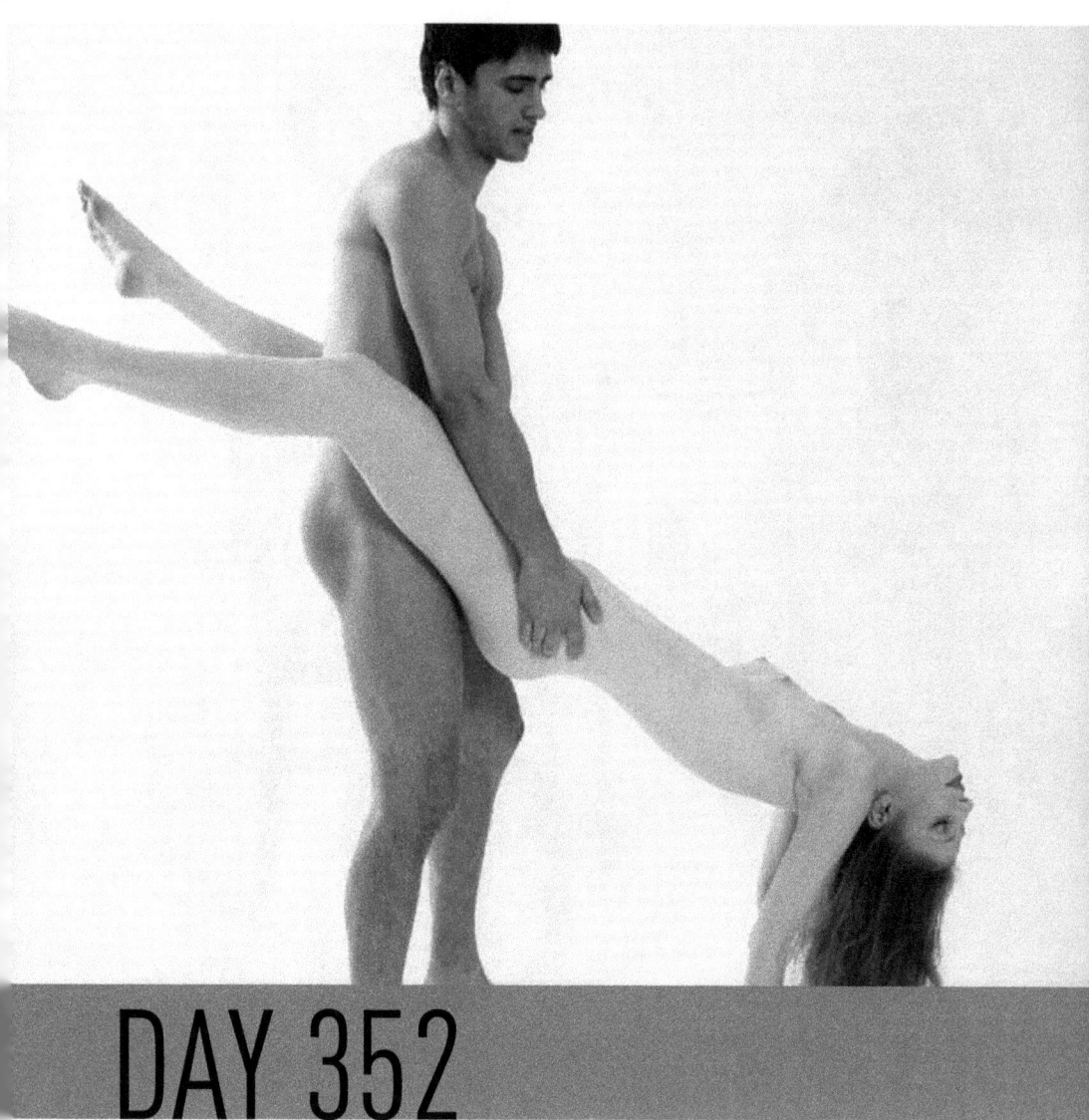

DAY 352

HOE MOTION

He lifts his partner at the waist as she brings her legs around him. She extends backwards supporting herself on her hands. He enters her and has a wonderful view of her face and breasts.

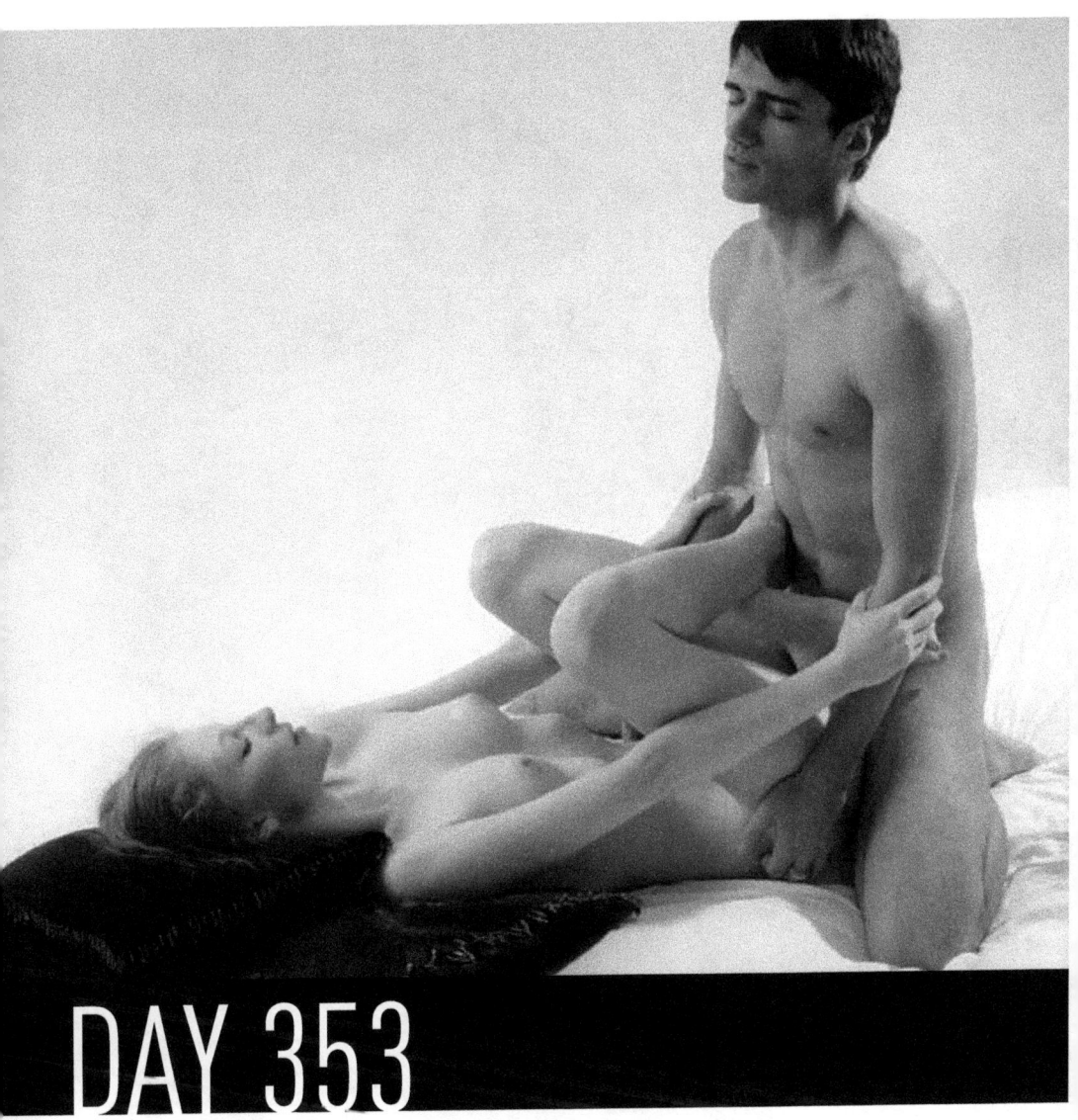

DAY 353

THE LUSTY LOTUS

Who's to say you can't practice yoga in bed? In this case, the woman gets into the lotus position while on her back. He penetrates his partner while sitting back on his legs.

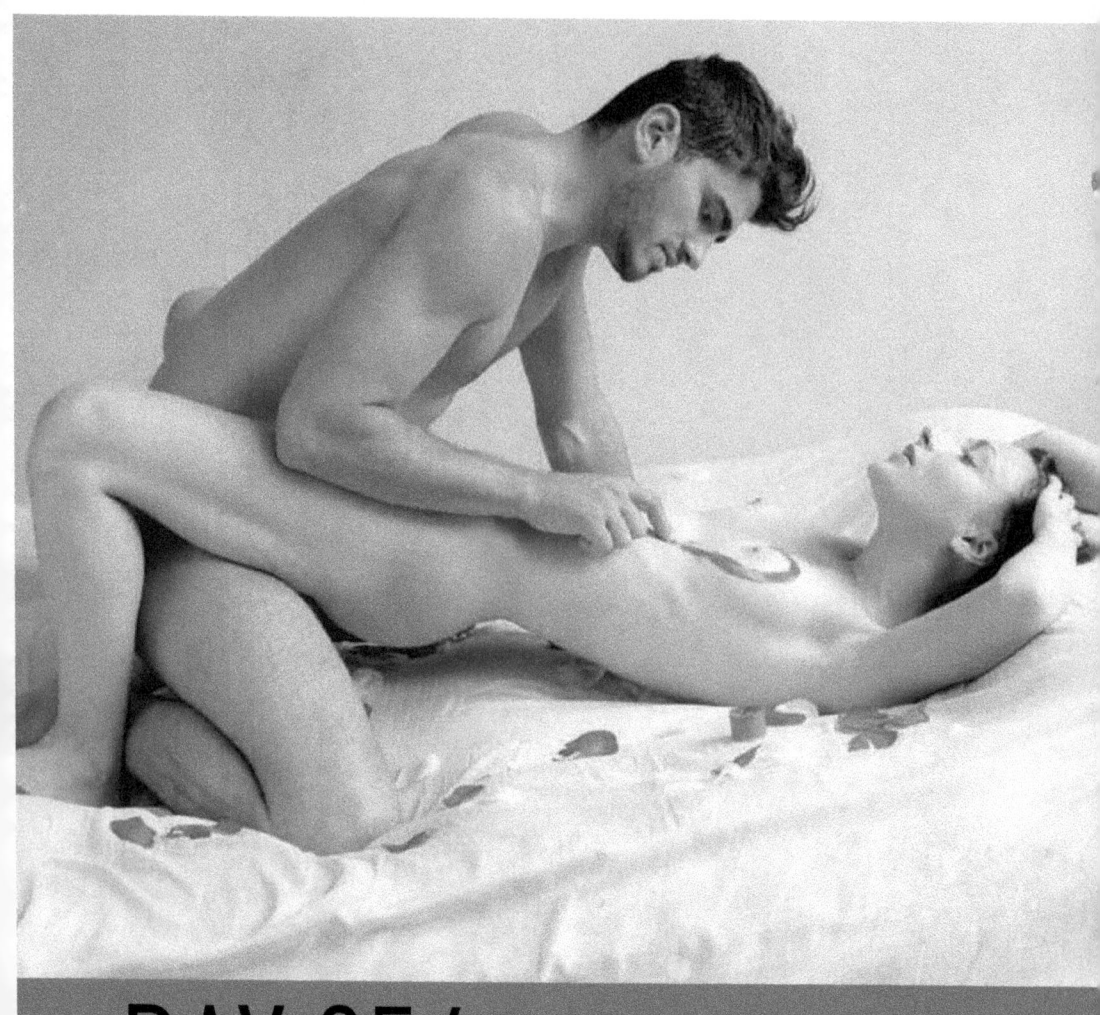

DAY 354

CROSS MY HEART

She lies back with her legs hooked over her lover's thighs as he swirls edible body paint over her chest. As he penetrates her from a kneeling position, he can lick his creation clean.

DAY 355

MR. CLEAN

You don't have to be dirty to enjoy this one. From a standing position, the man runs a soapy pouf sponge over his lover's breasts. She responds by lifting a leg and wrapping it around his thigh. As he enters her, the warm suds run between them.

DAY 356

THE WASH 'N' BLOW

As the lovers clean each other off after a night of body-painting passion, the woman drops to her knees to give her partner's penis some very personal attention. He can then return the favor.

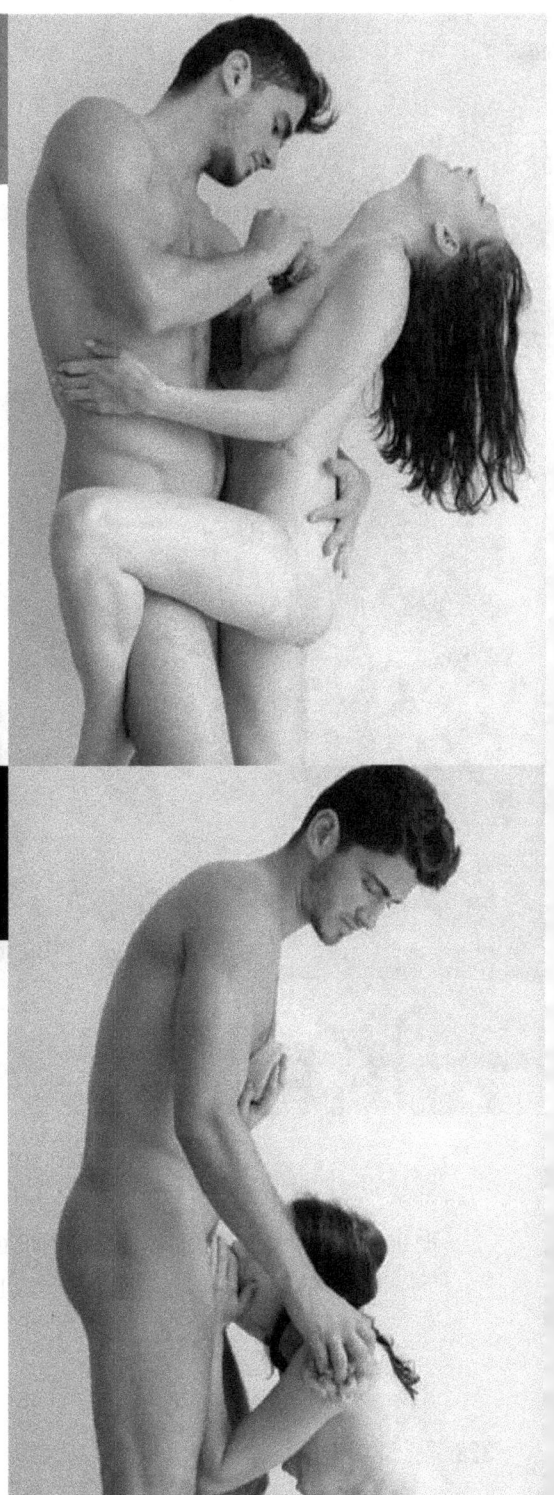

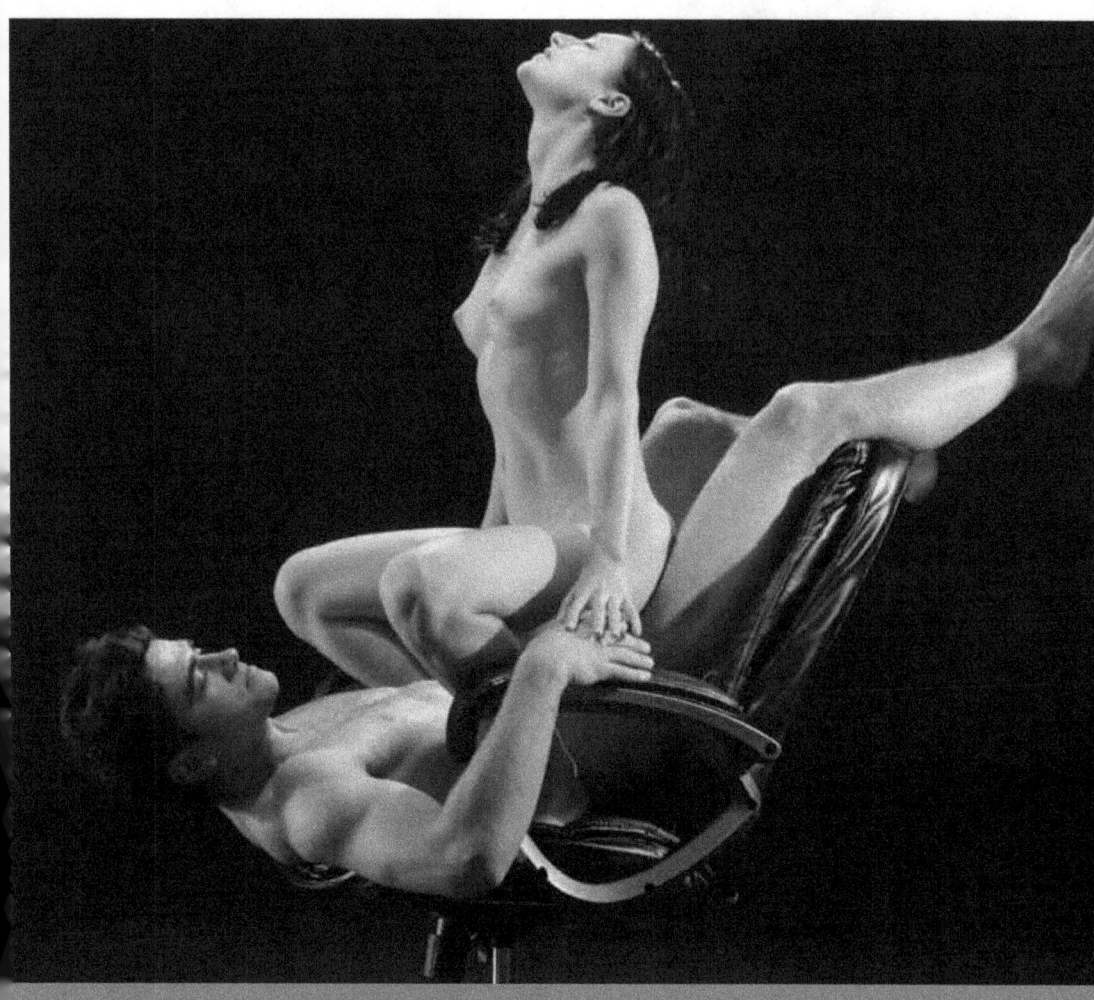

DAY 357

HOPPING SPREE

He lies backwards in a chair as she crouches over him and slowly lowers her lubed anus onto his penis. Once she's nice and comfortable, she's free to hop until he pops.

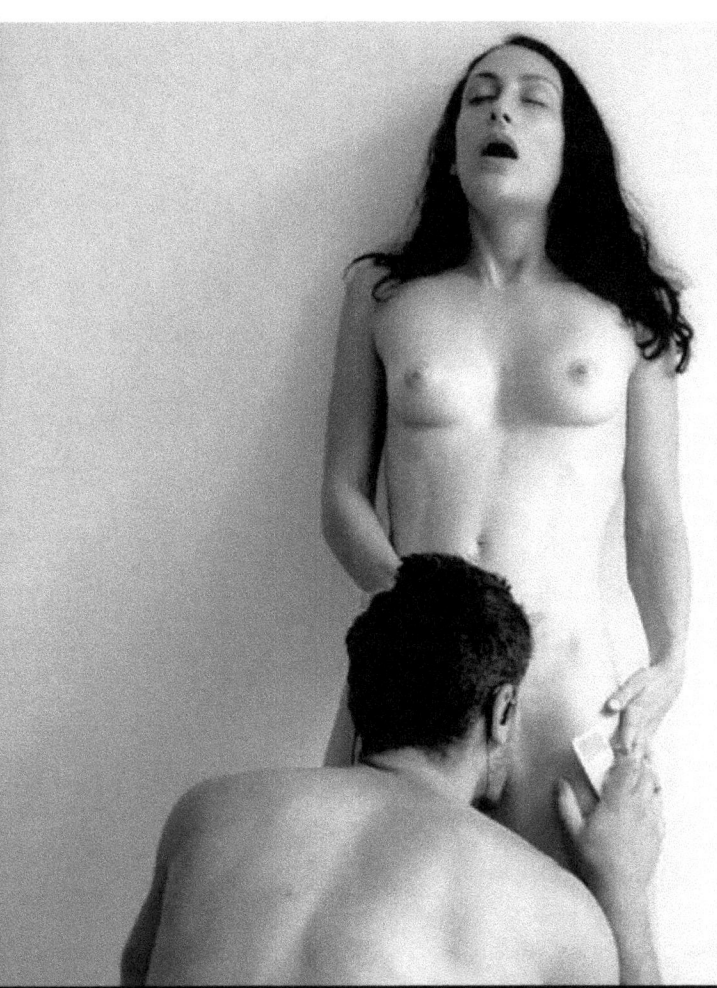

DAY 358

HUM'S THE WORD

A little music can be a great mood-setter when it comes to sex. In this case, it's a key component. As the man performs oral on his lover he amps up the sensation by humming along to one of his favorite songs.

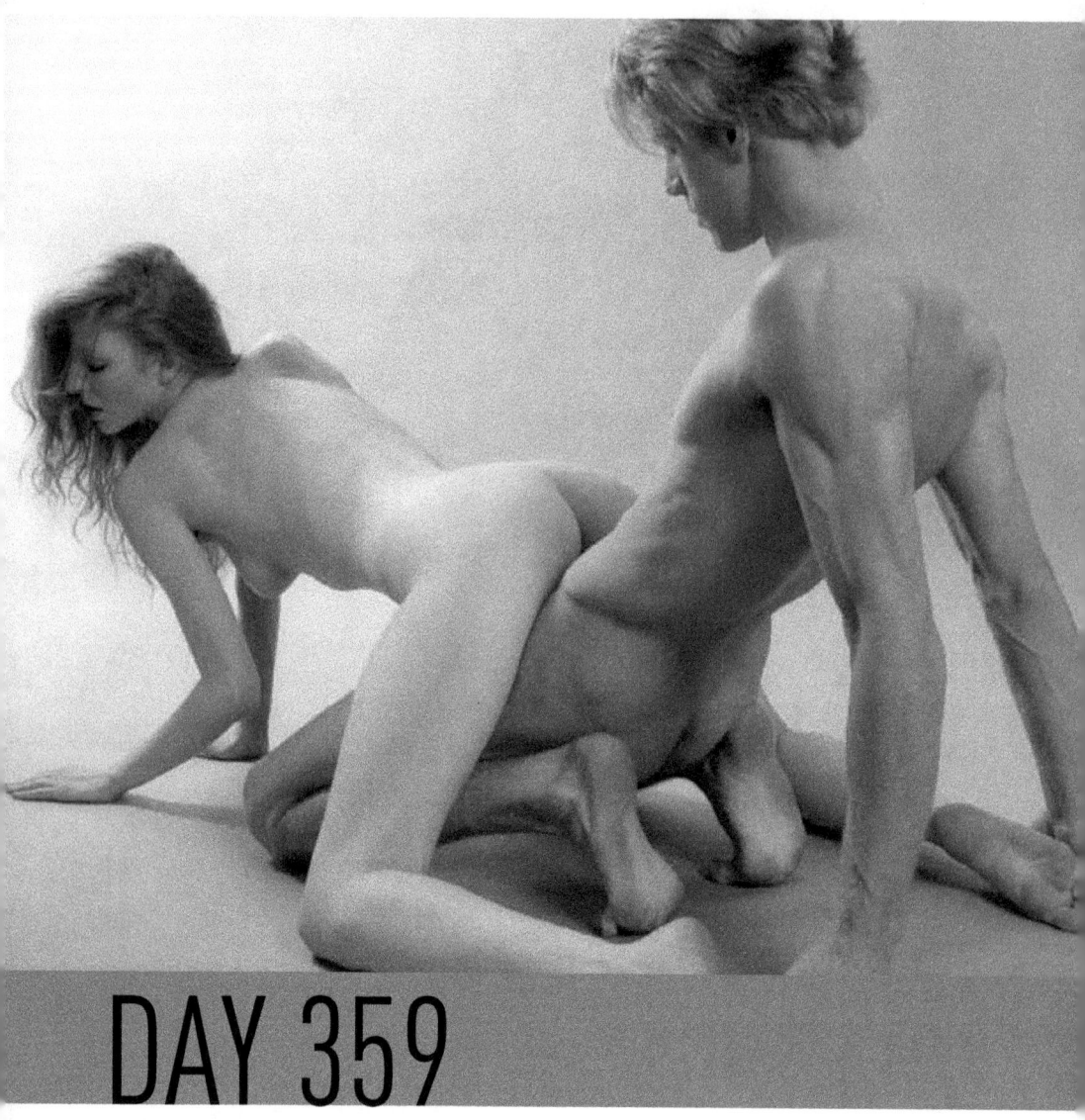

DAY 359

PARALLEL PARKING

The woman gets into a doggy position with her knees spread wide apart. Her lover enters her from behind with his back arched and hands on the floor for support and leverage. Pulling forward and backing in was never so much fun.

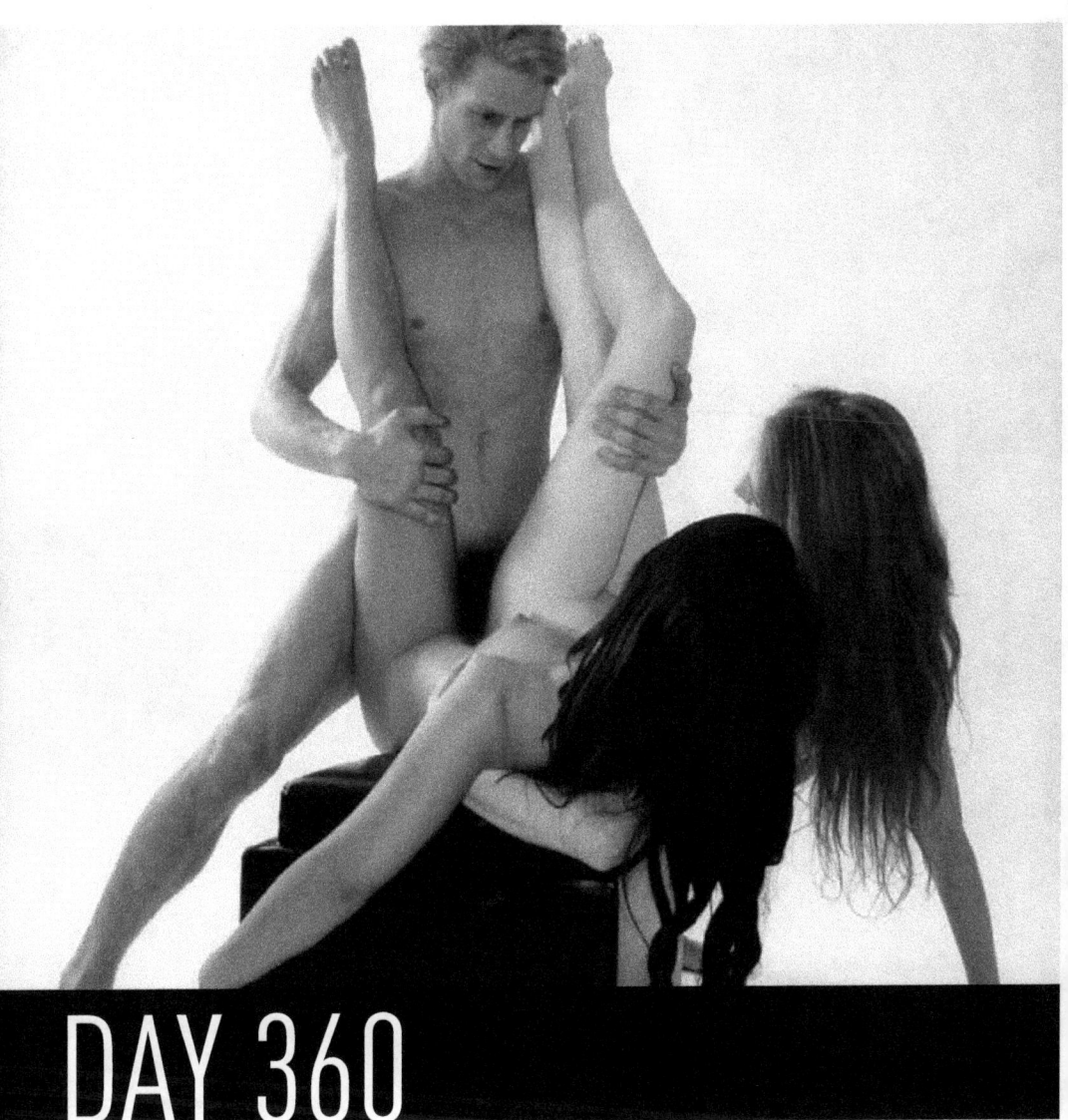

DAY 360

THE HOMEGIRL HANG

In this tricky position one woman leans back across an ottoman while the other strikes a similar pose by hanging onto her friend and placing one hand down to the floor. They both raise their legs up against their partner as he takes turns entering each of them. If you're a leg man, you'll love this one.

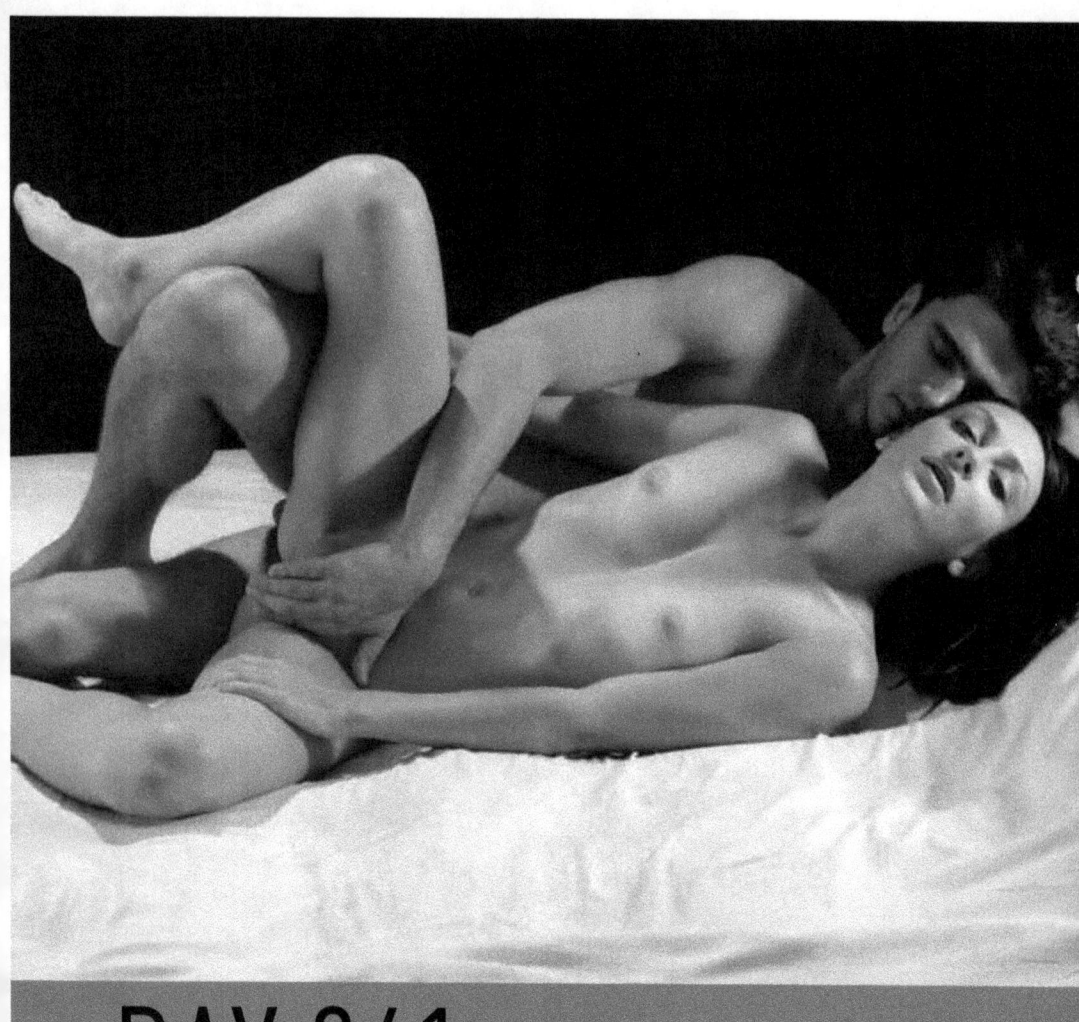

DAY 361

GO FOR STROKE

The man and the woman lie on their sides as she hooks one of her legs over his. As he enters her anus he brings his hand around to stroke her clitoris and finger her vagina.

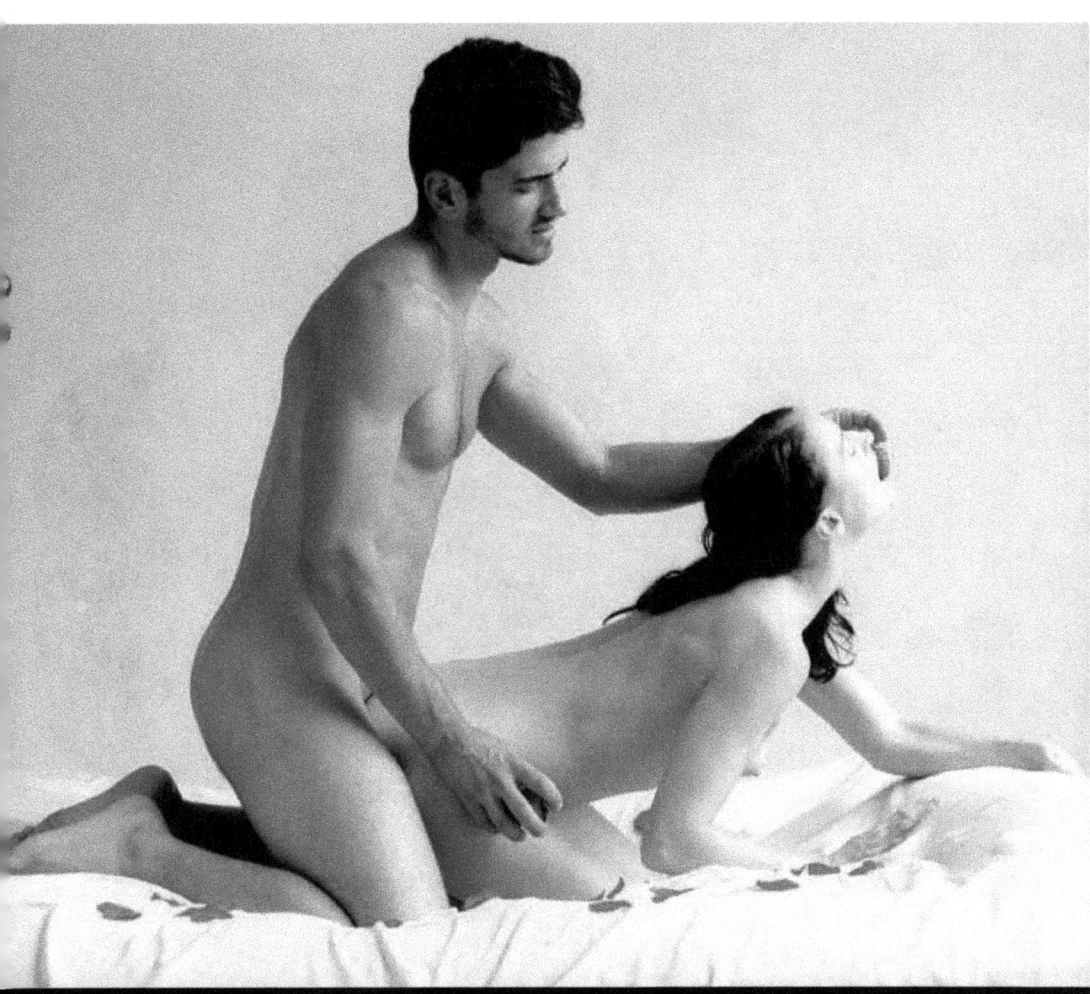

DAY 362

DOGGIE TREAT

The couple place themselves in a doggie position as he penetrates her from behind. She samples the berry he offers as he takes the bitten piece and runs it down the length of her back, only to taste that sweet trail with his tongue.

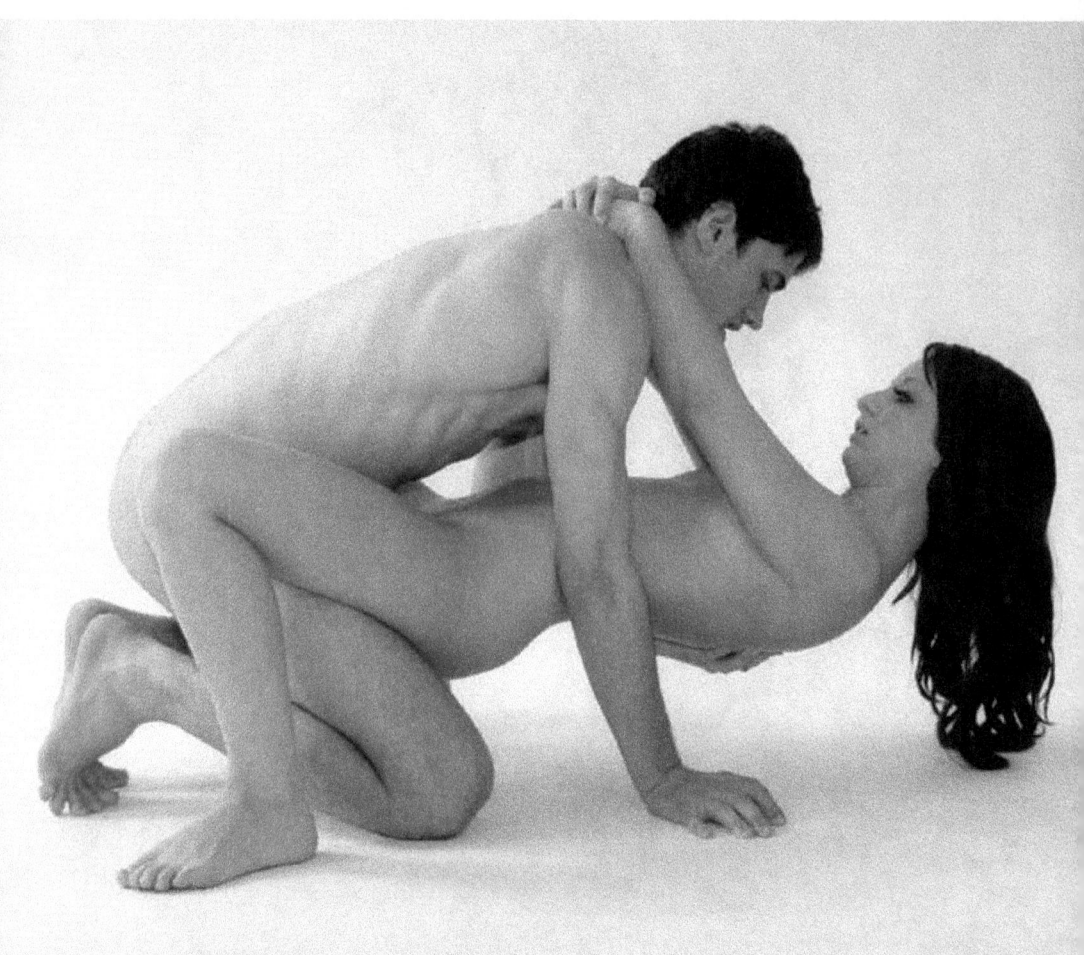

DAY 363

THE LOWDOWN

She likes things down and dirty, and she's going to take him with her. The woman starts on the floor but easily shifts into bridge position by pulling herself up to meet her kneeling lover. He enters her as she sways from side to side.

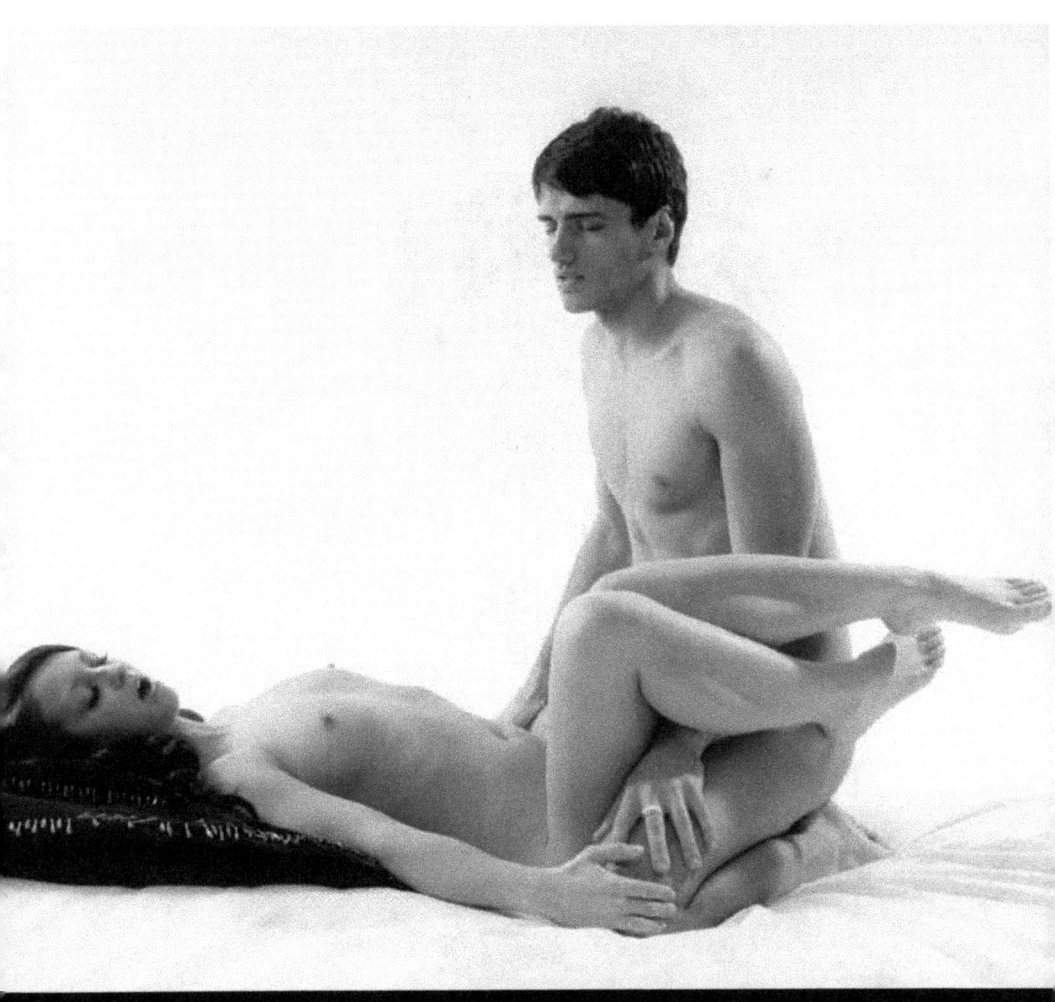

DAY 364

SPLENDID SPRINTER

She lies back and brings her legs up as her lover penetrates her from a kneeling position. She shifts her legs out to the side and pumps them back and forth as though she's running the 50-yard dash.

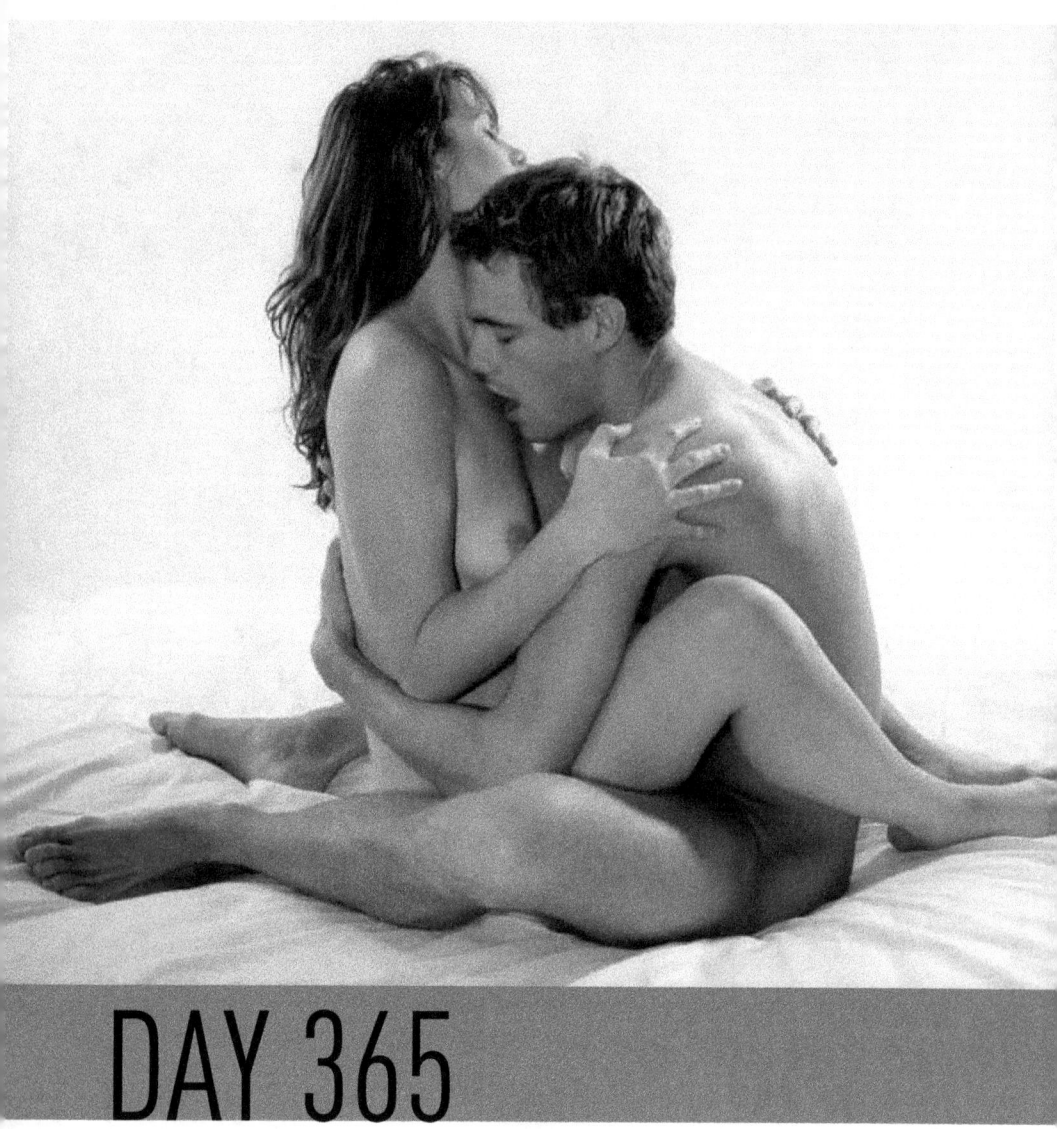

DAY 365

ENDLESS EMBRACE

The lovers sit facing each other, with his legs outside of hers. He's able to enter her deeply, but this one is all about the eyes and all-around, up-close, all-over physical contact

LES CONVULSIONS

DE PARIS

*Le Cacheux
B 12 R 91
n° 2580*

LES CONVULSIONS DE PARIS

4 volumes in-16, à 3 fr. 50

TOME PREMIER
LES PRISONS PENDANT LA COMMUNE.

TOME TROISIÈME
LES SAUVETAGES PENDANT LA COMMUNE

TOME QUATRIÈME
LA COMMUNE A L'HOTEL DE VILLE

---

407. — Imprimerie A. Lahure, rue de Fleurus, 9, à Paris.

MAXIME DU CAMP

DE L'ACADÉMIE FRANÇAISE

LES CONVULSIONS

DE PARIS

> Nous allons voir des scènes auprès desquelles les passées n'ont été que des verdures et des pastourilles.
> CARDINAL DE RETZ.

CINQUIÈME ÉDITION

TOME DEUXIÈME

EPISODES DE LA COMMUNE

PARIS
LIBRAIRIE HACHETTE ET Cⁱᵉ
79, BOULEVARD SAINT-GERMAIN, 79

1884

Droits de propriété et de traduction réservés